The South African Herbal Pharmacopoeia

The South African Herbal Pharmacopoeia

Monographs of Medicinal and Aromatic Plants

Edited by

Alvaro Viljoen
Department of Pharmaceutical Sciences, Tshwane University of Technology, Pretoria, South Africa
SAMRC Herbal Drugs Research Unit, Faculty of Science, Tshwane University of Technology, Pretoria, South Africa

Maxleene Sandasi
Department of Pharmaceutical Sciences, Tshwane University of Technology, Pretoria, South Africa
SAMRC Herbal Drugs Research Unit, Faculty of Science, Tshwane University of Technology, Pretoria, South Africa

Gerda Fouche
Chemistry Department, University of Pretoria, Pretoria, South Africa

Sandra Combrinck
Department of Pharmaceutical Sciences, Tshwane University of Technology, Pretoria, South Africa

Ilze Vermaak
Department of Pharmaceutical Sciences, Tshwane University of Technology, Pretoria, South Africa
SAMRC Herbal Drugs Research Unit, Faculty of Science, Tshwane University of Technology, Pretoria, South Africa

ELSEVIER
ACADEMIC PRESS
An imprint of Elsevier

Academic Press is an imprint of Elsevier
125 London Wall, London EC2Y 5AS, United Kingdom
525 B Street, Suite 1650, San Diego, CA 92101, United States
50 Hampshire Street, 5th Floor, Cambridge, MA 02139, United States
The Boulevard, Langford Lane, Kidlington, Oxford OX5 1GB, United Kingdom

ISBN: 978-0-323-99794-2

For information on all Academic Press publications
visit our website at https://www.elsevier.com/books-and-journals

Publisher: Andre G. Wolff
Editorial Project Manager: Barbara Makinster
Production Project Manager: Punithavathy Govindaradjane
Cover Designer: Greg Harris

Typeset by STRAIVE, India

Contents

Contributors

Chinedu Anokwuru
Department of Pharmaceutical Sciences, Tshwane University of Technology, Pretoria, South Africa

Kokoette Bassey
Department of Pharmaceutical Sciences, Tshwane University of Technology, Pretoria, South Africa

Thomas Brendler
Department of Botany and Plant Biotechnology, University of Johannesburg, Johannesburg, South Africa; Plantaphile, Collingswood, New Jersey, United States

Weiyang Chen
Department of Pharmaceutical Sciences, Tshwane University of Technology, Pretoria, South Africa

Sandra Combrinck
Department of Pharmaceutical Sciences, Tshwane University of Technology, Pretoria, South Africa

Gill Enslin
Department of Pharmaceutical Sciences, Tshwane University of Technology, Pretoria, South Africa

Gerda Fouche
Chemistry Department, University of Pretoria, Pretoria, South Africa

Thomas Idowu
Department of Pharmaceutical Sciences, Tshwane University of Technology, Pretoria, South Africa

Elizabeth Joubert
Plant Bioactives Group, Post-Harvest and Agro-Processing Technologies, Agricultural Research Council (Infruitec Nietvoorbij), Stellenbosch, South Africa

Guy Kamatou
Department of Pharmaceutical Sciences, Tshwane University of Technology, Pretoria, South Africa

Sowesa Kanama
Department of Pharmaceutical Sciences, Tshwane University of Technology, Pretoria, South Africa

Baatile Komane
Department of Pharmaceutical Sciences, Tshwane University of Technology, Pretoria, South Africa

Carmen Leonard
Department of Pharmaceutical Sciences, Tshwane University of Technology, Pretoria, South Africa

Lefa Lerotholi
Department of Pharmaceutical Sciences, Tshwane University of Technology, Pretoria, South Africa

Felix Makolo
Department of Pharmaceutical Sciences, Tshwane University of Technology, Pretoria, South Africa

Faith Malope
Department of Pharmaceutical Sciences, Tshwane University of Technology, Pretoria, South Africa

Nontobeko Mncwangi
Department of Pharmaceutical Sciences, Tshwane University of Technology, Pretoria, South Africa

Nduvho Mulaudzi
Department of Pharmaceutical Sciences, Tshwane University of Technology, Pretoria, South Africa

Baudry Nsuala
Department of Pharmaceutical Sciences, Tshwane University of Technology, Pretoria, South Africa

Emmanuel Rubegeta
Department of Pharmaceutical Sciences, Tshwane University of Technology, Pretoria, South Africa

Maxleene Sandasi
Department of Pharmaceutical Sciences; SAMRC Herbal Drugs Research Unit, Faculty of Science, Tshwane University of Technology, Pretoria, South Africa

Khotso Serabele
Department of Pharmaceutical Sciences, Tshwane University of Technology, Pretoria, South Africa

Zimkhitha Sotenjwa
Department of Pharmaceutical Sciences, Tshwane University of Technology, Pretoria, South Africa

Ilze Vermaak
Department of Pharmaceutical Sciences; SAMRC Herbal Drugs Research Unit, Faculty of Science, Tshwane University of Technology, Pretoria, South Africa

Alvaro Viljoen
Department of Pharmaceutical Sciences; SAMRC Herbal Drugs Research Unit, Faculty of Science, Tshwane University of Technology, Pretoria, South Africa

Acknowledgements

There are many people who helped bring this book to fruition, and we are grateful to all of them. We owe our gratitude to Sandie Burrows for completing the botanical illustrations and Lara Cocciuti for the distribution maps. All photographs were taken by AM Viljoen with the following exceptions; Cover and back page: Jan Vlok, *Adansonia*: Sandy Van Vuuren (a, b, d), Braam Van Wyk (c), *Artemisia*: Sandy Van Vuuren (b), *Aspalathus*: Elizabeth Joubert (a), *Athrixia*: Braam Van Wyk (a), *Cyclopia*: Braam Van Wyk (a), Elizabeth Joubert (b, c), *Eriocephalus*: Pietersarel de Bruyn (a, b, d), *Harpagophytum*: Ziets Zietsman (a, c), *Helichrysum odoratissimum*: John Burrows (b), John Manning (a), *Helichrysum petiolare*: Sandy Van Vuuren (a, b, c), *Hypoxis*: Braam Van Wyk (a), *Leonotis*: Braam Van Wyk (d), *Lessertia*: Braam Van Wyk (b), *Mesembryanthemum*: Sandy Van Vuuren (b, c, d), *Pelargonium sidoides*: Ulrich Feiter (a), Sandy Van Vuuren (b, c, d), *Prunus*: Braam Van Wyk (a, b), *Sclerocarya*: Braam Van Wyk (a, b, c, d), *Siphonochilus*: Sandy Van Vuuren (b, c), *Terminalia*: Braam Van Wyk (a, b, c) and *Xysmalobium*: SAplants, CC BY-SA 4.0, via Wikimedia Commons.

The plant material used in the Phytochemistry section was obtained from various sources, and we acknowledge the following people for their contribution: Sarah Venter and Baatile Komane (*Adansonia digitata*), Lindsey Chicken (*Agathosma betulina*), John Burrows (Buffelskloof) (*Athrixia phylicoides*), Pietersarel de Bruyn (HERBS-APLENTY) (*Pelargonium graveolens*), Jan Vlok (*Helichrysum odoratissimum*), Ulrich Feiter (Parceval Pty Ltd) (*Lessertia frutescens* and *Pelargonium sidoides*), HG&H Pharmaceuticals (*Mesembryanthemum tortuosum*), Roger Stewart (*Siphonochilus aethiopicus* and *Warburgia salutaris*), Peter Straughan (*Warburgia salutaris),* and The Kalahari Hoodia Growers (Namibia), Conrad Geldenhuys, Nico Laubscher, Marietjie Stander, Kobus Engelbrecht and Adolf Joubert for providing *Hoodia gordonii*.

We are also thankful to the following people for assisting with analytical aspects: Thandazile Mavimbela and Joanet Maree (*Agathosma betulina* and *Pelargonium sidoides* method development, respectively), Andrew Marston, Emmanuel Shikanga, Felix Makolo, Sushil Chaudhary and Thomas Idowu (isolation of some compounds). Gerhard Niemand is thanked for supplying diosphenol, and Lizette Joubert for the standards used in the monographs of *Aspalathus* and *Cyclopia*.

Introduction

1 The therapeutic properties of plants

1.1 Historical use of plants for holistic health and well-being

The use of medicinal plants has been proven by historians all over the world, to be as old as mankind itself. Sufficient archaeological evidence, in the form of written records and monuments, indicates that plant usage for healing purposes dates back to prehistoric times. Petrovska (2012) comprehensively provides a historical overview of events, outlining archaeological sources from as old as 5000 years ago, with the first discovery of a Sumerian clay slab from Nagpur, which had a record of 12 drug preparations from 250 medicinal plants. The Chinese 'Pen T'Sao' written in 2500 BC, documents 365 drugs from dried parts of medicinal plants, while various Indian holy books provide a record of medicinal plants, many of which are currently used as spices. Among the sources recorded over millennia is the prominent work of Theophrastus, the 'father of botany', who founded Botanical Science (371–287 AD) through documenting and classifying 500 medicinal plants known at that time. Dioscorides, the 'father of pharmacognosy', produced *De Materia Medica* approximately in 77 AD, describing the basic materia medica known up to the late Middle Ages and the Renaissance. In his work, he recorded 657 drugs of plant origin, describing the botanical features, occurrence/location, modes of collection and preparation, and therapeutic indications, among other aspects. These and other historical sources have provided invaluable knowledge that is still applied in various traditional medicine systems, as well as in modern drug development.

Although not as well documented as the abovementioned examples, Africa's medicinal plant use dates back many millennia, prior to the colonial era, however, records are sparse (Hammel, 2019). It is known that medicinal plants have always been a fundamental component of the traditional health care of Africa's indigenous tribes. The indigenous knowledge includes plant identification by vernacular names and morphological features, occurrence, useful plant parts, harvesting practices, therapeutic indications, modes of administration, and dosage. This knowledge was passed on orally through generations within a household, tribe, or community (Mahomoodally, 2013). Without physical records, it is possible that crucial parts of this information may have been distorted or lost between generations, hence a growing need exists to document ethnobotanical information on historical and modern-day plant use in African traditional medicine systems.

1.2 The healing properties of medicinal plants

The majority of plants have healing properties harboured in different plant parts, which can cure, soothe, or prevent various human and animal diseases and conditions. The source of these healing properties lies in the molecules that plants synthesise and accumulate to enhance their own survival. These molecules, otherwise known as secondary metabolites, include volatile oils, alkaloids, glycosides, terpenes, flavonoids and resins, among others. Secondary metabolites enable plants to inhibit or withstand parasitic, fungal, bacterial and viral infections, herbivory, other competing plants, as well as insect attacks. The ability of plants to regenerate following physical damage is an indication of underlying healing powers within this natural resource. Since ancient times, plants have been used to ease suffering as a result of acute or chronic illness, decontaminate surfaces and air, and for cleansing rituals. Many developing countries use medicinal plants as the mainstay of primary health care, particularly in rural areas, however, the practice is now widely accepted as an alternative to modern medicine in peri-urban and urban areas (Duri, 2009; Mwitwa, 2009). Ethnobotanical studies have shown that people from different parts of the world and varying cultures use the same plants to treat the same disease conditions. Some of the well-known traditional practices that make use of medicinal plants include Ayurveda, ancient Iranian medicine, Ifá, Islamic medicine, muti, Siddha medicine, traditional Chinese medicine, and Unani, among others. The inclusion of medicinal plants into the complementary and alternative medicine (CAM) system in developed countries indicates global acceptance of the healing potential of medicinal plants.

1.3 Plants as sources of therapeutic compounds for drug development

A vast range of plant secondary metabolites have medicinal properties, which has motivated researchers to tap into this rich resource for drug development. Contemporary science has proven that several groups of phytochemicals have various applications in disease management, resulting in a number of plant-based drugs being included in modern pharmacotherapy. Extensive research is currently underway to screen and test plant extracts and compounds against a range of pharmacological targets, particularly for the management of chronic and other diseases that have proven difficult to treat with conventional medicines. Some of the plant-based compounds that are currently exploited for potential health benefits include bitters, which can be used to improve appetite and strengthen the digestive system by stimulating the salivary glands.[a] Plant polysaccharides are useful in the management of dry and irritated skin and mucous membranes, due to their ability to produce mucilage or gum. Essential oils have a range of applications in respiratory tract infections, as antiseptics and disinfectants, which can be linked to traditional uses. Alkaloids, cardiac glycosides, phenols, pro-anthocyanins, flavonoids, minerals and vitamins have the potential for development into useful pharmaceutical products for disease management.[a] To date, a range of phytopharmaceuticals with various medicinal claims is available on both formal and informal markets as alternatives to conventional medicines.

[a] https://www.fs.fed.us/wildflowers/ethnobotany/medicinal/ingredients.shtml.

2 The South African scenario

2.1 Biodiversity and indigenous knowledge

South Africa is renowned for her diversity of fauna and flora. The country is listed as one of 25 biodiversity hotspots by Conservation International, a non-profit environmental organisation (Washington DC) (CI, 2005). This status was afforded because the ecology has been largely preserved, a large number of endemic plant species have been recorded, and the indigenous species and communities associated with these ecosystems are well represented. An estimated 24,300 plant taxa occur in southern Africa, and as many as 4000 of these are used in traditional medicine and cultural practices (Helwig, 2005; WHO, 2008). Although this flora represents a tenth of the global species, they occur on only 2.5% of the earth's land surface area (Germishuizen and Meyer, 2003). The Cape Floral Kingdom (Flora Capensis) is recognised internationally as one of the six floral kingdoms of the world. Although it is the smallest, it encompasses almost 9000 species of seed plants, which are mostly endemic (Manning and Goldblatt, 2012). Traditional medicine is widely used on the African continent. As many as 80% of the African population make use of indigenous medicines to treat minor and serious ailments (Mulholland and Drewes, 2004; Mulholland, 2005). The reasons for this practice are varied and include the unaffordability of registered drugs, cultural traditions, distance from clinics and pharmacies, and personal preference. Approximately 70% of all South Africans have consulted a Traditional Health Practitioner, of which there are 200,000 in the country (Kale, 1995). For a large proportion of the population, these practitioners are their only source of primary health care.

2.2 The regulatory framework of South Africa

Over the past two decades, the use of medicinal plants has been regulated through legislation proposed by the designated authorities in South Africa. The National Environmental Management: Biodiversity Act No. 10 (NEMBA) was adopted in 2004, with the aim of regulating the exploitation of herbal drugs and other biological resources. In 2008, the Bioprospecting, Access and Benefit Sharing (BABS) regulations came into effect, to ensure fair and equitable sharing of profits and other benefits resulting from bioprospecting involving indigenous knowledge and natural resources. The Biodiversity Act encompasses the sustainable use of indigenous resources and the protection of vulnerable species and ecosystems. Until 2013, natural health products were largely unregulated. However, amendments to the General Regulations were made in 2013, in terms of the Medicines and Related Substances Control Act, 1965 (Act 101 of 1965), to regulate products that are classified as complementary medicines. These include natural health products, although specific African traditional medicines are excluded. In February 2017, the South African Health Products Regulatory Authority (SAHPRA) was legally established as a Schedule 3A Public Entity in terms of the Public Finance Management Act (PFMA), 1999 (Act 1 of 1999) to fulfil specific responsibilities on behalf of the national government. The SAHPRA regulations pertain to all herbal medicinal products that are packaged as pharmaceutical dosage forms (capsules, tablets, etc.) or marketed as natural health products. These regulations are aimed at promoting the safety, efficacy and quality of the production and sale of complementary medicines as per guidelines. The Department of Health recognises the role of African Traditional Medicines, the potential and benefits of which have been integrated into the National Drug Policy of South Africa.

2.3 Commercialisation of South African plants

Traditional markets selling a large diversity of herbal drugs in their natural form, are widespread throughout South Africa (Street et al., 2008). These unprocessed drugs have considerable value and form an important part of the informal economy. However, despite the popularity of these traditional medicines, very few have been developed for the formal market. An extensive review by Van Wyk (2008) indicated that four species are well established globally, namely *Pelargonium sidoides* (for the treatment of infections of the upper respiratory tract), the indigenous herbal tea, rooibos (*Aspalathus linearis*), *Harpagophytum procumbens* (used for the relief of joint pain and mild digestive disorders), and marula (*Sclerocarya birrea*), used as food and cosmetic. Other commercialised species including, *Aloe ferox, Xysmalobium undulatum, Agathosma betulina* and *Hypoxis hemerocallidea*, have been well researched. An increased interest in herbal drugs is reflected by a marked increase in the number of patents filed, particularly for *Adansonia, Cyclopia, Mesembryanthemum* and *Lessertia* (*Sutherlandia*) species. Although extensively researched, several promising species remain only semi-commercialised. These include *Hoodia gordonii*, used as an appetite suppressant to treat obesity, *Sclerochiton ilicifolius*, containing a high intensity non-carbohydrate natural sweetener, *Lippia javanica*, used as a repellent for mosquitoes, and *Elephantorrhiza elephantina* that is applied to alleviate baldness. Most of the mentioned species are the topic of chapters in this book. Only a fraction of the wild-harvested plants reaches the formal market, despite approximately 1000 species being actively marketed in the informal sector. This is partly due to the lack of scientific data, which support and encourage commercialisation of specific species. Furthermore, insufficient knowledge of the raw plant material, lack of standardisation protocols, and phytochemical variation within a species, are additional factors that hamper the commercialisation of South African medicinal plants.

3 Quality control of herbal drugs

3.1 Role of quality control in ensuring safety and efficacy of herbal drugs

Although the quality control (QC) of Western medicines is considered non-negotiable, this aspect of herbal drugs was neglected for too long, largely due to a lack of regulation, and loopholes in the classification of herbal products, with the majority being marketed as supplements or nutraceuticals. However, QC, aimed at ensuring the consistency, safety and efficacy of herbal products, underpin their continued use by consumers. Quality control encompasses several aspects, of which the authentication of the plant material is crucially important (Mahomoodally, 2013). This is accomplished through macro- and/or microscope examination, or by chemical analysis (WHO, 2011). Species verification is of particular importance when related species with similar morphological characters can be easily confused, or when the plant material is costly, and cheaper, more readily available plant material can be used as a substitute (Tankeu et al., 2016). Once raw materials are powdered, taxonomic assessment is ruled out, and only chemical, genetic or anatomic methods can be relied upon for species identification. An assessment of the purity of the raw materials, which is linked to the safety of the product, is a second important step in QC. Purity determination is needed to establish the presence of foreign material, pesticides, bacteria, fungal toxins and/or potentially toxic metals (Busse, 2000; WHO, 2011) that may be naturally present, or result from incorrect harvesting and storage procedures. Finally, chemical analysis is needed to ensure that the content of distinctive markers or active ingredients conforms to the required levels, so that the recommended dosage consistently delivers the same amount of active ingredients (Busse, 2000). To achieve this, the development of in-house specifications and testing parameters by producers of herbal products is necessary in most cases (Folashade et al., 2012). These involve the evaluation of physicochemical properties and spectrophotometric, spectroscopic and/or chromatographic methods of analysis. Information provided in this book can assist with both species verification and the assessment of the chemical composition of the selected species.

3.2 Challenges specific to the quality control of herbal drugs

There are several challenges that hamper the development of QC protocols for herbal drugs. Plants produce an elaborate array of inter-linked secondary metabolites. The therapeutic benefits of the plant or its extract are determined by the specific and relative concentrations of active constituents (Busse, 2000). However, the active constituent(s) is often unknown, and/or pure reference standards may not be available commercially (Li et al., 2008). It may also be difficult to identify specific active ingredients, since loss of activity can occur during purification (Abdelgaleil et al., 2020). This arises from the elimination of compounds that play an additive, or even synergistic role, as the isolation proceeds. In such cases, marker compounds or visual patterns that display certain features, are used as a reference for qualitative and quantitative purposes. As opposed to cultivated material, which is generally more controlled, raw materials collected from the wild are often characterised by extensive chemical variation, arising from genetic traits, environmental conditions, as well as the phenotypic stage of the plant (Street et al., 2008). Different chemotypes within a species may display different bio-activities (Wink, 2003). The chemical fingerprint established as a reference should therefore correspond to the desired efficacy. Although tailor-made QC methods can be developed through research that takes phytochemical variability into account, these methods can often not be implemented by industry. Instead, simple, rapid analytical methods that require less sophisticated instrumentation are more practical in these settings.

3.3 Analytical techniques used in the quality control of herbal drugs

High-performance- (HPLC) or ultra-performance liquid chromatography (UPLC) coupled to ultraviolet/visible (UV/vis) light detection (such as photodiode array (PDA) detection) and/or mass spectrometry (MS) are techniques generally used for the analysis of botanical extracts dominated by non-volatile compounds (Alaerts et al., 2010). The chemical profiles of volatile constituents, for example, those present in essential oils, are obtained using gas chromatography (GC) with flame ionisation detection (FID) and/or MS, which facilitates the identification of compounds, even in the absence of authentic standards. For industrial environments, the development of thin-layer chromatography (TLC) methods is more appropriate. However, high-performance TLC (HPTLC), a semi-automated form of TLC, provides better resolution and reproducibility (Sagi et al., 2015). These planar techniques provide a visual fingerprint, with or without derivatisation of the compounds, which can be assessed quickly and compared to a reference fingerprint. Nuclear magnetic resonance spectroscopy has also been applied to obtain chemical fingerprints of plant extracts, thereby bypassing the limitations of the detectors used in chromatographic analysis (Zhao et al., 2018). Nevertheless, GC–MS and LC-UV/MS remain the preferred techniques for analysis of raw materials intended for herbal drugs, since complete separation and unequivocal identification of compounds in a mixture can be accomplished. Vibrational spectroscopy harnessing either near-infrared (NIR) or mid-infrared (MIR) radiation, has gained popularity as a QC technique and is particularly suited to industrial environments (Tankeu et al., 2016).

3.4 Typical workflow to develop QC methods for herbal drugs

It is challenging to develop QC methods that consider natural chemotypic variation for species where the active constituents are unknown. The starting point is to harvest as many samples of the selected species as possible, representing the same, and different sources or geographical origins (Sotenjwa et al., 2020). After authentication of the plant material, the extraction solvent is optimised. Solvent selection depends on the traditional use of the plant, or on the chemical class targeted. The extracts are then analysed using the technique of choice, and the data aligned (usually by using spectral data from UPLC–MS or GC–MS) for chemometric analysis. The large dataset generated is used to construct multivariate models, for example by applying principal component analysis or hierarchical cluster analysis. Patterns and trends in the data are evident in the generated scores plot. Subsequent construction of discriminant analysis models allows marker compounds (active or not) associated with each of the groups observed on the scores plot to be revealed (Bansal et al.,

2014; Sotenjwa et al., 2020). Such models can also be used to predict the group that best matches new raw materials tested against the model. Marker compounds can be targeted for isolation, and their structures elucidated, for use as reference standards. Typically, random samples from each cluster are tested in various *in vitro* and/or *in vivo* models to link the bio-activities to the chemical profiles. Software is also available for chemometric analysis of HPTLC images of samples (Fichou et al., 2016). The chemical fingerprints of selected species obtained using UPLC-PDA/MS, GC-FID/MS, HPTLC, and vibrational spectroscopy, provided in this book, can be used as a starting point to develop such models. Finally, the safety of samples reflecting different profiles should be established through *in vivo* testing.

4 The value of monographs and pharmacopoeias

4.1 The concept of monographs and pharmacopoeias

According to the World Health Organisation, which developed a document regarding Good Pharmacopoeial Practices (GPhP), the core function of a pharmacopoeia is *to protect public health by making available public standards to help ensure the quality of medicines* (WHO, 2015). Several documents contain medical knowledge and herbal remedies that are more than 3000 years old and date back to ancient Egypt. However, *De Materia Medica* is arguably perhaps the first example of a 'Pharmacopoeia'. This work originated from Greece and Rome during the 1st century BC and contained the known herbal remedies of the time, as well as their methods of preparation. The oldest known compilation of traditional Chinese materia medica, *Shen-nung Pen-ts'ao Ching*, dates back to the 2nd millennium AD. In Europe, several pharmacopoeias were prepared at the beginning of the 16th century. The first Indian Pharmacopoeia was completed in 1844, while the Russian Pharmacopoeia dates back to 1866. The Mexican, Japanese, Argentinean and Brazilian pharmacopoeias were published in 1846, 1886, 1898 and 1929, respectively. The United States Pharmacopoeia (USP) (1820) and the British Pharmacopoeia (BP) (1858), first recognised the need for pharmacopoeial harmonisation and standardisation to produce consistent standards for medicines. Other efforts at harmonisation followed and are still underway. The WHO published the International Pharmacopoeia to achieve wide global harmonisation of quality specifications for selected pharmaceutical products, excipients and dosage forms. The ultimate goal of this pharmacopoeia is to provide quality control specifications, to assist in providing global access to quality medicines. However, the International Pharmacopoeia only has legal status when the designated authority introduces it into appropriate legislation (Wiggins and Albanese, 2019). One of the goals included in the mandate of the WHO when it was established in 1948, was the publication of The International Pharmacopoeia. After several meetings and discussions on harmonisation, the goal became the development of Good Pharmacopoeial Practices (GPhP), to encourage harmonisation facilitated by the WHO. The Pharmacopoeial Discussion Group (PDG) defined harmonisation as *when a pharmaceutical substance or product tested by the document's harmonised procedure yields the same results and the same accept/reject decision is reached* (WHO, 2015).

Pharmaceutical monographs have been well-established and contain specific information pertaining to a pharmaceutical substance (active pharmaceutical ingredient) or finished pharmaceutical products. The WHO published four volumes of 'WHO Monographs on selected Medicinal Plants', which collectively contain 118 monographs on commonly used medicinal plants. The selection for inclusion is based on meeting two major criteria: (1) they must be in common use in at least two WHO Regions, and (2) there must be sufficient scientific data available to satisfy the requirements of the various sections in the monograph format. It is important to note that these monographs are not considered pharmacopoeial, but that their purpose is to: (1) provide scientific information on the safety, efficacy and quality control/quality assurance of widely used medicinal plants, to facilitate their appropriate use in WHO's Member States, (2) to provide models to assist WHO Member States in developing their own monographs or formularies for these and other herbal medicines, and (3) to facilitate information exchange among WHO's member states (WHO, 2009).

Herbal pharmacopoeias represent qualitative and therapeutic monographs on herbal medicines. According to Alamgir (2017), a herbal monograph is defined as *a document that defines a botanical drug and provides information that allows for its proper identification. It contains the basic description including nomenclature, part used, constituents, range of application, contraindications and side effects, incompatibilities with other medications, dosage, use and action of the herb*. The intention of a herbal pharmacopoeia is to promote the responsible use of herbal medicines with the highest possible degree of efficacy and safety, through the development of standards of identity, purity and analysis for botanicals. It should include a review of traditional and scientific data regarding the efficacy and safety of the herbal drug and its constituents. Several herbal pharmacopoeias have now been published.

4.2 Towards standardisation of African traditional medicines through monographs

The WHO (2019) Index of World Pharmacopoeias and Pharmacopoeial Authorities lists more than 40 pharmacopoeias used in various countries. For Africa, sadly only two Pharmacopoeias are listed: the African Pharmacopoeia Volumes 1 and 2 (published in 1985 and 1986, respectively) and the African Herbal Pharmacopoeia (AfrHP) 1st edition, 2010. The AfrHP produced by the Association for African Medicinal Plants Standards contains monographs on 51 African medicinal species. Information on nomenclature, botanical description, distribution, ethnobotany, chemistry, quality control markers and test methods, pharmacology, safety data, therapeutic information, market data, regulatory status in various countries, future prospects for development, and references are included (Blumenthal, 2011). In his review of the African Herbal Pharmacopoeia, the founder and executive director of the American Botanical Council, Mark Blumenthal (2011) stated that African medicinal herbs have gained significant popularity in the United States of America and elsewhere as traditional medicines, natural health products, dietary supplements and food supplements. Due to this popularity, the need for enhanced quality control of raw materials becomes inevitable. He provided several important examples of African medicinal plants that are well-known globally, including *A. linearis*, *Cryptolepis sanguinolenta*, *Griffonia simplicifolia*, *H. procumbens*, *Kigelia africana*, *Pelargonium sidoides*, *Prunus africana* and *Mesembryanthemum tortuosum*. Several of these plant species are indigenous to South Africa and have been included in this book.

In South Africa, various efforts to produce herbal monographs have been undertaken each containing different information aimed at a specific audience. For example, Scott and Springfield (2004) developed a set of monographs for 60 South African plant species used as traditional medicines. These monographs contained brief information on the synonyms and vernacular names, a macroscopic and crude drug description, geographical distribution, quality standards including identity tests, purity tests, assay method where available, information on major chemical constituents, adverse reactions, dosage etc. Each monograph publication builds towards establishing a complete set of monograph data for the immense number of medicinal plant species used in South Africa. As more research is published, it is important to update these monographs so that they contain the most comprehensive information.

Paramount to safety, is the quality of plant material. The first step towards producing a quality product is to confirm the identity of a plant species. Therefore, one of the key parts of a monograph is the identification of plant species. In addition to comprehensive literature reviews, this book provides analytical data to assist in confirming the identity of plant species through high-performance thin-layer chromatography, liquid chromatography coupled to mass spectrometry, gas chromatography coupled to mass spectrometry, where applicable, and MIR spectroscopic data.

References

Abdelgaleil, S., Saad, M., Ariefta, N., Shiono, Y., 2020. S. Afr. J. Bot., 128:35–41.

Alaerts, G., Dejaegher, B., Smeyers-Verbeke, J., Van der Heyden, Y., 2010. Comb. Chem. High Throughput Screen., 13 (10):900–922.

Alamgir, A.N.M., 2017. Therapeutic Use of Medicinal Plants and Their Extracts, vol. 1. Springer, Cham, Switzerland, pp. 295–353.

Bansal, A., Chhabra, V., Rawal, R.K., Sharma, S., 2014. J. Pharm. Anal., 4:223–233.

Blumenthal, M., 2011. HerbalGram, 90:71.

Busse, W., 2000. Drug Inf. J., 34:15–23.

CI (Conservation International), 2005. A Nonprofit Environmental Organization based in Washington DC. https://www.conservation.org.

Duri, J.Z., 2009. Consultancy Report Prepared for WWF Southern Africa Regional Programme Office. Harare, Zimbabwe.

Fichou, D., Ristivojević, P., Morlock, G.E., 2016. Anal. Chem., 88:12494–12501.

Folashade, O., Omoregie, H., Ochogu, P., 2012. Int. J. Bifurcation Chaos Appl. Sci. Eng., 4:101–112.

Germishuizen, G., Meyer, N., 2003. Plants of Southern Africa: An Annotated Checklist. Southern African Botanical Diversity Network, Strelitzia 14, Pretoria, South Africa.

Hammel, T., 2019. African farmers and medicinal plant experts. In: Shaping Natural History and Settler Society. Palgrave Macmillan, Cham, Switzerland.

Helwig, D., 2005. African traditional medicines. In: Alternative Medicine Encyclopedia. Cham, Switzerland.

Kale, R., 1995. BMJ, 310 (6988):1182–1185.

Li, S., Han, Q., Qiao, C., Song, J., Cheng, C.L., Xu, H., 2008. Chin. Med., 3:1–16.

Mahomoodally, M.F., 2013. Evid. Based Complement. Alternat. Med., 2013, Art. No. 617459.

Manning, J., Goldblatt, P., 2012. Plants of the Great Cape Floristic Region 1: The Core Cape Flora, Strelitzia 29. South African National Biodiversity Institute, Pretoria, South Africa.

Mulholland, D.A., 2005. J. Ethnopharmacol., 100:124–126.

Mulholland, D.A., Drewes, S.E., 2004. Phytochemistry, 65:769–782.

Mwitwa, J., 2009. Consultancy Report Prepared for WWF Southern Africa Regional Programme Office. Lusaka, Zambia.

Petrovska, B.B., 2012. Pharmacogn. Rev., 6 (11):1–5.

Sagi, S., Avula, B., Wang, Y., Khan, I., 2015. Planta Med., 81 (5), Art. No. PA21.

Scott, G., Springfield, E.P., 2004. Pharmaceutical Monographs for 60 South African Plant Species used as Traditional Medicines. South African National Biodiversity Institute (SANBI). http://pza.sanbi.org/information-library/medicinal-monographs/1102/2004.

Sotenjwa, V.Z., Chen, W., Veale, C.G.L., Anokwuru, C.P., Tankeu, S.Y., Combrinck, S., Kamatou, G.P.P., Viljoen, A.M., 2020. Fitoterapia, 147, Art. No. 104740.

Street, R.A., Stirk, W.A., Van Staden, J., 2008. J. Ethnopharmacol., 119:705–710.

Tankeu, S., Vermaak, I., Chen, W., Sandasi, M., Viljoen, A., 2016. Phytochemistry, 122:213–222.

Van Wyk, B.E., 2008. J. Ethnopharmacol., 119:342–355.

WHO, 2008. Traditional Medicine. Fact Sheet No. 134. http://www.who.int/mediacentre/factsheets/2003/fs134/en/.

WHO, 2009. WHO Monographs on Selected Medicinal Plants, vol. 4. https://www.who.int/medicines/areas/traditional/SelectMonoVol4.pdf.

WHO, 2011. World Health Organisation Report: Quality Control Methods for Herbal Materials. http://www.who.int/iris/handle/10665/44479.

WHO, 2015. World Health Organisation Expert Committee on Specifications for Pharmaceutical Preparations. Fiftieth Report. Good Pharmacopoeial Practices. https://www.who.int/medicines/publications/pharmprep/WHO_TRS_996_annex01.pdf.

WHO, 2019. World Health Organisation. Index of Pharmacopoeias. https://www.who.int/medicines/areas/quality_safety/quality_assurance/resources/index-of-pharmacopoeias_may_2019.pdf?ua=1.

Wiggins, J.M., Albanese, J.A., 2019. Pharmaceutical Technology. Regulatory Sourcebook. https://cdn.sanity.io/files/0vv8moc6/pharmtech/3920f12347b47bcf1f2c41d60a34b7706307bec6.pdf/PTebook0919_PharmacopeiaCompendia_History_watermark.pdf.

Wink, M., 2003. Phytochemistry, 64:3–19.

Zhao, J., Khan, I.A., Combrinck, S., Sandasi, M., Chen, W., Viljoen, A.M., 2018. Phytochemistry, 152:191–203.

CHAPTER

Adansonia digitata

1

Baatile Komane[a], Guy Kamatou[a], Nduvho Mulaudzi[a], Ilze Vermaak[a,b] and Gerda Fouche[c]

[a]*Department of Pharmaceutical Sciences, Tshwane University of Technology, Pretoria, South Africa*

[b]*SAMRC Herbal Drugs Research Unit, Faculty of Science, Tshwane University of Technology, Pretoria, South Africa*

[c]*Chemistry Department, University of Pretoria, Pretoria, South Africa*

Abstract

Adansonia digitata L. (Malvaceae), commonly known as 'baobab', is a large, seasonal tree distributed in many parts of Africa. It is more prevalent in Botswana, Namibia, Zimbabwe, Malawi, Mozambique, South Africa, Mali, the Ivory Coast, Senegal, Cameroon, Uganda, Kenya and Tanzania. Baobab is a very important non-timber forest product (NTFP) and contributes to the livelihoods of the African people. Various parts of the tree are used in African traditional medicine in the treatment of numerous ailments such as tuberculosis, malaria, fever, diarrhoea, microbial infections, anaemia and toothache. In addition, various plant parts are used as sources of food. The seed oil is applied topically as medicine or cosmetic. Several in vitro and in vivo pharmacological activities, including antimicrobial, anti-oxidant, anti-inflammatory, antimalarial and antidiabetic have been noted. Much research has been done on the nutritive value of the fruit pulp, seed kernels and seed oil. Chromatography techniques, such as semi-automated high-performance thin-layer chromatography (HPTLC), ultra-performance liquid chromatography coupled to mass spectrometry (UPLC–MS), and gas chromatography coupled to mass spectrometry (GC–MS), were used to determine the chemical profiles of A. digitata fruit pulp and seed oil. Several compounds, including procyanidin dimer I, epicatechin, procyanidin dimer II, kaempferol glycoside I and kaempferol glycoside II, were identified in the fruit pulp using UPLC–MS, whilst palmitic acid, stearic acid, linoleic acid and oleic acid were the major fatty acids detected in the seed oil, following esterification and analysis using GC–MS. The presence of some of the compounds was confirmed using HPTLC under 366 nm radiation.

Keywords: *Adansonia digitata*, Baobab, Seed oil, Fruit pulp, Fatty acids, HPTLC, UPLC–MS, GC–MS, MIR spectroscopy

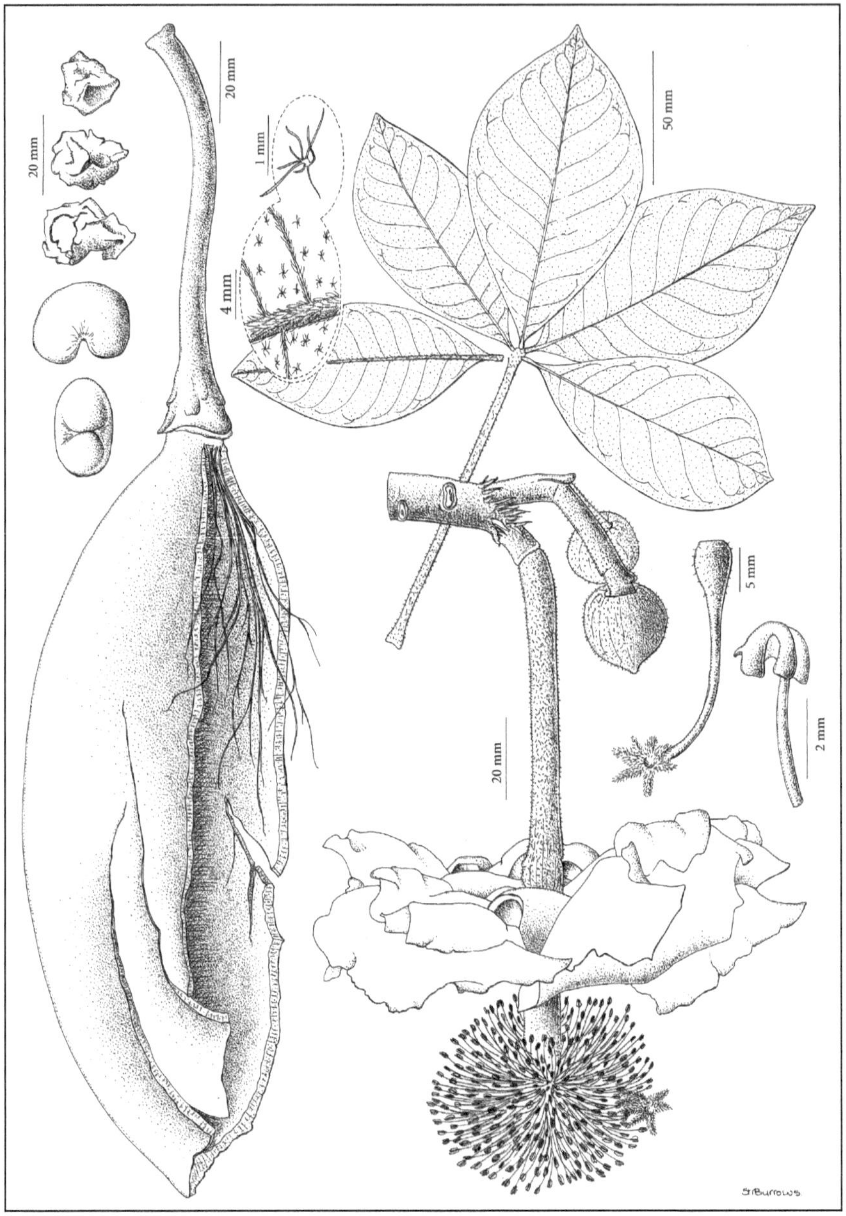
20 mm
20 mm
1 mm
4 mm
50 mm
5 mm
20 mm
2 mm
S.Burrows

Part A: General overview

1. Synonyms

Adansonia situla (Lour.) Spreng., *Adansonia integrifolia* Raf., *Adansonia baobab* Gaertn., *Adansonia scutula* Steud., *Adansonia sphaerocarpa* A.Chev., *Adansonia somalensis* Chiov., *Adansonia sulcata* A.Chev., *Ophelus sitularius* Lour., *Baobab digitata* (L.) Kuntze.[a]

2. Common name(s)

Cream of Tartar tree, baobab, lemonade tree, monkey-bread tree (English); '*kremetartboom*' (Afrikaans); '*umShimulu*', '*isimuku*', '*isiMuhu*' (isiZulu); '*mowana*' (Setswana); '*ximuwu*' (Xitsonga); '*muvhuyu*' (Tshivenda).[a]

3. Conservation status

Least concern.[a]

4. Botany

Adansonia digitata L. (baobab) is an iconic large tree, indigenous to Africa. The baobab tree is referred to as 'arbre a palabre', meaning a place where the village elders meet to resolve matters. The genus name '*Adansonia*' comes from the French surgeon, Michel Adanson (1727–1806) (SANBI, 2017) whilst the species name '*digitata*' refers to the shape of the leaves that appear hand-like with fingers resembling protrusions. The baobab tree belongs to the Malvaceae family, but it was previously associated with the Bombacaceae family. The trees are generally known as the upside-down trees, because the branches resemble a root system. The tree is considered the largest succulent plant in the world, with a height of up to 25 m. The stem, which reaches 28 m in circumference, gives rise to thick tapering branches (A). A thick bark covers the stem, which may be 50–100 mm thick. The bark is normally smooth, greyish-brown in colour and can be folded and seamed in different ways due to years of growth. The leaves are hand-sized and divided into 5–7 finger-like leaflets (B) (SANBI, 2017). Baobab is a deciduous tree with leaves that fall off during the winter and appear again in late spring or early summer. Large, sweetly scented, white, pendulous flowers (up to 200 mm in diameter) (C) emerge from large round buds on long drooping stalks in the late afternoon during the early summer season. The flowers last for 24 h before turning brown and smelling unpleasant, with

[a] Red List of South African Plants (http://redlist.sanbi.org).

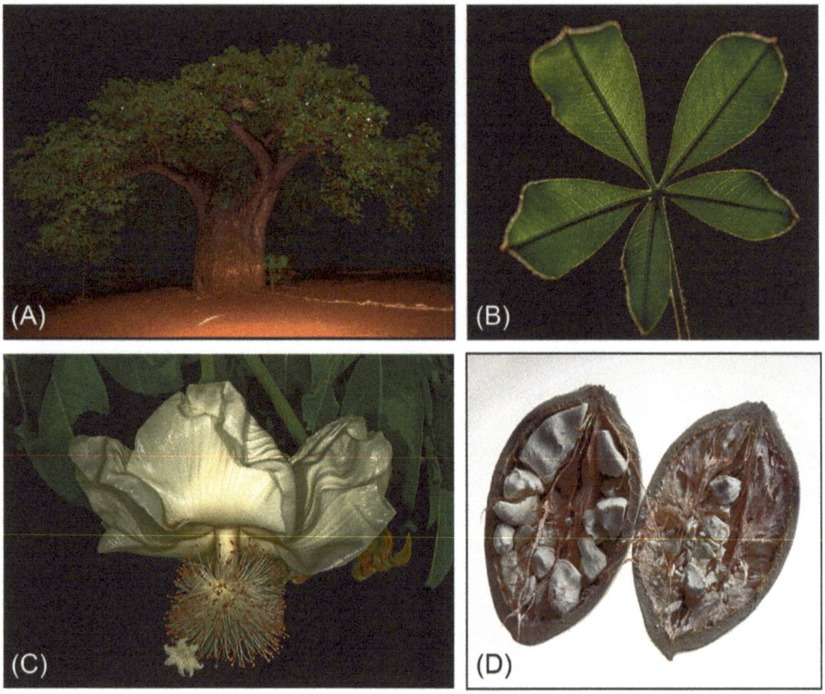

Adansonia digitata tree with thick tapering branches (A), finger-like leaflets (B), pendulous flowers (C) and a large egg-shaped fruit (D).

pollination facilitated by fruit bats taking place at night. The baobab fruit resembles a large egg-shaped capsule (often > 120 mm), covered with yellowish-brown hairs (SANBI, 2017). It consists of a woody, hard outer shell, with a powdery, dry substance inside that covers the black, hard, kidney-shaped seeds (D). The tree is slow-growing, mainly due to the low rainfall in the areas where it grows.

5. Geographical distribution

Adansonia digitata is indigenous to Africa and commonly found in Botswana, Namibia, Zimbabwe, Malawi, Mozambique and South Africa. In West Africa, it is found in Benin, Mali, the Ivory Coast, Senegal, Cameroon and Burkina Faso. In East Africa, the plant is common in Uganda, Kenya and Tanzania (Watt and Breyer-Brandwijk, 1962; Lamien-Meda et al., 2008). Furthermore, baobab trees grow in other tropical African countries, where suitable habitat occurs. It is restricted to dry, hot woodland with well drained, stony soils and frost-free areas that receive low rainfall. In South Africa, it is mostly found in the Limpopo and Mpumalanga provinces. However, it can be cultivated in areas of higher rainfall provided the winter season is mild and frost-free.

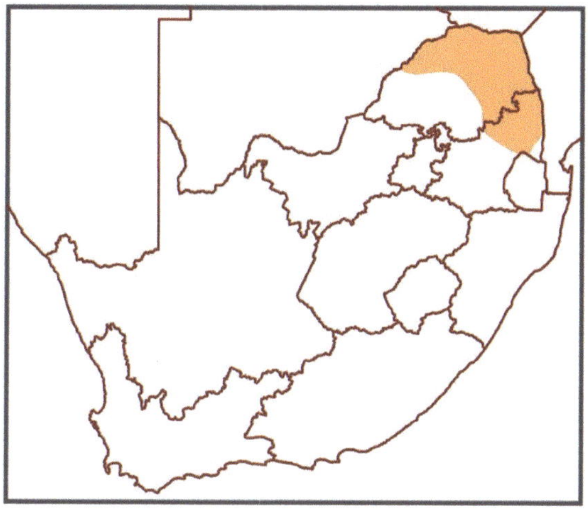

Geographical distribution of *Adansonia digitata* in South Africa.

6. Ethnopharmacology

Almost all parts of the tree are used in traditional medicine in Africa. The bark, leaves and seeds of the tree are used as a panacea to treat many diseases, but specific documented uses include the treatment of tuberculosis, malaria, fever, diarrhoea, microbial infections, anaemia, toothache and dysentery (Watt and Breyer-Brandwijk, 1962; Van Wyk and Gericke, 2000; Kamatou et al., 2011). Wickens (1982) reported that the leaves of baobab are used in Nigeria to overcome fever. The leaves of the baobab tree are reported to treat urinary tract infections, internal pain, otitis, insect bites and Guinea worm infestation, and are used as a tonic (Sidibe and Williams, 2002). The leaves are also used as an astringent and to alleviate excessive sweating (Watt and Breyer-Brandwijk, 1962). People infected with malarial parasites consume a mash containing dried baobab bark as a febrifuge to treat the fever associated with the infection (Wickens and Lowe, 2008). Other uses of the baobab include: tannin from the tree bark is used for curing leather; the fresh leaves are cooked and consumed as vegetables and are used as appetisers and as seasoning; from the bark fibre, rope, cloth and cordage are created; pulp is used for making paper from the harvested tree; glue is made from the pollen grains of the flowers; and the seed oil is used for topical treatment of skin ailments or as a cosmetic (Wickens, 1982; Van Wyk et al., 1997; Sidibe and Williams, 2002). The baobab is one of the most popular plant species utilised by Bapedi traditional healers across Limpopo Province in South Africa for treating sinusitis and related symptoms (Semenya and Maroyi, 2018a). It is also used by traditional healers to treat cancer (Segun et al., 2018).

The output of a survey conducted by Semenya and Maroyi (2018b) positioned *A. digitata*, *Catha edulis*, *Lasiosiphon caffer* and *Zanthoxylum capense* as Bapedi traditional healers' keystone species on the basis of the utility and application in the treatment of various ailments. Local people often harvest the bark on the lower part of the trunk to retrieve the strong fibre, which is used to make useful items such as ropes, mats, fishing nets, lines, clothing and sacks. Other uses of the bark include fodder during drought and feed for chickens (Lisao et al., 2017). Although the bark is often heavily stripped by elephants and people, the trees do not suffer from ringbarking as ordinary trees do, and have the ability to produce a new layer of bark and continue growing. The wood of the baobab is light yellow in colour, and soft and spongy in texture. It has been recorded that the wood has been used for making boxes, although not a commonly used practice. The seed oil of the tree has been used to produce soaps, lubricants, toothpaste, and for the topical treatment of various conditions such as varicose veins, muscle spasms and wounds. It is applied as a moisturiser for hair and skin hydration, and in treatment of dandruff and for nail conditions (Zimba et al., 2005; Nkafamiya et al., 2007; Chindo et al., 2010). Sidibe and Williams (2002) reported that baobab seed oil is used to treat skin ailments and is used for cosmetic applications. Local traditional uses of *A. digitata* amongst the Ovambo, Herero, Masubiya and San groups in northern Namibia showed that baobab uses go beyond merely the provision of food and medicine, but extend to spiritual needs. The value of bark is considered high amongst all ethnic groups, with the fruit as the most useful part of the plant.

7. Commercialisation

Many people in Africa derive an income from non-timber forest products (NTFPs). The baobab is considered an important commercial NTFP and is highly sought after in several market segments, for example botanical remedies (France, Germany and the Netherlands), beverages and food (France, Germany and the Netherlands), as well as natural cosmetics and nutraceuticals (United States, EU and Japan) (Kamatou et al., 2011). The baobab fruit is high in vitamin C and the powder can be used as a thickener, due to its high fibre and pectin content. It is therefore an ideal candidate for the functional food market. The oil extracted from baobab seeds is used by the cosmetic industry as an ingredient of healthcare and skincare products (Sidibe and Williams, 2002; UNCTAD, 2005). As the baobab fruit pulp has excellent anti-oxidant properties, it is therefore sought after as an ingredient in anti-ageing products (UNCTAD, 2005; IFAD, 2008). Non-profit community-based organisations, such as PhytoTrade Africa, play a major role in the baobab market in terms of the supply chain and marketing development of NTFPs. Baobab fruits are harvested in the rural areas of Zimbabwe and Malawi, and processing involves seed separation from the pulp. The pulp is then graded by particle size and sold as raw material. The seeds are processed into oil that is sold to cosmetic companies (UNCTAD, 2005; IFAD, 2008). On the 25th of July 2009, baobab dried fruit pulp (BDFP) was afforded the Generally Regarded as Safe (GRAS) status by the United States Food and Drug Administration (USFDA), for use as an ingredient in fruit cereal bars and blended fruit drinks, at levels of up to 15% and 10%, respectively (USFDA, 2009). The European Commission subsequently authorised the import of baobab fruit pulp as a novel food (Addy, 2009; Buchmann et al., 2010).

The phytochemical composition and properties of the baobab have led to its inclusion in various patent applications. The first patent application, granted on 26 September 1905, describes the process of producing a pulp-like mass through alkali treatment of the inner bark or the fibre of the monkey-bread tree. This mass can then be pressed or cast into any form before drying, to manufacture objects such as pulleys, buttons, pedestals and handles for tools, etc. (Geipel, 1905). Since then, patents have mostly focused on nutritional and dermatological applications. One patent documented that an extract or component of the baobab can be used for the care, treatment and prophylaxis of skin diseases and disorders, particularly of inflammatory reactions in animals and humans (Engels, 2009a). The baobab is also included as an ingredient of a nutraceutical product containing *Cyclanthera pedata* (Caigua), *Borojoa patinoi* (Borojo) and *Aframomum melegueta* (Grains of paradise) to promote well-being and to provide nutritional value, as an aid in preventative health management. According to the latter patent, this combination can be used as a dietary supplement in the form of powder, or sprinkled over food, as a capsule, a food additive or a ready-to-drink juice. The baobab is described as an intestinal regulator in the case of gastric disorders because it is a good source of micronutrients, vitamin C, and soluble fibres with pro- and prebiotic effects (Shatkina and Gurevich, 2010). Another invention focused on the baobab as an animal food additive to provide high-value food supplements, or food that counteracts malnutrition and is also tasty (Engels, 2009b). Various food products and postharvest treatments utilising the pulp were reported by Chipurura and Muchuweti (2013). A yoghurt product, with all the optimum sensory responses, was developed by a combination of baobab pulp, sugar and a stabiliser. Demands for baobab fruit and derivatives on the global organic market have increased rapidly, leading to concerns that this may negatively affect subsistence users, particularly in areas where there is an existing high dependence on these products, such as West Africa. In contrast to this, the baobab fruit is regarded as 'underutilised', and commercialisation would help reduce poverty in the southern parts of Africa. Harvesters are mostly women (98%), many of whom are uneducated (70%) and unemployed (98%). The majority of the harvesters (68%) were involved in informal occupations (55%) and received social grants, which contributed 18% and 35% to their total annual income, respectively. The direct-use and trade value of NTFPs contributed 33% and 14% to the annual income, of which the baobab fruit contributed 4% and 38%, respectively. The baobab fruit was the only NTFP that had a higher income value (4×) than direct-use value. The cash earned was used to invest in small businesses and buy food (73%), suggesting a move towards a cash economy away from subsistence (Venter and Witkowski, 2013).

In Europe, a wide range of products is available, encompassing more than 300 baobab products (Gebauer et al., 2014). In Germany, ready-made foodstuffs containing baobab, including sandwich spreads, soft drinks, cereal bars, chocolates and sweets, can be purchased. In addition, a diverse range of cosmetic and pharmaceutical products with baobab extracts is available on the market. Indoor pot plants, baobab seeds and saplings for cultivation and planting are sold. In Senegal, baobab bonsai seedlings are prepared for the European market. Baobab fruits are mainly harvested in Africa from wild stands. The baobab fruit is sold locally in urban areas or processed into a pulp that is either exported or sold to national confectionery companies (Wynberg et al., 2015). Since the early 1990s, local residents in Zimbabwe have produced and exported crafts made from baobab fibre to South Africa. Before this, harvesting was mostly for local consumption, with select members of the Gumbu tribe being skilled artisans for fibre crafting, with young boys and women involved in collecting leaves and fruits, with some of the fruit taken to open markets in urban areas. The baobab seed oil is very valuable, as it is exported for use in the cosmetic industry (Wynberg et al., 2015). In 2005, commercialisation of the seed oil started in South Africa, specifically in the Vhembe Municipal District in the northern region of Venda, where seeds were sold locally and oil was extracted from the seeds (Venter and Witkowski, 2010). The seed oil extracted from the baobab fruit is sold internationally and is very popular in the cosmetics industry (Munthali et al., 2012). The baobab is regarded as the highest earner of all NTFPs in the region, with an approximate annual income of up to US $1 billion for producer countries (RTFP, 2007). Locally, incomes are far more meagre, with households earning between US $350 and US $1500 per year from indirect or direct involvement in the baobab trade (Luckert et al., 2014). In South Africa, a complex regulatory framework for baobab exists due to the Government's view that the use of baobab in cosmetic and food products constitutes bioprospecting, which has led to an unworkable situation (Wynberg and Laird, 2014). Modiba et al. (2014) reported experimental results showing that it is feasible to produce biodiesel from baobab oil using sodium methoxide as a homogenous catalyst in a one-step transesterification process. Results also showed that important fuel properties of biodiesel from baobab oil met the specifications of the American Society for Testing and Materials (ASTM) and European standards.

8. Pharmacological evaluation

8.1 *In vitro* studies

8.1.1 Antifungal, antibacterial and anti-oxidant activity

Many scientific studies have been carried out on the baobab to determine its antimicrobial activities against pathogens that cause infections in both humans and animals. Yagoub (2008) investigated the antibacterial activity of petroleum ether, ethanol and aqueous extracts of *A. digitata* (whole plant) against *Escherichia coli* isolated from water and urine. The results showed that the ethanol extract inhibited bacterial growth, with the inhibition zones ranging from 20–30 mm, depending on the concentration tested. The susceptibility of the micro-organisms to the extracts was compared with selected antibiotics (Yagoub, 2008). Masola et al. (2009) investigated the antimicrobial activity of baobab plant parts (root and stem barks) against yeast, and Gram-negative and Gram-positive bacteria, and reported that the ethanolic and aqueous root and stem bark extracts inhibited the growth of various micro-organisms with minimum inhibitory concentrations (MICs) ranging from 1.5–6 mg/mL. The methanol, dichloromethane and hydro-ethanolic extracts from the stem bark of *A. digitata* have been tested for their antifungal, antibacterial and anti-oxidant activities. Sporulation inhibition of 70% was observed, whilst mycelial inhibition was < 40%, with MICs ranging from 0.039–2.5 mg/mL (Lagnika et al., 2012). A study by Gahane and Kogje (2013) assessed the potential of methanolic extracts of edible parts of the baobab, such as the stem (MESt), leaf (MEL), seed (MESe) and fruit pulp (MEFP) in terms of antibacterial and anti-oxidant activity. None or small inhibition zones were observed, indicating low sensitivity of the bacteria. The calculated half maximal inhibitory concentration (IC_{50}) values of 23 µg/mL (MEL), 22 µg/mL (MESt), 94 µg/mL (MESe) and 50 µg/mL (MEFP) were calculated for edible parts of *A. digitata* in the 2,2-diphenyl-1-picrylhydrazyl (DPPH) radical assay, indicating strong anti-oxidant activity.

The discovery of more efficient and new antibacterial agents is required due to the resistance of many bacteria to antibiotics, also referred to as multi-drug resistant (MDR) bacteria. The antibacterial effects of *A. digitata* were investigated, and the results indicated that the extracts exhibited good activity towards 81.48% of the 27 bacteria tested (Djeussi et al., 2013). The MDR isolates and various strains were tested for their susceptibilities to the extracts and the reference compound, chloramphenicol. Within the tested concentrations (8–1024 µg/mL), *A. digitata* exhibited low antibacterial activity against the bacteria tested (Seukep et al., 2013). In the lethality assay, stem bark and leaf essential oils yielded lethal concentration 50 (LC_{50}) values of 1932 and 1750 µg/mL, respectively. The study suggested that the essential oil can be used as an alternative antimicrobial agent to synthetic chemicals in the preservation of fresh tomato fruits. *In vitro* antifungal activity was observed for the methanol extract of *A. digitata* against *Rhizoctonia solani*, the causal agent of *Rhizoctonia* root rot of maize (Rashad et al., 2018). An eco-friendly, simple and cost effective method was reported by Kumar et al. (2015) for the synthesis of silver nanoparticles (AgNPs) from *A. digitata* leaf extract. Antimicrobial tests showed that the nanoparticles exhibited a broad range of antimicrobial efficacy against clinically isolated pathogenic micro-organisms. In another study, an alternative, efficient method for the large-scale production of AgNPs from *A. digitata* fruit pulp extract was documented (Kumar et al., 2016). It was shown through Fourier Transform Infrared (FTIR) spectroscopic analysis that proteins and phenols are mainly responsible for the stabilisation and reduction of nanoparticles. *Adansonia digitata* pulp extract was considered a good source for the reduction of AgNPs and acted as a benign antimicrobial agent.

Phytochemical evaluation of the extract of *A. digitata* was conducted using standard protocols to determine the total flavonoid and total phenolic content of the extract. Hydroxyl radical (•OH) scavenging activity, DPPH, and the reductive potential and ability of the extracts to chelate ferrous ions, were evaluated. The methanolic extract exhibited the highest flavonoid and phenolic content with 4.68 ± 0.00 µg/mL of quercetin equivalent (QE) and 2.15 ± 0.01 µg/mL of tannic acid equivalent (TAE), respectively. The aqueous extract yielded the highest ferric reducing anti-oxidant power (FRAP) value and the lowest IC_{50} values of 20.45 mg/mL, for hydroxyl radical scavenging activity. The IC_{50} values of DPPH radical scavenging activities were 14.62 and

18.22 mg/mL and ferrous-ion chelating activities were 28.95 and 38.75 mg/mL for the methanolic and aqueous extracts, respectively. The differences in ferrous-ion, DPPH and hydroxyl radical scavenging activities of methanolic and aqueous extracts were significant, with the methanolic extract displaying the highest anti-oxidant activity (Adeoye et al., 2016a). The maximum anti-oxidant activity of the baobab in terms of Trolox equivalent anti-oxidant capacity (TEAC), was $1.52 \times 10^3 \pm 17.1$ mg TEAC/100 g fresh weight (FW) for 2,2′-azinobis-(3-ethylenebenzothiazoline)-6-sulphonic acid (ABTS) assay, $2.81 \times 10^3 \pm 92.8$ mg TEAC/100 g FW for FRAP and 50.9% ± 0.43% for DPPH. Thermal pasteurisation (72 °C, 15 s) retained vitamin C content with an extended half-life under refrigeration temperature (6 °C). Correlation was shown between the anti-oxidant activity and bioactive compounds, and the anti-oxidant activity fluctuated during storage (Tembo et al., 2017). Microwave techniques and maceration were used to prepare ethanol, water and 50% ethanol extracts of *A. digitata* (Hussain et al., 2019). The fruit pulp of *A. digitata* showed variable anti-oxidant, phenolic content and enzyme inhibition capacity linked to the method of extraction and solvent type used. Microwave extraction resulted in the highest polyphenolic content (66.40 ± 0.32 mg GAE/g) extracted using 50% ethanol, whilst anthocyanidin (2.37 ± 0.06 mg GAE/g) and flavonoid (42.15 ± 0.12 mg QE/g) content was highest using water as solvent. The highest anti-oxidant activity in all five assays used was observed for the ethanol extract prepared using maceration. The microwave extraction technique recorded high anti-oxidant activity of a 50% ethanol extract. The highest acetycholine esterase (AChE) inhibition activity was recorded when 50% ethanol was used as solvent with maceration.

A study was conducted to evaluate the anti-oxidant activity and identify the phytochemicals in baobab fruit pulp (Ismail et al., 2019b). The best solvents for anti-oxidant activity and total phenolic content (TPC) were defined: 50% methanol for DPPH activity and 80% acetone was the best solvent for TPC, with a high correlation between anti-oxidant activity and phenolic content. The seed oil quality parameters were determined as 4.08 mEq/kg, 86 g/100 g and 188 mg/g for the peroxide value, iodine value and saponification value, respectively. The oil content of the kernel (23%) was higher than that of the hulls that contained 5.4% oil. The kernel oil contained substantial quantities of potassium, calcium and magnesium, which were determined as 2339, 4116 and 1629 mg/kg, respectively. The fatty acid profile indicated that palmitic acid was the major saturated acid, whereas linoleic and oleic acids were the major unsaturated fatty acids. The oil also exhibited good anti-oxidant activity, probably due to its high TPC. The fruit pulp extracts of twelve edible, wild fruits were investigated for their anti-oxidant, antimicrobial and cytotoxic activities. Methanol extracts of the pulps were tested against five micro-organisms (*Streptococcus pyogenes, Salmonella typhi, Bacillus cereus, Prevotella intermedia*, and *Klebsiella pneumoniae*). The fruit pulp extracts exhibited different antimicrobial activities, with significant antimicrobial activity against *Salmonella typhi*. None of the fruit pulp extracts were toxic (Tshikalange et al., 2017). The African baobab fruit produces natural compounds that can extend the shelf-life and preserve fruit quality, and these were determined to be several bioactive anti-oxidants, with ascorbic acid being the major component. The African baobab extract (100 mg/mL), in combination with *Sporidiobolus pararoseus* Y16, significantly inhibited the growth of *Penicillium expansum* infection when compared with either the African baobab or yeast alone, during storage at either 20 °C for 30 days or at 4 °C for 30 days, followed by 20 °C for 15 days (Abdelhai et al., 2019).

The ethyl acetate extract of *A. digitata* was found to exhibit potent anti-oxidant activity (IC_{50} = 0.2 µg/mL) in a hydroxyl radical scavenging assay (Kinghorn et al., 2011). Three compounds were isolated from this extract, previously identified as procyanidin B2, epicatechin and procyanidin B5, with IC_{50} values obtained in the hydroxyl radical scavenging assay of 0.59, 0.30 and 0.05 µg/mL, respectively, compared with the positive control, quercetin (IC_{50} = 0.04 µg/mL). Lamien-Meda et al. (2008) determined the anti-oxidant activity of the fresh ripe fruit of *A. digitata* as 1000 mg AEAC/100 g (ascorbic acid equivalent anti-oxidant capacity). Brady (2011) found that the anti-oxidant capacity of the lipophilic extract of fruit pulp (3.32 mg ascorbic acid equivavalent) was lower than that of the hydrophilic extract of fruit pulp (7.65 mg ascorbic acid equivalent/g). Carlson et al. (2010) also confirmed that the anti-oxidant potential of the baobab varies according to the plant part used. The anti-oxidant content of dried leaves was almost five times higher (48.1 mmol/100 g) than that of fruit pulp. The anti-oxidant content of the dried leaves and fruit of baobab was higher than that of mango (1.7 mmol/100 g), orange (0.9 mmol/100 g), papaya (0.6 mmol/100 g) and apple (3.8 mmol/100 g). Vertuani et al. (2002) also compared the anti-oxidant activity of baobab to other fruits and showed that the fruit pulp of the baobab exhibited potent anti-oxidant activity corresponding to 6–7 mmol/g of Trolox® equivalent, compared to the fruit pulps of strawberry (0.90 mmol/g), orange (0.1 mmol/g), kiwi (0.34 mmol/g) and apple (0.16 mmol/g). Nhukarume et al. (2010) researched the capacity of solvent extracts of various fruits to inhibit the peroxidation of lipids, and the data revealed a significant difference in the activity of the beverage extracts, with *A. digitata* having the highest activity. The order of activity was *A. digitata* > ascorbic acid > *Citrus sinensis* (orange) > *Strychnos spinosa* > *Parinari curatellifolia*. Besco et al. (2007) investigated the anti-oxidant activity of baobab red fibre and the lipid soluble-, ascorbic acid- and the water-soluble anti-oxidant capacities. The results revealed significant anti-oxidant capacity of the lipid-soluble baobab red fibre (508.0 ± 0.008 µmol/g, Trolox® equivalent). The same pattern was observed for the water-soluble anti-oxidant capacity, corresponding to the activity expressed as µmol/g equivalents of ascorbic acid for each gram, with the ascorbic acid equivalents of the baobab red fibre exceptionally high (386.0 µmol/g). In the same study, it was shown that the integral anti-oxidant capacity of baobab red fibre (1617.3 µmol/g) was significantly higher (66 times) compared to that of orange pulp (24.3 µmol/g).

8.1.2 *Trypanosoma* inhibition

The capacity of the bark and leaves of *A. digitata* to reduce the mobility of *Trypanosoma brucei* (causing sleeping sickness) was investigated using four different solvent extracts (chloroform, petroleum ether, methanol and water). The time at which mobility stopped ranged between 25 and 45 min for the leaves, whilst for the root bark, the mobility ceased between 10 and 45 min, for extracts tested at 2 mg/mL (Atawodi, 2005). In another study, the *in vitro* trypanocidal activity of the baobab was microscopically investigated against *T. congolense* and *T. brucei brucei*, which cause nagana in animals. The methanol root extract showed a good effect on motility after 55 and 50 min for *T. congolense* and *T. brucei brucei*, respectively (Atawodi et al., 2003).

8.1.3 Antidiabetic activity

Blanching of the leaves of the baobab caused a significant decrease in the phenolic acid and flavonoid contents; reducing power; $ABTS^{*+}$ and DPPH* scavenging ability; and Fe^{2+}-induced lipid peroxidation inhibitory capacity of the extract. Similarly, the inhibitory effect of the extract of the baobab on the activities of α-glucosidase, α-amylase and aldose reductase was significantly reduced due to blanching (Irondi et al., 2017). Extracts of fruit pulps from *A. digitata*, obtained from three markets, were evaluated for their anti-oxidant activity, TPC and α-glucosidase inhibition (Braca et al., 2018). Baobab fruit pulps were found to be rich in flavonol glycosides and procyanidins, with the major constituent identified as tiliroside. A profile of the baobab fruits similar to that of the leaves was obtained, and all fruit pulp extracts exerted high α-glucosidase inhibition and anti-oxidant activity compared to the acarbose standard.

8.1.4 Antiviral and anti-HIV/AIDS activity

Adansonia digitata has been investigated for its antiviral activity. Fruit pulp, leaves and seeds were extracted with three different solvents: methanol, water and dimethyl sulphoxide (DMSO) (Vimalanathan and Hudson, 2009). The extracts were compared quantitatively for their ability to inhibit the respiratory syncytial virus. In addition, their effects on cytokine secretion (IL-8 and IL-6) in human epithelial cell cultures and antiviral MIC values were established against the herpes simplex virus and the influenza virus. The influenza virus was found to be the most susceptible, whilst the leaf extracts displayed the most potent antiviral properties, especially the DMSO extracts. Significant activity was also seen for the seed and pulp extracts. Several of the extracts, particularly the leaf extracts, were active as cytokine modulators, some being anti-inflammatory and others pro-inflammatory. Anani et al. (2000) investigated the antiviral activity of several plants against the sindbis, herpes simplex and polio viruses. The baobab leaf extract was found to have the most potent effect. The antiviral activity of *A. digitata* fruit pulp, leaves and seeds extracted with DMSO, water and methanol was researched by Vimalanathan and Hudson (2009). The study was conducted using the serial dilution method against the herpes simplex virus, influenza virus and respiratory syncytial virus. The respiratory syncytial virus was resistant, whilst the influenza virus was highly susceptible. The most promising activity against the influenza virus was observed for the leaf extract, with MIC values of 2.8 μg/mL for water and 0.12 μg/mL for the DMSO extract. The leaf extract was also active against the herpes simplex virus (HSV) (MIC value: 1.0–11.7 μg/mL), whilst the seed and pulp displayed much lower activity (MIC value > 72.5 μg/mL). Furthermore, the anti-HSV activity was markedly enhanced by light, especially long wavelength UV, although good 'dark' antiviral activity was also observed. All the extracts contained antiviral photosensitisers (Hudson et al., 2000; Vimalanathan and Hudson, 2009).

The aerial parts of *A. digitata* were successively extracted by gradient solvents (Ateya et al., 2016). The resulting extracts were bioassayed and significant activities observed: adenovirus type-7, 56.6% (MeOH extract) and 66.6% (water extract), HepG2 cytotoxicity (IC_{50} 19.3 μg/mL *vs* 24.46 μg/mL for doxorubicin), analgesic (82.5% *vs* 79.6% for standard aspirin), as well as anti-inflammatory activity (61.5% *vs* 59.5% for indomethacin). The methanolic root bark extract of *A. digitata* was evaluated for its antiviral properties against 175 specific antibodies by treating it with embryonated chicken eggs (ECEs) infected with a Newcastle disease virus (NDV) strain (Sulaiman et al., 2011). After 2 h of exposure of the virus to eight different concentrations of the extract, followed by 24 h incubation, mortality was observed. The 100 ED_{50} concentration of the virus and the highest concentration of the extract were inoculated as positive and negative controls, respectively. All eggs inoculated with 2 and 5 mg/mL virus/extract suspensions, as well as the virus alone, died 72 h post inoculation, with no mortality amongst those inoculated with 200 and 250 mg/mL extract/virus suspensions, as well as those inoculated with the extract alone. Anti-HIV-1 reverse transcriptase activity was recorded for *A. digitata* and an IC_{50} value of 2.3 μg/mL was obtained (Chinsembu, 2019).

8.1.5 Anti-inflammatory activity

Extracts of *A. digitata* were evaluated for genotoxicity using the Ames test, both without and with S9 metabolic activation against *Salmonella typhimurium* tester strain TA98. The extracts were also tested to determine their anti-inflammatory activity against the cyclooxygenase (COX-1 and COX-2) enzymes. The highest anti-inflammatory activities were observed for the petroleum ether and dichloromethane extracts of *A. digitata* bark in both COX-1 and COX-2 assays at a concentration of 250 mg/mL (Mulaudzi et al., 2013). The methanol extract of *A. digitata* leaf (MEAD) was investigated for its anti-inflammatory and anti-oxidant effects because of its inhibition of NO production and high polyphenol concentration. The potency of MEAD was 10.2 times higher than that of vitamin C at eliminating peroxyl radicals in the oxygen radical absorbance capacity (ORAC) assay. It also displayed a strong reactive oxygen species (ROS) scavenging effect in the DPPH assay and significantly inhibited iNOS activity (IC_{50} value of 28.6 μg/mL) in lipopolysaccharide (LPS)-stimulated RAW 264.7 cells. In addition, MEAD inhibited NF-κB translocation from the cytosol to the nucleus and IκBα degradation in LPS-induced RAW 264.7 cells without significant cytotoxic effects, as confirmed in the 3-(4, 5-dimethylthiazol-2-yl)-2,5-diphenyltetrazolium bromide (MTT) assay. The study revealed that MEAD inhibited anti-inflammatory iNOS expression, which may be related to the elimination of peroxyl radicals and thus the inhibition of IκBα-mediated

NF-κBκB signal transduction (Ayele et al., 2013). The polysaccharide isolated from *A. digitata* mainly consisted of glucose and fructose (1:8) with a molecular weight of $\pm 5.3 \times 10^4$ Da. Ibrahim et al. (2014) showed that *A. digitata* demonstrated potential anti-oxidant activity in a concentration-dependent manner. At concentrations of 300 and 600 μg/mL, *A. digitata* exhibited 100% effect as a chelator for the superoxide radical, metal and hydrogen peroxide, and inhibited both nitric oxide formation (96%) and lipid peroxidation (100%). The anti-inflammatory activities of the polysaccharide at different concentrations were assessed in the COX inhibition assay. Both enzymes (COX-1 and COX-2) were inhibited by the polysaccharide; the inhibition of COX-2 was higher than COX-1 inhibition at all concentrations tested. The 15-lipoxygenase (LOX) inhibitory activity of *A. digitata* was examined using the ferrous oxidation-xylenol orange assay method (Dzoyarchem et al., 2014). All the extracts displayed some 15-LOX inhibitory activity, ranging from 32.9% to 78.64%. The fruit of *A. digitata* had the highest anti-oxidant capacity i.e. IC_{50} values of 9.16 and 8.15 μg/mL in the ABTS and DPPH assays, respectively; the highest concentrations of total phenolics (237.68 mg GAE/g) and total flavonoids (16.14 mg GAE/g), as well as a TEAC of 0.75 in the FRAP assay. Good correlations were observed between ABTS and DPPH values, and between total flavonoids and phenolics.

8.1.6 Immunomodulating properties

Arabinogalactan proteins (AGP) derived from plants were determined as dermatologically and immunologically active compounds (Zahid et al., 2017). An *in vitro* system was used to investigate AGP extracted from baobab seeds for their biological effects on the HaCaT keratinocyte cell line. Real-time quantitative reverse transcription-polymerase chain reaction (qRT-PCR) analysis showed that AGP induced a substantial overexpression of TLR-5, hBD-2 and IL1-α genes. The results showed that plant-derived AGP could also modulate skin innate immune responses, already known to control plant defensive processes.

8.1.7 Antimalarial activity

The methanol extract of *A. digitata* was evaluated for *in vitro* antimalarial activity using a multiresistant strain of *Plasmodium falciparum* K1. Ajaiyeoba et al. (2004) reported that the extract did not exhibit any significant activity (IC_{50} value of 429.9 μg/mL). Köhler et al. (2002) investigated the antiplasmodial activity of an aqueous extract of baobab pulp against the chloroquine-resistant and -sensitive strains of *P. falciparum*; low activity was observed with an IC_{50} value > 50 μg/mL.

8.1.8 Other activities

A study was conducted to investigate the use of *A. digitata* mucilage in a formulation of matrix tablets, as well as the *in vitro* mechanism and kinetics of drug delivery using aminophylline as positive control (Builders et al., 2007). The drug-release retardation efficiency of *A. digitata* mucilage at equal polymer concentrations was less than that of hydroxypropyl methylcellulose, but higher than those of plasma concentration in simulated gastrointestinal fluid and simulated intestinal fluid. It was deduced that the mechanism of release of aminophylline from *A. digitata* mucilage in hydroxypropyl methylcellulose was by diffusion. The methanol extracts, as well as the aqueous- and organic-soluble partitioning materials of barks and leaves of *A. digitata* were evaluated for thrombolytic, anti-oxidant, membrane-stabilising, cytotoxic, antimicrobial, antidiarrhoeal and analgesic activities (Tahia et al., 2015). The carbon tetrachloride-soluble partition fraction of the leaves caused a 48.11% clot lysis in the assay for thrombolytic activity of human blood clots. In the DPPH free radical scavenging assay, the aqueous soluble materials of leaves and bark exhibited a potent free radical scavenging activity, with IC_{50} values of 7.70 and 2.21 µg/mL, respectively, whilst the crude extract of leaves and their petroleum ether soluble fraction showed significant lethality to brine shrimps having LC_{50} values of 6.99 and 0.284 µg/mL, respectively (Tahia et al., 2015). In the membrane-stabilising assay, the aqueous- and carbon tetrachloride-soluble fractions of the methanol extract from the leaves inhibited 16.03% and 61.52% hypotonic heat- and solution-induced haemolysis of red blood cells, respectively. The methanolic extracts of bark and leaves of *A. digitata* revealed significant peripheral and central analgesic activity at 400 and 200 mg/kg body weight (bw). The crude extract of the leaves of *A. digitata* also displayed mild antibacterial and significant antidiarrhoeal activities (Tahia et al., 2015).

8.2 *In vivo* studies and clinical trials

8.2.1 Antimalarial activity

Aqueous and organic extracts of *A. digitata* which is used for the treatment of malaria in traditional health systems of the Msambweni people in Kenya, were evaluated for brine shrimp lethality and antimalarial activity against *Plasmodium berghei* (Musila et al., 2013). The water extract of the stem bark of *A. digitata* displayed a high chemosuppression (460%) of parasitaemia in a murine model of *Plasmodium berghei* infection. No toxicity was observed to brine shrimps for the organic and aqueous extracts of *A. digitata*. Sesquiterpene lactones and saponins were present in organic extracts, but absent in aqueous extracts of *A. digitata*. The therapeutic effects of the methanolic and aqueous extracts of *A. digitata* stem bark were investigated *in vivo* against established infection in chloroquine-sensitive *Plasmodium berghei*-infected mice (Adeoye and Bewaji, 2015). Two doses (400 and 200 mg/kg bw) of methanolic and aqueous stem bark extracts were administered orally to albino mice. Significant dose-dependent chemosuppressive effects were exerted for the extracts (both dosages) at different levels of the infection. It was shown that the 400 mg/kg bw dose was more effective with respect to the parasite clearance than the lower dose of 200 mg/kg bw. Significant chemosuppression was observed for the methanolic extract at a dose of 400 mg/kg bw, and significant mean survival time was recorded in the extract-treated group when compared to the control. Another study (Adeoye et al., 2016b) investigated the prophylactic and suppressive potential of flavonoid-rich extracts of *A. digitata* stem bark in *Plasmodium berghei*-infected mice. Doses of 200 or 400 mg/kg bw, of extract were administered to albino mice for five consecutive days. The data revealed a dose-dependent chemosupression in the extract-treated groups, with the

400 mg/kg bw dose exhibiting better parasite clearance than the 200 mg/kg bw dose. The study demonstrated that a flavonoid-rich extract of *A. digitata* stem bark has potent antimalarial properties and caused a mutual delay in parasitaemia.

In another study, the efficacy of *A. digitata* stem bark extract was examined for its remediation effect, after malaria infection was established, and for its ability to protect against experimental malaria (Adeoye and Bewaji, 2018). Mice were transfected intraperitoneally with a chloroquine-susceptible strain of *Plasmodium berghei*-infected erythrocytes. Significant dose-dependent increases were observed for percentage clearance/chemosupression and packed cell volume (PCV), as well as a significant decrease in the percentage parasitaemia at the two doses of the extracts administered after established infection. Potent chemosuppressive activity was observed for the methanolic extract. The extract further significantly increased the level of superoxide dismutase and catalase activity, as well as the level of glutathione (GSH), with a reduction in the degree of tissue peroxidation. Administration of the extract after established infection reduced TNF-α concentrations and serum CRP, as well as tissue alkaline phosphatase (ALP) and serum activity. Adeoye and Bewaji (2019) investigated the efficacy of *A. digitata* stem bark extract on renal and haematological changes in established *Plasmodium berghei* infection in mice. The white blood cell (WBC) count, haemoglobin (Hb) content and cell differentials were examined. The extracts showed a significant dose-dependent increase in percentage chemosupression and PCV, and a significant decrease in percentage parasitaemia at the two doses tested after established infection. A significant decrease in neutrophils, haemoglobin content, mean corpuscular haemoglobin concentration (MCHC) and lymphocytes was noted in the control group. The extract significantly reduced platelets, WBC, mean corpuscular haemoglobin (MCH), monocyte count and mean cell volume (MCV). Administration of the extract after established infection significantly reduced the Na^+, creatinine, Ca^{2+}, K^+ and Cl^- concentrations.

8.2.2 Antidepressant activity

The methanol extract of the stem bark of *A. digitata* (MEAD) was evaluated for chronic unpredictable mild stress (CUMS) and the mechanism responsible for its antidepressant activity researched (Shehu et al., 2019). On CUMS-induced depression, MEAD significantly and dose-dependently increased sucrose consumption, increased the line-crossing activity, increased the novelty exploration time in the novelty object recognition test, reversed weight loss, and decreased the duration of immobility. The results from the study showed that MEAD ameliorated CUMS-induced depressive-like behaviour, and the effect was possibly mediated *via* the neurotrophic, neuroendocrine and oxidative stress pathways.

8.2.3 Analgesic and antipyretic activity

The aqueous extract of the fruit of *A. digitata* was evaluated *in vivo* for analgesic activity in mice. Activity was demonstrated 2 h after administration of the extract (Ramadan et al., 1994). At a dose of 800 mg/kg, the reaction time was noted at 15.4 min in comparison to the negative control (10.2 min). The petroleum ether extract from the seed oil of *A. digitata* exhibited analgesic activity with the tail flick response (6.1 s), and the response was not statistically different from the positive control, aspirin (Khan et al., 2006). The antipyretic activity of *A. digitata* extract was investigated using 20 rats. Hyperthermia was induced by subcutaneous injection of a yeast suspension (12%) and the temperature of the rats was monitored (Ramadan et al., 1994). Results demonstrated that the baobab extract exhibited antipyretic activity, as the rectal temperature of the rats decreased (37.3 °C) compared to the initial temperature of 38.6 °C, after 4 h of treatment, at a concentration of 800 mg/kg. *Adansonia digitata* was assessed for analgesic effects at doses of 50, 100 and 200 mg/kg bw by tail flick, acetic acid-induced writhing and hot plate analgesic models (Mumtaz et al., 2017). No acute oral toxicity was observed for the extracts at doses of 50–3000 mg/kg bw. The extract of *A. digitata* (orally administered) demonstrated analgesic activity by a decrease in writhe counts. A significant increase was observed in the latency period in the hot plate analgesic test when compared to the standard drug, diclofenac sodium (50 mg/kg). Furthermore, in a tail-flick test at doses of 50, 100 and 200 mg/kg bw, the extracts exhibited significant analgesic activity, which was dose-dependent when compared to the control group. Another study demonstrated the analgesic effect of a water extract of the bark of *A. digitata* using Wistar rats (Owoyele and Bakare, 2018). Oral administration of a dose of 25, 50, 100 or 200 mg/kg of the aqueous extracts of *A. digitata* were evaluated, as well as 5 mg/kg of indomethacin (reference group) and 10 mL/kg of normal saline (control group). Animals treated with the water bark extract of *A. digitata* exhibited significantly prolonged response time to thermal stimuli (4.42 ± 0.11 s) compared to the control group (3.29 ± 0.29 s). Animals administered with the aqueous bark extract showed a significant reduction in paw-licking time (47.88 ± 3.48–40.80 ± 3.85 s) at the early phase compared to the control group (91.51 ± 7.32 s) in the formalin paw-licking test. In the late phase, the water bark extract significantly reduced the paw-licking time (43.57 ± 2.6–25.49 ± 3.46 s) compared to the control group (66.31 ± 5.04 s). Bakare et al. (2019) investigated the effects of *A. digitata* bark extract on sciatic nerve ligated induced neuropathic pain. An increase in the pain threshold was observed on the hot plate, as well as the cold- and hot-immersion test, with extract treatment. Interestingly, a decrease in systemic prostaglandin E2 occurred simultaneously with a strengthened oxidative defence system. In contrast, extract-propranolol, -hexamethonium, or -prazosin, or -atropine co-treatments in induced neuropathic rats suggested no involvement of nicotinic, muscarinic, α-1 or β-receptors in the analgesic action of the extract. However, a weaker oxidative defence system was observed, based on the oxidative markers measured.

8.2.4 Hepatoprotective properties

The hepatoprotective activity of an aqueous extract of the fruit pulp towards chemical-induced toxicity using carbon tetrachloride (CCl_4) was investigated *in vivo* in rats by Al-Qarawi et al. (2003). The data obtained from the study clearly revealed that the extract exhibited significant hepatoprotective properties. The liver protective activity of *A. digitata* extract was 87%, 77% and 76% for alkaline phosphatase (ALP), aspartate transferase (AST) and alanine transferase (ALT) activity, respectively, when the extract was administered at the start of the CCl_4 test. The results indicated that consumption of *A. digitata* fruit may play an important role in resistance to liver damage in areas where the baobab is consumed. It was reported that the protective effect could be due to β-sitosterol, triterpenoids, β-amyrin palmitate and/or ursolic acid and α-amyrin present in the fruit, although the mechanism of action was not established (Al-Qarawi et al., 2003). The effect of baobab seed oil on drug-metabolising enzymes (cyclopropenoid fatty acids) were evaluated in rats fed either with heated baobab seed oil (0.046% cyclopropenoid fatty acids) or baobab seed oil (1.27% cyclopropenoid fatty acids in the diet) (Andrianaivo-Rafehivola et al., 1995). Retarded growth was seen with rats fed baobab oil, when compared to other groups of animals. Cytochrome P-450 content, as well as NADH cytochrome C reductase and NADPH cytochrome C reductase activities, were decreased with the relative liver weights markedly increased. The methanol extract of *A. digitata* (fruit pulp) was investigated for its hepatoprotective activity against liver damage induced by acetaminophen in rats (Hanafy et al., 2016). The researchers demonstrated that treatment of the rats with the methanol extract, prior to administration of acetaminophen, significantly reduced the disturbance in liver function. Liver functions were measured by the assessment of total bilirubin, total protein, ALT, ALP, AST and anti-oxidant markers, as well as oxidative stress parameters. Results from the study showed significant protective effects of *A. digitata* extract towards acetaminophen-induced hepatotoxicity. The extract exerted this protection through amelioration of lipid peroxidation by its scavenging activity of free radicals, and therefore enhancement of the anti-oxidant defence system. In another study (Adegoke et al., 2017), the protective role of an orally administered methanol leaf extract of *A. digitata* on sodium arsenite (SA)-induced hepatotoxicity and clastogenicity in male Wistar rats was evaluated. Rats were divided into six groups, with groups 2–6 receiving the extract (250 or 500 mg/kg bw) and/or sodium arsenite at 2.5 mg/kg bw, and group 1 receiving distilled water and a normal diet (negative control). Statistically significant increases were observed in lipid peroxidation and the number of micronucleated polychromatic erythrocytes in the sodium arsenite group, as compared with the treated and negative control groups. Histological analyses revealed that the methanol leaf extract-treated groups showed mild portal congestion and cellular infiltration with periportal cellular infiltration by mononuclear cells.

8.2.5 Immunomodulating properties

The immunomodulatory activities of different plant parts of *A. digitata* were investigated using a delayed-type hypersensitivity rat model. Sharma and Rangari (2016) demonstrated that the extracts exhibited significant increases in the delayed-type hypersensitivity reaction, indicating the ability of *A. digitata* to stimulate T-cells. The extract further produced a significant increase in phagocytic index by rapid removal of carbon particles from the bloodstream, and also increased sheep red blood cell-induced antibody titre in immunosuppressed rats. The data indicated that the methanol extracts of the root bark, leaf and fruit pulp of *A. digitata* may have potential as immunomodulatory agents.

8.2.6 Antidiabetic and anti-oxidative stress effects

Published research indicated that the baobab fruit extract has potential for reducing the glycaemic response (GR) and the inhibition of starch digestion was observed with water extract (66%) as well as the MeOH extract (56.6%) (Coe et al., 2013). Six extracts of baobab, from different locations in Africa, were investigated for their polyphenol content and anti-oxidant activities. The baobab extract at different doses was used to bake white bread, to determine the optimal dose for reducing sugar release and starch breakdown from the bread. The baobab extract was consumed in solution as both a high-dose (37 g) and a low-dose (18.5 g) aqueous drink in 250 mL of water along with white bread. Satiety, GR and postprandial energy expenditure were measured in the study. The baobab fruit extract added to white bread at a concentration of 1.88% significantly reduced rapidly digestible starch from the white bread samples. The baobab fruit extract also significantly reduced GR at both high and low doses, although there were no significant effects on energy expenditure and satiety. The growth performance of guinea fowl keets fed with baobab seed cake was investigated by Mwale et al. (2008). Their diet consisted of different concentrations of the baobab seed cake (0%, 10% and 15%). High body weight gain and feed intake were observed with 0% and 5% of baobab seed cake added to their diet (Mwale et al., 2008). The ethanolic extract of the bark of baobab was evaluated for antilipidaemic and antihyperglycaemic activities in alloxan-induced diabetic female rats (Bhargav et al., 2009). Baobab bark extract was given orally to diabetic rats for 7 days at doses of 250 or 500 mg/kg bw, with glipizide (500 μg/kg bw) as the control antidiabetic drug. The bark extract exhibited hypoglycaemic activity, as reflected by a 26.7% and 35.9% decrease in plasma glucose levels and an 11.3% and 32% increase in glycogenesis for the two doses, respectively. In addition, the extracts significantly decreased hepatic lipid and plasma profiles, indicating that the solvent extract of the stem bark of *A. digitata* exhibited hypolipidaemic and antidiabetic effects on type I diabetic animals (Bhargav et al., 2009). Research showed positive implications for the use of baobab for maintaining weight and reducing hunger (Garvey et al., 2017). In a randomised crossover, single-blinded study, healthy participants ($n = 20$) were administered a smoothie with baobab extract (15 g), or a control smoothie. Hunger was reduced after the consumption of the test smoothie, and results demonstrated a positive effect on weight maintenance.

The hypolipidaemic and hyperglycaemic effects of a methanolic extract of *A. digitata* leaves (200 and 400 mg/kg) were evaluated in diabetic rats (Ebaid et al., 2019). Treatment with the extract caused a signifcant reduction in the glycosylated haemoglobin, blood glucose, triglycerides, cholesterol, interleukin 6 (IL-6), tumour necrosis factor-alpha (TNF-α), low-density lipoprotein (LDL) and malondialdehyde (MDA) levels by 30.4%–66.0%, as compared to the diabetic group after the 6th week of treatment. The leaf extract also caused a decline in red blood cell (RBC) count, high-density lipoprotein (HDL) level, packed cell volume (PCV %), haemoglobin level and erythropoietin concentrations in diabetic rats by 31.0%–220.68% with respect to the diabetic group. The extract reduced the level of GSH and maintained the level of catalase (CAT), anti-oxidant enzymes and superoxide dismutase (SOD) in the diabetic rats. Ebaid et al. (2019) also reported the reduction of the WBC count in the STZ-induced diabetic rats. Hyperlipidaemia is a key factor related to the development of ischaemic heart disease. An intervention trial was conducted to investigate the effects of *A. digitata*, containing 6% soluble fibre and 56% pectin based on dry weight, on serum lipids amongst a population of hyperlipidaemic patients (Gadour et al., 2017). In addition to 30mg of baobab, a 20mg tablet of atorvastatin was given daily to participants for a period of 28days, whilst the control group received atorvastatin only. A noteworthy reduction in the levels of triglycerides (78.13 *vs* 57.44%) and total cholesterol (120.06 *vs* 49.06%) was seen in the intervention group compared to the control group.

8.2.7 Anti-inflammatory activity

The anti-inflammatory activity of the fruit of baobab, extracted with hot water, was evaluated *in vivo* using the rat paw formalin-induced oedema test (Vimalanathan and Hudson, 2009). The extract administered at a dose of 400 and 800mg/kg inhibited formalin-induced oedema. The mean swelling of the foot was 1.81 and 1.75mm for 400 and 800mg/kg, respectively, after 24h, in comparison to the negative control (6.35mm) (Ramadan et al., 1994). The aqueous leaf extract and the DMSO fruit pulp extract exhibited significant inhibition of cytokine IL-8.

8.2.8 Insecticidal activity

Pellets of *A. digitata* leaves were produced, and smoke from the pellets was assayed for repellency and toxicity against adult (0–7-days old) *Musca domestica* (housefly), *Anopheles gambiae* (African malaria mosquito) and *Periplaneta americana* (American cockroach) insects. The smoke caused the death of *M. domestica* and *Anopheles gambiae*, but not *P. americana*. The median lethal dose for *M. domestica* was 0.46, 0.52 and 0.46g, for pellets containing 0, 0.01 and 0.05g of d-allethrin, respectively, whilst for *Anopheles gambiae* it was 0.47, 0.50 and 0.20g (Denloye et al., 2006).

8.2.9 Antidiarrhoeal effects

The flesh of the fruit of the baobab tree is eaten raw as a treatment for dysentery and diarrhoea. The effect of the traditional medicine was evaluated in a clinical study in Senegal, and the *Adansonia* fruit was compared with oral rehydration therapy (ORT), with 82 children in each group. No significant differences were observed between the two treatments in terms of increase in weight and duration of diarrhoea, thus confirming the efficacy of baobab (Palombo, 2006). The astringent constituents of the fruit may be responsible for the effect, although the high levels of tartaric acid can lead to gastrointestinal irritation if large quantities of fruit are consumed. In another clinical study, the effect of a baobab fruit solution was compared to the World Health Organisation (WHO) standard solution in the treatment of children with acute diarrhoea (6-months old, a total of 161). The data showed that the WHO solution was superior to the solution of *A. digitata* in terms of duration of weight gain, diarrhoea and rehydration (Tal-Dia et al., 1997). An *in vivo* study to evaluate the antidiarrhoeal property of the methanol extract of the fruit of baobab was conducted in rats and mice (Suleiman et al., 2014). The acute oral toxicity (LD_{50}) of the extract was also calculated, whilst the antidiarrhoeal effect of different doses of the extract was examined in both rats and mice. The effect of the extract at doses of 300, 700 and 1000 mg/kg were evaluated against magnesium sulphate-induced gastrointestinal motility test, intestinal transit time, and castor oil-induced diarrhoea in mice. The methanol extract did not exhibit any toxic effect in mice at doses of up to 5000 mg/kg. At doses of 300 and 700 mg/kg, the extract significantly decreased intestinal transit time in mice. Furthermore, the extract at doses of 300, 700 and 1000 mg/kg, significantly lowered diarrhoea induced by castor oil and magnesium sulphate in mice. The extract produced a similar significant effect of enteropooling caused by castor oil in rats, and the antidiarrhoeal effect was reported to be dose-dependent.

8.2.10 Cardioprotective effects

The role of *A. digitata* fruit pulp was investigated against isoproterenol (ISP)-induced myocardial oxidative stress in rats by demonstrating the changes in some anti-oxidant enzymes, tissue cardiac markers, monocyte chemo-attractant protein-1 (MCP-1), myeloperoxidase (MPO), interleukin-1β (IL-1β), serum corticosterone, collagen-1 and galectin-3 (Ghoneim et al., 2016). The activities of non-enzymatic anti-oxidant and enzymatic anti-oxidant glutathione peroxidase (GPX) reduced GSH in the heart tissue. Male albino rats were divided into four groups of ten animals each. Group IV received baobab fruit pulp; Group III included myocardial oxidative animals and received baobab fruit pulp (200 μg/rat/day) for 4 weeks; Group II animals received isoproterenol (ISP) (85 mg/kg bw intraperitonealy to develop myocardial injury), whilst Group I served as the normal control group. The results showed an isoproterenol-induced increase in levels of cardiac marker enzymes [lactate dehydrogenase (LDH), creatine kinase MB (CK-MB) and aspartate aminotransferase (AST)], MCP-1, IL-1ß, collagen, MPO and galectin-3, with a concomitant decrease in the activities of GSH and GPX in heart tissue, as well as a decrease in serum corticosterone levels (Ghoneim et al., 2016). Baobab fruit pulp affected all the parameters and brought them back to normal level in ISP-induced myocardial infarction in rats. Histopathological examination of the heart tissue of ISP-administered model rats showed congestion in the blood vessels and infiltration of inflammatory cells. Treatment with baobab fruit pulp (200 μg/rat/day) resulted in no inflammatory cell infiltration and normal myocardial structure in heart tissue.

8.2.11 Food, dietary supplements, nutraceuticals

Fruit pulp, seed/kernels

Magaia et al. (2013b) reported the content of minerals, dietary fibre and select organic acids in the kernels and pulp of wild fruits. The content of insoluble fibres in the pulps of *A. digitata* ranged from 2.6 to 45.8 g/100 g and that of soluble fibre ranged from 4.3 to 65.6 g/100 g. In the kernels, the content of insoluble fibre ranged from 14.7 to 20.9 g/100 g and that of soluble fibre from 8.4 to 42.6 g/100 g, with citric acid present in all fruits at concentrations up to 25.7 g/kg. Analysis of the kernels of *A. digitata* revealed high concentrations of iron, calcium, zinc and magnesium. The concentration of vitamin C in fruit pulp is high and can range from 2.8 to 3 g/kg (Vertuani et al., 2002). Other researchers confirmed the high vitamin C content (280–300 mg/100 g), seven to ten times more than that in oranges (51 mg/100 g), in the fruit pulp (Manfredini et al., 2002; Rahul et al., 2015). The fruit pulp contains no starch, but contains sugars and is rich in pectin. The pulp is used as a sauce for food and as a drink, as a substitute for cream of tartar in baking and as a fermenting agent in local brewing. One study reported that the consumption of 40 g of baobab pulp provides 100% of the recommended daily intake of vitamin C in pregnant women (19–30 years) (Chadare et al., 2009). The calcium (Ca) content reported in the fruit pulp varies according to the origin of the samples. Brady (2011) noted a Ca content of 344.2 mg/100 g sample, which differs from that reported by Osman (2004), 295.0 mg/100 g. Similar results were seen for the levels of K in fruit pulp: 1240.0 mg/100 g reported by Osman (2004) compared to 1578.5 mg/100 g reported by Brady (2011). The oil is used in food preparation for paste/sauce and the seeds are eaten roasted/raw and are rich in protein (Osman, 2004). Baobab fruit pulp and oil contain several vitamins that are essential for skin care (Nkafamiya et al., 2007). These include vitamin E (anti-ageing and anti-oxidant effects) (Nyam et al., 2009); vitamin A and omega-3 and omega-6 essential fats (cell renewal and rejuvenation) and vitamin D3, which decreases blood pressure and increases calcium absorption in the elderly (Wasserman, 2004).

The nutritive, chemical and antinutritive values of baobab seed flour were reported in a study by Adubiaro et al. (2012). The seeds were found to contain a moderately high content of carbohydrate (21.9%) and a very high content of protein (48.3%). The most abundant mineral in the seed flour was found to be K (536 mg/100 g), followed by Mg (352 mg/100 g). The least abundant minerals were Zn (3.40 mg/100 g), Cu (4.26 mg/100 g) and Mn (5.23 mg/100 g). When compared with the recommended values, the ratios of Ca/P, Na/K and Ca/Mg in seed flour comply. A feeding trial was done in broiler chickens to determine the effect of graded levels of baobab seed meal on cost benefit and growth performance. Baobab seed meal was included in the diets at 0%, 10%, 20%, 30% and 40% levels designated as diets 1, 2, 3, 4 and 5, respectively. At the starter phase, daily weight gain (30.36–36.16 g), feed intake (65.18–71.73 g) and feed conversion ratio (1.96–2.39) were not significantly affected by the dietary treatments. However, at the finisher phase, the weight gain (37.23–55.00 g) and daily feed intake (133.40–148.40 g) were significantly affected. The birds fed diet 5 gained the least weight (33.80 g) and birds fed the 20% diet gained the most (44.55 g). Results showed that baobab seed meal can be included into broiler chicken diets at up to 30% of the feed without any adverse effect on performance, whilst reducing feed cost (Sarven Bale et al., 2013). In another 28-day feeding study, 150-day old Anak broiler chicks were used to evaluate the effect of quantitative substitution of raw baobab seed meal (RBSM) for soyabean meal (Saulawa et al., 2014). The birds were grouped into five treatment groups of 0, 5, 10, 15 and 20 levels of inclusion of raw baobab seed meal (RBSM). Data of productive performance indicated significant differences for all the parameters considered.

Final body weight and feed intake increased with an increase in the level of inclusion of the test ingredient. Inclusion of RBSM (10%) gave the best productive performance of the inclusion levels tested. It was concluded that 10% RBSM can be used in a starter diet for broiler chicks without any negative effect on productive performance.

Baobab seed was investigated as a substitute for coffee and roasted at temperatures of 100 °C, 120 °C and 150 °C for 30 min, milled and sieved (Olaitan et al., 2014). The roasted seeds were evaluated, and samples of baobab were blended with spices (ginger and cloves, at 0.5%) and oven dried for 30 min at different temperatures. Results revealed that the group roasted for 30 min at 150 °C with spices was the most generally accepted sample for a baobab seed coffee-like beverage. The bacterial count and total mould decreased as the roasting temperature increased. Mineral, caffeine, antinutrient and vitamin content determinations were done on the most preferred sample, with fresh baobab seed flour serving as the control. Results indicated that roasting for 30 min at 150 °C significantly increased the carbohydrate, protein, ash, crude fibre, Ca, P, Mg and K content, but significantly decreased the fat, moisture, energy, Fe, caffeine, phytate, oxalate, saponin and tannin content of the sample. To enable resource-poor populations in southern Africa to benefit from a functional food, a probiotic dairy product was developed on the basis of a traditional dish called 'mutandabota' (Mpofu et al., 2014). The process involved the boiling of raw cow milk, with subsequent cooling to ambient temperature (25 °C). Dry pulp from the fruit of the baobab tree was then added to the milk at a concentration of 4% (w/v). The mixture was inoculated with the probiotic *Lactobacillus rhamnosus yoba* and left to ferment for 24 h, whilst monitoring the bacterial culture growth. Final ingredients were then added to produce probiotic '*mutandabota*' that contained 7% (w/v) sugar and 14% (w/v) baobab fruit pulp in dairy milk. Baobab fruit pulp at 4% promoted the growth of *L. rhamnosus yoba* with a maximal specific growth rate (μmax) of 0.6 ± 0.2/h at 30 °C. The developed technology has potential to be used for the delivery of probiotics. De Lucia et al. (2015) showed that the prebiotic action of baobab fruit is not due to the presence of fructo-oligosaccharides, but is probably due to the presence of other components in the fruit e.g. flavonoids or monosaccharides largely represented in the soluble fraction (glucose, sucrose and fructose), as reported by Parkar et al. (2008). These components may have an impact on colonic health and influence the microflora, being able to bring the micro-organisms from the lag phase to the exponential phase of growth (Tzounis et al., 2008). Magaia and Skog (2017) showed that *A. digitata* kernels are rich in unsaturated fatty acids (32%). The dominating fatty acids in the kernels were linoleic, palmitic and oleic acid; varying from 25.7% to 34.9% of the total fatty acid content. *Adansonia digitata* kernels contained the two essential fatty acids, namely linolenic acid (2%) and linoleic acid (around 30%). The protein content of kernels was 35%, with glutamic acid as the most abundant amino acid, comprising more than 20% of the protein. *Adansonia digitata* kernels can provide cheap, good sources of protein, especially when combined with foods with high lysine content as the essential amino acids content in the kernels compared favourably with the requirements stated by the WHO. The main constituent identified in the insoluble fraction of *A. digitata* kernels was glucose.

Seed and pulp composition and mineral element concentration were researched using inductively coupled plasma-atomic emission spectroscopy (ICP-AES) and AOAC 1984 methods. The results indicated significant variations in pulp protein, moisture, ash, fibre and elemental content of African samples (Muthai et al., 2017). The highest mean pulp crude fibre (8.68 g $100\,g^{-1}$ dw) was recorded in Kenya. Malawian pulp samples contained, on average, the most Ca (4300 mg/kg), K (22.2 mg/g), Na (1000 mg/kg), Mg (2300 mg/kg) and P (1100 mg/kg). Kenyan pulp samples had the highest Mn (27.2 μg/g) and Fe (57.4 μg/g) content, whilst samples from Mali contained the least Mn (8.6 μg/g) and Fe (13.1 μg/g). The mean seed Ca content was the lowest (2000 mg/kg) in Kenyan samples and the highest (3200 mg/kg) in samples from Malawi. Overall, baobab seeds and fruit pulp contained significant amounts of nutritionally essential minerals and components, but the concentrations varied depending on the origin.

Leaves, flowers, roots/tubers

Baobab provides hunger relief in many parts of Africa. It is a multisource food tree with edible parts available for several months of the year, and the fruit and leaves, in particular, can be preserved and stored (Rashford, 2018). A number of studies identified the leaves of the baobab as a good source of essential nutrients (Nordeide et al., 1996; Chadare et al., 2009; Rashford, 2018). The leaves are rich in vitamins, especially vitamins A and C, and contain a number of essential amino acids, including lysine, which is often limited in the diet of people who consume little meat; and contain protein and iron (Fe). The leaves are estimated to contain three to five times more Ca (307–2640 mg/100 g dw) than milk (Brady, 2011). Phytochemicals and minerals present in baobab root tubers indicate their medicinal and nutritional value (Kamanula et al., 2018). Calcium (69.39 mg/100 g) and magnesium (44.16 mg/100 g) levels are the highest in baobab root tubers. Pakenham (2004) commented: 'If you needed fresh salad you could eat both the elegant white flowers and the pale green foliage'. Aitken (1951) reported that the leaves are sometimes crushed in water with sugar to make an unusual and refreshing beverage.

Oil cakes

Baobab oil cakes (BOC) were examined for their amino acid and mineral content. To determine the *in situ* rumen degradability of crude protein (CP) and dry matter (DM) from the oil cakes, polyester bags were used to incubate triplicate subsamples of each oil cake in the ventral rumen of cannulated mid-lactating Holstein cows for a period of 2, 4, 8, 16, 24 or 48 h. Apparently, BOC can be used as a supplement for fibre, as well as being a source of K and Ca in ruminant diets. An inadequate availability of feed ingredients significantly contributes to reduced animal production, Nkosi et al. (2019) recommended the use of BOC in ruminants after evaluation of nitrogen digestion, growth performance and carcass characteristics in these ruminants yielded satisfactory results.

8.2.12 Other activities

Baobab seed oil is popularly included as a functional ingredient in cosmetic products. After topical application to the skin of healthy adult female Caucasian participants ($n=20$), a 2× magnifying lamp was used for visual analysis, whilst for monitoring and evaluation of the irritancy level, transepidermal water loss (TEWL) and hydration level of the skin, Chromameter®, Aquaflux® and Corneometer® instruments, respectively, were used. In addition, Aquaflux® and Corneometer® instruments were used to assess occlusive effects. The moisture efficacy test showed a reduced transepidermal water loss and an improved capacitance moisture retention for all test products (baobab oil, Vaseline® Intensive Care lotion, liquid paraffin and Vaseline®). The occlusivity wipe-off test showed a decreased transepidermal water loss (TEWL) and an increased moisture hydration (Komane et al., 2017). Chika et al. (2019) investigated the effect of an aqueous methanolic root bark of *A. digitata* on the oestrous cycle of female Wistar rats. Forty mature Wistar female rats (weighing 135 ± 28 g) with regular oestrous cycles were administered extracts, whilst the control group received distilled water of equal volume. Results indicated that the extracts at 150 and 300 mg/kg bw prolonged the occurrence of diestrus and proestrus, and produced atretic cyst-like ovaries at the higher dose. The water extract of baobab inhibited ethanol-induced gastric ulceration in rats (Karumi et al., 2008). Pretreatment with *A. digitata* (given orally at 150–600 mg/kg) caused a significant dose-dependent increase both in preventative ratio and percentage ulcer reduction. These effects were thought to be related to the astringent, anti-oxidant and flavonoid properties of the extract.

8.3 Safety

A low acute toxicity (LD_{50} 8000 mg/kg) following parenteral administration of a fruit pulp extract was reported by Ramadan et al. (1994). Extracts prepared using a variety of solvents (water, methanol and DMSO) and plant parts (leaves, seeds or fruits) caused cytotoxicity in Vero monkey kidney cells ranging from 130 µg/mL (leaves) to ≈1900 µg/mL (fruit pulp, MIC_{100} values) (Vimalanathan and Hudson, 2009). The Ames test indicated that baobab extracts were non-mutagenic towards *Salmonella typhimurium* strain TA98 (Mulaudzi et al., 2013). The safety of baobab seed oil was assessed on female Caucasian participants and the results indicated that the irritancy of sodium lauryl sulphate (SLS), the positive control, in the patch test differed significantly for both baobab seed oil and de-ionised water, but the difference between the irritancy of baobab seed oil and de-ionised water was not significant. It was concluded that baobab seed oil is non-irritant (Komane et al., 2017). The oil does not burn the skin when applied and is non-sensitising and non-irritating (Wren and Stucki, 2003).

9. Phytochemistry

9.1 Essential oil

The yields of the hydro-distilled essential oil from the stem bark and leaves of *A. digitata* were found to be 0.403% and 0.302%, whilst 40 and 23 compounds were identified, respectively (Kayode et al., 2018). The classes of compounds identified were: alkene alcohols, hydrocarbons, cyclic ketonic ethers, amides, terpenoids and esters. 8-Dimethyl-2-(1-methylethenyl) (8.20%), tetramethyl-2-hexadecen-1-ol (26.31%), tetracosane (6.54%), tetratetracontane (5.59%) and heptacosane (5.81%) were the major compounds identfied in the leaf essential oil (Kayode et al., 2018). Dominant compounds of the stem bark essential oil were: cyclopentane (8.81%), octadecane (9.30%), 1-octadecanesulphonyl chloride (8.73%), eicosane (8.34%), heptadecane (8.50%) and tetracosan (7.12%).

9.2 Seed oil

Pressing of the seeds, followed by filtration, yielded semifluid, golden-yellow, slightly scented oil. The Baobab Fruit Company reported that the oil contains mono-unsaturated (36%), saturated (33%) and polyunsaturated (31%) fatty acids, with oleic and palmitic acids as the major constituents of the oil (Andrianaivo-Rafehivola et al., 1993). β-Sitosterol (≈80% of the total sterols) is one of the major sterol constituents present in baobab seed oil. Other sterols include stigmasterol (2.9%) and campesterol (8.3%). Baobab oil is deeply nourishing, highly penetrating, and softens dry skin, similar to avocado oil (PhytoTrade Africa, n.d.). Several vitamins, including vitamins D, A, E and omega 3 and 6 essential fatty acids (vitamin 'F') are present in baobab oil (Nkafamiya et al., 2007). Vitamin E is a superior anti-oxidant, with an anti-ageing effect, whilst vitamins 'F' and A are polyunsaturated fatty acids, directly implicated in the renewal and rejuvenation of cell membranes. Wasserman (2004) reported that baobab oil is a natural source of vitamin D3, which decreases blood pressure and increases Ca absorption. The fatty acid content and profiles of baobab seed oils harvested from several wild populations in sub-Saharan Africa were investigated, and the influence of geographical region and provenance on the profiles were assessed in a study by Muthai et al. (2019). The seed oil contained 32%–38% mono-unsaturated fatty acids (MUFA), 17%–22% saturated fatty acids (SFA) and 22%–26% polyunsaturated fatty acids (PUFA). Linoleic acid (C18:2) and oleic acid (C18:1) were the dominant PUFA and MUFA, respectively, in the oil, whilst palmitic acid (C16:0) was the most abundant SFA. Gas chromatography coupled to mass spectrometry (GC–MS) was used to detect compounds, including cholesterol, campesterol, isofucosterol, stigmasterol, β-sitosterol and tocopherol (δ, γ, β and α) in the seed oil (Bianchini et al., 1982). Squalene (39.5%) and *n*-alkanes (57.3%), were found to be the major hydrocarbons in the seed oil. Fatty acids detected in the seed oil include oleic and linoleic acids in high concentration, as well as smaller amounts of linolenic, palmitic, arachidic and stearic acids (Sidibe and Williams, 2002; Osman, 2004; Nkafamiya et al., 2007).

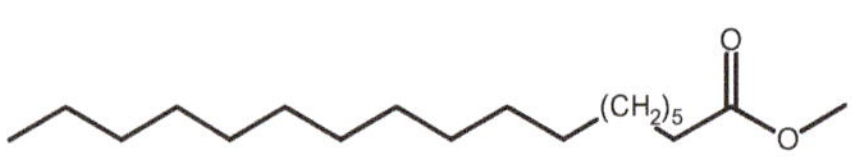

Stearic acid methyl ester

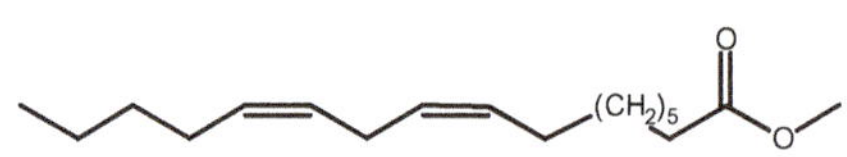

Linoleic acid methyl ester

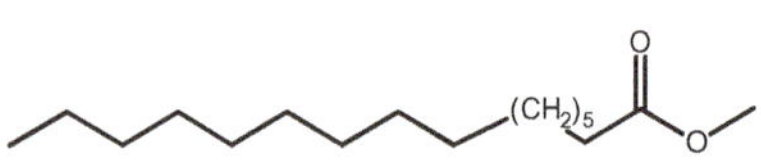

Palmitic acid methyl ester

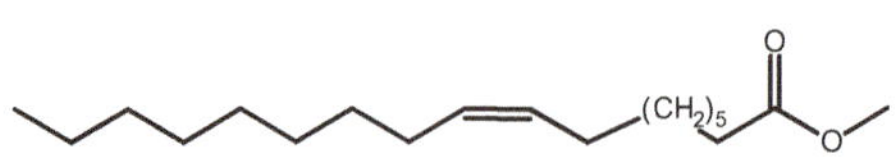

Oleic acid methyl ester

9.3 Fruit

In the early 1950s, the fruit pulp was analysed and the presence of organic acids such as tartaric, citric, malic, ascorbic and succinic acid reported. The pulp represents 14%–28% of the total fruit weight (Soloviev et al., 2004). The fruit pulp was found to contain large amounts of crude fibre (≈ 11.2%) and carbohydrates (≈ 70%), with a low concentrations of protein (≈ 2.2%), ash (≈ 5.7%), and almost no fat (≈ 0.4%) (Lockett et al., 2002). A number of amino acids from fruit pulp, for example arginine, alanine, glycine, methionine, lysine, serine, proline and valine (Glew et al., 1997), vitamins from leaves and/or fruit pulp (A, B1, C, B2 and B3) (UNCTAD, 2005) and minerals from fruit pulp (Fe, Cu, K, Mn, Mg, P, Na and Zn) have been identified (Glew et al., 1997). Ten aromatic compounds, including nonanal and isopropyl myristate, were identified in the fruit pulp using GC–MS (Cisse et al., 2009). Several compounds have been isolated from the pericarp using column chromatography and include epicatechin-(4β → 8)-epicatechin, (−)-epicatechin, epicatechin-(4β → 6)-epicatechin, epicatechin-(4β → 8)-epicatechin-(4β → 8)-epicatechin and epicatechin-(2β → O → 7,4β → 8)-epicatechin (Shahat, 2006). Tembo et al. (2017) studied baobab pulp and showed that it contained high levels of vitamin C (AA + DHA) [466 ± 2.5 mg/100 g fresh weight (FW)], procyanidin B2 (533 ± 22.6 mg/100 g FW), (−)-epicatechin (43.0 ± 3.0 mg/100 g FW) and gallic acid (68.5 ± 12.4 mg/100 g FW). They also reported a maximum TPC of $1.89 \times 10^3 \pm 1.61$ mg GAE/100 g FW. Ismail et al. (2019a) conducted a study to identify the phytochemicals in *A. digitata* using liquid chromatography–mass spectrometry (LC–MS)/quadrupole time-of-flight (QToF) detection, and also investigated the effect of solvents on the phenolic compound content. Forty-six compounds representing phenolic acids, proanthocyanidins, saponins and flavonols were identified using LC–MS analysis. Six iridoid glycosides, four hydroxycinnamic acid glycosides and three phenylethanoid glycosides were isolated by Li et al. (2017) from the dried baobab fruit pulp. Their structures were determined by means of spectroscopic analyses, using ^{1}H and ^{13}C NMR and two-dimensional experiments and high-resolution mass spectrometry (HRMS). An ultra-high performance liquid chromatography-high-resolution accurate mass spectrometry (UHPLC–HRAM–MS) method was employed to conduct further analysis of the chemical compositions of the hydro-alcohol baobab fruit pulp extract. Iridoid glycosides, hydroxycinnamic acid glycosides and phenylethanoid glycosides were found to be the major components in baobab fruit pulp.

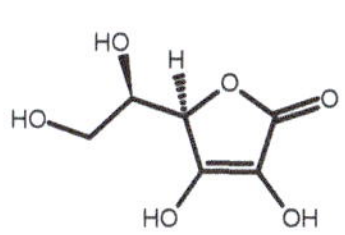

Ascorbic acid (Vitamin C)

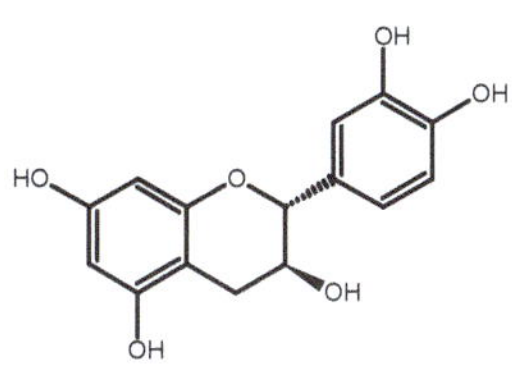

Catechin

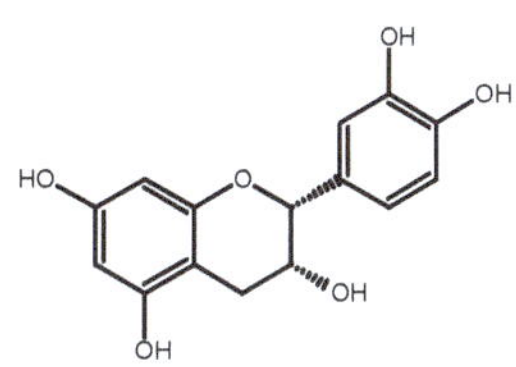

Epicatechin

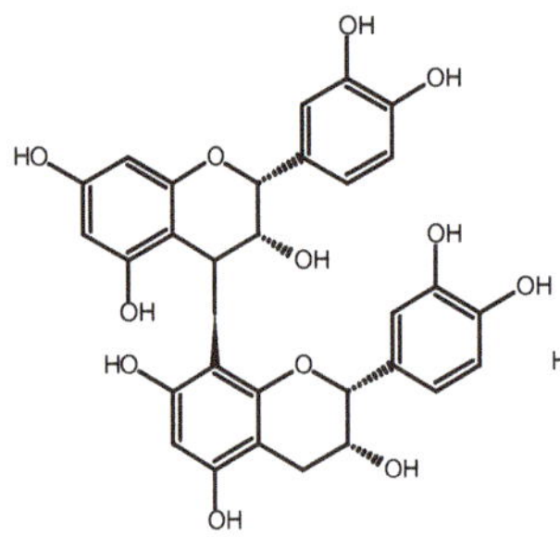

Procyanidin dimer I

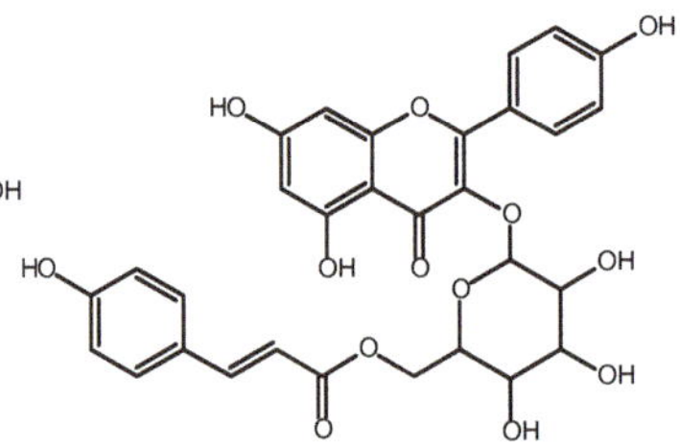

Kaempferol glucoside I and II

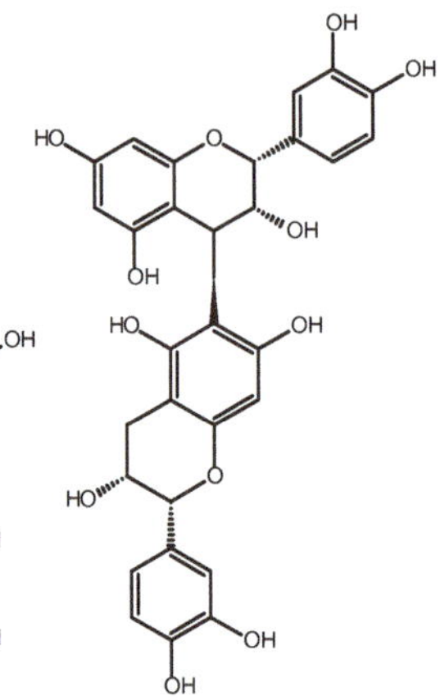

Procyanidin dimer II

9.4 Leaves

The elemental, phytochemical and proximate analyses of stored, shade and sun-dried leaves of baobab were conducted by Ogbaga et al. (2018). They reported that the leaves contain phytochemicals such as saponins, glycosides, flavonoids and steroids, whilst tannins, alkaloids and resins were not detected. The leaves are also an important source of minerals such as Cu, Zn, Mn and Fe. In addition, they are rich in crude protein, fibre, ash and nitrogen. The presence of uronic acid groups was confirmed *via* Fourier Transform Infrared (FTIR) spectral studies of the polysaccharides (Nwokocha and Williams, 2016).

9.5 Roots

3,3′,4′-Trihydroxy-flavan-4-one-7-*O*-α-L-rhamnopyranoside, 3,7-dihydroxy-flavan-4-one-5-*O*-β-D-galactopyranosyl-(1 → 4)-β-D-glucapyroside and quercetin-7-*O*-β-D-xylopyranoside were isolated from the roots of *A. digitata* (Chauhan et al., 1984, 1987; Shukla et al., 2001).

Part B: Chemical profiling and quality control

10. Chromatography analysis

10.1 High-performance thin-layer chromatography (HPTLC) fingerprint analysis

General instrumentation: A CAMAG HPTLC instrument consisting of an automatic TLC sampler (ATS 4), automatic developing chamber (ADC 2), CAMAG TLC Visualizer 2, CAMAG derivatiser and TLC plate heater. *HPTLC plates:* Silica gel glass plates 60 F_{254} (Merck).

10.1.1 Fruit pulp analysis

Plant part: Fruit pulp, methanol extract. *Sample application:* Application volume of 2 μL pulp extract (100 mg/mL) and standards (1 mg/mL) spotted as 10 mm bands. Plates developed in a 20×10×4 cm glass twin-trough chamber to a migration distance of 70 mm. *Tank saturation:* 20 min at 15 °C and 33% RH, with 25 mL of mobile phase. *Mobile phase:* Ethyl acetate: water: formic acid (16:1:1 v/v/v). *Derivatisation:* *p*-Anisaldehyde prepared by mixing 0.5 mL *p*-anisaldehyde with 85 mL methanol, 10 mL glacial acetic acid, and 5 mL sulphuric acid. The plate was sprayed with 3 mL of anisaldehyde reagent, followed by heating the plate for 3 min at 100 °C and then visualised. *Visualisation:* The plate was viewed under white reflectance and under 254 nm radiation.

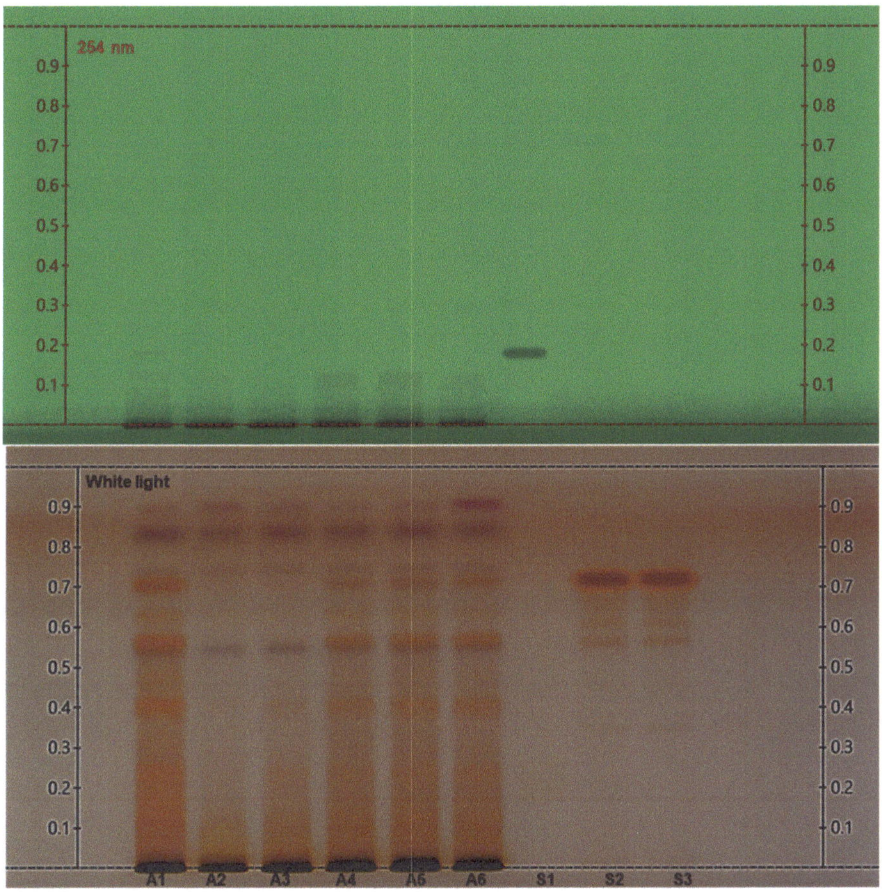

HPTLC plate of *Adansonia digitata* fruit pulp methanol extracts (A1–A6) and the standards (S1–S3). The samples are characterised by a grey band for ascorbic acid (S1) (R_f=0.17) under 254 nm radiation and two brown bands for catechin (S2) (R_f=0.70) and epicatechin (S3) (R_f=0.70), respectively, under white reflectance.

10.1.2 Seed oil analysis

Plant part: Seed oil, cold press. *Sample application:* Application volume of 2 µL oil (25 µL/mL in toluene) and standards (25 µL/mL in hexane) spotted as 10 mm bands. Plates developed in a 20 × 10 × 4 cm glass twin-trough chamber to a migration distance of 70 mm. *Tank saturation:* 20 min at 15 °C and 33% RH, with 25 mL of mobile phase. *Mobile phase:* Toluene: ethyl acetate (95:5 v/v). *Derivatisation: p*-Anisaldehyde prepared by mixing 0.5 mL *p*-anisaldehyde with 85 mL methanol, 10 mL glacial acetic acid and 5 mL sulphuric acid. The plate was sprayed with 3 mL of anisaldehyde reagent, followed by heating the plate for 3 min at 100 °C and then visualised. *Visualisation:* The plate was viewed under white reflectance.

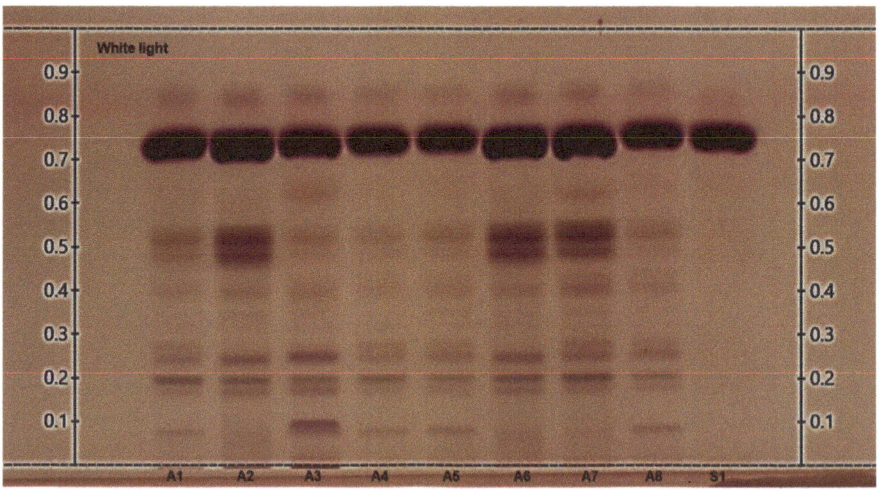

HPTLC plate of *Adansonia digitata* seed oils (A1–A8) and the standard (S1). The samples are characterised by a purple band for linoleic acid (S1) (R_f=0.75).

10.2 Ultra-performance liquid chromatography (UPLC) analysis

General instrumentation: Waters Acquity Ultra-Performance Liquid Chromatography system with PDA detector combined with a Xevo G2QToF mass spectrometer (Waters, United States). *Plant part:* Fruit pulp, methanol extract. *Sample application:* Injection volume of 2.0 µL (full-loop injection) at 1 mg/mL concentration. *Column:* CORTECS UPLC C_{18} column (150 mm × 2.1 mm, i.d., 1.6 µm particle size, Waters). *Mobile phase:* 0.1% formic acid in water (solvent A) and acetonitrile (solvent B). *Analysis conditions:* Gradient elution at a flow rate of 0.3 mL/min, initially 95% A: 5% B, held for 0.5 min, then changed to 80% A: 20% B in 1.5 min, to 20% A: 80% B in 8 min, to 5% A: 95% B in 5 min and returning to the initial ratio in 0.5 min, equilibrating the system for 2.5 min, total run time 18 min. *Mass spectrometry:* ESI^- (negative ionisation mode), N_2 used as the desolvation gas, desolvation temperature 350 °C at a flow rate of 500 L/h and source temperature of 100 °C. Capillary and cone voltages, 2500 and 45 V, respectively. Data collected between *m/z* 100 and 1200.

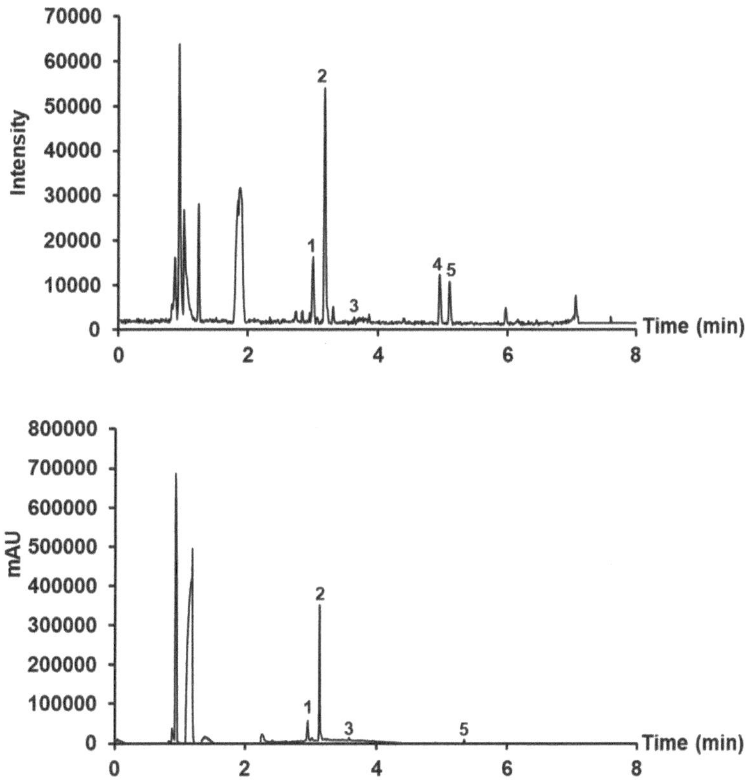

UPLC–ToF–MS ESI$^-$ (upper) and PDA (lower) chromatograms of *Adansonia digitata* pulp methanol extract. [1] = procyanidin dimer I *m/z* 577.1139, [2] = epicatechin *m/z* 289.0560, [3] = procyanidin dimer II *m/z* 557.1125, [4] = kaempferol glycoside I *m/z* 593.1095 and [5] = kaempferol glycoside II *m/z* 593.1089.

10.3 Gas chromatography (GC) analysis

General instrumentation: An Agilent 6860 N chromatograph (Agilent Technologies, Hanova, United States) fitted with a flame ionisation detector and a mass spectrometer. *Column:* HP-Innowax, 60 m × 250 μm × 0.25 μm (polyethylene glycol column, Agilent Technologies, Hanova, United States). *Plant part:* Seed oil. *Sample application:* The fatty acid methyl esters were prepared using the modified method of Ross and Harynuk (2010). Injection volume 1 μL (split) at 20% (v/v) in hexane, split ratio: 1:194 and inlet temperature 250 °C. *Analysis conditions:* Helium carrier gas, flow rate: 1.0 mL/min, pressure: 23.48 psi. Starting oven temperature at 80 °C for 2 min, then increasing at a rate of 10 °C/min to 240 °C. *Mass spectrometry conditions:* Chromatograms obtained on electron impact at 70 eV on an Agilent 5973 mass selective detector, scanning range: *m/z* 35 to 550 (Agilent Technologies, Hanova, United States). *Identification:* Authentic standards, NIST®, Mass Finder®.

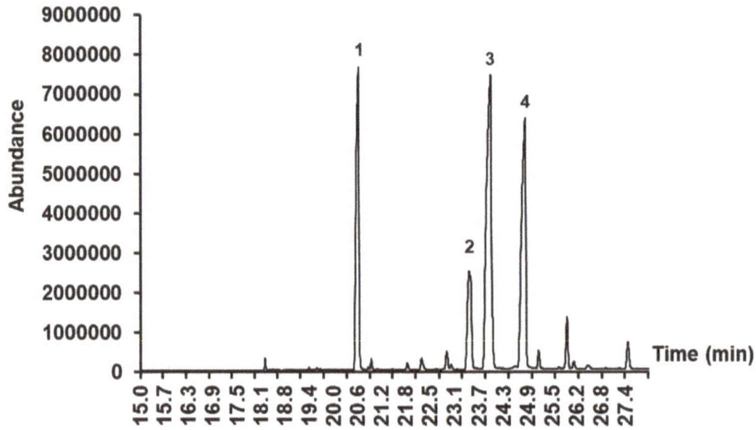

Total ion chromatograms (TIC) of *Adansonia digitata* seed oil indicating major compounds. [1] = Palmitic acid methyl ester (R_t 20.65, *m/z* 270.2559), [2] = stearic acid methyl ester (R_t 23.60, *m/z* 298.2872), [3] = oleic acid methyl ester (R_t 24.05, *m/z* 296.2715) and [4] = linoleic acid methyl ester (R_t 24.90, *m/z* 294.5959).

11. Mid-infrared (MIR) spectroscopy analysis

General instrumentation: Alpha-P Bruker spectrometer, mounted with an attenuated total reflectance (ATR) diamond crystal. *Spectral acquisition:* Spectrum obtained in the absorbance mode, with a spectral resolution of 4 cm^{-1} over the range 4000–550 cm^{-1} and captured using OPUS 6.5 software.

11.1 Fruit pulp analysis

Plant part: Fruit pulp. *Sample preparation:* Powdered fruit pulp sieved (< 500 μm) and placed directly onto the surface of the diamond crystal.

11.2 Seed oil analysis

Plant part: Seed oil. *Sample preparation:* Cold pressed oil, placed directly onto the surface of the diamond crystal.

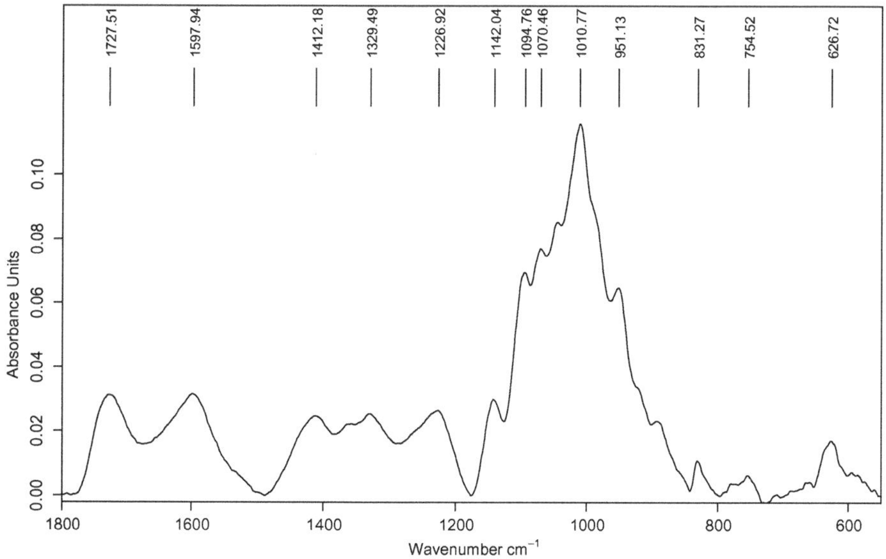

Mid-infrared spectrum of *Adansonia digitata* fruit pulp displaying the fingerprint region (1800–550 cm^{1}).

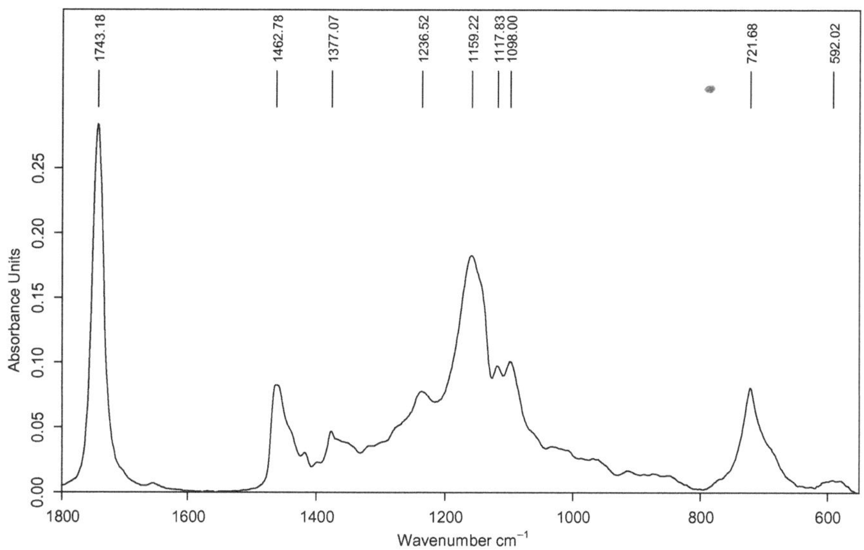

Mid-infrared spectrum of *Adansonia digitata* seed oil displaying the fingerprint region (1800–550 cm^{1}).

References

Abdelhai, M.H., Tahir, H.E., Zhang, Q., Yang, Q., Ahima, J., Zhang, X., Zhang, H., 2019. Biol. Control, 134:87–94.

Addy, R., 2009. Baobab Fruit Approved as Food Ingredient in US. Available from: http://www.nutraingredients-usa.com/content/view/print/2595742009.

Adegoke, A.M., Gbadegesin, M.A., Odunola, O.A., 2017. Pharmacogn. Res., 9:7–11.

Adeoye, A.O., Bewaji, C.O., 2015. J. Biol. Sci., 15:78–84.

Adeoye, A.O., Bewaji, C.O., 2018. J. Ethnopharmacol., 210:31–38.

Adeoye, A.O., Bewaji, C.O., 2019. Comp. Clin. Path., https://doi.org/10.1007/s00580-019-02972-5.

Adeoye, A.O., Boligon Aline, A., Athayde Margareth, L., Bewaji Clement, O., 2016a. Int. J. Pharmacogn. Phytochem. Res., 8:1951–1958.

Adeoye, A.O., Komolafe Kayode, C., Olatunde Moses, D., 2016b. Res. J. Med. Plant, 10:254–260.

Adubiaro, H.O., Olaofe, O., Akintayo, E.T., Babalola, O.-O., 2012. Adv. J. Food Sci. Technol., 3:228–232.

Aitken, R.B., 1951. Nat. Hist., 60:456–462.

Ajaiyeoba, E., Ashidi, J., Abiodun, O., Okpako, L., Ogbole, O., Akinboye, D., Falade, C., Bolaji, O., Gbotosho, G., Falade, M., Itiola, O., Houghton, P., Wright, C., Oduola, A., 2004. Pharm. Biol., 42:588–591.

Al-Qarawi, A.A., Al-Damegh, M.A., El-Mougy, S.A., 2003. J. Herb. Spices Med. Plant., 10:1–6.

Anani, K., Hudson, J.B., De Souza, C., Akpaganal, K., Tower, G.H.N., Amason, J.T., Gbeassor, M., 2000. Pharm. Biol., 38:40–45.

Andrianaivo-Rafehivola, A.A., Blond, J.P., Cao, J., Gaydou, E.E., Bezard, J., 1993. J. Nutr. Biochem., 4:92–96.

Andrianaivo-Rafehivola, A.A., Siess, M.-H., Gaydou, E.M., 1995. Food Chem. Toxicol., 33:377–382.

Atawodi, S.E., 2005. Afr. J. Biotechnol., 4:177–182.

Atawodi, S.E., Bulus, T., Ibrahim, S., Ameh, D.A., Nok, A.J., Mamman, M., Galadima, M., 2003. Afr. J. Biotechnol., 2:317–321.

Ateya, A., Ammar, N., El-Eraky, W., El-Senousy, W., El Awdan, S., Amer, A., 2016. Int. J. Pharmacogn. Phytochem. Res., 8:499–504.

Ayele, Y., Kim, J.-A., Park, E., Kim, Y.-J., Retta, N., Dessie, G., Rhee, S.-K., Koh, K., Nam, K.-W., Kim, H.S., 2013. Biomol. Ther., 21:146–152.

Bakare, A.O., Oyewole, A.L., Owoyele, B.V., 2019. Orient. Pharm. Exp. Med., https://doi.org/10.1007/s13596-019-00373-1.

Besco, E., Braccioli, E., Vertuani, S., Ziosi, P., Brazzo, F., Bruni, R., Sacchetti, G., Manfredini, S., 2007. Food Chem., 102:1352–1356.

Bhargav, B., Rupal, A.V., Reddy, A.S., Narasimhacharya, A.V.R.L., 2009. J. Cell Tissue Res., 9:1879–1882.

Bianchini, J.-P., Ralaimanarivo, A., Gaydou, E.M., Waegell, B., 1982. Phytochemistry, 21:1981–1987.

Braca, A., Sinisgalli, C., De Leo, M., Muscatello, B., Cioni, P.L., Milella, L., Ostuni, A., Giani, S., Sanogo, R., 2018. Molecules, 23 (12), Art. No. 3104, https://doi.org/10.3390/molecules23123104.

Brady, O., 2011. The Characterisation and Bioactivity Determination of *Adansonia digitata* L. Baobab Fruit Pulp, for Commercial Product Development. Bachelor of Science Dublin Institute of Technology, Ireland.

Buchmann, C., Prehsler, S., Hartl, A., Vogl, C.R., 2010. Ecol. Food Nutr., 49:145–172.

Builders, P.F., Okeke, U., Egieye, A.S., 2007. J. Phytomed. Ther., 12:22–30.

Carlson, M.H., Halvorsen, B.L., Holte, K., Bøhn, S.K., Dragland, S., Sampson, L., Willey, C., Senoo, H., Umezono, Y., Sanada, C., Barikmo, I., Berhe, N., Willett, W.C., Phillips, K.M., Jacobs, D.R., Blomhoff, R., 2010. Nutr. J., 9:3.

Chadare, F.J., Linnemann, A.R., Hounhouigan, J.D., Nout, M.J.R., van Boekel, M.A.J.S., 2009. Crit. Rev. Food Sci. Nutr., 49:254–274.

Chauhan, J.S., Cahturvedi, R., Kumar, S., 1984. Planta Med., 50:113.

Chauhan, J.S., Kumar, S., Cahturvedi, R., 1987. Nat. Acad. Sci. Lett., 10:177–179.

Chika, C., Ifeyinwa, N., Azubuike, U., David, O., 2019. Asian Pac. J. Reprod., 8:75–82.

Chindo, I.Y., Gushit, J.S., Olotu, P.N., Mugana, J., Takbal, D.N., 2010. J. Am. Sci., 6:990–994.

Chinsembu, K.C., 2019. Braz. J. Pharmacogn., https://doi.org/10.1016/j.bjp.2018.10.006.

Chipurura, B., Muchuweti, M., 2013. Int. J. Postharvest Technol., 3:392-402.

Cisse, M., Sakho, M., Dornier, M., Mar Diop, C., Reynes, M., Sock, O., 2009. Fruits, 64:19–34.

Coe, S.A., Clegg, M., Armengol, M., Ryan, L., 2013. Nutr. Res., 33:888–896.

De Lucia, D., Manfredini, S., Bernardi, T., Vertuani, S., 2015. Food Anal. Methods, 8:32–39.

Denloye, A.A.B., Teslim, K.O., Fasasi, O.A., 2006. J. Entomol., 3:9–15.

Djeussi, D.E., Noumedem, J.A.K., Seukep, J.A., Fankam, A.G., Voukeng, I.K., Tankeo, S.B., Nkuete, A.H.L., Kuete, V., 2013. BMC Complement. Altern. Med., 13, Art. No. 164, https://doi.org/10.1186/1472-6882-13-164.

Dzoyarchem, J.P., Kuete, V., McGaw, L.J., Eloff, J.N., 2014. J. Ethnopharmacol., 156:1–8.

Ebaid, H., Bashandy, S.A.E., Alhazza, I.M., Hassan, I., Al-Tamimi, J., 2019. BioMed Res. Int., Art. No. 2835152, https://doi.org/10.1155/2019/2835152.

Engels, P., 2009a. Use of a Component or Extract From the Baobab Plant for Skin Diseases. Patent WO/2009/115216.

Engels, P., 2009b. Use of Parts of the Baobab Plant as Animal Food or as Additive in Animal Food. US Patent 2009/0258112 A1.

FDA (U.S. Food and Drug Administration), 2009. Agency Response Letter GRAS Notice No. GRN 000273. Available from: http://www.fda.gov/Food/FoodIngredientsPackaging/GenerallyRecognizedasSafeGRAS/GRASListings/ucm174945.htm2009.

Gadour, M.O., Khidir, H.B., Adam, I., Gasim, G.I., 2017. J. Herb. Med., 8:14–16.

Gahane, R.N., Kogje, K.K., 2013. Acta Hortic., 972:55–60.

Garvey, R., Clegg, M., Coe, S., 2017. Nutr. Health, 23:83–86.

Gebauer, J., Assem, A., Busch, E., Hardtmann, S., Möckel, D., Krebs, F., Ziegler, T., Wichern, F., Wiehle, M., Kehlenbeck, K., 2014. Erwerbs-Obstbau, 56:9–24.

Geipel, A., 1905. Process for Manufacturing Plastic Mass. US Patent 800,563.

Ghoneim, M.A.M., Hassan, A.I., Mahmoud, M.G., Asker, M.S., 2016. Anim. Biotechnol., 27:84–95.

Glew, R.H., Vanderjagt, D.J., Lockett, C., Grivetti, L.E., Smith, G.C., Pastuszyn, A., Millson, M., 1997. J. Food Compos. Anal., 10:205–217.

Hanafy, A., Aldawsari, H.M., Badr, J.M., Ibrahim, A.K., Abdel-Hady, S.E.-S., 2016. Evid. Based Complement. Altern. Med., 2016, Art. No. 4579149, https://doi.org/10.1155/2016/4579149.

Hudson, J.B., Anani, K., Lee, M.K., De Souza, C., Arnason, J.T., Gbeassor, M., 2000. Pharm. Biol., 38:46–50.
Hussain, Z.T.E., Yagi, S., Mahomoodally, M.F., Mohammed, I., Zengin, G., 2019. S. Afr. J. Bot., https://doi.org/10.1016/j.sajb.2019.01.034.
Ibrahim, A.Y., Mahmoud, M.G., Asker, M.M.S., 2014. Int. J. Pharm. Sci. Rev. Res., 25:174–182.
IFAD, 2008. Gender and Non-Timber Forest Products. Promoting Food Security and Economic Empowerment. International Fund for Agricultural Development (IFAD). Available from: http://www.ifad.org/gender/pub/timber.pdf.
Irondi, E.A., Akintunde, J.K., Agboola, S.O., Boligon, A.A., Athayde, M.L., 2017. Food Sci. Nutr., 5:233–242.
Ismail, B.B., Guo, M., Pu, Y., Wang, W., Ye, X., Liu, D., 2019a. Ultrason. Sonochem., 52:257–267.
Ismail, B.B., Pu, Y., Guo, M., Ma, X., Liu, D., 2019b. Food Chem., 277:279–288.
Kamanula, M., Munthali, C.R.Y., Dziwapo, A., Kamanula, J.F., 2018. Malawi Med. J., 30:250–255.
Kamatou, G.P.P., Vermaak, I., Viljoen, A.M., 2011. S. Afr. J. Bot., 77:908–919.
Karumi, Y., Augustine, A.I., Umar, I.A., 2008. J. Biol. Sci., 8:225–228.
Kayode, R.M., Azubuike, C.U., Laba, S.A., Dauda, A.O., Balogun, M.A., Ajala, S.A., 2018. LWT, 93:58–63.
Khan, M., Shingare, M.S., Zafar, R., Ramesh, D., Siddiqui, A.R., 2006. Ind. J. Nat. Prod., 22:20–21.
Kinghorn, A.D., Chai, H.-B., Sung, C.K., Keller, W.J., 2011. Fitoterapia, 82:71–79.
Köhler, I., Jenett-Siems, K., Kraft, C., Siems, K., Abbiw, D., Bienzle, U., Eich, E., 2002. Z. Naturforsch. C, 57, 1022–1027.
Komane, B.M., Vermaak, I., Kamatou, G.P.P., Summers, B., Viljoen, A.M., 2017. Braz. J. Pharmacogn., 27:1–8.
Kumar, C.M.K., Yugandhar, P., Savithramma, N., 2015. J. Appl. Pharm. Sci., 5:82–89.
Kumar, C.M.K., Yugandhar, P., Savithramma, N., 2016. J. Intercult. Ethnopharmacol., 5:79–85.
Lagnika, L., Amoussa, M., Adjovi, Y., Sanni, A., 2012. J. Pharmacogn. Phytother., 4:44–52.
Lamien-Meda, A., Lamien, C.E., Compaoré, M.M.Y., Meda, R.N.T., Kiendrebeogo, M., Zeba, B., Millogo, J.F., Nacoulma, O.G., 2008. Molecules, 13:581–594.
Li, X.-N., Sun, J., Shi, H., Yu, L.L., Ridge, C.D., Mazzola, E.P., Okunji, C., Iwu, M.M., Michel, T.K., Chen, P., 2017. Food Res. Int., 99:755–761.
Lisao, K., Geldenhuys, C.J., Chirwa, P.W., 2017. S. Afr. J. Bot., 113:449–456.
Lockett, C.T., Calvert, C.C., Grivetti, L.E., 2002. Int. J. Food Sci. Nutr., 51:195–208.
Luckert, K.M., Nemarundwe, N., Gibbs, L., Grundy, I., Hauer, D., Maruzane, D., Shackleton, S., Sithole, J., 2014. Contribution of baobab production activities to household livelihoods. A case study in Zimbabwe. In: Cunningham, B.A., Campbell, M.B., Luckert, K.M. (Eds.), Bark Use, Management, and Commerce in Africa. Advances in Economic Botany, vol. 17, Chapter 14. The New York Botanical Garden Press, New York, USA.
Magaia, T.L.J., Skog, K., 2017. Afr. J. Food Agr. Nutr. Develop., 17:12441–12454.
Magaia, T., Uamusse, A., Sjöholm, I., Skog, K., 2013b. Springerplus, 2:1–8.
Manfredini, S., Vertuani, S., Buzzoni, V., 2002. *Adansonia digitata*. Il baobab farmacista. L'integratore Nutrizionale, 5:25–29.
Masola, S.N., Mosha, R.D., Wambura, P.N., 2009. Afr. J. Biotechnol., 8:5076–5083.
Modiba, E., Osifo, P., Rutto, H., 2014. Ind. Crop. Prod., 59:50–54.
Mpofu, A., Linnemann, A.R., Sybesma, W., Kort, R., Nout, M.J.R., Smid, E.J., 2014. J. Dairy Sci., 97:2591–2599.

Mulaudzi, R.B., Ndhlala, A.R., Kulkarni, M.G., Finnie, J.F., Staden, J.V., 2013. J. Ethnopharmacol., 146:173–179.

Mumtaz, T., Rizwani, G.H., Shareef, H., 2017. Pak. J. Pharm. Sci., 30:1657–1663.

Munthali, C.R.Y., Chirwa, P.W., Akinnifesi, F.K., 2012. Agrofor. Syst., 85:271–290.

Musila, M.F., Dossaji, S.F., Nguta, J.M., Lukhoba, C.W., Munyao, J.M., 2013. J. Ethnopharmacol., 146:557–561.

Muthai, K.U., Karori, M.S., Muchugi, A., Indieka, A.S., Dembele, C., Mng'omba, S., Jamnadass, R., 2017. Food Sci. Nutr., 5:1116–1129.

Muthai, U.K., Indieka, A.S., Muchugi, A., Karori, S.M., Mng'omba, S., Ky-Dembele, C., Jamnadass, R., 2019. S. Afr. J. Bot., 123:1–8.

Mwale, M., Mupangwa, J.F., Mapiye, C., Saina, H., Chimvuramahwe, J., 2008. Int. J. Poult. Sci., 7:429–432.

Nhukarume, L., Chikwambi, Z., Muchuweti, M., Chipurura, B., 2010. J. Food Biochem., 34:207–221.

Nkafamiya, I., Osemeahon, S., Dahiru, D., Umaru, H., 2007. Afr. J. Biotechnol., 6:756–759.

Nkosi, B.D., Phenya, J.S.M., Malebana, I.M.M., Muya, M.C., Motiang, M.D., 2019. Trop. Anim. Health Prod., https://doi.org/10.1007/s11250-019-01896-0.

Nordeide, M.B., Hatloy, A., Folling, M., Lied, E., Osbaug, A., 1996. Int. J. Food Sci. Nutr., 47:455–468.

Nwokocha, L.M., Williams, P.A., 2016. Food Hydrocoll., 58:29–34.

Nyam, K.L., Tan, C.P., Lai, O.M., Long, K., Che Man, Y.B., 2009. LWT - Food Sci. Technol., 42:1396–1403.

Ogbaga, C.C., Nuruddeen, F.A., Alonge, O.O., Nwagbara, O.F., 2018. 13th International Conference on Electronics, Computer and Computation, ICECCO 2017, 2018 January, pp. 1–5.

Olaitan, N.I., Eke, M.O., Aitiya, E., 2014. Adv. J. Food Sci. Technol., 6:1050–1055.

Osman, M.A., 2004. Plant Foods Hum. Nutr., 59:29–33.

Owoyele, B.V., Bakare, A.O., 2018. Biomed. Pharmacother., 97:209–212.

Pakenham, T., 2004. The Remarkable Baobab. Jonathan Ball Publishers, Johannesburg, South Africa.

Palombo, E.A., 2006. Phytother. Res., 20:717–724.

Parkar, S.G., Stevenson, D.E., Skinner, M.A., 2008. Int. J. Food Microbiol., 124:295–298.

PhytoTrade Africa Baobab Oil. Available from: http://www.phytotradeafrica.com/products/BaobabOil.htm.

Rahul, J., Jain, M.K., Singh, S.P., Kamal, R.K., Anuradha, N., Gupta, A.K., Mrityunjay, S.K., 2015. Asian Pac. J. Trop. Biomed., 5:79–84.

Ramadan, A., Harraz, F.M., El-Mougy, S.A., 1994. Fitoterapia, LXV:418–422.

Rashad, Y.M., Aseel, D.G., Hafez, E.E., 2018. Phytopathol. Mediterr., 57:73–88.

Rashford, J., 2018. Econ. Bot., 72:478–495.

Regional Trade Facilitation Programme, 2007. New Brief No. 2, Regional Trade Facilitation Programme. http://www.rtfp.org.

Ross, A.D., Harynuk, J.J., 2010. Anal. Methods, 2:1176–1179.

Sarven Bale, J., Pam Mancha, Y., Sanusi, M., Dass Doma, U., 2013. Int. J. Poult. Sci., 12:273–276.

Saulawa, L.A., Ukachukwu, S.N., Onwudike, O.C., Garba, M.G., Aruwayo, A., 2014. Int. J. Poult. Sci., 13:335–339.

Segun, P.A., Ogbole, O.O., Ajaiyeoba, E.O., 2018. J. Herb. Med., 14:68–75.

Semenya, S.S., Maroyi, A., 2018a. J. Appl. Bot. Food Qual., 91:287–295.

Semenya, S.S., Maroyi, A., 2018b. Med. Plants, 10:320–339.
Seukep, J.A., Fankam, A.G., Djeussi, D.E., Voukeng, I.K., Tankeo, S.B., Noumdem, J.A.K., Kuete, A.H.L.N., Kuete, V., 2013. Springerplus, 2:1–8.
Shahat, A.A., 2006. Pharm. Biol., 44:445–450.
Sharma, A., Rangari, V., 2016. Trop. J. Pharm. Res., 15:1923–1927.
Shatkina, R., Gurevich, S.D., 2010. Nutraceutical Composition. US Patent 2010/0136064 A1.
Shehu, A., Magaji, M.G., Yau, J., Ahmed, A., 2019. J. Basic Clin. Physiol. Pharmacol., 30 (3), Art. No. 20180153, https://doi.org/10.1515/jbcpp-2018-0153.
Shukla, Y.N., Dubey, S., Jain, S.P., Kumar, S., 2001. J. Med. Arom. Plant Sci., 23:429–434.
Sidibe, M., Williams, J.T., 2002. Baobab–*Adansonia digitata*. Fruits for the Future 4. International Centre for Underutilised Crops, Southampton, UK.
Soloviev, P., Niang, T.D., Gaye, A., Totte, A., 2004. Fruits, 59:109–119.
South African National Biodiversity Institute (SANBI), 2017. Andrew Hankey, Walter Sisulu National Botanical Garden. Available from: http://pza.sanbi.org/adansonia-digitata.
Sulaiman, L.K., Oladele, O.A., Shittu, I.A., Emikpe, B.O., Oladokun, A.T., Meseko, C.A., 2011. Afr. J. Biotechnol., 10:4256–4258.
Suleiman, M.M., Mamman, M., Hassan, I., Garba, S., Kawu, M.U., Kobo, P.I., 2014. Vet. World, 7:496–500.
Tahia, F., Majumder, P., Sikder, M.A.A., Rashid, M.A., 2015. Dhaka Univ. J. Pharm. Sci., 14:157–162.
Tal-Dia, A., Toure, K., Sarr, O., Sarr, M., Cisse, M.F., Garnier, P., Wone, I., 1997. Dakar Méd., 42:68–73.
Tembo, D.T., Holmes, M.J., Marshall, L.J., 2017. J. Food Compos. Anal., 58:40–51.
Tshikalange, T.E., Modishane, D.C., Tabit, F.T., 2017. J. Herbs Spices Med. Plants, 23:68–76.
Tzounis, X., Vulevic, J., Kuhnle, G.G.C., George, T., Leonczak, J., Gibson, G.R., Kwik-Uribe, C., Spencer, J.P.E., 2008. Br. J. Nutr., 99:782–792.
UNCTAD (United Nations Conference on Trade and Development), 2005. Market Brief in the European Union for Selected Natural Ingredients Derived From Native Species. *Adansonia digitata* L. Baobab. Available from: http://www.biotrade.org/ResourcesPublications/biotradebrief-baobab.pdf.
Van Wyk, B.-E., Gericke, N., 2000. People's Plants—A Guide to Useful Plants of Southern Africa. Briza Publications, Pretoria, South Africa.
Van Wyk, B.-E., Van Oudtshoorn, B., Gericke, N., 1997. Medicinal Plants of South Africa. Briza Publications, Pretoria, South Africa.
Venter, S.M., Witkowski, T.F., 2010. For. Ecol. Manag., 259:294–300.
Venter, S.M., Witkowski, E.T.F., 2013. Agrofor. Syst., 87:159–172.
Vertuani, S., Braccioli, E., Buzzoni, V., Manfredini, S., 2002. Acta Phytother., 2:86–91.
Vimalanathan, S., Hudson, J.B., 2009. J. Med. Plant Res., 3:576–582.
Wasserman, R.H., 2004. J. Nutr., 134:3137–3139.
Watt, J.M., Breyer-Brandwijk, M.G., 1962. The Medicinal and Poisonous Plants of Southern and Eastern Africa, second ed. E. & S. Livingstone Ltd, Edinburgh and London, UK.
Wickens, G.E., 1982. The baobab, Africa's upside-down tree. Kew Bull., 37:171–202.
Wickens, G.E., Lowe, P., 2008. The Baobabs: Pachycauls of Africa. Madagascar and Australia. Springer, UK.
Wren, S., Stucki, A., 2003. Int. J. Aromather., 23:71–81.
Wynberg, R., Laird, S., 2014. Access and Benefit Sharing for Baobab Fruit and Oil in South Africa. Unpublished report PhytoTrade Africa, Harare, Zimbabwe.

Wynberg, R., Laird, S., Van Niekerk, J., Kozanayi, W., 2015. Soc. Nat. Resour., 28:559–574.
Yagoub, S.O., 2008. Res. J. Microbiol., 3:193–197.
Zahid, A., Despres, J., Benard, M., Nguema-Ona, E., Leprince, J., Vaudry, D., Rihouey, C., Vicré-Gibouin, M., Driouich, A., Follet-Gueye, M.-L., 2017. J. Cell. Physiol., 232:2558–2568.
Zimba, N., Wren, S., Stucki, A., 2005. Int. J. Aromather., 15:177–182.

CHAPTER

Agathosma betulina

2

Maxleene Sandasi[a,b], Guy Kamatou[a], Weiyang Chen[a] and Nduvho Mulaudzi[a]

[a]*Department of Pharmaceutical Sciences, Tshwane University of Technology, Pretoria, South Africa*

[b]*SAMRC Herbal Drugs Research Unit, Faculty of Science, Tshwane University of Technology, Pretoria, South Africa*

Abstract

Agathosma betulina (P.J. Bergius) Pillans (Rutaceae), commonly referred to as 'buchu', is an evergreen, fragrant shrub that grows up to 2 m in height and is naturally distributed in the Western Cape Province of South Africa. The leaves are aromatic and, upon distillation, produce a golden oil, with a strong-sweetish, peppermint-like scent. Buchu oil is a flavour enhancer in foods and beverages, and a fragrance material in perfumes. Traditionally, the plant is used to treat cholera, indigestion, constipation, prostatitis, rheumatism, fever, respiratory and urinary tract infections, as well as for disinfecting wounds and relieving menstrual cramps. Agathosma betulina is commercially marketed as fresh or dried leaves, tinctures, herbal water and essential oils. This monograph is a record of the ethnobotany, phytochemistry, in vitro and in vivo biological properties of the plant, as well as its toxicity profile. Furthermore, chemical profiling was performed using semi-automated high-performance thin-layer chromatography (HPTLC), ultra-performance liquid chromatography coupled to mass spectrometry (UPLC–MS), gas chromatography coupled to mass spectrometry (GC–MS) and flame ionisation detection. Isomenthone, diosphenol, limonene, menthone, pulegone, pseudo-diosphenol, 8-mercapto-p-menthan-3-one, 8-acetylthio-p-menthan-3-one, 8-methylthio-p-menthan-3-one, 4-hydroxydiosphenol and 1-hydroxydiosphenol were the predominant compounds in the essential oil, as determined by GC–MS analysis. The marker compounds in the non-volatile fraction were identified as diosmin, hesperidin and rutin, based on both HPTLC and UPLC–MS analysis.

Keywords: *Agathosma betulina*, Buchu, Essential oil, HPTLC, GC–MS, UPLC–MS, MIR spectroscopy, Diosphenol, Hesperidin, Rutin

The South African Herbal Pharmacopoeia. https://doi.org/10.1016/B978-0-323-99794-2.00019-2

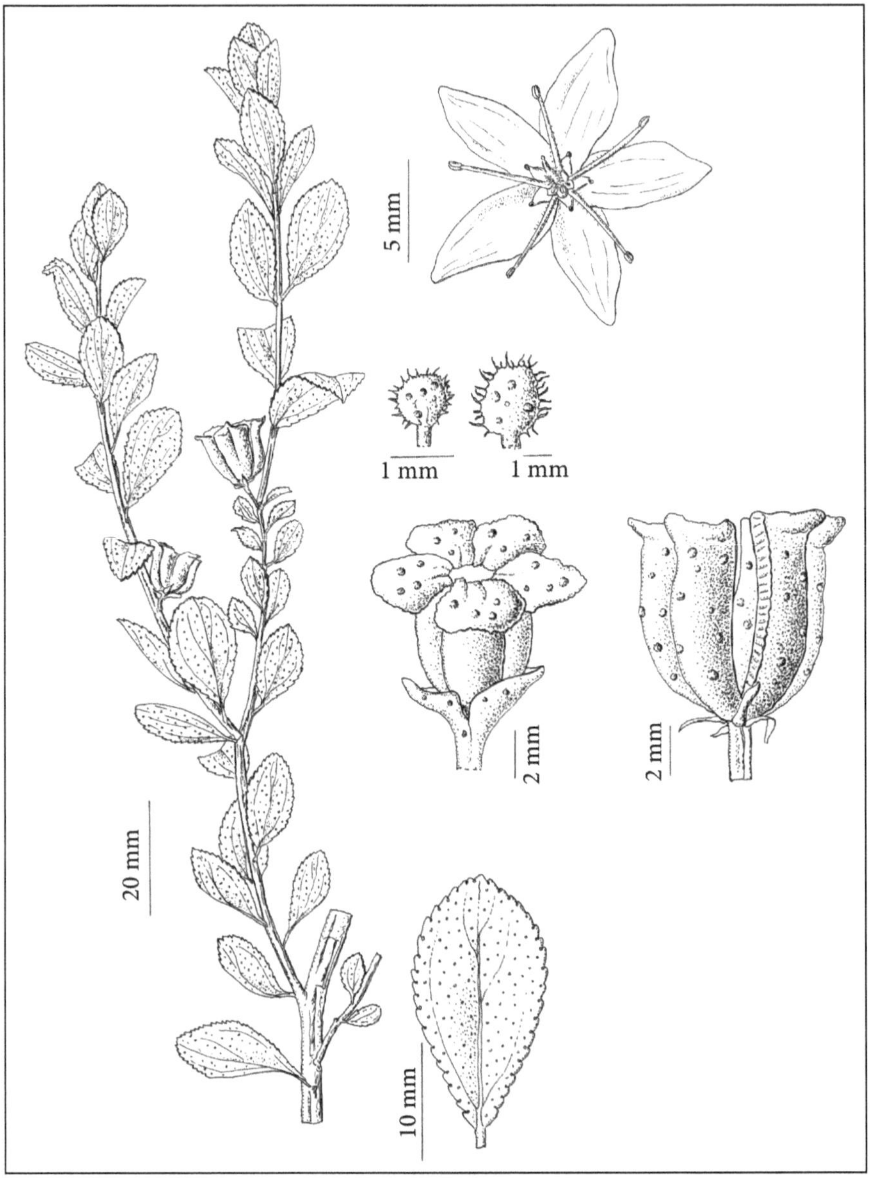
5 mm
1 mm
1 mm
2 mm
2 mm
20 mm
10 mm

Part A: General overview

1. Synonyms

Barosma betulina Bartl. & H.L.Wendl., *Bucco betulina* Roem. & Schult., *Diosma betulina* Thunb., *Diosma crenata* Lodd. (later homonym), not of L. (1759), *Hartogia betulina* P.J.Bergius.[a]

2. Common name(s)

Buchu (Khoi, English), round-leaf, oval-leaf and short-leaf buchu (English), '*ibuchu*' (isiXhosa), '*boegoe*', '*rondeblaarbuchu*', '*bergboegoe*' (Afrikaans).[a]

3. Conservation status

Least concern.[a]

4. Botany

Agathosma betulina (P.J.Bergius) Pillans is an evergreen, resprouting, fragrant shrub that grows up to 2 m in height. The leaves are round, small and broad, growing up to 20 mm in length. They are pale green and glossy with finely toothed margins and a strong rounded apex, which curves backwards (A). Leaf surfaces are scattered with round, pellucid oil glands that are mostly visible on the margins and lower surfaces (C). The leaves are aromatic and the oil is golden in colour, with a strong-sweetish, peppermint-like odour. The flowers are solitary, five-petalled, star-shaped and open, and the flower colour varies from white to pink, to pale purple (B). New shoots have distinctive red-flushed stems. The plant also produces brownish fruits that are five-chambered (Spreeth, 1976). The aerial parts of the plant, particularly the leaves, are harvested (D) and prepared using various methods for medicinal purposes.

5. Geographical distribution

Agathosma betulina is endemic to the mountainous areas of the Western Cape Province of South Africa. The distribution of *A. betulina* expands from the Cederberg mountains, situated east of the towns of Citrusdal and Clanwilliam, to the Groot Winterhoek mountains, including the Piketberg mountain (Goldblatt and Manning, 2000). It is particularly well adapted to dry conditions and can be found in fynbos habitats on rocky sandstone slopes at altitudes of 300–700 m above sea level.

[a] Red List of South African Plants (http://redlist.sanbi.org).

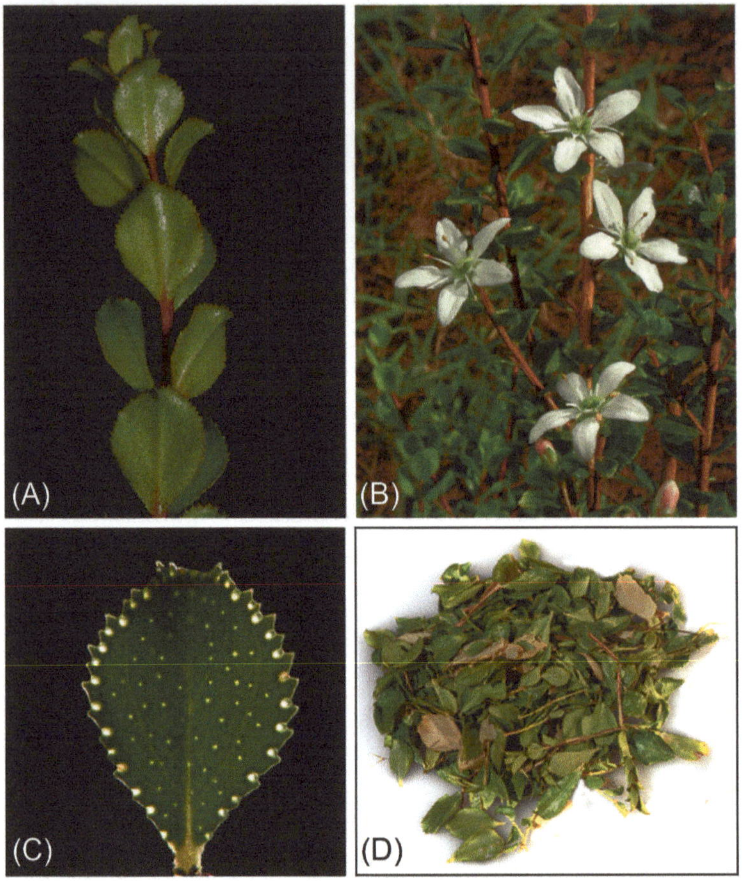

Agathosma betulina plant with pale green leaves that curve backwards (A), star-shaped open flowers (B), leaf displaying finely toothed margins and round pellucid oil glands (C) and dried aerial parts (D).

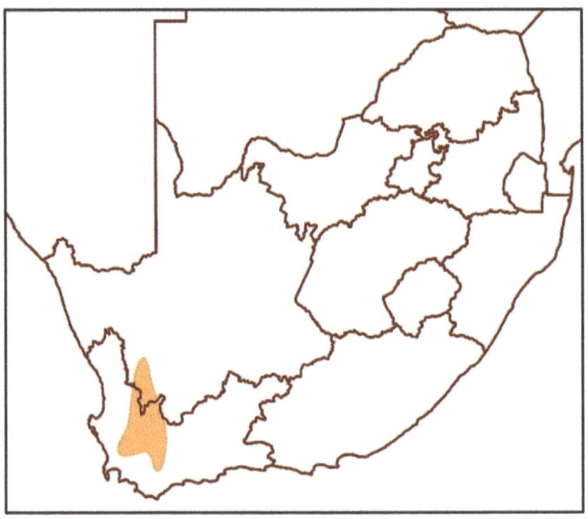

Geographical distribution of *Agathosma betulina* in South Africa.

6. Ethnopharmacology

Agathosma betulina is an important part of the Khoi-San culture and it is still used in the Cape region as a general tonic and medicine. The indigenous people first introduced buchu in the mid-17th century as a medicinal plant to the European settlers in the Cape (Low, 2007). The aerial parts of the plant, particularly the leaves, were chewed to cure stomach ailments including cholera. Buchu tea was used as a general tonic and stomachic to increase appetite. The plant is prepared as an infusion, tincture or as '*boegoebrandewyn*' (buchu brandy) for disinfecting wounds and relieving menstrual cramps (Watt and Breyer-Brandwijk, 1962; Van Wyk et al., 1997). Other traditional uses of buchu include liniment, diuretic, treatment of kidney and urinary tract infections (UTIs), haematuria and prostatitis, rheumatism, relief of calculus and arthritis, indigestion, constipation, fevers, colds and flu, coughs, gout and bruises (Watt and Breyer-Brandwijk, 1962; Van Wyk et al., 1997; Simpson, 1998; Swerdlow, 2000). *Agathosma* species have also been used for cosmetic purposes. The San lubricated their bodies to keep their skin soft and moist in the dry desert climate. The topical application (plant mixed with fat) displays antibacterial, antifungal, insect repellent and deodorant effects, and thus promotes the general well-being of the body (Van Wyk et al., 1997). Buchu is popularly used to treat renal disorders, including infections of the bladder, urinary tract, kidneys and chest complaints (Van Wyk and Wink, 2004).

7. Commercialisation

There are a variety of products on the market prepared from buchu, of which the therapeutic effect is claimed to be due to the non-volatile components. These include teas, capsules, tablets, gels and herbal water. *Agathosma betulina* is one of the earliest and best-known exported medicinal plants from South Africa. Whilst the use of buchu as a medicine became customary amongst Cape Settlers and Africans alike, it was only in 1821 that buchu formally entered the international market. Buchu leaves were harvested, dried and baled in South Africa and exported to Europe and America, where they were processed into tinctures, teas and ointments. Bales of buchu were famously aboard the Titanic on its first and final voyage in 1912 (Encyclopedia Titanica, 2003). Commercialisation of the plant has seen cultivation of buchu in the dry regions between Citrusdal, Paarl and Piketberg in the Western Cape Province. The effect of pH on growth, mineral content and essential oil quality of *A. betulina*, grown under controlled conditions, was evaluated (Ntwana et al., 2013). Growth and highest biomass accumulation were achieved for the acidic treatments, indicating that the plant grows well under acidic conditions, with the best pH in the range between 4 and 5. Approximately 20,000 plants can be planted per hectare with an oil yield of approximately 1%. The volumes of production, domestic consumption and export are estimated at 300, 50 and 250 tons per year, respectively. A micropropagation protocol was developed for *A. betulina*, and a technique developed to enhance the biosynthesis of some of the bioactive compounds in the plant (Witbooi et al., 2017). *In vitro* seed germination produced healthy seedlings that can be transplanted *ex vitro*. Biosynthesis of certain compounds in *Agathosma* was induced by a plant growth regulator application. The use of micropropagation techniques and enhancement of bioactive compounds in the plant can be an efficient means to meet the high demand for this sought-after crop. The value of the essential oil can be improved by removing potentially unstable compounds, such as monoterpene hydrocarbons. This was demonstrated by Madzimbamuto et al. (2016) in a deterpenation process. Based on the solubility differences between limonene and the oxygenated terpenes, it was shown that the deterpenation of *Agathosma* essential oils can be done using supercritical CO_2 fractionation. Economically, *Agathosma* is a high-value crop that is marketed in various forms such as fresh leaf, dry leaf, tinctures and buchu water, a by-product of hydro-distillation. Lubbe and Verpoorte (2011) reported the price of buchu at $56/kg for cultivated material. The oil and seed have been reported to sell on international markets (Moolla and Viljoen, 2008). The essential oil is not only used for medicinal purposes, but also as a flavour fixative in the food industry (Coetzee et al., 1999). In the United States, buchu volatile oil is approved for culinary use with concentrations usually up to about 0.002% (Complementary Medicines, 2003). The oil is used as a flavourant, enhancing fruity flavours such as blackcurrant notes in food and beverages. The oil is also used as a fragrance material, imparting minty, camphoraceous scents to perfumes and colognes (Simpson, 1998; Turpie et al., 2003; Van Wyk and Wink, 2004). Buchu is an active ingredient of Fluidex® and Odrinil® complementary medicines used for the relief of premenstrual blotting (Swerdlow, 2000).

8. Pharmacological evaluation

8.1 *In vitro* studies

Several *in vitro* studies have been conducted to investigate the anti-infective properties of *A. betulina* using the agar well diffusion and microplate dilution assays. Non-volatile extracts demonstrated good antimicrobial activity against a range of human pathogens, including Gram-positive, Gram-negative bacteria and fungal pathogens (Viljoen et al., 2006; Moolla et al., 2007). The antimicrobial activity of the hydro-distilled essential oils and methanol:dichloromethane (1:1) extracts of *A. betulina* was evaluated using the minimum inhibitory concentration (MIC) values, as determined using the microplate dilution assay in studies performed by Moolla et al. (2007) and Viljoen et al. (2006). Both the extract and the essential oil were active against the four pathogens tested (*Staphylococcus aureus*, *Bacillus cereus*, *Klebsiella pneumoniae* and *Candida albicans*). The extract exhibited antimicrobial activity against the pathogens, with MIC values between 2 and 4 mg/mL. In another study, moderate to poor antimicrobial activity was also observed for the essential oil (Lis-Balchin et al., 2001). Sandasi (2008) re-investigated the *in vitro* antimicrobial activity of *A. betulina* extracts (water, dichloromethane:methanol (1:1 v/v) and methanol) towards seven pathogenic micro-organisms. The dichloromethane:methanol (1:1 v/v) extracts displayed moderate activity with MIC values between 3 and 6 mg/mL.

The effect of *A. betulina* extracts on the growth and development of biofilms was demonstrated using the crystal violet (CV) assay. The extracts showed good inhibition of biofilm formation, but the inhibition of growth and development of an established biofilm was poor (Sandasi, 2008). The ethanolic leaf extract of *A. betulina* exhibited antibacterial activity against some urinary tract pathogens, including *Escherichia coli*, *K. pneumoniae*, *Proteus mirabilis*, *Pseudomonas aeruginosa*, *S. aureus*, *Staphylococcus saprophyticus* and *Enterococcus faecalis* (Geetha et al., 2012). An aqueous extract of *A. betulina* leaves exhibited antitubercular activity against *Mycobacterium tuberculosis* H37Rv at 25 µg/mL (Famewo et al., 2017). Further interactive antimicrobial and toxicity profiles *of A. betulina* (essential oil, aqueous and organic extracts) with the conventional antimicrobial, ciprofloxacin, against *E. coli* provided a notable synergistic profile. The identified synergistic interactions could possibly lead to more effective treatment of UTIs and reverse the resistance of *E. coli* towards ciprofloxacin (Hübsch et al., 2014). Activation of *A. betulina* antimicrobial constituents, following exposure to simulated intestinal fluid, was demonstrated during dissolution studies (Viljoen et al., 2007; Vermaak et al., 2009). Crude water and methanol extracts were prepared and exposed to simulated gastric and intestinal fluids, and the products were subsequently screened for antimicrobial activity towards *S. aureus*, *E. faecalis*, *E. coli* and *Proteus vulgaris*. The results demonstrated that the simulated intestinal fluid product exhibited enhanced antimicrobial activity compared to the gastric fluid product. Viljoen et al. (2007) used the *in vitro* Caco-2-cell model to predict the absorption and bioavailability of the extracts. The results revealed that compounds present in the crude water extract were able to permeate the Caco-2 cell monolayer (≈ 100% transport).

Agathosma betulina oil was also investigated for *in vitro* spasmolytic activity on smooth muscle using guinea-pig ileum (Lis-Balchin et al., 2001). At high concentrations, the oil had an initial spasmogenic activity, followed by spasmolysis. In the presence of the phosphodiesterase inhibitor rolipram, the spasmolytic action of *A. betulina* was significantly increased. The results suggested a mode of action for the oil involving cyclic adenosine monophosphate. In addition, *A. betulina* appeared to block calcium channels. Another *in vitro* study confirmed anti-oxidative, weak antimicrobial, and also anti-inflammatory effects (Latté, 2010). *Agathosma betulina* extracts and essential oils demonstrated weak anti-oxidant capacity using the 2,2-diphenyl-1-picrylhydrazyl radical (DPPH) assay. In the 2,2-azino-*bis*(3-ethylbenzothiazoline-6-sulphonic acid) (ABTS) assay, the extracts displayed good anti-oxidant activity (IC_{50} value of 37.75 ± 0.54 µg/mL), which was attributed to the presence of flavonoids in the non-volatile fraction (Moolla et al., 2007; Moolla and Viljoen, 2008). The oil of *A. betulina* demonstrated good anti-inflammatory activity with an IC_{50} value of 50.37 ± 1.87 µg/mL, using the 5-lipoxygenase assay (Viljoen et al., 2006; Moolla et al., 2007). In another study, the ethanolic extract of *A. betulina* inhibited cyclooxygenase-2 (COX-2)-catalysed prostaglandin biosynthesis by 25% (Steenkamp et al., 2006).

8.2 *In vivo* studies and clinical trials

The ethanolic extract and essential oil of *A. betulina* exhibited analgesic and anti-inflammatory properties in formalin- and albumin-induced rat paw oedema models, respectively (Chiguvare, 2015; Chiguvare et al., 2016). The analgesic properties of synthesised silver nanoparticles (Ag-NPs) showed significant inhibition of pain as compared to aspirin, a standard analgesic drug at a dosage of 200 mg/kg. The combined plant extract and Ag-NPs was found to be more effective in pain management than both the aspirin and the extract alone. A clinical study documented the efficacy of topical *Agathosma* oil to treat pain and swelling on an exercise-induced damaged muscle. A study undertaken at the Research Unit of Exercise and Sports Medicine, University of Cape Town in South Africa, evaluated the efficacy of the oil applied topically to treat pain resulting from muscle damage. The results from the double-blind placebo-controlled trial indicated that the group treated three times daily with *Agathosma* gel presented with a reduction in swelling that may be ascribed to the anti-inflammatory properties associated with the oil (Lambert et al., 2002).

8.3 Safety

In vitro toxicity studies using the 3-(4,5 dimethylthiazol-2-yl)-2,5-diphenyltetrazolium bromine (MTT) assay have demonstrated that the essential oil of buchu is highly toxic (IC_{50} values of < 0.0001 µg/mL), whilst the non-volatile extracts are non-toxic (IC_{50} values > 100 µg/mL) (Viljoen et al., 2006; Moolla et al., 2007). The toxicity of the essential oil can be attributed to the hepatotoxic compound *cis*-isopulegone, which occurs in relatively low levels in *A. betulina. In vitro* toxicological studies indicate DNA damage and pro-oxidative effects for some leaf extracts (Latté, 2010). When the combinations of ciprofloxacin with *A. betulina* were tested for toxicity, none of the combinations were found to be toxic, with no mortality and a cell viability of no less than 100% recorded for both the brine shrimp lethality assay (BSLA) and MTT assay (Hübsch et al., 2014).

9. Phytochemistry

9.1 Volatile constituents

The essential oil yield ranges between 1.5% and 2.5% dry weight. The volatile fraction has been well researched due to its widespread application in the flavour and fragrance industries. A typical essential oil profile of *A. betulina* is characterised by isomenthone, diosphenol, limonene, menthone, pulegone, pseudo-diosphenol, 8-mercapto-*p*-menthan-3-one, 8-acetylthio-*p*-menthan-3-one, 8-methylthio-*p*-menthan-3-one, 4-hydroxydiosphenol and 1-hydroxydiosphenol

(Van Wyk, 2011). The minor sulphur-containing compounds are responsible for the blackcurrant odour of the oil (Collins et al., 1996). Köpke et al. (1992) reported the simultaneous and direct stereo-analysis of the aroma-active flavour compounds, 8-mercapto-*p*-menthan-3-one and 3-oxo-*p*-menthane-8-thiol acetate; the stereoisomers of the latter were identified by ^{1}H and ^{13}C nuclear magnetic resonance (NMR) spectroscopy and gas chromatography coupled to mass spectrometry (GC–MS). *Agathosma betulina* has a higher content of 8-mercapto-*p*-menthan-3-one than 8-acetylthio-*p*-menthan-3-one and the *cis*-8-mercapto-*p*-menthan-3-one content is higher than that of the *trans*-isomer. Two chemotypes of *A. betulina* have been reported: a diosphenol chemotype characterised by high levels of diosphenol and low levels of isomenthone (<29%), and an isomenthone chemotype characterised by high isomenthone (>31%) and low diosphenol levels (Fluck et al., 1961; Lamparsky and Schudel, 1971; Kaiser et al., 1975; Collins et al., 1996; Posthumus et al., 1996; Viljoen et al., 2006).

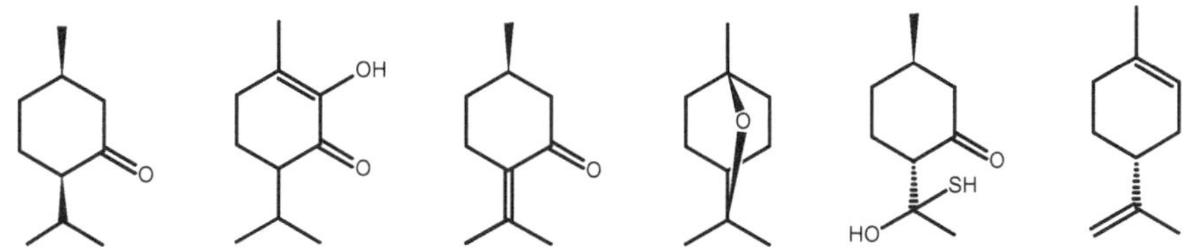

Isomenthone | Diosphenol | Pulegone | 1,8-Cineole | 8-Mercapto-*p*-menthan-3-one | Limonene

9.2 Non-volatile constituents

The non-volatile fraction of *A. betulina* is not well studied; however, phytochemical screening of the ethanol extract revealed the presence of glycosides, proteins, tannins, alkaloids, flavonoids and saponins (Chiguvare et al., 2016). The following three flavonoids have been identified in the methanol extract; rutin, diosmin and hesperidin (British Pharmaceutical Codex, 1963; British Herbal Medicine Association, 1996). The two main flavonoids (diosmin and hesperidin) were identified in the leaves and also in commercial tablets, using a reversed-phase high-performance liquid chromatography (HPLC) method (El-Shafae and El-Domiaty, 2001).

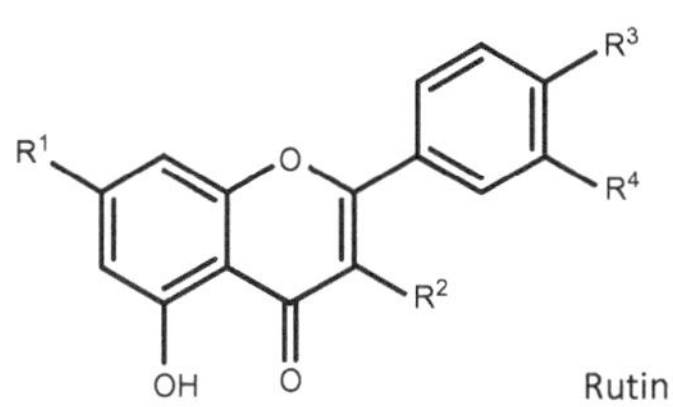

Rutin: R^1=OH, R^2=rutinoside, R^3=OH, R^4=OH
Diosmin: R^1=rutinoside, R^2=H, R^3=OMe, R^4=OH
Hesperidin: R^1=rutinoside, R^2=2H, R^3=OMe, R^4=OH

Part B: Chemical profiling and quality control

10. Chromatography analysis

10.1 High-performance thin-layer chromatography (HPTLC) fingerprint analysis

General instrumentation: A CAMAG HPTLC instrument consisting of an automatic TLC sampler (ATS 4), automatic developing chamber (ADC 2), CAMAG TLC Visualizer 2, CAMAG derivatiser and TLC plate heater. *HPTLC plates:* Silica gel glass plates 60 F_{254} (Merck).

10.1.1 Non-volatile fraction analysis

Plant part: Aerial parts, methanol extract. *Sample application:* Application volume of 2 µL methanol extract (100 mg/mL) and standards (1 mg/mL) spotted as 10 mm bands. Plates developed in a 20 × 10 × 4 cm glass twin-trough chamber to a migration distance of 70 mm. *Tank saturation:* 20 min at 20.8 °C and 30.4% RH, with 25 mL of mobile phase. *Mobile phase:* Ethyl acetate: water: formic acid (12:1:1 v/v/v). *Derivatisation:* Natural Product reagent and polyethylene glycol reagent. The plate was sprayed with 3 mL of the reagent mixture, heated for 3 min at 100 °C on a TLC plate heater, and then visualised. *Visualisation:* The plate was viewed under 366 nm fluorescent light.

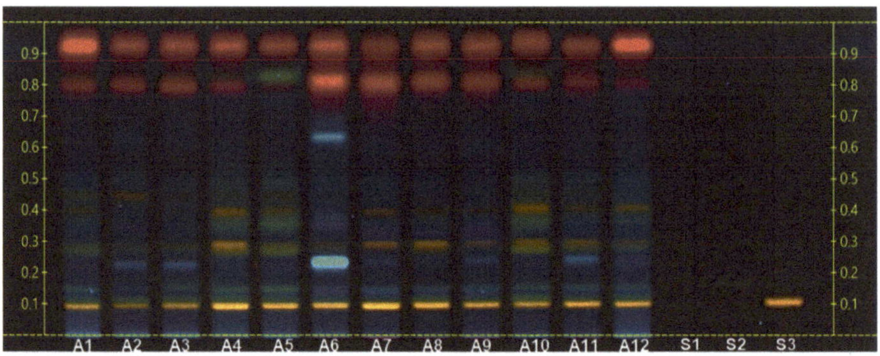

HPTLC plate of *Agathosma betulina* methanol extracts (n = 12) (A1–A12) and the standards (S1–S3). The samples are characterised by a grey band for diosmin (S1) (R_f = 0.12), a yellow band for hesperidin (S2) (R_f = 0.16) and an orange band for rutin (S3) (R_f = 0.10) under 366 nm radiation.

10.1.2 Essential oil analysis

Plant part: Aerial parts, essential oil. *Sample application:* Application volume of 2 µL essential oil (25 µL/mL in toluene) and standards (1 mg/mL in methanol) spotted as 10 mm bands. Plates developed in a 20 × 10 × 4 cm glass twin-trough chamber to a migration distance of 70 mm. *Tank saturation:* 20 min at 15 °C and 45% RH, with 25 mL of mobile phase. *Mobile phase:* Neat dichloromethane. *Derivatisation:* *p*-Anisaldehyde/sulphuric acid. The plate was sprayed with 3 mL of the reagent and heated for 3 min at 100 °C on a TLC plate heater and visualised. *Visualisation:* The plate was viewed under 254 nm fluorescent light before derivatisation, and under white reflectance after derivatisation.

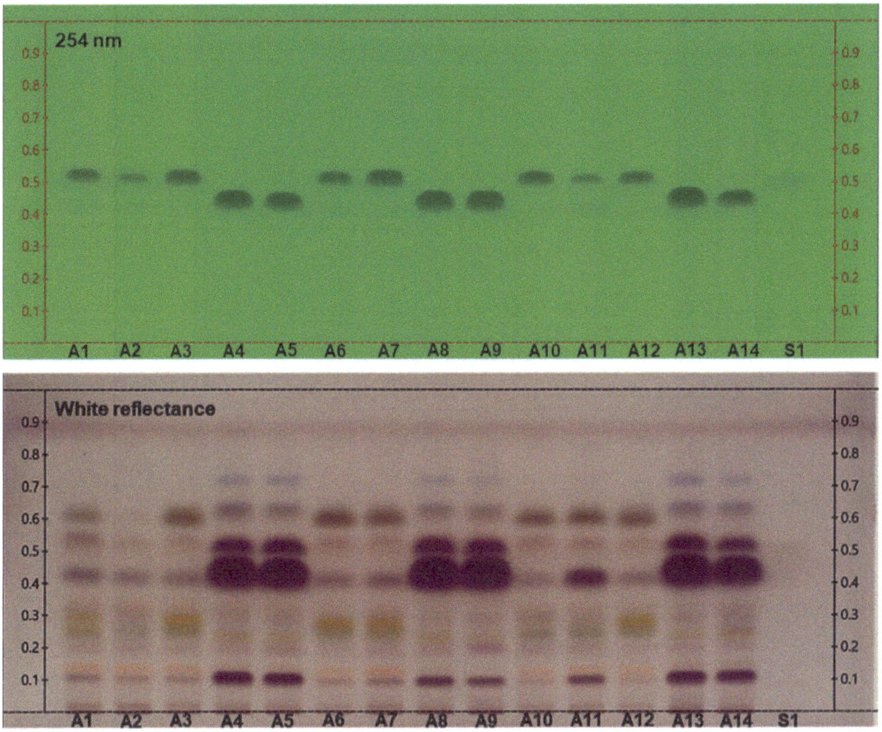

The HPTLC plate of *Agathosma betulina* essential oil ($n = 14$) (A1–A14) and the standard diosphenol (S1) characterised by a bold black band at $R_f = 0.51$ under 254 nm radiation.

10.2 Ultra-performance liquid chromatography (UPLC) analysis

General instrumentation: Waters Acquity Ultra-Performance Liquid Chromatography system with photodiode array (PDA) detector combined with a Xevo G2QToF mass spectrometer (Waters, United States). *Plant part:* Aerial parts, methanol extract. *Sample application:* Injection volume of 1.0 µL (full-loop injection) at 1 mg/mL. *Column:* Acquity UPLC BEH C_{18} column (150 mm × 2.1 mm, i.d., 1.7 µm particle size, Waters). *Mobile phase:* 0.1% formic acid in water (solvent A) and acetonitrile (solvent B). *Analysis conditions:* Gradient elution at flow rate: 0.4 mL/min, changing as follows: 90% A: 10% B to 65% A: 35% B in 3.5 min, to 50% A: 50% B in 3 min, to 10% A: 90% B in 1 min, keeping for 1 min and back to the initial ratio in 1 min, equilibrating the system for 2.5 min, total run time 12 min. *Mass spectrometry*: ESI^+ (positive ionisation mode), N_2 used as desolvation gas, desolvation temperature 400 °C at a flow rate of 600 L/h and source temperature at 100 °C. Capillary and cone voltages, 3500 and 55 V, respectively. Data collected between *m/z* 100 and 1200.

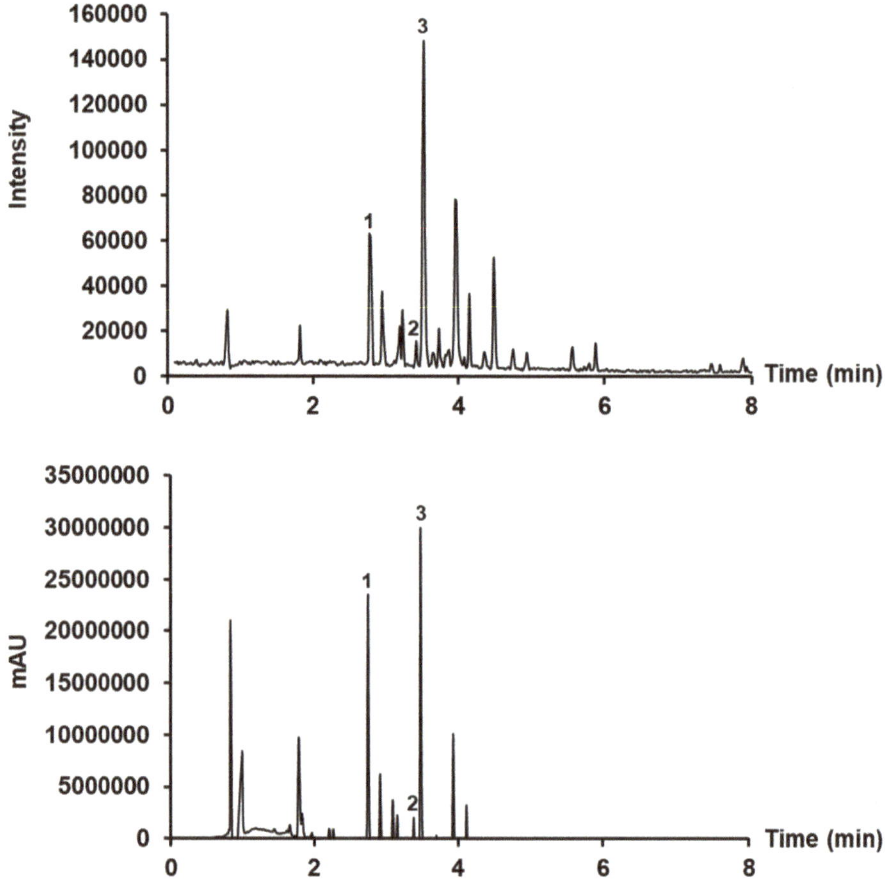

UPLC–ToF–MS ESI^+ (upper) and PDA (lower) chromatograms of *Agathosma betulina* methanol extract. [1] = rutin *m/z* 611.1583, [2] = diosmin *m/z* 609.1797, [3] = hesperidin *m/z* 611.1957.

10.3 Gas chromatography (GC) analysis

General instrumentation: An Agilent 6860N chromatograph (Agilent Technologies, Hanova, United States) fitted with a flame ionisation detector and a mass spectrometer. *Column:* HP-Innowax, 60 m × 250 μm × 0.25 μm (polyethylene glycol column, Agilent

Technologies, Hanova, United States). *Plant part:* Aerial parts, essential oil. *Sample application:* Injection volume of 1 μL (split) at 20% (v/v) in hexane. *Analysis conditions:* Inlet temperature 250 °C, split ratio: 1:200, helium carrier gas, flow rate: 1.2 mL/min, pressure: 24.79 psi. Starting oven temperature at 60 °C and then rising to 220 °C at 4 °C/min, holding for 10 min and increased to 240 °C at 1 °C/min. *Mass spectrometry conditions:* Chromatograms obtained on electron impact at 70 eV on an Agilent 5973 mass selective detector, scanning range: *m/z* 35 to 550 (Agilent Technologies, Hanova, United States). *Identification:* Authentic standards, NIST® and Mass Finder®.

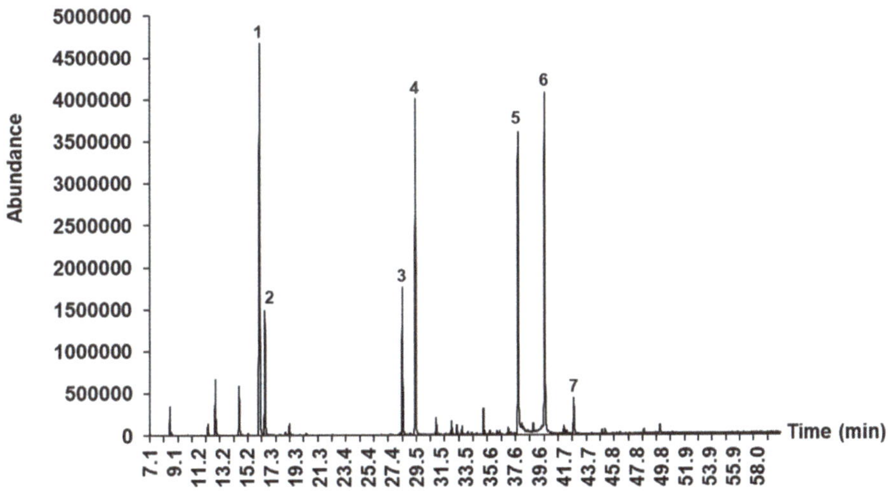

Total ion chromatogram (TIC) of *Agathosma betulina* essential oil indicating major compounds. [1] = limonene (R_t 16.31, *m/z* 136.1252), [2] = 1,8-cineole (R_t 16.74, *m/z* 154.1357), [3] = menthone (R_t 28.28, *m/z* 154.1357), [4] = isomenthone (R_t 29.39, *m/z* 154.1352), [5] = pseudo-diosphenol (R_t 37.88, *m/z* 168.2360), [6] = diosphenol (R_t 40.07, *m/z* 168.2360), [7] = 8-mercapto-menthan-3-one (R_t 42.49, *m/z* 186.3130).

11. Mid-infrared (MIR) spectroscopy analysis

General instrumentation: Alpha-P Bruker spectrometer, mounted with an attenuated total reflectance (ATR) diamond crystal. *Spectral acquisition:* Spectrum obtained in the absorbance mode, with a spectral resolution of 4 cm^{-1} over the range 4000–550 cm^{-1} and captured using OPUS 6.5 software.

11.1 Powder analysis

Plant part: Aerial parts. *Sample preparation:* Aerial parts powdered, sieved (<500 μm) and placed directly onto the surface of the diamond crystal.

11.2 Essential oil analysis

Plant part: Aerial parts, essential oil. *Sample preparation:* Aerial parts, hydro-distillation to obtain essential oil, placed directly onto the surface of the diamond crystal.

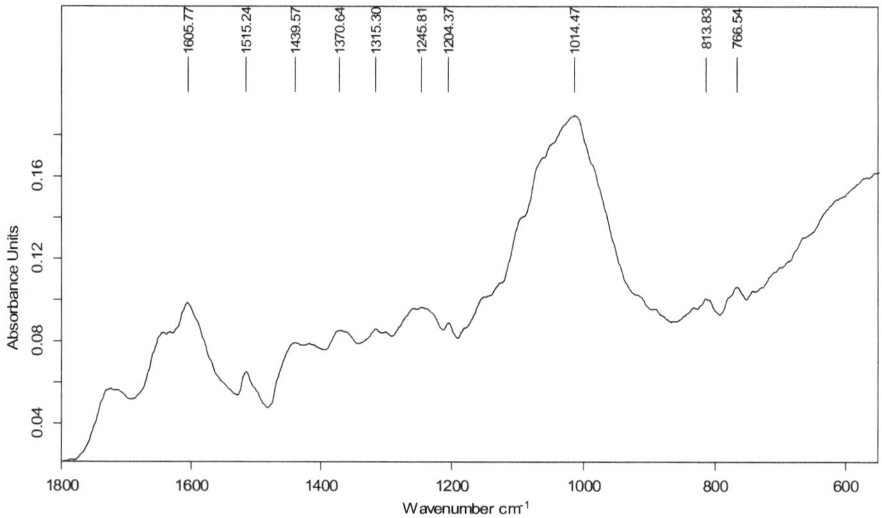

Mid-infrared spectrum of *Agathosma betulina* powder displaying the fingerprint region (1800–550 cm^{-1}).

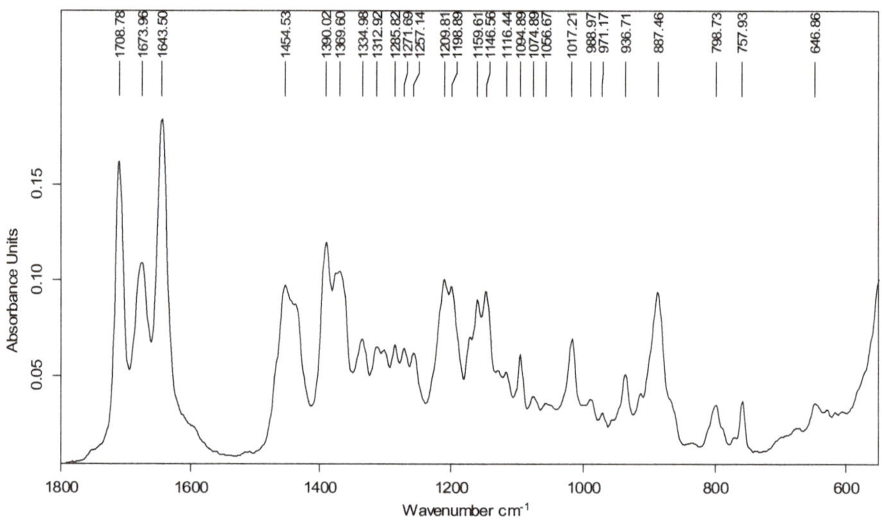

Mid-infrared spectrum of *Agathosma betulina* essential oil displaying the fingerprint region (1800–550 cm^{-1}).

References

British Herbal Medicine Association, 1996. Buchu. In: British Herbal Pharmacopoeia. Biddles Ltd, King's Lynn, UK, pp. 46–47.

British Pharmaceutical Codex, 1963. Pharmaceutical Society of Great Britain. Lund Humphries, London, UK.

Chiguvare, H., 2015. Phytochemical Analyses, Synthesis of Silver Nanoparticles From *Filipendula ulmaria* (L.) Maxim. and *Agathosma betulina* (Berg.) Pillans and Their Bioassays. PhD thesis. University of Fort Hare, Alice, South Africa.

Chiguvare, H., Oyedeji, O.O., Matewu, R., Aremu, O., Oyemitan, I.A., Oyedeji, A.O., Nkeh-Chungag, B.N., Songca, S.P., Mohan, S., Oluwafemi, O.S., 2016. Molecules, 21:774.

Coetzee, C., Jefthas, E., Reinten, E., 1999. Indigenous plant genetic resources of South Africa. In: Janick, J. (Ed.), Perspectives on New Crops and Uses. ASHS Press, Alexandria, Virginia, USA, pp. 160–163.

Collins, N.F., Graven, E.H., Van Beek, T.A., Lelyveld, G.P., 1996. J. Essent. Oil Res., 8:229–235.

Complementary Medicines—UK. Mintel International Group Ltd. April 2003. Medicines Act Leaflet (MAL) 8. A Guide to the Status Under the Medicines Act of Borderline Products for Human Use. Medicines Control Agency, London, UK.

El-Shafae, A.M., El-Domiaty, M.M., 2001. J. Pharm. Biomed. Anal., 26:539–545.

Encyclopedia Titanica, 2003. Cargo Manifest. Available from: http://www.encyclopedia-titanica.org/cargo-manifest.html.

Famewo, E.B., Clarke, A.M., Wiid, I., Ngwane, A., Van Helden, P., Afolayan, A.J., 2017. Afr. Health Sci., 17:780–789.

Fluck, A.A.J., Mitchell, W.M., Perry, H.M., 1961. J. Sci. Food Agric., 12:290–292.

Geetha, R.V., Roy, A., Lakshmi, T., 2012. Int. J. Pharm. Sci. Rev. Res., 14:94–97.

Goldblatt, P., Manning, J.C., 2000. Cape Plants: A Conspectus of the Cape Flora of South Africa. National Botanical Institute of South Africa, Pretoria, South Africa.

Hübsch, Z., Van Zyl, R.L., Cock, I.E., Van Vuuren, S.F., 2014. S. Afr. J. Bot., 93:185–197.

Kaiser, R., Lamparsky, D., Schudel, P., 1975. J. Agric. Food Chem., 23:943–950.

Köpke, T., Schmarr, H.-G., Mosandl, A., 1992. Flavour Fragr. J., 7:205–211.

Lambert, M.I., Burgess, T., Noakes, T.D., 2002. Available from: https://www.buchulife.com/sites/default/files/Research.

Lamparsky, D., Schudel, P., 1971. Tetrahedron Lett., 36:3323–3326.

Latté, K.P., 2010. Phytothérapie, 31:164–170.

Lis-Balchin, M., Hart, S., Simpson, E., 2001. J. Pharm. Pharmacol., 53:579–582.

Low, C.H., 2007. Environ. Hist., 13:333–361.

Lubbe, A., Verpoorte, R., 2011. Ind. Crop. Prod., 34:785–801.

Madzimbamuto, T.F.N., Schwarz, C.E., Knoetze, J.H., 2016. J. Supercrit. Fluids, 107:612–623.

Moolla, A., Van Vuuren, S.F., Van Zyl, R.L., Viljoen, A.M., 2007. S. Afr. J. Bot., 73:88–592.

Moolla, A., Viljoen, A.M., 2008. J. Ethnopharmacol., 119:413–419.

Ntwana, B., Agenbag, G.A., Langenhoven, P., 2013. S. Afr. J. Plant Soil., 30:107–112.

Posthumus, M.A., Van Beek, T.A., Collins, N.F., Graven, E.H., 1996. J. Essent. Oil Res., 8: 223–228.

Sandasi, M., 2008. The Effect of Plant Extracts on Microbial Biofilm Formation and Development. MTech dissertation, Tshwane University of Technology, Pretoria, South Africa.

Simpson, D., 1998. Scott. Med. J., 43:189–191.

Spreeth, A.D., 1976. S. Afr. J. Bot., 42:109–119.
Steenkamp, V., Gouws, M.C., Gulumian, M., Elgorashi, E.E., Van Staden, J., 2006. J. Ethnopharmacol., 103:71–75.
Swerdlow, J.L., 2000. Nature's Medicine: Plants That Heal. National Geographic Society, Washington D.C., USA.
Turpie, J.K., Heydenrych, B.J., Lamberth, S.J., 2003. Biol. Conserv., 112:233–251.
Van Wyk, B.-E., 2011. S. Afr. J. Bot., 77:812–829.
Van Wyk, B.-E., Van Oudtshoorn, B., Gericke, N., 1997. Medicinal Plants of South Africa. Briza Publications, Pretoria, South Africa.
Van Wyk, B.-E., Wink, M., 2004. Medicinal Plants of the World. Briza Publications, Pretoria, South Africa.
Viljoen, A.M., Moolla, A., Van Vuuren, S.F., Van Zyl, R.L., Baser, K.H.C., Demirci, B., Özek, T., 2006. J. Essent. Oil Res., 18:2–16.
Viljoen, A.M., Vermaak, I., Hamman, J., Huang, M., Van Vuuren, S., Du Plessis, J., 2007. S. Afr. J. Bot., 73:319–320.
Vermaak, I., Viljoen, A.M., Hamman, J.H., Van Vuuren, S.F., 2009. S. Afr. J. Bot., 75:594–599.
Watt, J.M., Breyer-Brandwijk, M.G., 1962. The Medicinal and Poisonous Plants of Southern and Eastern Africa, second ed. E. & S. Livingstone Ltd, Edinburgh and London, UK.
Witbooi, H., Okem, A., Makunga, N.P., Kambizi, L., 2017. S. Afr. J. Bot., 111:283–290.

CHAPTER

Aloe ferox

3

Alvaro Viljoen[a,b], Weiyang Chen[a], Nduvho Mulaudzi[a] and Gerda Fouche[c]
[a]*Department of Pharmaceutical Sciences, Tshwane University of Technology, Pretoria, South Africa*
[b]*SAMRC Herbal Drugs Research Unit, Faculty of Science, Tshwane University of Technology, Pretoria, South Africa*
[c]*Chemistry Department, University of Pretoria, Pretoria, South Africa*

Abstract

Aloe ferox Mill. (Asphodelaceae), commonly known as 'Cape aloe', is indigenous to South Africa, occurring in the Free State, Eastern Cape and KwaZulu-Natal provinces. It is an arborescent perennial plant that reaches 2–3 m in height with leaves arranged in a rosette, characterised by bright red or yellow-orange flowers. Cape aloe is well known for its medicinal properties, which clarifies its long history of use to alleviate sinusitis, arthritis, conjunctivitis, sores, open wounds, ulcers, burns, skin conditions and inflammation-related disorders. Aloe ferox is a highly valued plant and has a number of commercial applications in the natural health, pharmaceutical, cosmetic and food industries. Some in vitro and in vivo activities, including laxative, skin and wound-healing, anti-oxidant, anti-inflammatory and anticancer effects, have been extensively investigated. The permeation-enhancing effects of A. ferox were demonstrated in both in vitro and in vivo assays. The leaf comprises two distinct parts, the inner leaf gel that contains polysaccharides and the exudate consisting of chromones and anthrones. Using a semi-automated high-performance thin-layer chromatography (HPTLC) system and ultra-performance liquid chromatography coupled to mass spectrometry (UPLC–MS) in under 3 min, the chemical profiles of A. ferox leaf exudates were obtained. Both HPTLC and UPLC–MS profiles confirmed the presence of marker compounds aloesin, aloeresin A and aloin A and B in all the tested methanol extract samples.

Keywords: *Aloe ferox*, Cape aloe, Leaf gel, Polysaccharides, Chromones, Anthrones, HPTLC, UPLC–MS, MIR spectroscopy

The South African Herbal Pharmacopoeia. https://doi.org/10.1016/B978-0-323-99794-2.00006-4

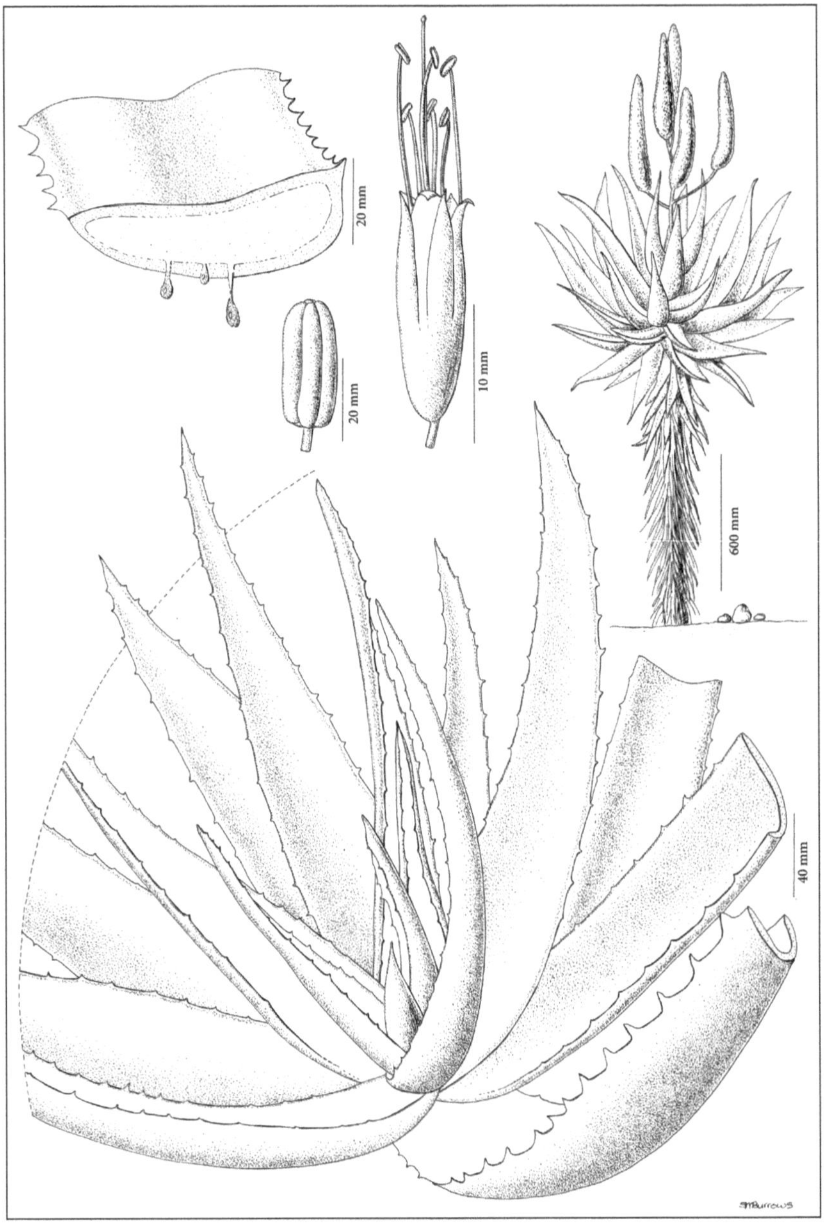
20 mm
20 mm
10 mm
600 mm
40 mm

Part A: General overview

1. Synonyms

Aloe ferox Mill. var. *galpinii* (Baker) Reynolds, *Aloe candelabrum* A.Berger, *A. ferox* Mill. var. *incurva* Baker, *Aloe perfoliata* L. var. *epsilon* L., *Aloe galpinii* Baker, *A. perfoliata* L. var. *theta* (Mill.) Aiton, *A. perfoliata* L. var. *gamma* L., *A. perfoliata* Thunb., *A. perfoliata* L. var. *zeta* Willd., *Aloe subferox* Spreng., *Aloe pseudo-ferox* Salm-Dyck, *Aloe supralaevis* Haw. var. *erythrocarpa* A.Berger, *Aloe supralaevis* Haw., *Pachidendron pseudo-ferox* (Salm-Dyck) Haw., *Pachidendron ferox* (Mill.) Haw., *Pachidendron supralaeve* (Haw.) Haw.[a]

2. Common name(s)

Cape aloe, tap aloe, red aloe, bitter aloe (English), '*bergaalwyn*', '*bitteraalwyn*', '*Kaapse aalwyn*', '*tapaalwyn*' (Afrikaans), '*ikhala*' (isiXhosa), '*inhlaba*' (isiZulu), '*umhlaba*' (Sesotho).[a]

3. Conservation status

Not threatened, least concern.[a]

4. Botany

Aloe ferox Mill., commonly known as 'Cape aloe' is one of approximately 160 *Aloe* species indigenous to South Africa. The species name '*ferox*', which means 'fierce' or 'warlike', refers to the spiny-edged leaves. *Aloe ferox* is an arborescent perennial plant with a robust single stem (2–3 m in height) and is characterised by bright red, yellow–orange or rarely white flowers, crowned by a large rosette of numerous leaves, which are glaucous and oval lanceolate in a spiral arrangement (A) (Van Wyk and Smith, 2014). The old leaves remain after they have dried, forming a 'petticoat' on the stem. The leaves are a dull green, sometimes with a slightly blue appearance. They may also have a reddish tinge. The flowers are carried in a large candelabra-like flower-head (B). There are usually between five and eight branches, each carrying a spikelike head of many flowers. Flowering occurs between May and August, but in colder parts of the country this may be delayed until September. This aloe forms a beautiful display and attracts many bird species, such as sunbirds, weavers, glossy starlings and mousebirds. In natural areas, monkeys and baboons will raid the aloes for nectar. Figure (C) shows the cross-section of the aloe leaf displaying the rind and the inner pulp. The leaves are stacked in a circular arrangement (D) to 'tap' the leaf exudate, which is processed into aloe bitters.

[a] Red List of South African Plants (http://redlist.sanbi.org).

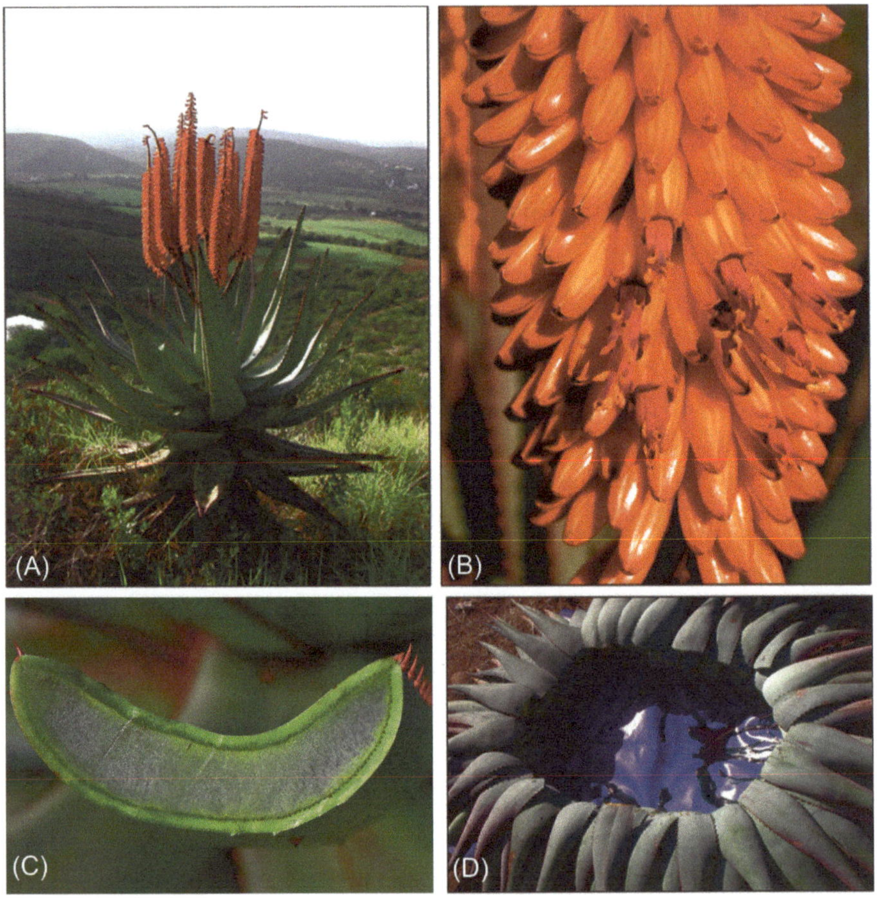

Succulent *Aloe ferox* plant (A) with characteristic bright orange–red flowers (B), a cross-section of aloe leaf (C), and aloe leaves stacked in a circular arrangement (D).

5. Geographical distribution

Although *A. ferox* is not endemic to South Africa, it has a wide distribution range of over 1000 km. It occurs in the Free State, Eastern Cape and KwaZulu-Natal provinces from southern KwaZulu-Natal in the north to Swellendam in the south, and inland to the southern Free State and Lesotho (Raimondo et al., 2012). The plant grows in a large selection of habitats ranging from inaccessible mountain ridges to easily accessible valleys, which ensures the survival of the species in nature, even if agricultural development has decreased its range on cultivated lands (Newton and Vaughan, 1996). It occurs commonly in very large numbers on rocky hill slopes,

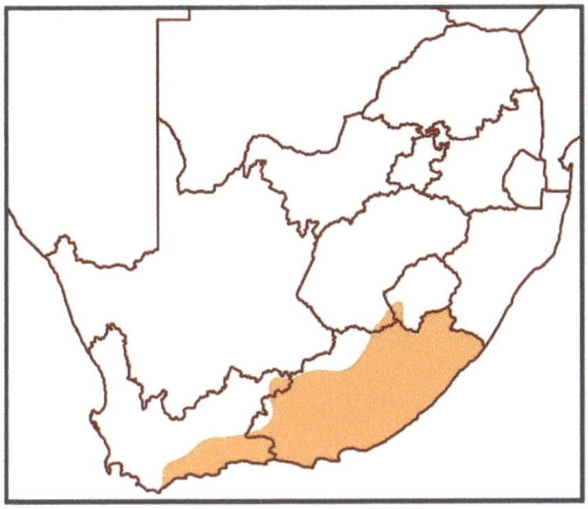

Geographical distribution of *Aloe ferox* in South Africa.

where it displays a stunning winter picture. In the southern and eastern Cape, it is found on the edges of the Karoo and in the southwestern Cape it occurs in grassy fynbos. *Aloe ferox* can be found in both open and bushy areas. Depending on the local climatic conditions, the plants can differ physically from area to area.

6. Ethnopharmacology

Aloe ferox is well-known for its medicinal properties. A number of ethnomedicinal applications of the leaf exudate of *A. ferox* are known in southern Africa, for example, to alleviate sinusitis, arthritis, and conjunctivitis, eye ailments and ophthalmia, by applying the sap of the leaf as eye drops (Chen et al., 2012). The bitter powdered fraction is administered as a dusting powder to open wounds, and to dress venereal ulcers and traditional scarifications (Van Wyk and Gericke, 2000). Powdered Cape aloe is mixed with Vaseline® and applied topically to treat shingles and herpes. Leaf and stem decoctions are used as emetics, and leaf decoctions are applied to venereal sores or gargled for a sore throat (Chen et al., 2012). Crushed or split fresh leaves are administered on sores, open wounds, ulcers and burns in humans, and used in livestock to treat injuries and sores (Van Wyk and Gericke, 2000). The roots and leaves of *A. ferox* are also taken internally to treat dermatitis, eczema and acne. *Aloe ferox* has long been used to treat a number of skin conditions including skin burns, cancer and psoriasis (Van Wyk et al., 2009), as well as for the treatment of inflammation-related injuries (Van Wyk and Gericke, 2000). *Aloe ferox* is also used to treat various infections, such as internal parasites and sexually transmitted infections. In the Eastern Cape Province of South Africa, it is generally used for syphilis and gonorrhoea (Grace et al., 2008). Roots or leaves boiled in water are used to alleviate stress and hypertension, and parts of the plant are applied to the eyes and skin, nose, or ears (Hutchings, 1989). Grace et al. (2008) reported the use of *A. ferox* to treat impotence in men and infertility in women. The sap, mixed with fodder, is used as a purgative for cattle in South Africa (Watt and Breyer-Brandwijk, 1962). Leaf preparations are used for washing hair and are also used as a 'blood purifier' for the treatment of acne, in low doses (Watt and Breyer-Brandwijk, 1962). The bitter yellow juice found just below the skin has been used for a long time in certain parts of South Africa as a renewable resource. Aloe lump, the black, hard, resinous part, is used as a laxative, as well as for the treatment of arthritis. The gel-like flesh from the inside of the leaves is known to have wound-healing properties and is used as an ingredient in cosmetic products. Other traditional uses include the treatment of stomach ailments, diabetes, constipation, as a blood purifier, treatment of retained placenta, for sores and wounds, and as a veterinary medicine (Nortje and Van Wyk, 2015).

7. Commercialisation

Aloe ferox is considered as the first plant exported from South Africa (18th century), since it was well-known by colonists at the Cape of Good Hope as a traditional medicine (Hodge, 1953). Today, it is South Africa's leading wild-harvested commercial plant species (Melin, 2009). Between 1981 and 1994, the total export of *A. ferox* was 4549 tons, based on annual reports, with the largest amount exported to Japan, Germany, Italy and Argentina (Chen et al., 2012). In 1976, the first commercial plantations of *A. ferox* were established by Dr. Muller on Vinklaagte farm in the Western Cape near Albertinia. Currently, aloe is cultivated in different areas of the Western Cape Province, including Albertinia and Uniondale and in the Swellendam region. In the latter region, propagation and cultivation is mainly for the landscaping and nursery markets. Processing of *A. ferox* gel on an industrial scale started with the construction of a factory in the early 1990s in Albertinia. *Aloe ferox* grows abundantly in the Western and Eastern Cape provinces, where historically, processing and harvesting centred in these areas (Melin, 2009). Nearly all of the raw materials are wild-crafted (wild-harvested), although small plantations have been established, mostly to allow irrigation during drought, as well as for ease of harvesting. Bitters from *A. ferox* are used as laxatives in South Africa with an estimated export value of US $1.2 million in 1996 and close to US $2 million in 2008 (Dickson, 2008). Kleinschmidt (2004) documented the health benefits of fortified food products and beverages containing the leaf parenchyma of *A. ferox*, although *A. vera* products available internationally are difficult to compete with. Botha (1994) described a patented process for the production of drinks from aloe polysaccharides. *Aloe ferox*, *A. barbadensis* and some hybrids were approved by the United States Food and Drug Administration (US FDA, 2010) for inclusion in over-the-counter drugs, as a natural flavouring agent in food, and as dietary supplements. Aloe is also listed as a permitted natural source for food flavouring by the Council of Europe. This category means that aloe can be added to foodstuffs; however, it indicates that insufficient information is available for an adequate assessment of potential toxicity (Barnes et al., 2007). Blumenstein-Stahl et al. (2005) filed a patent regarding a food product containing aloe that can be taken as a supplement for the hydration of the skin. In addition, aloe is utilised as the key ingredient in a composition (orally administered) for weight management by reducing appetite (Buchwald-Werner, 2008). Some of the best-selling herbal products in South Africa contain *A. ferox* as an ingredient, for example Schweden-bitter® and LENNON Lewensessens (Van Wyk et al., 2009).

Gel preparations that are commercially available were proven to be effective in improving cases of eczema and for healing certain chronic leg ulcers, as well as for providing significant relief from acute sunburn (Van Wyk and Gericke, 2000). Aloe gel is added to cosmetic products, such as moisturisers, cleansers, shampoos, sunburn screens and suntan lotions. Aloesin in *Aloe* is effective as a pigmentation-altering agent for therapeutic and cosmetic applications (Chen et al., 2012). In addition, *A. ferox* is used as an intestinal permeation-enhancing vehicle for poorly permeable drugs. Historically, the aloe industry was centred in the Albertinia-Gouritz River region, but it expanded some time ago to the Eastern Cape and other regions (Chen et al., 2012). Independent entrepreneurs from rural communities in South Africa are involved in the aloe-tapping industry. The commercialisation of the gel and aloe tapping are indirectly connected as the products are closely linked in terms of processing and manufacturing (Standards South Africa, 2007). South Africa is considered the largest exporter of wild-harvested aloe bitters, in either powdered or crystalline form. An estimated 400 tons of aloe bitters are produced by the harvesting of 10 million plants. Value adding is done mostly at export destinations in the form of producing beverages or cosmetics (Melin, 2009). Botha (1994) reported that the production of aloe drinks from polysaccharides has become the most lucrative and important part of the local aloe-manufacturing industry. *Aloe ferox* is a highly valued plant and has a number of commercial applications in the natural health, pharmaceutical, cosmetic and food industries. Aloe tapping is the livelihood of numerous rural communities, but if this industry is formalised through trade and co-operative agreements, it may have a huge poverty-alleviation effect (Melin, 2009). The cosmetic industry has indicated an interest in *A. ferox* gel. Chen et al. (2012) in their review quote an internet site which states '*a skin care routine without Super Aloe Gel is incomplete*'. According to this website, the gel should be applied all over the body and face to repair the skin, to heal insect bites, cuts, burns and wounds, and to enhance the complexion (Chen et al., 2012). It also indicates that the gel contains at least 130 medicinal agents with analgesic, anti-inflammatory, calming, germicidal, antiseptic, antiviral, antitumour and antiparasitic effects. The website collates numerous scientific studies and traditional uses reported for *A. ferox* and its compounds.

8. Pharmacological evaluation

8.1 *In vitro* studies

8.1.1 Laxative effects

Aloe ferox is known for its potent cathartic and laxative effects, which are ascribed to the presence of anthraquinones and, specifically, aloe emodin (Steenkamp and Stewart, 2007). The anthrone-*C*-glycosides (aloin B and A) should be stable in the acidic medium of the stomach, with the sugar moiety of the molecules blocking absorption within the upper part of the gastrointestinal tract and subsequent detoxification in the liver. This protection in the intestine allows the anthrone-*C*-glycosides to reach the site of action in the rectum and colon. When the molecules reach the large intestine, they act as prodrugs, releasing the aglycones that have a laxative effect through bacterial breakdown (Breimer and Baars, 1976).

8.1.2 Skin and wound-healing effects

Aloe ferox exhibits wound-healing effects and different mechanisms have been suggested, such as increased epithelial cell migration, keeping the wound moist, reduction in inflammation and more rapid maturation of collagen (Reynolds and Dweck, 1999). The key constituents responsible for the wound-healing property have been shown to be mucilaginous polysaccharides within the leaf pulp of aloe. Barrantes and Guinea (2003) reported that *A. ferox* enriched with aloins inhibited metalloprotease and collagenase activities, which can reduce collagen connective tissue. Skin hyperpigmentation originates from the overproduction of epidermal melanin, caused by the action of tyrosinase. It was demonstrated that the compounds arbutin and aloesin inhibited tyrosinase activity in a synergistic manner (Jin et al., 1999). When L-tyrosine was employed as a substrate, the ethanol leaf extracts of *A. ferox*, at a concentration of 500 μg/mL, exhibited 60% inhibition of tyrosinase activity (Mapunya et al., 2012). The whole leaf and gel of *A. ferox* demonstrated better wound-healing activity compared to untreated keratinocytes. Very low toxicity was seen in the 3-[4,5-dimethylthiazole-2-yl]-2,5-diphenyltetrazolium bromide (MTT) assay, indicating that the whole leaf and gel of *A. ferox* exhibited negligible toxicity towards cultured human keratinocyte (HaCaT) cells (Fox et al., 2017).

8.1.3 Anti-oxidant activity

Aloe ferox demonstrated good anti-oxidant activity in both the ferric reducing anti-oxidant power (FRAP) assay, as well as the oxygen radical absorbance capacity (ORAC) assay (Loots et al., 2007). Most of the polyphenols/phenolic acids, alkaloids and indoles identified in *A. ferox* are reported to have anti-oxidant activity and, therefore, contribute to the FRAP and ORAC activities of the extracts of Cape aloe. *Aloe ferox* demonstrated superior anti-oxidant activity when compared to grape seed extracts and green tea (Jones et al., 2002). Frum and Viljoen (2006) demonstrated that the methanol extract of *A. ferox* leaves exhibited significant anti-oxidant activity in the 2,2-diphenyl-1-picrylhydrazyl (DPPH) assay, with an IC_{50} value of 19.11 ± 0.10 mg/L. A patent application was filed by Jia and Farrow (2003) describing the purification and identification of 7-hydroxychromones, which inhibited the production of reactive oxygen species (ROS) and free radical generation, thus treating and preventing ROS-mediated conditions and other diseases associated with oxidative processes. The anti-oxidant properties of the acetone, ethanol, water and methanol extracts of *A. ferox* were determined spectrophotometrically, and the results indicated significant radical scavenging activity of the methanol and ethanol extracts, with lower anti-oxidant activities recorded for the aqueous and acetone extracts (Wintola and Afolayan, 2011). In another study, extracts of *A. ferox* exhibited good anti-oxidant activity when tested in the FRAP and DPPH radical scavenging assays (Thibane et al., 2018).

8.1.4 Anti-inflammatory activity

Aloe ferox possesses anti-inflammatory properties, and inhibited cyclooxygenase-1 (COX-1) activity, when 53 methanolic extracts of different *Aloe* species were screened (Lindsey et al., 2002). Fawole et al. (2010) reported good anti-inflammatory activity (COX-1) for ethanol and dichloromethane leaf extracts, being 96% and 95% inhibition at 0.25 µg/µL, respectively, whilst moderate anti-oxidant activity (DPPH radical scavenging activity) was observed for the 50% aqueous methanol extract (EC_{50} of 10.45 µg/mL). The ethanol extract (95%) exhibited significant anti-inflammatory activity as well as anti-*Propionibacterium acnes* properties, implying that *A. ferox* can be considered a potential source of acne treatment (Jeong and Kim, 2017).

8.1.5 Anticancer activity

A compound isolated from Cape aloe, namely emodin, showed selective activity towards neuro-ectodermal tumours, with no toxicity in normal cells (Pecere et al., 2000). The mechanism of emodin was investigated by Pecere et al. (2003), and specific drug uptake by neuro-ectodermal tumours was demonstrated that resulted in cell death. Koyama et al. (2001) reported the role of emodin in the emergence of cancer and demonstrated the inhibitory effect on the activation of Epstein–Barr virus with a log IC_{50} value of 2.656. Fenig et al. (2004) also demonstrated the combined effect of the chemotherapeutic agent cisplatinol (5-fluorouracil, doxorubicin) and aloe emodin on the proliferation of an adhering variant cell line of Merkel cell carcinoma. The growth-inhibiting effect on Ehrlich ascites tumour cells (EATC) was investigated employing constituents isolated from Cape aloe (Kametani et al., 2007a). Significant effects observed from the experiments suggested synergistic effects of chromone compounds, such as 7-hydroxy-2,5-dimethylchromone and aloe emodin. Decreased retinoblastoma protein phosphorylation was demonstrated to be the mode of action. Due to a 'hypercoagulable state' often observed with cancer patients, medications having both anticoagulant and antithrombotic activity would be beneficial. Kee et al. (2008) demonstrated that the water extract of *A. ferox* exhibited anticoagulant activity and an IC_{50} value of 7.74 mg/mL was obtained in the thrombin-induced clotting time assay.

8.1.6 Antimicrobial activity

The microplate dilution method was used to evaluate the antibacterial activity of chrysophanol, emodin and aloin A, isolated from *A. ferox*. Chrysophanol only displayed activity against *Staphylococcus epidermidis*, *Bacillus subtilis* and *Escherichia coli*, whilst aloin A and emodin exhibited activity against all the test organisms (*B. subtilis, Bacillus cereus, Staphylococcus epidermidis, Staphylococcus aureus, Shigella sonnei* and *E. coli*) (Kambizi et al., 2004). Coopoosamy and Magwa (2006) reported that aloin A and emodin demonstrated antibacterial activity with minimum inhibitory concentration (MIC) values ranging from 250 µg/mL against *Shigella sonnei* and *Staphylococcus epidermidis*, to 62.5 µg/mL against *E. coli* and *B. subtilis*. Antifungal activity of *A. ferox* juice against *Trichophyton* spp., which causes thrush and athlete's foot, was reported (Soeda et al., 1966). The compound, aloin as well as the methanol extract of Cape aloe, yielded MICs of 0.1 and 0.5 mg/mL, respectively, towards *Neisseria gonorrhoeae*, indicating moderate activity. Aloin showed poor activity (MIC 5 mg/mL) against *Candida albicans*, whilst the methanol extract was inactive (MIC 20 mg/mL) (Kambizi and Afolayan, 2008). Afolayan et al. (2002) reported fungicidal activity for the acetone extract of *A. ferox* (10 mg/mL) against five fungi using the agar dilution method. *Aloe ferox* is topically applied to sores caused by viral infections, such as herpes, warts and shingles (Van Wyk and Gericke, 2000). *In vitro* antiviral activity was reported by Kambizi et al. (2007) using *A. ferox* against herpes simplex virus type 1 (HSV-1). Activity at a concentration of 1 mg/mL was demonstrated for water extracts with no cytotoxic effects. Zapata et al. (2013) proved that aloin is one of the key components of Cape aloe linked to its antifungal activity, and experiments show that *A. ferox* affects the growth of artificially inoculated fungi on the leaves. Another study (Ghuman et al., 2016) in KwaZulu-Natal Province, South Africa, investigated the phenolic content, antimicrobial efficacies and cytotoxic effects of 11 plant extracts commonly used in traditional medicine for wound-healing and treating skin conditions. *Aloe ferox* was one of three extracts that exhibited significant activity against most of the fungal and bacterial strains tested. No cytotoxicity was observed. The extract contained high levels of flavonoids, total phenolics and tannins.

8.1.7 Antimalarial activity

Thirty-four *Aloe* species and their major constituents were examined for their antiplasmodial activity by Van Zyl and Viljoen (2002), using the titrated [^{3}H]-hypoxanthine incorporation assay. It was reported that a number of methanol extracts reduced *Plasmodium falciparum* growth by 50% at concentrations ranging from 32 to 77 µg/mL. *In vitro* screening of 134 plant species for their activities towards the *P. falciparum* strain D10, using the parasite lactate dehydrogenase (pLDH) assay, was conducted by Clarkson et al. (2004). The water extracts did not exhibit activity, but the organic extract (methanol:dichloromethane (1:1)) of *A. ferox* revealed good antiplasmodial activity (IC_{50} = 8 µg/mL).

8.1.8 Permeation-enhancing effect

Kai et al. (2002) investigated the effect of emodin anthrone on poorly permeable and water-soluble compounds, for example 5(6)-carboxyfluorescein (CF), in rat colonic mucosa, using an Ussing-type chamber. Aloin B and A can be converted into emodin under aerobic conditions, and into emodin anthrone under anaerobic conditions, through an enzymatic redox reaction involving rat intestinal microflora. Emodin anthrone significantly increased the permeation of CF in a dose-dependent manner. The enhanced permeability was significantly suppressed by pyrilamine, a histamine H1 receptor antagonist, ketotifen, a mast cell stabiliser and an inhibitor of protein kinase, but not by cimetidine, a histamine H2 receptor antagonist. The electrical resistance of the membrane was reduced to 30% by emodin anthrone, but the lactate dehydrogenase activity was not significantly different from that of the control. The mechanism proposed for the enhancement of permeation was that aloe emodin anthrone stimulated mast cells within the colonic mucosa with the release of histamine that binds to the H1 receptor. H1 receptor activation activated the intracellular protein kinase C route with enhanced permeability of poorly permeable and water-soluble drugs *via* opening of tight junctions in the rat colonic membrane (Kai et al., 2002). The effects of gel and leaf material from *Aloe* species (*A. ferox* and *A. vera*) were compared with that of the precipitated polysaccharides derived from these materials, on the transepithelial electrical resistance (TEER), as well as on the transport of atenolol, a model compound in the apical-to-basolateral direction across rat intestinal tissue. All the materials tested caused a significant reduction in the TEER compared to the control group, indicating their ability to open tight junctions between adjacent epithelial cells (Beneke et al., 2012).

8.1.9 Other activities

The water extract of *A. ferox* was examined for *in vitro* anthelmintic activity on the larvae and eggs of the nematode parasite, *Haemonchus contortus*. The extracts caused total inhibition of larval development at 2.5 mg/mL, and egg hatch inhibition at 20 mg/mL (Maphosa et al., 2010). The dichloromethane leaf extract of *A. ferox* affected 98% mosquito mortality and can possibly be used as an insecticide against *Anopheles arabiensis* (Mavundza et al., 2014). When subjected to a dose-dependent bioassay, the extract yielded an EC_{50} of 4.92 mg/mL.

8.2 *In vivo* studies and clinical trials

8.2.1 Laxative effects

Izzo et al. (1999) investigated the effect of nitric oxide (NO) on aloe-induced diarrhoea in a rat model. The data indicated that aloe inhibited the basal calcium-dependent NO synthesis activity with reduction of diarrhoeal effects. Wintola et al. (2010) examined the toxicological effect of the water extract of *A. ferox* in loperamide-induced constipated rats. The data revealed that *A. ferox* can be considered safe as an oral remedy to relieve constipation. A patent, filed in 2004, described a suppository to be used as a laxative, containing aloe bitters. Zolotariov and Zolotariov (2004) stated in the patent that it may be used for the treatment of bacterial infections and haemorrhoids of the anus, as an anti-allergic agent, anti-inflammatory agent, and as a wound-healing promoter. Aloe fibres have been shown to be a regulator of lower bowel function, together with kaolin and/or bentonite in a patent application for the treatment of irritable bowel syndrome (IBS). The leaves cut by aloe tappers (from which the bitter sap has been drained) are used to produce an aloe powder. The leaves are sliced thinly and the remaining bitter sap removed, before they are sun-dried, and then milled into a so-called whole-leaf powder. The powder is used in a formulation in a ratio of 70%–30%, with kaolin/bentonite constituting the balance, and finally formulated into tablets or granules. This formulation has been recommended for use in end-stage AIDS patients with chronic diarrhoea, in addition to IBS treatment (Taylor, 2003).

8.2.2 Skin, wound-healing and antidiabetic effects

A mouse model of atopic dermatitis (AD) was employed to compare the activities of topically applied gel extracts of *A. vera* to that of *A. ferox* (Finberg et al., 2015). Both *Aloe* species inhibited serum IgE levels and the cutaneous inflammatory response in the rats, but the extract of *A. ferox* was superior to that of *A. vera* in reducing IgE levels. It can therefore be concluded from the results that the gel of *A. ferox*, applied topically, is a proven safe alternative to topical corticosteroids and antihistamines for the treatment of patients suffering from recurring chronic AD. A patent application comprising Cape aloe gel and benzoyl peroxide demonstrated the positive effects of the gel on the irritation caused by the application of benzoyl peroxide. It was shown that the blend can reduce skin irritation, thereby enabling the use of higher concentrations of benzoyl peroxide (20%) with superior clinical efficacy and limited side effects (Gruber, 1986). Results from a rat study demonstrated that emodin promoted the repair of excisional wounds *via* the stimulation of tissue regeneration (Tang et al., 2007). Farkas (1963) described, with reference to a patient, the healing properties of topically applied polyuronide derived from *A. ferox* in the treatment of burns and open wounds. It detoxified the damaged surface area, and showed anaesthetic and analgesic activities, with the formation of new tissue (granulation) that filled the wound (Farkas, 1963). The leaf juice of *A. ferox* was evaluated for skin repair and wound-healing using an animal model with additional safety evaluation. The data revealed that the aloe juice improved wound closure and inhibited microbial growth selectively. No side effects or any dermal toxicity were seen during the experiments (Jia et al., 2008). Choi et al. (2002) demonstrated that aloesin inhibited hyperpigmentation in human skin after ultraviolet (UV) radiation, in a dose-dependent manner, and that co-treatment with arbutin and aloesin indicated an additive effect. Aloesin is included in a patent application focusing on cosmetic formulation and/or a Cape aloe extract containing at least 40% aloesin, to be applied as a sunscreen to the hair or skin. Aloesin effectively protects against solar radiation, as it absorbs light, specifically in the ultraviolet B (UVB) region, with an absorption peak at 296 nm (Grollier et al., 1987). In an antihyperpigmentation formulation, a higher concentration of aloesin should be beneficial. A patent was filed by Steenkamp et al. (2008) describing the hydrolytic conversion of aloeresin A to aloesin, which can be used to increase the levels of aloesin from the sap *via* extraction. The commercial application and value of the aloe bitters or sap is therefore extended (Steenkamp et al., 2008).

Antidiabetic effects of extracts of aloe have been investigated and reported by a number of researchers, incorporating both human and animal models. Aloe juices, extracts or compounds have been shown to be linked to a reduction in insulin resistance (Pérez et al., 2007), reduced hyperglycaemia and adipogenesis in mice (Kong et al., 2010), improved glucose tolerance in type II diabetes rodent models (Kim et al., 2009), decreased glycated haemoglobin in patients with metabolic syndrome/prediabetes (Devaraj et al., 2008), as well as reversal of obesity in rats (Sibuyi et al., 2007). The compound aloesin from *A. ferox* is considered to be one of the active ingredients with regard to the antidiabetic effect of *Aloe* (Devaraj et al., 2008). Some data indicated that aloesin is poorly absorbed in the gastrointestinal tract of rats (Park et al., 2009), but that the compound may possibly be degraded by microflora in the gut to produce the aglycone, although no enzyme or intestinal organism in the human was identified to be responsible for the cleavage (Che et al., 1991). A 90-day study with aloesin showed no side effects at a high dose of 1000 mg/kg body weight per day. Urinary ketones were detected in the urine of aloesin-treated animals, as a result of the near-quantitative excretion of the parent compound, which contained ketone moieties (Lynch et al., 2011). This finding was not due to endogenously produced ketones, which would demonstrate a ketogenic state. The no-observed-adverse-effect level (NOAEL) was calculated as 1000 mg/kg body weight per day. Another study investigated the antidiabetic activity of ethanol extracts of the leaf gel of *A. ferox* in a streptozotocin (STZ)-induced type II diabetes rat model (Loots et al., 2011). *Aloe ferox* demonstrated a moderate increase in serum insulin, together with slight corrections in high-density lipoprotein-cholesterol (HDL-C) and alkaline phosphatase (ALP), without any changes to the values of end-point plasma glucose.

8.2.3 Anti-inflammatory activity

Speranza et al. (2005) reported *in vivo* reduction (39%) of an oedematous response induced by croton oil in the mouse ear for the compound aloeresin I (1 μmol/cm^2) isolated from *A. ferox*. This potency is comparable to that of aloesin, but higher than that of indomethacin and aloeresin H (0.3 μmol/cm^2) (Speranza et al., 2005). Mwale and Masika (2014) investigated the anti-inflammatory activity of the water extract of *A. ferox* (whole leaf) and at doses of 400 mg/kg, the extract demonstrated analgesic and anti-inflammatory effects. Formaldehyde- and carrageenan-induced rat-paw oedema was inhibited by 89.3% and 78.2%, respectively. The analgesic activity was 88.2% in the acetic acid test and 67.3% and 57.1% in phase 2 and 1 of the formalin test, respectively. *Aloe ferox* and constituents isolated from the extracts are included in a medicinal patent formulation for the treatment of a number of diseases such as minor wounds, arthritis and sport injuries, due to topical counter-irritant and analgesic properties (Squires, 2010).

8.2.4 Antimicrobial activity

Zolotariov and Zolotariov (2004) filed a patent application for the topical anti-inflammatory and antibacterial properties of Cape aloe embodied in a laxative suppository preparation for use against bacterial infections and haemorrhoids of the anus. Aloe compounds and extracts are also part of a multicomponent preparation for treatment oral mucositis with anti-inflammatory action on mouth ulcers, as well as antibacterial effects against wound-infecting bacteria (Sekharam and Sekharam, 2007).

8.2.5 Permeation-enhancing effects

Several patent applications have been filed for *Aloe* compositions with penetration-enhancing effects. Meyer et al. (2007) described the transdermal delivery of an opioid analgesic in one patent application, and in another, Fischer et al. (2003) demonstrated the topical application of a local anaesthetic. In both applications, the *Aloe* composition included any of several *Aloe* species, including *A. ferox*, that can be formulated into a transdermal permeation-enhancing agent.

8.2.6 Other activities

Constipation is the most common gastrointestinal complaint all over the world, and this is a risk factor for colorectal cancer. An *in vivo* study in Wistar rats evaluated the efficacy of an aqueous leaf extract of *A. ferox* to combat loperamide-induced constipation (Wintola et al., 2010). The extract resulted in increased faecal volume, improved intestinal motility, and normalisation of the body weight of the rats, indicative of the laxative activity of Cape aloe, with the 200 mg/kg body weight of the extract showing the best effect. In another study (Mwale and Masika, 2014), the anthelmintic efficacy of *A. ferox* in village chickens was investigated. Extracts of *A. ferox* (200 mg/kg) were fed to chickens infected with *Heterakis gallinarum*. The results revealed a worm count reduction of 85%, indicating good efficacy.

8.3 Safety

A number of single-case reports noted hypersensitivity and allergic conditions related to the use of aloe preparations (Ernst, 2000). Wang et al. (2003) showed that a 2-*O*′-*p*-coumaroyl derivative and 8-*C*-D-glucopyranosyl-7-hydroxy-5-methylchromone-2-carboxylic acid, which are structurally related to aloeresin A and aloesin present in *Aloe*, caused severe vomiting in a South African patient who had administered the remedy to ‘clean’ his stomach. These compounds may be the result of oxidative degradation during the preparation of the tea from an *Aloe* species, or may even occur during its storage. Another case involved a 47-year-old man from Soweto, South Africa, that developed liver dysfunction and acute oliguric renal failure after ingestion of a herbal remedy containing Cape aloe (Luyckx et al., 2002). A 28-year-old Turkish man also reported multiorgan toxicity after ingestion of a mixture of herbs, containing *Rosmarinus officinalis*, *Pimpinella anisum*, *Matricaria chamomilla*, *A. ferox* and Swedish syrup. The man presented with a sore throat, dyspnoea, vomiting, nausea, leg muscle cramps and fatigue, within 30 min after ingestion. Clinical tests showed acute renal failure due to acute hepatitis-like hepatotoxicity, rhabdomyolysis, angio-oedema and cardiotoxicity (Berrin et al., 2006). A report by Andersen (2007) indicated no ocular and acute dermal toxicity of an *A. ferox* leaf extract tested in New Zealand white rabbits. Some studies revealed that the mechanism of aloe-induced toxicity, and thus the key compounds responsible for the toxicity, are apoptosis-inducing anthraquinones, such as aloin and aloe emodin. These constituents are present in the outer leaf and sap of the plant and not in the inner gel of the aloes (Eshun and He, 2004). Lee et al. (2006) demonstrated that aloe emodin-induced apoptosis, through a P53-dependent pathway, altered the cell cycle, and involved affected mitochondria and ROS. Aloin has also been proven to change the cell cycle at the M phase, and to cause apoptosis *via* inhibition of the cell cycle through down-regulation of cyclin B1 (Esmat et al., 2006). Aloin also induced dose-dependent apoptosis through the mitochondria in Jurkat cells (Buenz, 2008). Mello et al. (2008) researched possible toxicological properties of a formulation containing *Rheum palmatum*, *Gentiana lutea*, *A. ferox*, *Atropa belladona*, *Cynara scolymus*, *Baccharis trimera* and *Paumus boldus*, when administered orally to New Zealand rabbits. The data revealed that this formulation could be considered relatively innocuous. The toxicological properties of a water extract of the leaves of *A. ferox* were assessed at 50, 100 and 200 mg/kg body weight over a period of 7 days, for kidney and liver function indices, as well as haematological parameters in loperamide-induced constipated rats. The extract did not significantly affect kidney function indices and the liver and kidney body weight ratio, as well as serum levels of uric acid, creatinine, urea, and potassium and calcium ions, at any of the dosages tested. The haematological analysis data also indicated that the extracts had no significant effect on the haematological parameters. The results of the study infer that *A. ferox* may be safe when administered orally for constipation. In general, the extract compared favourably with that of a recommended drug, Senokot®, for the treatment of constipation (Wintola et al., 2011). Celestino et al. (2013) reported that *A. ferox* has laxative properties, with no toxicity observed, as the LD_{50} could not be calculated in the experiments, and is possibly higher than 5.0 g/kg.

9. Phytochemistry

9.1 Volatile constituents

Magwa et al. (2006) investigated the chemical composition of the volatile oil of *A. ferox* obtained by prolonged hydro-distillation, and subsequent gas chromatography coupled to mass spectrometry (GC–MS) analysis. Twenty-one compounds were reported in total, with the key constituents identified as 3-cyclohexane-1-heptanol (7.3%), 3,6-octatriene (23.9%), 1,3-cyclopentadiene (4.1%), bornylene (5.2%) and 5-methyl-3-heptanol (3.9%).

9.2 Non-volatile constituents

9.2.1 Chromones

Almost all of the chromones isolated from *A. ferox* are derivatives of 8-*C*-glucosyl-7-hydroxy-5-methyl-2-propyl-4-chromone. The differences in structure depend on methylation of the hydroxyl group at the C_7 position, the degree of oxidation in the propyl sidechain, and esterification of the glucose moiety (Reynolds, 2004). Furoaloesone was identified as a chromone derivative in which the 7-hydroxyl group is cyclised into a furan ring at position C_8 of the chromone ring. Speranza et al. (1993a) reported a 7-hydroxy-5-methyl-chromone with a methyl group on the C_2 position. Haynes et al. (1970) reported the compound, aloesin, for the first time. This chromone is regarded as the parent compound of the aloe chromones and is widespread throughout the genus. Speranza et al. (1988) identified isoaloeresin A, a 2′-*p*-coumaric acid ester of aloesin, as a minor component of Cape aloe. Speranza et al. (2005) also identified aloeresin D (7-methyl-ether, 2″-*O*-(4-hydroxy-*E*-cinnamoyl)), aloeresin C (2′-*p*-coumaroyl-7-glucosylaloesin), 2-acetonyl-7-hydroxy-8-(3-hydroxyacetonyl)-5-methylchromone, 8-acetyl-1,2-dihydro-6,9-dihydroxy-1-(4-hydroxyphenyl)-7-methyl-3H-naphtho[2,1-*b*]pyran-3-one, aloeresin I (2″-*O*-(4-hydroxy-*E*-cinnamoyl)) and 2-acetonyl-8-(2-furoylmethyl)-7-hydroxy-5-methylchromone from Cape aloe. Manitto et al. (2003) isolated a novel constituent, aloeresin H, from the leaves of *A. ferox*. Aloeresin H is considered to be the first C,C-diglucoside identified in commercial samples of *Aloe*, and its polyketide origin can be demonstrated as a two-chain condensation.

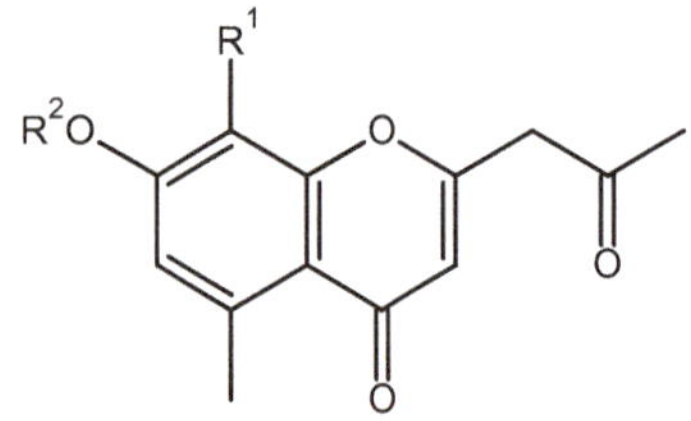

Aloeresin A: R^2 = H; R^1 =

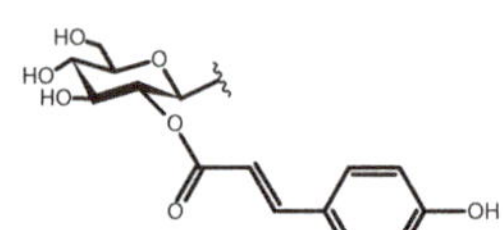

Aloesin: R^2 = H; R^1 =

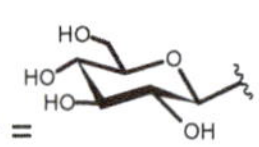

9.2.2 Anthraquinones and anthrones

Two types of anthraquinones (aloesaponarin I-type and chrysophanol-type) were demonstrated to be present in the roots of *A. ferox*. The chrysophanol-type anthraquinones were found to occur both in roots and in leaves, whilst the aloesaponarin I-type were present only in the roots. Van Wyk et al. (1995b) investigated root samples of *Aloe* species (172 in total) and demonstrated that constituents isolated from the roots were very different to those isolated from the leaves of the plant. Preanthraquinones and anthraquinones detected in the roots have chemotaxonomic significance in the genus *Aloe*. Research indicated that these compounds are derived through two parallel routes of the polyketide pathway, resulting in 1,8-dihydroxy- and 1-methyl-8-hydroxyanthraquinones (Dagne et al., 1994). Koyama et al. (1994) used paper chromatography to isolate aloe emodin from

A. ferox. Deoxyerythrolaccin, a 6-hydroxy derivative of aloesaponarin II, has been isolated and identified from *A. ferox* (Koyama et al., 1994). Ultra-high-performance liquid chromatography coupled to mass spectrometry (UHPLC–MS) was employed as an accurate, ultrafast and sensitive method for the quantification of anthrones (aloin B and A) and chromones (aloesin and aloeresin A) in *A. ferox* exudates (101 samples; Kanama et al., 2015). Four chemical markers were determined and the quantitative results revealed high levels of aloesin (111.8–561.8 μg/mg) and aloeresin A (129.0–371.6 μg/mg), but low levels of aloin B (18.4–149.7 μg/mg) and aloin A (21.3–133.4 μg/mg).

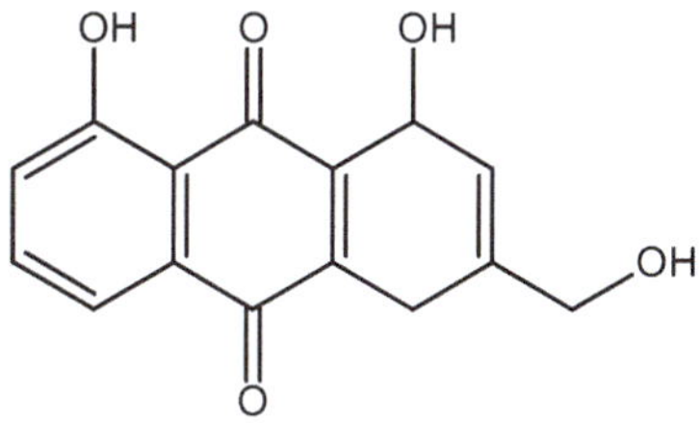

Aloe-emodin

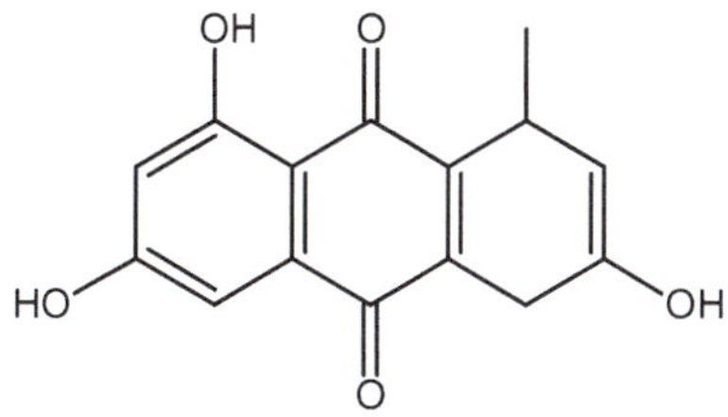

Deoxyerythrolaccin

9.2.3 Anthrone-C-glycosides

Two main parts can be distinguished in aloe leaf, namely an inner clear pulp and an outer green rind. Within the green rind, aloe bitters are found in the aloin cells (canals) situated adjacent to the vascular bundles. The major compounds detected in fresh aloe bitters are aloesin, aloeresin A and aloin, representing 70%–97% of total dry weight, in a ratio of approximately 3:4:2, respectively (Van Wyk et al., 2009). The inner clear pulp contains the slightly viscous gel, which is usually used for moisturising effects and as an emollient, with major constituents fructose, glucose, quinic acid and malic acid (Chen et al., 2012). Aloe bitters contain anthrone-*C*-glycosides, usually represented by aloin B and A, together known as barbaloin or aloin. These anthrone-*C*-glycosides are mostly responsible for the purgative and bitter properties (Dagne et al., 2000). The content of aloe bitters can vary and some reports indicate up to 10% barbaloin/aloin, but Van Wyk et al. (1995a) determined levels ranging between 10% and 30% in natural populations, with around 20% in good-quality commercial products. The compound, 5-hydroxyaloin A, is typical of *A. ferox* (Rauwald and Beil, 1993). Aloinosides B and A, two stereo-isomeric 15-*O*-rhamnosides of aloin, have been reported from *A. ferox* (Rauwald, 1990). Gao et al. (2004) determined that aloinoside B can be metabolised to isobarbaloin, barbaloin/aloin and a hydroxyl metabolite by rat intestinal bacteria. Eight compounds from the extract of *A. ferox* were separated using high-performance countercurrent chromatography (HPCCC). Aloeresin C, aloesin, aloeresin A, aloin B, 5-hydroxyaloin, aloin A, aloinoside B and aloinoside A were isolated employing the solvent system *n*-butanol: ethyl acetate: water (1.5:3.5:5, v/v/v) (Adhami and Viljoen, 2015).

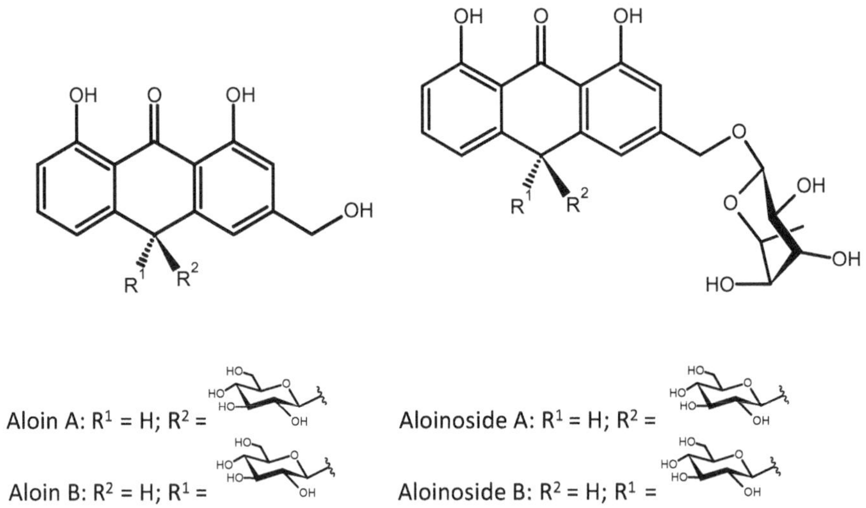

9.2.4 Other phenolic compounds

Methyl-*p*-coumarate was isolated from Cape aloe by Graf and Alexa (1982). Speranza et al. (1993b) isolated feralolide, a minor dimer constituent, from *A. ferox*, consisting of 6,8-dihydroxy-isocoumarin and 2,4-dihydroxyacetophenone joined by a methylene bridge (Speranza et al., 1993b). In addition, three derivatives of 5,6,7,8-tetrahydro-anthracene, identified as 1-methyltetralins, were isolated from *A. ferox*. Various other compounds based on the tetralin and naphthalene nuclei have been identified from Cape aloe. Speranza et al. (1991) first isolated and identified feroxidin as 3,6,8-trihydroxy1-methyltetralin (1,3,6-trihydroxy-8-methyl-5,6,7,8-tetrahydroanthracene) with a 6S,8S configuration, and thereafter feroxin B and feroxin A were reported (Speranza et al., 1992). Three naphtha [2,3-*c*] furans with structural similarity to a reduced iso-eleutherol were also reported from Cape aloe (Koyama et al., 1994). Kametani et al. (2007a,b) identified a number of compounds from the dichloromethane extract of *A. ferox*, including *p*-hydroxybenzaldehyde, aloe emodin, *p*-hydroxyacetophenone, 10-oxo-octadecanoic acid, pyrocatechol, methyl 10-hydroxyoctadecanoate, 10-hydroxyoctadecanoic acid, furoaloesone 7-hydroxy-2,5-dimethyl-chromone and 2-acetonyl-8-(2-furoylmethyl)-7-hydroxy-5-methyl-chromone. Since the traditional preparation of Cape aloe requires a long process involving several hours of boiling of the exudate over an open fire to evaporate the water and to solidify the extract, some of the compounds occurring in Cape aloe may be artefacts or process compounds (Dagne et al., 2000).

9.2.5 Miscellaneous compounds

The polysaccharide composition of *A. ferox* gel remains poorly explored, but differs markedly from that of *A. vera*. Mabusela et al. (1990) reported 14 distinct polysaccharide structures from the gel of *A. ferox*, mainly composed of rhamnogalacturonans or arabinogalactans. Nitrogen analysis of the extracts of the leaves indicated that the amino acid asparagine was the major constituent, together with alanine, glutamine and histidine (Ishikawa et al., 1987). Polysaccharides were identified from the skin juice, gel juice and flowers of *A. ferox*. Analysis revealed that skin juice contained 15 times the amount of polysaccharides than gel juice, therefore having possible industrial application as a source of polysaccharides. Further analysis of the fractions revealed the presence of key constituents, glucose, galactose and mannose, but the acidic flower polysaccharides also contained the two monosaccharides, xylose and rhamnose, with neutral skin juice polysaccharides containing glucose as the only monosaccharide. Chang et al. (2013) reported galacturonic acid as the only uronic acid detected in all acidic polysaccharides from different tissues. O'Brien et al. (2011) investigated the gel yields, leaf dimensions and gel compositions from samples obtained from different natural populations. The only free sugar detected in the gel from *A. ferox* was shown to be glucose, at concentrations of 0.1–0.4 mg/mL. Gel fingerprinting of monosaccharides, released after hydrolysis, can be employed to distinguish between *A. vera* and *A. ferox*. The former yielded only mannose, whilst the latter contained different combinations of galactose and glucose as key monosaccharides. The climatic conditions and the age of the plant affected the levels of flavonoids and polysaccharides (Hu et al., 2003).

Part B: Chemical profiling and quality control

10. Chromatography analysis

10.1 High-performance thin-layer chromatography (HPTLC) fingerprint analysis

General instrumentation: CAMAG HPTLC instrument consisting of an automatic TLC sampler (ATS 4), automatic developing chamber (ADC 2), CAMAG TLC Visualiser 2, CAMAG derivatiser and TLC plate heater. *HPTLC plates*: Silica gel glass plates 60 F_{254} (Merck). *Plant part*: Leaf exudate, methanol extract. *Sample application*: Application volume of 2 μL methanol extract (10 mg/mL) and standards

(1 mg/mL) spotted as 10 mm bands. Plates developed in a 20×10×4 cm glass twin-trough chamber to a migration distance of 70 mm. *Tank saturation*: 20 min at 15 °C and 45% RH, with 25 mL of mobile phase. *Mobile phase*: Ethyl acetate: acetonitrile: formic acid (6:2:1 v/v/v). *Derivatisation*: Potassium hydroxide in 96% methanol. The plate was sprayed with 3 mL of the reagent and heated for 3 min at 100 °C on a TLC plate heater, and visualised. *Visualisation*: The plate was viewed under 366 nm fluorescent light.

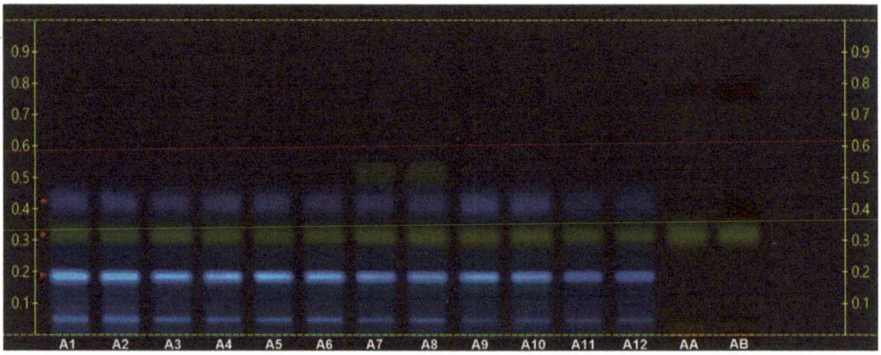

HPTLC plate of *Aloe ferox* leaf exudate from various localities (A1–12) and the standards aloin A (AA) and aloin B (AB). The samples are characterised by a blue band for aloesin (R_f=0.19), yellow bands for aloin A (R_f=0.32) and aloin B (R_f=0.32), and a strong blue band for aloeresin (R_f=0.42).

10.2 Ultra-performance liquid chromatography (UPLC) analysis

General instrumentation: Waters Acquity Ultra-Performance Liquid Chromatography system, with a photodiode array (PDA) detector, and combined with a Xevo G2QToF mass spectrometer (Waters, United States). *Plant part*: Leaf exudate, methanol extract. *Sample application*: Injection volume: 1.0 µL (full-loop injection) at 1 mg/mL. *Column*: Acquity UPLC BEH C_{18} column (50 mm×2.1 mm, i.d., 1.7 µm particle size, Waters). *Mobile phase*: 0.1% formic acid in water (solvent A) and acetonitrile (solvent B). *Analysis conditions*: Gradient elution at flow rate: 0.6 mL/min, changing as follows: 90% A: 10% B, change to 32% B in 2.5 min, returning to the initial ratio in 0.5 min, equilibrating the system for 1 min, total run time 4 min. *Mass spectrometry*: ESI^- (negative ionisation mode), N_2 used as desolvation gas, desolvation temperature 350 °C at a flow rate of 500 L/h and source temperature at 100 °C. Capillary and cone voltages, 2500 and 45 V, respectively. Data collected between *m/z* 100 and 1000.

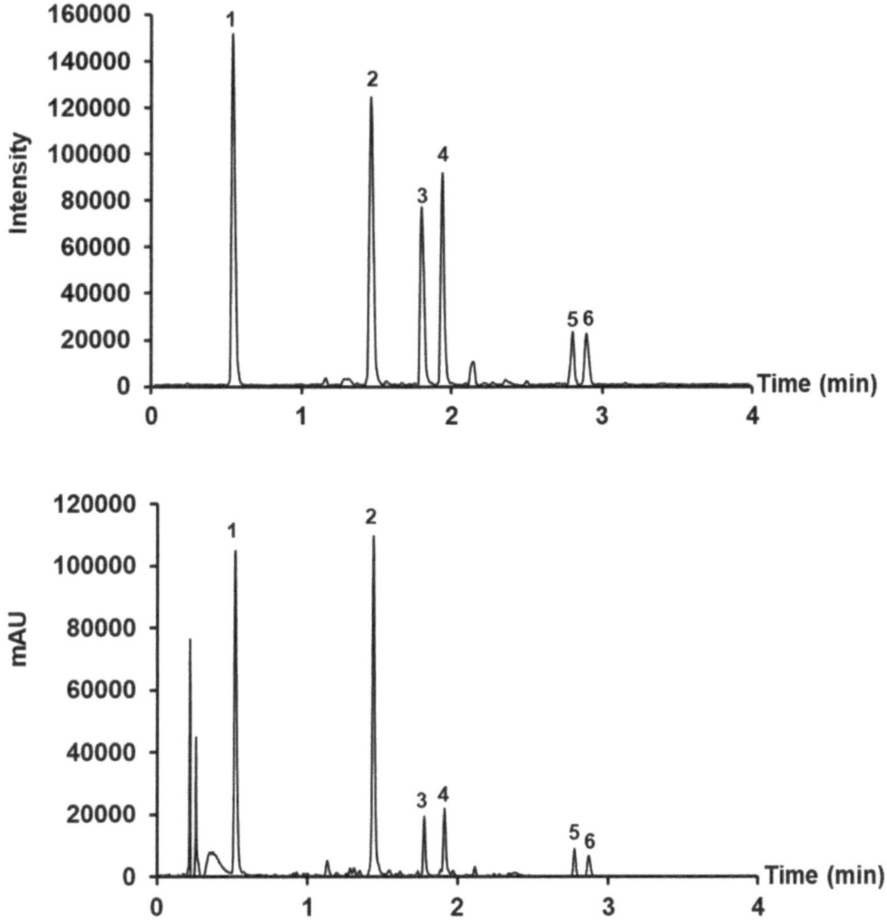

UPLC–ToF–MS ESI$^-$ (upper) and PDA (lower) chromatograms of *A. ferox* methanol extract. [1] = aloesin *m/z* 393.1178, [2] = aloeresin A *m/z* 539.1555, [3] = aloin B *m/z* 417.1176, [4] = aloin A *m/z* 417.1174, [5] = aloinoside B *m/z* 563.1532, [6] = aloinoside A *m/z* 563.1519.

11. Mid-infrared (MIR) spectroscopy analysis

General instrumentation: Alpha-P Bruker spectrometer mounted with an attenuated total reflectance (ATR) diamond crystal. *Spectral acquisition*: Spectrum obtained in the absorbance mode, with a spectral resolution of 4 cm^{-1} over the range 4000–550 cm^{-1} and captured using OPUS 6.5 software. *Plant part*: Leaf exudate powder. *Sample preparation*: Leaf exudate dried, powdered, sieved (< 500 µm), and placed directly onto the surface of the diamond crystal.

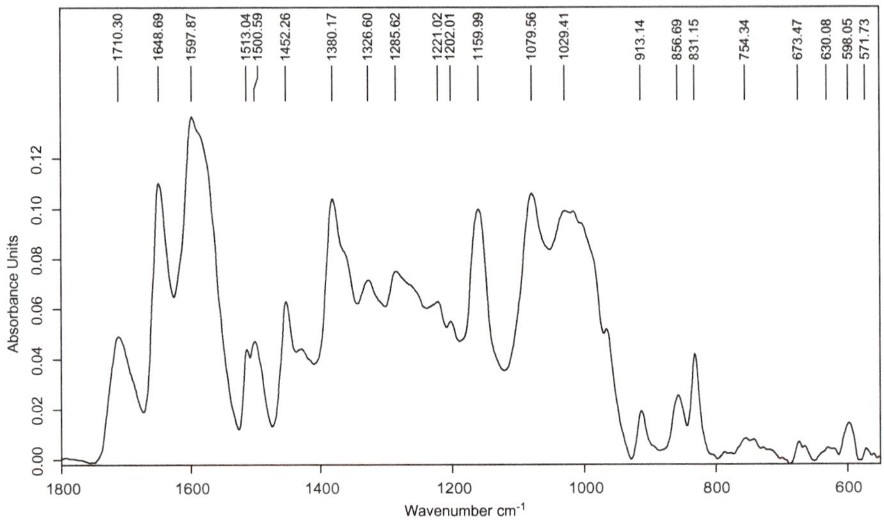

Mid-infrared spectrum of powdered *Aloe ferox* exudate displaying the fingerprint region (1800–550 cm^{-1}).

References

Adhami, H.R., Viljoen, A.M., 2015. Phytochem. Lett., 11:321–325.

Afolayan, A.J., Grierson, D.S., Kambizi, L., Madamombe, I., Masika, P.J., 2002. S. Afr. J. Bot., 68:72–76.

Andersen, F.A., 2007. Int. J. Toxicol., 26:1–50.

Barnes, J., Anderson, A.L., Phillipson, J.D., 2007. Herbal Medicines, third ed. Pharmaceutical Press, Grayslake, Illinois, USA.

Barrantes, E., Guinea, M., 2003. Life Sci., 72:843–850.

Beneke, C., Viljoen, A., Hamman, J., 2012. Sci. Pharm., 80:475–486.

Berrin, Y., Ali, O., Umut, S., Meltem, E., Murat, B., Barut, Y., 2006. Eur. J. Intern. Med., 17:130–132.

Blumenstein-Stahl, G., Podbielski, U., Fishcer, C.M., 2005. Compositions Suitable for Oral Administration and Kits Thereof for Hydrating Mammalian Skin European Patent EP 1,257,283.

Botha, M.C., 1994. Process for Extracting Polysaccharides From Plant Material South African Patent 941,581.

Breimer, D.D., Baars, A.J., 1976. Pharmacology, 14:30–47.

Buchwald-Werner, S., 2008. Composition of Extracts of *Aloe* for Oral Administration US Patent 2008/0220101 A1.

Buenz, E.J., 2008. Aloin induces apoptosis in Jurkat cells. Toxicol. In Vitro, 22:422–429.

Celestino, V.R.L., Maranhão, H.M.L., Vasconcelos, C.F.B., Lima, C.R., Medeiros, G.C.R., Araújo, A.V., Wanderley, A.G., 2013. Braz. J. Pharmacogn., 23:279–283.

Chang, X.-L., Xu, H., Wang, J.-J., Wang, W.-H., Feng, Y.-M., 2013. Food Sci. Technol. Res., 19:901–907.

Che, Q.M., Akao, T., Hattori, M., Kobashi, K., Namba, T., 1991. Chem. Pharm. Bull., 39:704–708.
Chen, W.Y., Van Wyk, B.-E., Vermaak, I., Viljoen, A.M., 2012. Phytochem. Lett., 5:1–12.
Choi, S., Park, Y.I., Lee, S.K., Kim, J.E., Chung, M.H., 2002. Clin. Exp. Dermatol., 27:513–515.
Clarkson, C., Maharaj, V.J., Crouch, N.R., Grace, O.M., Pillay, P., Matsabisa, M.G., Bhagwandin, N., Smith, P.J., Folb, P., 2004. J. Ethnopharmacol., 92:177–191.
Coopoosamy, R.M., Magwa, M.L., 2006. Afr. J. Biotechnol., 5:1092–1094.
Dagne, E., Yenesew, A., Asmellash, S., Demissew, S., Mavi, S., 1994. Phytochemistry, 35:401–406.
Dagne, E., Bisrat, D., Viljoen, A., Van Wyk, B.-E., 2000. Curr. Org. Chem., 4:1055–1078.
Devaraj, S., Jialal, R., Jialal, I., Rockwood, J., 2008. Planta Med., 74:32.
Dickson, B., 2008. Oryx, 42:548–553.
Ernst, E., 2000. Br. J. Dermatol., 143:923–929.
Eshun, K., He, Q., 2004. Crit. Rev. Food Sci. Nutr., 44:91–96.
Esmat, A.Y., Tomasetto, C., Rio, M.C., 2006. Cancer Biol. Ther., 5:97–103.
Farkas, A., 1963. Topical Medicament Including Polyuranide Derived From Aloe US Patent 3,103,466.
Fawole, O.A., Amoo, S.O., Ndhlala, A.R., Light, M.E., Finnie, J.F., Van Staden, J., 2010. J. Ethnopharmacol., 127:235–241.
Fenig, E., Nordenberg, J., Beery, E., Sulkes, J., Wasserman, L., 2004. Oncol. Rep., 11:213–217.
Finberg, M.J., Muntingh, G.L., van Rensburg, C.E.J., 2015. Inflammopharmacology, 23:337–341.
Fischer, W., Haber, P., Mason, P., 2003. Intradermal Penetration Agents for Topical Local Anesthetic Administration US Patent 2003/0138505 A1.
Fox, L.T., Mazumder, A., Dwivedi, A., Gerber, M., du Plessis, J., Hamman, J.H., 2017. J. Ethnopharmacol., 200:1–7.
Frum, Y., Viljoen, A.M., 2006. Skin Pharmacol. Physiol., 19:329–335.
Gao, J., Zhang, G., Dai, R., Bi, K., 2004. Pharm. Biol., 42:581–587.
Ghuman, S., Ncube, B., Finnie, J.F., McGaw, L.J., Coopoosamy, R.M., Van Staden, J., 2016. Front. Pharmacol., 7:320.
Grace, O.M., Simmonds, M.S.J., Smith, G.F., Van Wyk, A.E., 2008. J. Ethnopharmacol., 119:604–614.
Graf, E., Alexa, M., 1982. Arch. Pharm., 315:969–970.
Grollier, J.F., Lang, G., Forestier, S., Rosenbaum, G., 1987. Cosmetic Composition Containing Aloesin as an Agent for Protection Against Sunlight and Its Use for Skin and Hair Protection US Patent 4,656,029.
Gruber, M., 1986. Method of Reducing Skin Irritation From Benzoyl Peroxide US Patent 4,593,046.
Haynes, L.J., Henderson, J.I., Tyler, J.M., 1970. J. Chem. Soc. C, 2581–2586.
Hodge, W.H., 1953. Econ. Bot., 7:99–129.
Hu, Y., Xu, J., Hu, Q., 2003. J. Agric. Food Chem., 51:7788–7791.
Hutchings, A., 1989. Bothalia, 19:111–123.
Ishikawa, M., Yamamoto, M., Masui, T., 1987. Shizuoka-ken Eisei Kankyo Senta Hokoku, 30:25–30.
Izzo, A.A., Sautebin, L., Borrelli, F., Longo, R., Capasso, F., 1999. Eur. J. Pharmacol., 368:43–48.
Jeong, W.Y., Kim, K., 2017. J. Herb. Med., 9:53–59.
Jia, Q., Farrow, T.M., 2003. 7-Hydroxychromones Potent Anti-Oxidants US Patent α2003/0207818 A1.

Jia, Y.M., Zhao, G.D., Jia, J.C., 2008. J. Ethnopharmacol., 120:181–189.
Jin, Y.H., Lee, S.J., Chung, M.H., Park, J.H., Park, Y.I., Cho, T.H., Lee, S.K., 1999. Arch. Pharm. Res., 22:232–236.
Jones, K., Hughes, J., Hong, M., Jia, Q., Orndorff, S., 2002. Pigment Cell Res., 15:335–340.
Kai, M., Hayashi, K., Kaida, I., Aki, H., Yamamoto, M., 2002. Biol. Pharm. Bull., 25:1608–1613.
Kambizi, L., Afolayan, A.J., 2008. Afr. J. Biotechnol., 7:12–15.
Kambizi, L., Sultana, N., Afolayan, A., 2004. S. Afr. J. Sci., 42:636–639.
Kambizi, L., Goosen, B.M., Taylor, M.B., Afolayan, A.J., 2007. S. Afr. J. Sci., 103:359–360.
Kametani, S., Kojima-Yuasa, A., Kikuzaki, H., Kennedy, D.O., Honzawa, M., Matsui-Yuasa, I., 2007a. Biosci. Biotechnol. Biochem., 71:1220–1229.
Kametani, S., Oikawa, T., Kojima-Yuasa, A., Kennedy, D.O., Norikura, T., Honzawa, M., Matsui-Yuasa, I., 2007b. J. Nutr. Sci. Vitaminol., 53:540–546.
Kanama, S.K., Viljoen, A.M., Kamatou, G.P.P., Chen, W., Sandasi, M., Adhami, H.-R., Van Wyk, B.-E., 2015. Phytochem. Lett., 13:85–90.
Kee, N.L.A., Mnonopi, N., Davids, H., Naudé, R.J., Frost, C.L., 2008. Afr. J. Biotechnol., 7:217–223.
Kim, K., Kim, H., Kwon, J., Lee, S., Kong, H., Im, S.A., Lee, Y.H., Lee, Y.R., Oh, S.T., Jo, T.H., Park, Y.I., Lee, C.K., Kim, K., 2009. Phytomedicine, 16:856–863.
Kleinschmidt, B., 2004. Fruit Process., 14:194–198.
Kong, H., Lee, S., Shin, S., Kwon, J., Jo, T.H., Shin, E., Shim, K.-S., Park, Y.-I., Lee, C.-K., Kim, K., 2010. Biomol. Ther., 18:336–342.
Koyama, J., Ogura, T., Tagahara, K., 1994. Phytochemistry, 37:1147–1148.
Koyama, J., Morita, I., Tagahara, K., Ogatab, M., Mukainaka, T., Tokuda, H., Nishino, H., 2001. Cancer Lett., 170:15–18.
Lee, H.Z., Lin, C.J., Yang, W.H., Leung, W.C., Chang, S.P., 2006. Cancer Lett., 239:55–63.
Lindsey, K.L., Jager, A.K., Viljoen, A.M., 2002. S. Afr. J. Bot., 68:47.
Loots, D.T., Van Der Westhuizen, F.H., Botes, L., 2007. J. Agric. Food Chem., 55:6891–6896.
Loots, D.T., Pieters, M., Islam, M.S., Botes, L., 2011. S. Afr. J. Sci., 107:7–8.
Luyckx, V.A., Ballantine, R., Claeys, M., Cuyckens, F., Van den Heuvel, H., Cimanga, R.K., Vlietinck, A.J., De Broe, M.E., Katz, I.J., 2002. Am. J. Kidney Dis., 39:E13.
Lynch, B., Simon, R., Roberts, A., 2011. Regul. Toxicol. Pharmacol., 61:161–171.
Mabusela, W.T., Stephen, A.M., Botha, M.C., 1990. Phytochemistry, 29:3555–3558.
Magwa, M.L., Gundidza, M., Coopoosamy, R.M., Mayekiso, B., 2006. Afr. J. Biotechnol., 5:1652–1654.
Manitto, P., Speranza, G., Tommasi, N.D., Ortoleva, E., Morelli, C.F., 2003. Tetrahedron, 59:401–408.
Maphosa, V., Masika, P.J., Bizimenyera, E.S., Eloff, J.N., 2010. Trop. Anim. Health Prod., 42:301–307.
Mapunya, M.B., Nikolova, R.V., Lall, N., 2012. Evid. Based Complement. Alternat. Med., Art. No. 374017.
Mavundza, E.J., Maharaj, R., Chukwujekwu, J.C., Finnie, J.F., Van Staden, J., 2014. Malar. J., 13: Art. No. 173.
Melin, A., 2009. A Bitter Pill to Swallow: A Case Study of the Trade & Harvest of *Aloe ferox* in the Eastern Cape, South Africa. Available from: https://www.iccs.org.uk/wp-content/thesis/consci/2009/Melin.pdf.
Mello, J.R.B., Mello, F.B., Langeloh, A., 2008. Lat. Am. J. Pharm., 27:752–756.

Meyer, E., Altenschoepfer, P., Woess, A., McLeod, S., 2007. Transdermal Formulation Comprising an Opioid Analgesic and an Aloe Composition US Patent 2007/0077284 A1.
Mwale, M., Masika, P.J., 2014. Trop. Anim. Health Prod., 47:131–138.
Newton, D.J., Vaughan, H., 1996. South Africa's *Aloe ferox* Plant, Parts and Derivatives Industry. TRAFFIC East/Southern Africa, South Africa, pp. 61.
Nortje, J.M., Van Wyk, B.-E., 2015. J. Ethnopharmacol., 171:205–222.
O'Brien, C., Van Wyk, B.-E., Van Heerden, F.R., 2011. S. Afr. J. Bot., 77:988–995.
Park, M.Y., Kwon, H.J., Sung, M.K., 2009. Nutr. Res. Pract., 3:9–14.
Pecere, T., Gazzola, M.V., Mucignat, C., Parolin, C., Vecchia, F.D., Cavaggioni, A., Basso, G., Diaspro, A., Salvato, B., Carli, M., Palu, G., 2000. Cancer Res., 60:2800–2804.
Pecere, T., Sarinella, F., Salata, C., Gatto, B., Bet, A., Vecchia, F., Dalla, Diasprp, A., Caril, M., Palumbo, M., Palu, G., 2003. Int. J. Cancer, 106:836–847.
Pérez, Y.Y., Jiménez-Ferrer, E., Zamilpa, A., Hernández-Valencia, M., Alarcón-Aguilar, F.J., Tortoriello, J., Román-Ramos, R., 2007. Am. J. Med., 35:1037–1046.
Raimondo, D., Viok, J.H., Van Wyk, B.E., Van Jaarsveld, E., Victor, J.E., 2012. Aloe ferox Mill. National Assessment: Red List of South African Plants version 2013.
Rauwald, H.-W., 1990. PZ Wiss, 3:169–181.
Rauwald, H.-W., Beil, A., 1993. Z. Naturforsch., 48:1–4.
Reynolds, T., 2004. Aloe chemistry. In: Reynolds, T. (Ed.), Aloes: The Genus Aloe. CRC Press, Boca Raton/London/New York/Washington DC, USA, pp. 39–74.
Reynolds, T., Dweck, A.C., 1999. J. Ethnopharmacol., 68:3–37.
Sekharam, K.S., Sekharam, M.K., 2007. Therapeutic Compositions for the Prevention and Treatment of Mucositis and Mucosal Disorders US Patent 7,288,270B1.
Sibuyi, N.R.S., Katerere, D.R., Boboyi, T., Madiehe, A.M., 2007. S. Afr. J. Bot., 73:336.
Soeda, M., Otomo, M., Ome, M., Kawashima, K., 1966. Nippon Saikingaku Zasshi, 21:609–614.
Speranza, G., Martignoni, A., Manitto, P., 1988. J. Nat. Prod., 51:588–590.
Speranza, G., Manitto, P., Pezzuto, D., Monti, D., 1991. Chirality, 3:263–267.
Speranza, G., Manitto, P., Monti, D., Pezzuto, D., 1992. J. Nat. Prod., 55:723–729.
Speranza, G., Manitto, P., Cassara, P., Monti, D., 1993a. J. Nat. Prod., 56:1089–1094.
Speranza, G., Manitto, P., Cassara, P., Monti, D., 1993b. Phytochemistry, 33:175–178.
Speranza, G., Morelli, C.F., Tubaro, A., Altinier, G., Duri, L., Manitto, P., 2005. Planta Med., 71:79–81.
Squires, M.J., 2010. Medicinal Composition US Patent 2010/0303935 A1.
Standards South Africa, 2007. South African National Standard. Aloe Raw Material. SANS 368: 2007, first ed. Standards South Africa, Pretoria, South Africa, p. 26.
Steenkamp, V., Stewart, M.J., 2007. Pharm. Biol., 45:411–420.
Steenkamp, L.H., Mitra, R.K., Heggie, S.J., Phehane, V.N., 2008. Methods for Converting Aloeresin A to Aloesin US Patent 2008/0280348.
Tang, T., Yin, L.W., Yang, J., Shan, G., 2007. Eur. J. Pharmacol., 567:177–185.
Taylor, A., 2003. Preparation for Regulating Bowel Function European Patent EP 1 154 781 B1.
Thibane, V.S., Ndhlala, A.R., Abdelgadir, H.A., Finnie, J.F., Van Staden, J., 2018. S. Afr. J. Bot., 122:475–483.
US FDA, 2010. Part 172—Food additives permitted for direct addition to food for human consumption. Subpart F. Flavoring Agents and Related Substances. Section 172.510—Aloe. In: US Code of Federal Regulation (CFR). Title 21 Food and Drugs (Food and Drug Administration). Government Printing Office, Washington, DC.

Van Wyk, B.-E., Gericke, N., 2000. People's Plants. A Guide to Useful Plants of Southern Africa. Briza Publications, Pretoria, South Africa.
Van Wyk, B.-E., Smith, G.F., 2014. Guide to the Aloes of South Africa, third ed. Briza Publications, Pretoria, South Africa.
Van Wyk, B.-E., Van Rheede van Oudtshoorn, M.C.B., Smith, G.F., 1995a. Planta Med., 61:250–253.
Van Wyk, B.-E., Yenesew, A., Dagne, E., 1995b. Biochem. Syst. Ecol., 23:267–275.
Van Wyk, B.-E., Van Oudtshoorn, B., Gericke, N., 2009. Medicinal Plants of South Africa, second ed. Briza Publications, Pretoria, South Africa.
Van Zyl, R.L., Viljoen, A.M., 2002. S. Afr. J. Bot., 68:106–110.
Wang, W., Cuyckens, F., Van den Heuvel, H., Apers, S., Pieters, L., Steenkamp, V., Stewart, M.J., Luyckx, V.A., Claeys, M., 2003. Rapid Commun. Mass Spectrom., 17:49–55.
Watt, J.M., Breyer-Brandwijk, M.G., 1962. The Medicinal and Poisonous Plants of Southern and Eastern Africa, second ed. E. & S. Livingstone Ltd, Edinburgh and London, UK.
Wintola, O.A., Afolayan, A.J., 2011. Pharmacogn. Mag., 7:325–333.
Wintola, O.A., Sunmonu, T.O., Afolayan, A.J., 2010. BMC Gastroenterol., 10:95–99.
Wintola, O.A., Sunmonu, T.O., Afolayan, A.J., 2011. Hum. Exp. Toxicol., 30:425–431.
Zapata, P.J., Navarro, D., Guillén, F., Castillo, S., Martínez-Romero, D., Valero, D., Serrano, M., 2013. Ind. Crop. Prod., 42:223–230.
Zolotariov, E., Zolotariov, Z., 2004. Aloe Suppositories US Patent 2004/0265344 A1.

CHAPTER

Artemisia afra

4

Zimkhitha Sotenjwa[a], Alvaro Viljoen[a,b], Sandra Combrinck[a] and Guy Kamatou[a]

[a]*Department of Pharmaceutical Sciences, Tshwane University of Technology, Pretoria, South Africa*

[b]*SAMRC Herbal Drugs Research Unit, Faculty of Science, Tshwane University of Technology, Pretoria, South Africa*

Abstract

Artemisia afra Jacq. ex Willd. (Asteraceae), referred to as African wormwood, is an aromatic, perennial shrub that can grow up to 2 m in height. The finely divided leaves have a silver-green colour due to the presence of fine hairs. The plant is found in the mountainous regions of Africa, as far north as Ethiopia. In southern Africa, it occurs in Namibia, Zimbabwe, Swaziland (Eswatini), Lesotho and South Africa, where it is widespread and abundant. The plant is mainly used in the form of decoctions, infusions, poultices, or as an inhalant, to treat a range of ailments including coughs, colds, headaches, chills, colic, asthma, malaria, diabetes, influenza, convulsions, fever and rheumatism. In vitro and in vivo studies of the plant have indicated that it has promising antimicrobial, anti-oxidant, anti-inflammatory, antidiabetic and antimycobacterial activities. The essential oil composition has been reported to be highly variable, and several (artemisia ketone, 1,8-cineole, α-thujone, β-thujone, camphor and myrcenone) chemotypes have been described. Chemical profiles of A. afra essential oils, obtained by hydro-distillation were obtained using semi-automated high-performance thin-layer chromatography (HPTLC) and gas chromatography coupled to mass spectroscopy (GC–MS). The HPTLC plate, viewed under white light after derivatisation with anisaldehyde, confirms variation in the composition of the oils. The use of UPLC–MS for non-volatile qualitative analysis enabled the identification of scopolin, rutin, scopoletin, chrysoeriol, 3,5-di-O-caffeoylquinic acid and acacetin in the acetone:methanol extracts. The use of HPTLC indicated considerable variation in the phenolic compound composition of samples from different populations.

Keywords: *Artemisia afra*, African wormwood, Scopoletin, Acacetin, Thujone, UPLC–MS, GC–MS, HPTLC, MIR spectroscopy

The South African Herbal Pharmacopoeia. https://doi.org/10.1016/B978-0-323-99794-2.00016-7

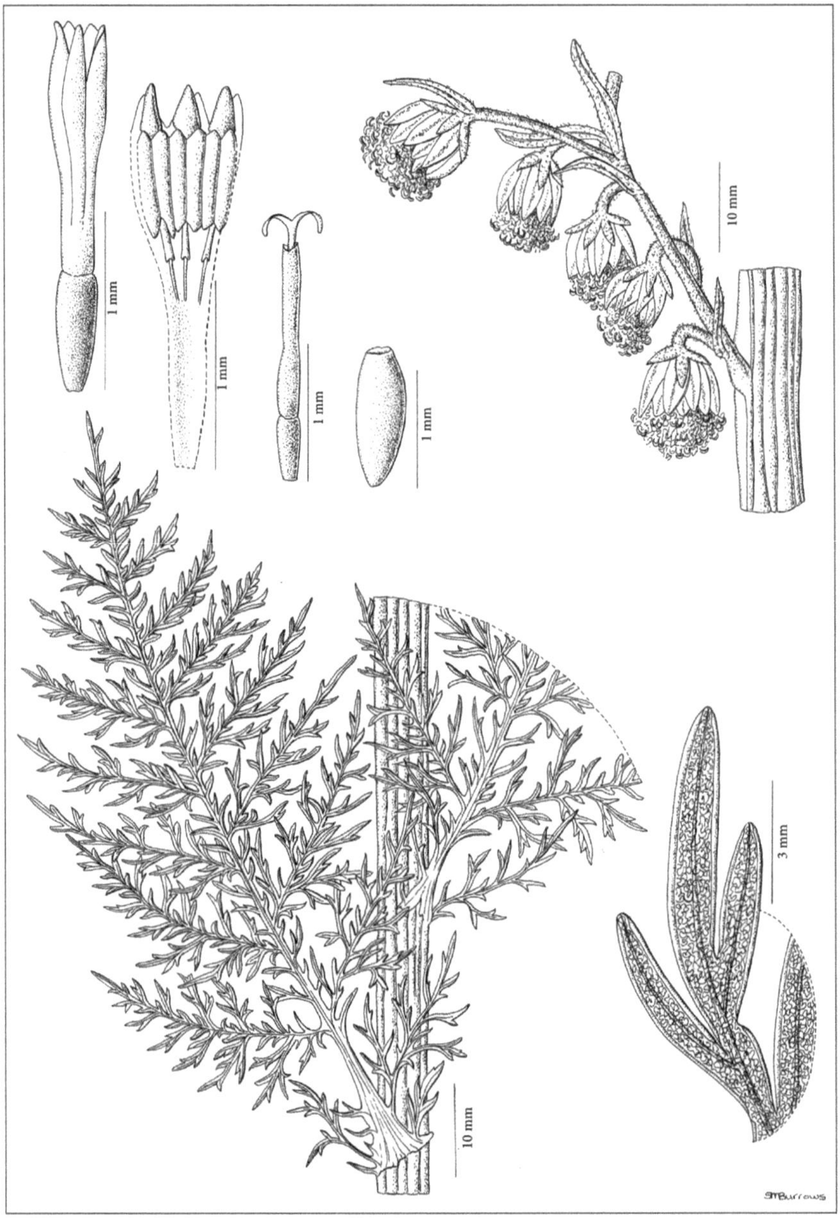
1 mm
1 mm
1 mm
1 mm
10 mm
10 mm
3 mm

Part A: General overview

1. Synonyms

Artemisia afra var. *afra*, *Artemisia afra* var. *friesiorum* Chiov.[a]

2. Common name(s)

African wormwood, wild wormwood (English); '*wilde-als*', '*wilde-alsies*', '*wildeal-sem*', '*bitterals*' (Afrikaans); '*umhlonyane*' (isiXhosa); '*mhlonyane*' (isiZulu); '*lengana*' (Sesotho); '*zengana*' (Southern Sotho).[a,b]

3. Conservation status

Least concern.[b]

4. Botany

The genus *Artemisia* consists of about 500 species that are distributed throughout the world. It is one of the largest genera in the family Asteraceae. The genus name is derived from the name of the Greek goddess of hunting, Artemis (Jackson, 1990), while the species name '*afra*' refers to Africa. The aromatic shrub reaches a height of 0.6–2.0 m, and releases a sweet odour when touched or cut. It has thick, woody stems at the base that become softer as they lengthen. The main stems are characterised by many side branches, which have conspicuous swollen ribs along their length. Finely divided soft, feathery leaves give the shrub a fern-like appearance (A). Mature leaves are about 8 cm long, 4 cm wide, and narrowly ovate (B and D). Although the adaxial leaf surfaces are dark green in colour, small white hairs covering the abaxial surfaces and stems impart a grey colour that is characteristic of the shrub. Individual creamy-yellow flowers are 3–4 mm in diameter, nodding and crowded at the tips of the branches (C). The three-angled and slightly curved fruit are silvery-white, and approximately 1 mm in length (Liu et al., 2009).

[a] World Flora Online (http://www.worldfloraonline.org).
[b] Red List of South African Plants (http://redlist.sanbi.org).

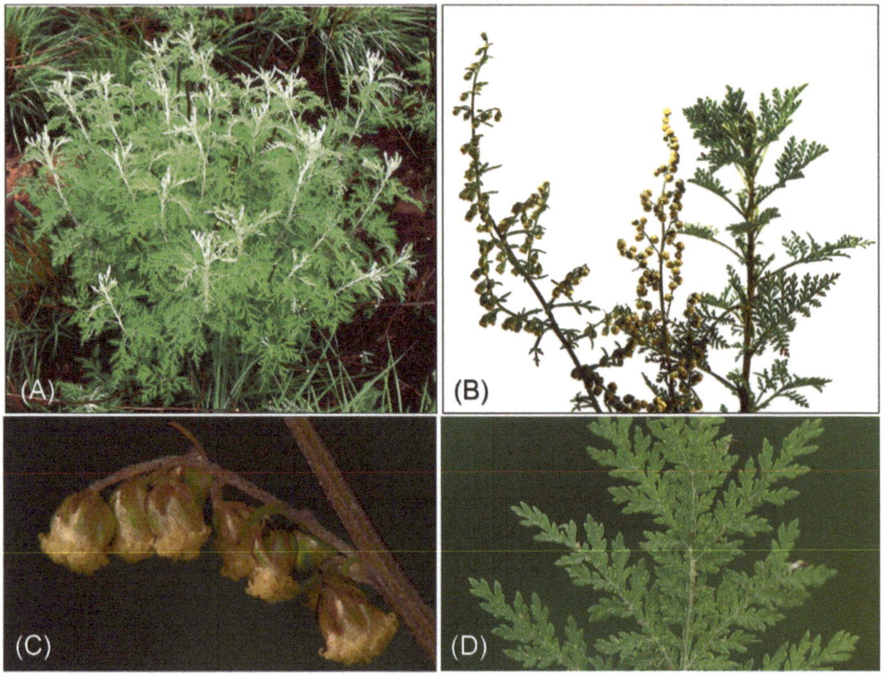

Artemisia afra in natural habitat (A), with woody stems that have many side branches (B), crowded yellow flowers at the tip of a branch (C) and finely divided leaves (D).

5. Geographical distribution

Artemisia afra grows abundantly and is widely distributed throughout South Africa, occurring in most of the provinces (Germishuizen et al., 2006). It is the only species

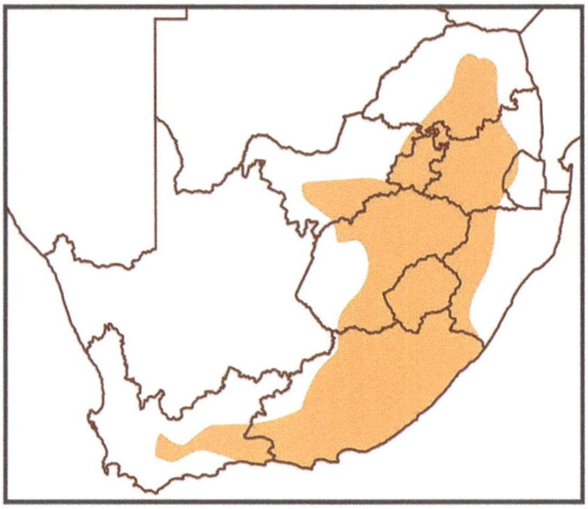

Geographical distribution of *Artemisia afra* in South Africa.

in this genus that is indigenous to southern Africa. *Artemisia afra* is found as far south as the Cederberg Mountains in the Cape, extending to neighbouring countries and northwards to tropical East Africa and Ethiopia. Wild plants occur from sea level to altitudes above 2400 m on damp slopes, along streams and on the edges of forests.

6. Ethnopharmacology

Artemisia afra is one of the best-known medicinal plants in South Africa, and is still used by people of all cultures. The plant is commonly used to relieve conditions of the upper and lower respiratory tract, including blocked nose, cough, bronchitis, cold, fever, infection of the throat and inflammation. Decoctions and infusions of the roots, stems and/or leaves are the most common forms, but treatments are also administered as enemas, poultices, body washes, lotions, smoke or snuff. Fresh leaves are inserted directly into the nostrils to treat sinusitis. Patients inhale steam generated by boiling leaves or use the decoction as a gargle (Watt and Breyer-Brandwijk, 1962; Van Wyk et al., 2009). Leaves are placed inside socks to comfort sweaty feet and to combat odour (Watt and Breyer-Brandwijk, 1962). A poultice prepared from the leaves is applied to reduce swelling caused by mumps, to relieve neuralgia, and is placed on the stomach of babies to treat colic. A tincture for colic is also made by soaking the leaves in brandy (Watt and Breyer-Brandwijk, 1962). Further uses include the treatment of loss of appetite, headache, earache, intestinal parasites and malaria. The leaves have a very bitter taste, and sugar or honey is often added to sweeten decoctions. Margaret Roberts (1990) lists many other alternative uses, which include the preparation of natural insecticidal sprays to repel moths and other insects. It is also used as a bitter tonic and appetite stimulant in the Cape region of South Africa (Rood, 1994).

7. Commercialisation

Brandy infused with *A. afra*, known as wilde-als brandy, is a popular medicine that is still in use and available commercially. Prof. Earle Graven first planted *A. afra* at Fort Hare University in the late 1980s, as part of a research project on essential oils (Graven et al., 1990). The South African Druggists established the first commercial plantation in South Africa in 1995 at Gouda in the Western Cape Province. Commercial products containing material with a low thujone content were developed under the brand names of Healer's Choice in 1996 (as a tincture) and Phyto Nova in 2002 (as tablets).

8. Pharmacological evaluation

8.1 *In vitro* studies

8.1.1 Antimicrobial activity

The antibacterial activity of essential oil, obtained by steam distillation from *A. afra*, was determined against a variety of strains (Graven et al., 1992). The essential oil caused growth inhibition of 15 species, with *Acinetobacter calcoaceticus*, *Beneckea natriegens*, *Brevibacterium linens*, *Brochothrix thermosphacta*, *Citrobacter freundii*, *Klebsiella pneumoniae* and *Serratia marcescens* reported as the most susceptible organisms. Rabe and Van Staden (1997) tested the antimicrobial activities of extracts of

A. afra against *Staphylococcus aureus*, *Staphylococcus epidermis* and *Bacillus subtilis*. The results indicated that the lowest minimum inhibitory concentration (MIC) was achieved against *S. aureus*. They also reported that the methanol extracts displayed a higher antibacterial activity than those prepared using water. The antimicrobial efficacy of essential oils of *A. afra*, *Pteronia incana* and *Rosmarinus officinalis* were compared against 41 microbial strains. All the oils tested displayed some activity, but those of *A. afra* and *R. officinalis* resulted in similar and better activity than that of *P. incana* (Mangena and Muyima, 1999). Using a challenge test, the possible use of essential oils, instead of synthetic preservatives, in cosmetic products was evaluated through an aqueous cream formulation (Muyima et al., 2002). Essential oils isolated from *A. afra*, *P. incana*, *Lavandula officinalis* and *R. officinalis* displayed remarkable antimicrobial activities against several common bacteria and fungi, and some environmental isolates. In general, the test micro-organisms were more susceptible to the oils when the challenge test was conducted using aqueous cream, compared to an agar medium. Of the essential oils tested, *A. afra* oil caused the largest reduction in the load of artificial contamination in the aqueous cream formulation within 2–7 days.

An apparatus, designed to simulate the burning process that occurs in a traditional setting, was used to capture the smoke fraction from *A. afra*, which was subsequently analysed and evaluated in a bio-assay (Braithwaite et al., 2008). Methanol and acetone extracts, as well as the essential oil, were prepared and tested together with the smoke fraction. Lower MIC values (0.26–0.52 mg/mL) were obtained for the inhalation extract, compared to the methanol extract (1.00–3.00 mg/mL) and the essential oil (8.00–16.00 mg/mL), which was inactive. The activities of *A. afra*, *Carpobrotus edulis* and *Tulbaghia violacea* were determined towards *Bacillus cereus*, *Escherichia coli*, *K. pneumoniae*, *S. aureus*, and a strain of *Mycobacterium aurum* A+, using a twofold microdilution bio-assay (Buwa and Afolayan, 2009). All the tested micro-organisms were susceptible to the extracts of *A. afra*. Water extracts of *A. afra* and *C. edulis* were the only ones that displayed activity against the *M. aurum* A+ strain. The antimicrobial activity of essential oils of *A. afra*, in combination with those of the medicinal aromatic plants *Agathosma betulina*, *Eucalyptus globulus* and *Osmitopsis asteriscoides*, was investigated. In most cases, individual oils displayed only moderate antimicrobial activity. However, several additive interactions were reported. The strongest synergistic interaction, with a fractional inhibitory concentration (FIC) of 0.5, was achieved towards *C. neoformans*, for the combination of eight parts of *A. afra* and two parts of *O. asteriscoides* (Suliman et al., 2010). No antagonistic interactions were evident.

Compounds isolated from the ethanol extract of *A. afra* were evaluated for antimicrobial activity towards *Actinomyces naeslundii*, *A. israelii* and *Streptococcus mutans* (Gram-positive bacteria), and against *Prevotella intermedia*, *Porphyromonas gingivalis* and *Aggregatibacter actinomycetemcomitans* (Gram-negative bacteria) and *Candida albicans* (fungus) (More et al., 2012). The growth of all the microbial species tested was inhibited by the crude extract over the concentration range 1.6–25 mg/mL. Compounds present in the plant were also tested and the three most active compounds were reported as scopoletin, betulinic acid and acacetin. Antagonistic interaction was identified for the aqueous extract of *A. afra* combined with ciprofloxacin against *E. coli*, which suggests possible impairment of the efficacy of the antibiotic in the treatment of gastro-intestinal complaints caused by the pathogen (Hübsch et al., 2014). Five popular medicinal plants from South Africa (*A. afra*, *Lippia javanica*, *O. asteriscoides*, *Croton gratissimus* and *Tetradenia riparia)* were tested against antibiotic-resistant bacterial strains (*Enterococcus faecalis*, *S. aureus*, *Bacillus cereus*, *K. pneumoniae*, *Acinetobacter baumannii*, *Pseudomonas aeruginosa*, *E. coli* and *S. marcescens*) and comparatively evaluated against ciprofloxacin as the standard drug (Van Vuuren and Muhlarhi, 2017). The general trend was that resistant strains were more susceptible to the organic extracts, followed by the essential oils, and were less susceptible to the antibiotics. *Artemisia afra* was found to be the most effective species against the resistant strains, followed by *T. riparia* and *O. asteriscoides*. The microdilution assay and bio-autography incorporating *p*-iodonitrotetrazolium violet (INT) as indicator were used to assess the antimycobacterial activity of acetone extracts of *A. afra* against *Mycobacterium smegmatis* ATCC 1441 (Masoko and Nxumalo, 2013). A moderate MIC of 0.39 mg/mL was reported.

8.1.2 Antimalarial activity

The dicholoromethane (DCM) extract of *A. afra* was found to display stronger antiplasmodial activity as measured using half maximal inhibitory concentration (IC_{50}) towards *Plasmodium falciparum* D10 ($IC_{50} = 5\,\mu g/mL$) than the corresponding DCM: methanol (1:1), methanol and water extracts, respectively (IC_{50} values of 7.3, 8.0 and $>100.0\,\mu g/mL$) (Clarkson et al., 2004). The infusion of *A. afra* is used traditionally to treat malaria throughout the southern parts of Africa, in much the same way as *A. annua* is used as an antimalarial in China (Liu et al., 2010). This prompted an investigation of the metabolic differences between *A. afra* and *A. annua* using multivariate data analysis. The antiplasmodial activity of extracts was tested against *P. falciparum* 3D7 (chloroquine-sensitive strain), with chloroquine, quinine and artemisinin applied as positive controls. Non-polar fractions of both *A. afra* and *A. annua* were active towards *P. falciparum*, but the tea infusion of *A. afra* was inactive. Multivariate data analysis using one-dimensional (1D) and two-dimensional (2D)-nuclear magnetic resonance (NMR) spectroscopy enabled the identification of 24 components of intermediate polarity in *A. afra*. Since the infusion of *A. afra* was inactive towards *P. falciparum*, metabolites associated with the differences in antimalarial activities between the two species could be identified for quality control purposes. In a separate study, *in vitro* screening of extracts prepared from eight selected plant species, including *A. afra*, was conducted against *P. falciparum* NF54 early- and late-stage gametocytes (Moyo et al., 2016). The parasite lactate dehydrogenase assay was applied to assess the *in vitro* inhibition of gametocyte viability. *Artemisia afra* was highly active towards both gametocyte stages, as reflected by IC_{50} values below $10\,\mu g/mL$. The activity of the plant species was significantly more pronounced towards late-stage gametocytes, compared to the early stages.

8.1.3 Anti-oxidant activity

The essential oils of *A. afra*, *A. abyssinica* and *Juniperus procera* were compared for their potential radical scavenging activities (Burits et al., 2001). Oils from all three species displayed anti-oxidant potential. The oils of *A. afra* and *J. procera* also acted as effective hydroxyl radical scavenging agents when assessed using the deoxyribose degradation assay. The *in vitro* assay for non-enzymatic lipid peroxidation in liposomes provided evidence of the anti-oxidant activity of the oils of *A. afra* and *J. procera* (Burits et al., 2001). The aqueous extract of the plant exhibited significant inhibition when tested in the 2,2-diphenyl-1-picryl-hydrazyl-hydrate (DPPH) and 2,2-azino-*bis*(3-ethylbenzothiazoline-6-sulphonic acid) (ABTS) assays, and demonstrated ferric reductive ability, in a concentration-dependent manner. The anti-oxidant activity of *A. afra* was attributed to an abundance of phenolic compounds, and the activity was similar to those of known standard anti-oxidants, including butylated hydroxytoluene, rutin and vitamin C (Sunmonu and Afolayan, 2012). The anti-oxidant activity of the ethanol extract and compounds from *A. afra* was also investigated by More et al. (2012). The extract displayed good anti-oxidant activity with an IC_{50} value of 22.2 μg/mL. Scopoletin, present in the extract, caused the transformation of the DPPH radical to its reduced form, with an IC_{50} value of 1.24 μg/mL, which was similar to that of vitamin C (1.22 μg/mL). The extract was only moderately toxic towards the McCoy fibroblast cell line (IC_{50} 16.95 μg/mL), while scopoletin was found to be non-toxic, as reflected by an IC_{50} value of 132.5 μg/mL.

8.1.4 Anticancer properties

Treurnicht (1997) investigated the cytotoxic activities of 16 South African plant species, and reported that the aqueous extracts of *A. afra* were cytotoxic towards HeLa, Vero, Jurkat E6.1, AA-2 and CEM-SS cells, at the high concentrations used in the assay. A DCM:methanol (1:1) extract of *A. afra* induced cytotoxicity against renal and breast cancer, and melanoma cells (Fouché et al., 2008). The mode of cell death caused by an ethanolic *A. afra* extract was investigated using U937 and HeLa cancer cells, with IC_{50} values of 18.21 and 31.88 μg/mL obtained, respectively (Spies et al., 2013). The aqueous extract was inactive, as reflected by an IC_{50} value of above 250 μg/mL. Following 12 h of treatment with *A. afra*, the G2/M phase of the cell cycle was found to have been delayed. Use of the TUNEL assay for DNA fragmentation confirmed apoptosis, together with results from fluorescent staining with Annexin V-FITC. Treatment with *A. afra* for 24 and 48 h, followed by JC-1 staining, revealed a decrease in mitochondrial membrane potential at 24 h. An ethanol extract of *A. afra* was reported to induce caspase-dependent apoptosis in a mitochondrial-dependent manner. Bio-assay-guided fractionation of the extract yielded isoalantolactone as an active component (Venables et al., 2016). Subsequent treatment of HeLa cancer cells with the isolated compound caused dose-dependent cytotoxicity. A low IC_{50} value of 8.15 ± 1.16 μM was achieved. Apoptosis was confirmed after 24 h of exposure to the compound. The TUNEL assay was used to detect DNA fragmentation, while Annexin V-FITC staining revealed the translocation of phosphatidylserine.

8.1.5 Anti-HIV and immunomodulating activity

Informal claims abound in Africa that *Artemisia* infusions are able to inhibit HIV. An infusion was found to be highly active towards the virus, with IC_{50} values as low as 2.0 µg/mL (Lubbe et al., 2012). Moreover, it was found that artemisinin (present in *A. annua*) was inactive at 25 µg/mL, while the chemically related species *A. afra* that does not contain artemisinin displayed a similar level of activity. This indicated that artemisinin has none, or a limited role in the observed activity. Even the highest concentration of the *A. afra* infusion tested did not induce observable cellular toxicity. This study was the first to provide *in vitro* evidence of anti-HIV activity of *A. annua*. The biological activities of leaf extracts of *A. afra*, prepared by sequential extraction with organic solvents (DCM and methanol), 50% aqueous ethanol and water at 50 °C and 100 °C, respectively, were tested using the complement fixation assay (Braünlich et al., 2018). Purified polysaccharide-rich fractions were found to display higher immunomodulating activity than the selected standard in the complement assay. Digestion of these polysaccharides with an *endo*-polygalacturonase enzyme yielded low-molecular-weight polymers with higher activity than that of the standard. It was deduced from these results that the health-promoting effects of this medicinal plant are probably associated with its immune-boosting properties.

8.1.6 Other activities

Artemisia afra was tested as an alternative treatment for the control of dermatophytes, associated with dandruff and related inflammatory conditions of the scalp (Muyima and Nkata, 2005). The antifungal activities of the essential oils of *A. afra*, *P. incana*, *L. officinalis* and *R. officinalis* were determined against eight dermal fungi and two yeast strains that included *Epidermophyton*, *Microsporum*, *Trichophyton* and *Malassezia* strains. Noteworthy antifungal activities were recorded for all four essential oils against the test organisms. The efficacy followed the order *A. afra* > *L. officinalis* > *R. officinalis* > *P. incana*. The $GABA_A$-benzodiazepine receptor-binding assay was applied to evaluate 35 plant species, including *A. afra* (Stafford et al., 2005). In this assay, the binding of ^{3}H-Ro 15–1788 (flumazenil) to the benzodiazepine site was measured. The $GABA_A$-benzodiazepine receptor complex plays a role in epilepsy, convulsions and sedation. Good dose-dependent activity was recorded for the ethanolic leaf extracts of *Arctopus echinatus*, *A. afra*, four *Helichrysum* species and *Mentha aquatica*. The effects of acetone and aqueous extracts prepared from *A. afra* on egg hatch, larval development and mortality of nematodes were determined (Molefe et al., 2012). Egg hatch and larval mortality were inhibited to some degree; however, the development of the larvae was completely inhibited at all concentrations. Gastro-intestinal nematodes of livestock were generally the most susceptible to the acetone extracts. These results validated the traditional use of *A. afra* and other species by the Basotho of the eastern Free State Province of South Africa in the management of internal parasites. The pulmonary effects of *A. afra* were evaluated in isolated perfused lungs (IPL) by Mjiqiza et al. (2013). They determined the effects of *A. afra* steam inhalation, nebulised luteolin and nebulised aqueous leaf extract on lung function, as well as the pulmonary disposition of intravenously (IV) administered luteolin, using a modified IPL assay. A significantly higher luteolin concentration was present in the extract compared to the crude dried leaves. It was found that nebulisation with the extract resulted in exposure to larger quantities of luteolin than luteolin nebulisation. In addition, inhaled *A. afra* steam, nebulised luteolin, and aqueous leaf extract and IV administered luteolin produced significant dose-dependent improvements in lung function. The greatest improvement resulted from nebulised *A. afra*.

8.2 *In vivo* studies and clinical trials

8.2.1 Cardiovascular activity

The cardiovascular effects of an aqueous extract of *A. afra*, as well as the effects of a mixture of long chain fatty esters ($C_{44}H_{88}O_2$) and scopoletin, isolated from *A. afra* were studied in a rabbit model (Guantai and Addae-Mensah, 1999). While the aqueous extract at 10–45 mg/kg body weight (bw) exerted a hypotensive effect, lower doses initially caused cardiostimulation, followed by cardiodepression. Higher doses acted mainly as cardiodepressants. Scopoletin, administered at a dose of 1.0–2.5 mg/kg, resulted in a dose-dependent decrease in inotropic activity, together with a reduction in chronotropic effects, particularly at higher doses. These results indicate that *A. afra* and its constituents should be further investigated for the management of hypertension and related conditions. The antihypertensive effect of an hydro-ethanolic extract of *A. afra* was studied in spontaneously hypertensive rats (Mungho et al., 2018). The extract exerted its greatest antihypertensive effects 2 and 4 h after treatment. The antihypertensive effect of *A. afra* was significantly higher than that of furosemide, 24 h after treatment.

8.2.2 Antidiabetic activity

The effects of oral administration of an aqueous leaf extract of *A. afra* on the pancreas of streptozotocin-induced diabetic rats were explored by Afolayan and Sunmonu (2011). They found that blood glucose levels were significantly reduced, with a simultaneous increase in serum insulin concentrations. In addition, a significant improvement in the anti-oxidant enzyme activities of glutathione peroxidase, glutathione reductase and superoxide dismutase was reported following treatment with the extract. The extracts normalised the increased pancreatic lipid peroxidation activity in the diabetic rats. These findings indicated that the herb probably exerts its antidiabetic activity through the regeneration of pancreatic β-cells, thereby stimulating the release of insulin. The increased levels of lipid peroxidation detected in the diabetic rat tissues were also returned to near normality after administration of the extract (Afolayan and Sunmonu, 2012). It appears that the *A. afra* extract plays a protective role in the tissues of diabetic individuals by reducing oxidative stress, which may be attributed to the many flavonoids produced by the plant. An *in vivo* trial using streptozotocin-induced diabetic rats was used to assess the hypoglycaemic activity and potential toxicity of an aqueous leaf extract of *A. afra* (Sunmonu and Afolayan, 2013). At a dose of 200 mg/kg bw, the hypoglycaemic action of the extract was similar to that of glibenclamide, a standard hypoglycaemic drug. The extract restored liver function indices and haematological parameters to normal levels at all concentrations tested, but kidney function was only normalised when the diabetic rats were administered 50 mg/kg extract. These findings demonstrated that *A. afra* not only has hypoglycaemic activity, but also affords protection to the liver and blood against injury caused by diabetes. However, Sunmonu and Afolayan (2013) warned that high concentrations of the extract may have detrimental effects on kidney function.

8.2.3 Antimycobacterial activity

Extracts of *A. afra* were investigated for their ability to control mycobacterial replication *in vivo*. It was found that bacterial replication of *Mycobacterium aurum* exposed to aqueous, methanol and DCM extracts of *A. afra* was inhibited only by the DCM extract (Ntutela et al., 2009). This activity was confirmed in dose-dependent studies against both *M. aurum* and *M. tuberculosis* with IC_{50} values of 270 and 290 µg/mL, respectively. It was found that the antimycobacterial activity was associated mostly with a fraction rich in sesquiterpene lactones, containing mainly artemin and arsubin, obtained through fractionation of the DCM extract. This fraction reduced the *in vitro* replication of *M. aurum* and *M. tuberculosis* in a dose-dependent manner, with IC_{50} values of 1.9 and 2.0 µg/mL, respectively, and an MIC of 10 µg/mL. After administration of the sesquiterpene lactone-rich fraction and the crude DCM extract to *M. tuberculosis*-infected mice at a tolerated dose of 1000 mg/kg bw for up to 26 weeks, the bactericidal activities were evaluated. The mycobacterial loads were compared to those of untreated, isoniazid/rifampin (INH/RIF)-treated, and aqueous extract-treated animals. Bacterial replication was not affected during treatment with the enriched fraction or the DCM extract, resulting in similar pulmonary and splenic bacilli burdens to those of untreated mice. However, INH/RIF treatment reduced *M. tuberculosis* infection to undetectable levels after only 8 weeks. It is noteworthy that, despite its inability to inhibit mycobacterial growth, the aqueous extract of *A. afra* regulated pulmonary inflammation in *M. tuberculosis*-infected mice during the early stage of infection.

8.2.4 Other effects

An investigation of the antitumour activity in mice, of fresh leaf extracts (50% ethanol) prepared from a variety of samples of *A. afra*, revealed no activity against Leuk-L-1210 and Sarcoma-WM256 (IM) lines (Charlson, 1980). Compounds with anti-oxidant activities present in the extract of *A. afra* demonstrated potential for the control of *Eimeria* infections, since coccidial infection is closely associated with lipid peroxidation of the intestinal mucosa (Naidoo et al., 2008). The *in vivo* anticoccidial activity of an *A. afra* extract was screened, using toltrazuril as the positive control. The extract (150 mg/kg) resulted in feed conversion ratios that were comparable to those resulting from toltrazuril, and higher than the untreated control. The effect of the herb on isoproterenol (ISO)-induced myocardial injury in rats was studied by Sunmonu and Afolayan (2010). An increase in serum marker enzymes (lactate dehydrogenase, aspartate transaminase, alanine transaminase and alkaline phosphatase) was prevented by a 30-day pretreatment of myocardial-injured rats with an aqueous leaf extract of *A. afra*, at 100 and 200 mg/kg bw. Following treatment with the aqueous extract, decreased and almost normal levels of glutathione reductase, glutathione peroxides, superoxide dismutase and glutathione were found in the heart of ISO-induced animals. The extract also reduced lipid peroxidation in the heart and improved the lipid profile, which had been altered by ISO. The effect was more pronounced at the higher dose (200 mg/kg) tested. These findings provide evidence of the cardioprotective effect of *A. afra* against ISO-induced myocardial injury. A study was conducted to investigate the potential of *A. afra* on growth and disease-resistance in *Oreochromis mossambicus* (Mbokane and Moyo, 2018). Triplicate groups of 45 fish were randomly fed (32.5 ± 1 g) with one of five specially formulated *A. afra*-based diets. Some of the groups exposed to *A. afra* exhibited higher phagocytosis and lysozyme activity than those fed the other diets. Fish on *A. afra*-based diets also had higher white blood cell counts. To evaluate disease resistance, fish representing each dietary treatment were injected with varying inoculum sizes (0.1×10^6, 1.5×10^6, 3×10^6 and 4×10^6 colony forming units/mL) of *Aeromonas hydrophila*. The higher relative percentage survival and survival rate of certain groups of *O. mossambicus* provided evidence that the immunity of the fish was boosted after ingesting *A. afra*-based diets.

8.3 Safety

The safety of *A. afra* has been a much debated issue due to the presence of thujone. According to The Merck Index (1989), the α-isomer of thujone (LD_{50} subcutaneous (s.c.) in mice: 87.5 mg/kg) is substantially more toxic than the β-isomer (LD_{50} s.c. in mice: 442.2 mg/kg). Aqueous extracts of the plant are used in traditional practice in South Africa. However, the poor solubility of thujone in water (Treurnicht, 1997) should limit the quantity of either isomer of thujone in an aqueous extract of *A. afra* to below the toxic level. Nevertheless, it would be judicious to avoid using the herb for extended periods (no more than 2 weeks). The "standard permitted proportion" of α- and/or β-thujone in food flavourings is 0.5 mg/kg in the UK and European community (Tisserand and Balacs, 1995). Mukinda and Syce (2007) reported acute intraperitoneal and oral half-maximal lethal dose (LD_{50}) values of 2.45 and 8.96 g/kg for aqueous *Artemisia* extract, respectively, in mice. To test the chronic effects, daily doses of 0.1 and 1.0 g/kg of aqueous extract were administered to rats over a period of 3 months. A low chronic toxicity potential was demonstrated, with no significant changes in organ weights and normal histopathological profiles, indicating the absence of morphological alterations. Acute toxicity effects of a hydro-ethanolic extract of *A. afra* were studied in Swiss albino mice. The plant extract was non-toxic with an LD_{50} greater than 5000 mg/kg bw. The collective results indicate that *A. afra* extract is not toxic when administered acutely, that it has a low chronic toxicity, and may even have a protective effect on the liver at high doses. However, in this study the concentration of thujone and the *Artemisia* chemotype were not mentioned. High doses of thujone have been reported to cause confusion, convulsions and even coma, but selected low-thujone clones that are available can circumvent the associated toxicity. The World Health Organization in the 1970's declared that the plant is unsafe for consumption (Oyedeji et al., 2009), but this decision should be re-evaluated taking new evidence into consideration. It remains one of the most popular medicinal plants in southern Africa, particularly during winter when influenza is widespread. The essential oils of *A. afra* were assayed for hatchability and lethality activities towards *Artemia salina* for 72 h (Adeogun et al., 2018). The LC_{50} values recorded for *A. salina* were 207 and 406 μg/mL for the essential oil from fresh leaves isolated by hydro-distillation (HD) and solvent-free microwave extraction (SFME), respectively, while the oils produced by HD and SFME of the dried leaves yielded LC_{50} values of 277 and 669 μg/mL, respectively.

9. Phytochemistry

9.1 Volatile constituents

The volatile constituents have been investigated by various researchers. Essential oil isolated from leaves of *A. afra* by hydro-distillation (1.5% yield) was analysed by gas chromatography (GC) and gas chromatography–mass spectrometry (GC–MS). Essential oil from Ethiopia was reported to contain artemisyl acetate as the major constituent (24.4%–32.1% of the total oil) (Worku and Rubiolo, 1996) while 1,8-cineole (67.4%), terpinen-4-ol (6.5%) and borneol (5.1%) were found to dominate Kenyan oil (Mwangi et al., 1995). Graven et al. (1990) reported that 1,8-cineole (50.1%), α-thujone (74.9%–75.3%), β-thujone (21.5%–22.4%) and camphor (27.9%) were the major compounds in the essential oil isolated from *A. afra*. However, in a later study by Graven et al. (1992), α- and β-thujone (52%), camphor (15%), 1,8-cineole (13%) and α-pinene (2%) were found to be the major constituents of steam-distilled volatile oil. These studies reveal the existence of other chemotypes within wild populations of *A. afra*. Many different techniques have been applied to isolate volatile organic metabolites from *A. afra*. These include HD, microwave-assisted extraction (MAE), ultrasound-assisted extraction (UAE) and liquid/supercritical CO_2 extraction (l-CO_2 and SC-CO_2). The results indicated that l-CO_2 and SC-CO_2 were the most effective (3.2%, v/w yield), followed by traditional HD (1.5%, v/w) and MAE (1.3%, v/w). The lowest yield was obtained when using UAE (0.7%, v/w). Liu et al. (2009) identified 131 compounds in the essential oil of *A. afra*. Viljoen et al. (2006) analysed essential oils, isolated through HD of the aerial parts, using GC–MS. The composition of the essential oils from 16 individual plants, representing four natural populations, was exceptionally variable. However, 1,8-cineole, α-thujone, β-thujone, camphor and borneol featured as the main components in many cases, together with chrysanthenyl acetate and other sesquiterpenoids. Hydrodistilled volatile oils from the aerial parts of *A. afra* were investigated by Vagionas et al. (2007). They identified 37 compounds, representing 95.3% of the total oil. Camphor (46.2%), α-thujone (15.2%), artemisia ketone (7.4%) and 1,8-cineole (4.2%) were reported as the main oil components.

The impact of drying methods, namely air, sun and oven drying on the quality and quantity of the essential oil of *A. afra* was studied by Asekun et al. (2007). The drying method used had a pronounced effect on the amount of essential oil obtained, since fresh, oven-dried, air-dried and sun-dried oils yielded 0.18%, 0.88%, 1.54%, and 1.88% oil, respectively. The essential oils contained mostly monoterpenoids (84.0%–96.3%) and to a lesser extent, sesquiterpenoids (0.1%–2.6%). Compounds responsible for the unique flavour of the herb, namely α- and β-thujone (39.8%–52.1%), camphor (8.2%–14.4%), 1,8-cineole (13.1%–21.8%) and borneol (2.7%–7.8%), were present in significant amounts in the oils obtained from the dried herb. The fresh oil contained artemisia ketone (6.9%), which was absent in oils from the dried material. It was concluded that the drying method did not have a significant effect on the monoterpenoid composition of the essential oils, although sun drying resulted in the lowest number of components (14), obtained at the highest percentage oil yield. The effects of various drying methods on the yield and chemical composition of the essential oil of *A. afra* were also studied by Ashafa and Pitso (2014). Their results indicated a higher essential oil yield from fresh than from dried leaves. In total, 65 compounds were identified, of which monoterpenoids were the most prominent. β-Thujone (60.5%, 60.6%, 54.6% and 49.4%), α-thujone (18.1%, 16.9%, 15.1% and 12.5%), 1,8-cineole (8.9%, 7.7%, 7.2% and 7.4%) and chrysanthenyl acetate (6.9%, 10.3%, 10.0% and 9.4%) were the major components of the fresh, air-, sun- and oven-dried material, respectively. Microwave drying was the only technique that resulted in a substantial change to the major components of the oil. Following this process, an oil free of 1,8-cineole and β-thujone, which is known to be toxic, was obtained. The essential oils isolated from both fresh and dried leaves of *A. afra* were also investigated by Adeogun et al. (2018), using HD and SFME, combined with GC–MS analysis. The most abundant compound was thujone, of which 32.0 and 30.0% was obtained from fresh leaves by HD and SFME methods, respectively, and in dried leaf, which contained 26.6 and 25.8%, by HD and SFME methods, respectively. The compositions of essential oils, isolated by HD from twigs sourced from various locations in the Eastern Cape, Free State and KwaZulu-Natal provinces, were determined using both gas chromatography with flame ionisation detection (GC-FID) and GC–MS. α-Thujone was the major component of the essential oils from *A. afra* from Philippolis (Free State) and Keiskammahoek (Eastern Cape) (62%–74%). These oils contained only low levels of camphor (≤0.1%–0.6%). In contrast, oil samples from plants originating from Gqumahshe, Hogsback (Eastern Cape) and Empangeni (KwaZulu Natal) had a low α-thujone content (3.7%–20.0%), while 1,8-cineole (13.0%–49.5%) and camphor (13.9%–21.2%) were the main compounds (Oyedeji et al., 2009). This study confirmed that not all essential oils from *A. afra* contain high concentrations of α- and β-thujone.

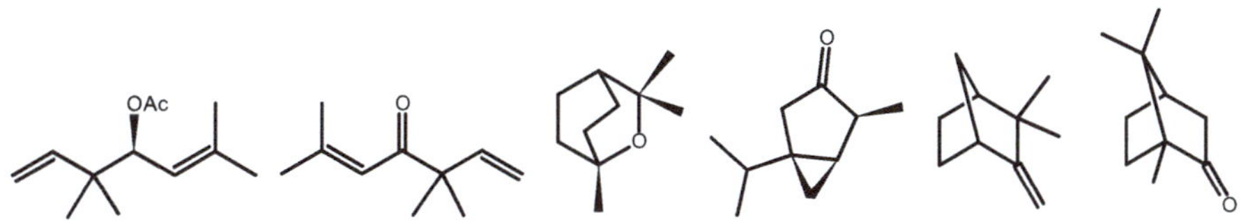

Artemisyl acetate Artemisia ketone 1,8-Cineole β-Thujone Camphene Camphor

9.2 Non-volatile constituents

Several coumarins have been isolated from *A. afra* (Bohlmann and Zdero, 1972). The flowerheads of the plant contain scopoletin, while the aerial parts contain umbelliferone derivatives. Silbernagel et al. (1990) isolated cerylcerotinate, a wax ester, the hydrocarbon nonacosane, and the triterpenes friedelin and α- and β-amyrin from the pentane leaf extract. A rapid and specific quantitative analytical method for the determination of flavonoids from the aerial parts was developed by Avula et al. (2009). Quantification of apigenin, chrysoeriol, tamarixetin, acacetin and genkwanin was described. *Artemisia afra* also afforded 10 new guaianolides and five glaucolides, as well as 12-hydroxy-α-cyperone (Jakupovic et al., 1988). High-field NMR spectroscopy and chemical transformations were used to elucidate their chemical structures. Isoalantolactone, a sesquiterpene lactone, was isolated from *A. afra* and the structure was confirmed using infrared (IR) spectroscopy, both 1D-and 2D-NMR, circular dichroism (CD) and mass spectrometry (Venables et al., 2016). Sequential extraction of the leaves with DCM, methanol, 50% aqueous ethanol and water at 50 °C and 100 °C, respectively, was used to identify polysaccharides in the leaves of *A. afra* (Braünlich et al., 2018). The monosaccharides were identified and linkage analyses were conducted for the relevant fractions. The extracts containing polysaccharides were purified by ion exchange chromatography, and further fractionated using gel filtration. Polysaccharides were found to be of the pectin type, with mostly structural features of arabinogalactan, rhamnogalacturonan and homogalacturonan. The presence of high levels of xylose as a monosaccharide constituent was highlighted as an unusual feature of some of these polysaccharides.

Sotenjwa et al. (2020) investigated chemical variation within the non-volatile constituents of *A. afra* samples representing 12 distinct populations, using ultra-performance liquid chromatography–mass spectrometry (UPLC–MS). Multivariate analysis revealed three groups, each characterised by marker compounds, which were isolated and identified using NMR spectroscopy, as the acacetin (Group 1), chrysoeriol (Group 2) and 3,5-di-*O*-caffeoylquinic acid and scopoletin (Group 3) groups. Rutin was also identified in the extracts. A high-performance thin-layer chromatography (HPTLC) method was described enabling retardation factors (R_f) and band colours, following derivatisation, to be used to identify marker compounds for quality control purposes. Chemical groupings within the samples were also confirmed using multivariate analysis of the data using an online application known as rTLC.

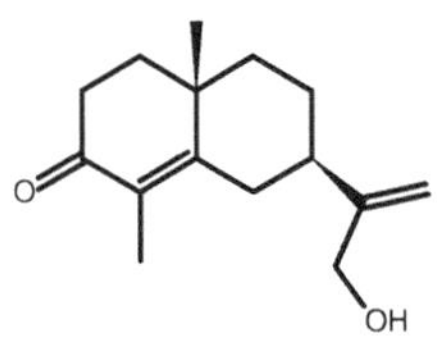

12-Hydroxy-α-cyperone

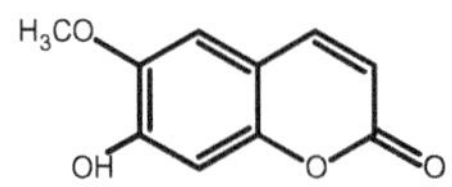

Scopoletin

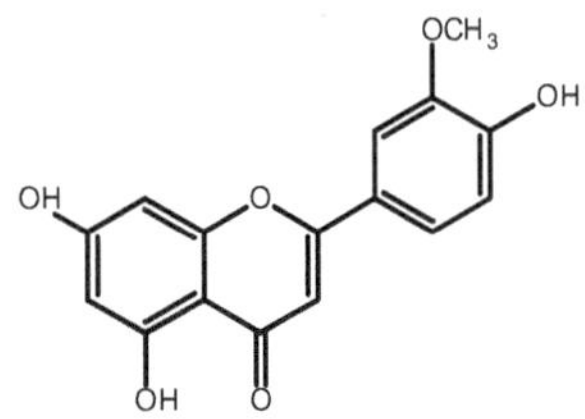

Chrysoeriol

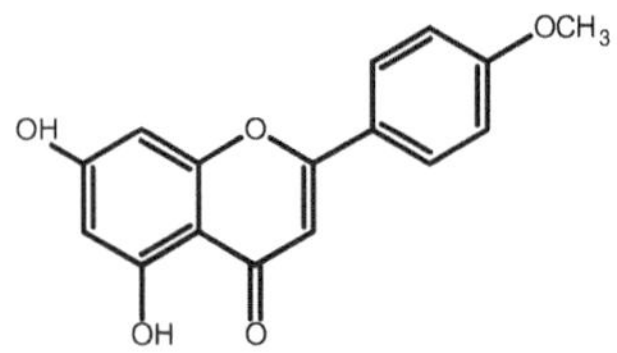

Acacetin

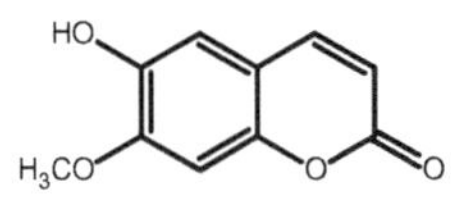

Iso-scopoletin

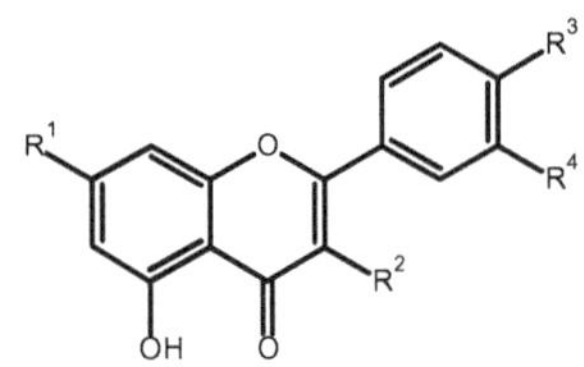

Rutin: R^1=OH, R^2=rutinoside, R^3=OH, R^4=OH

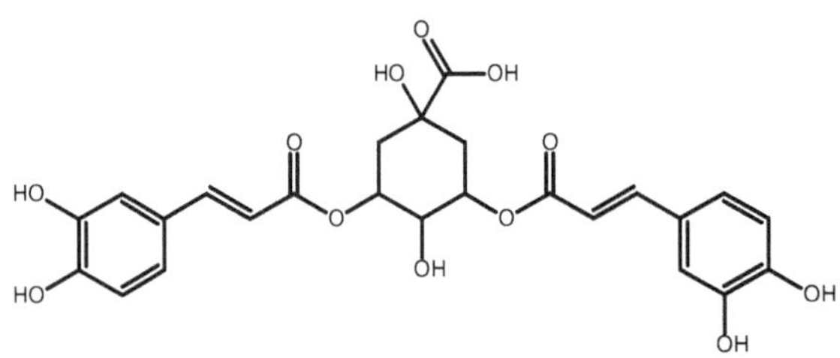

3,5-di-*O*-Caffeoylquinic acid

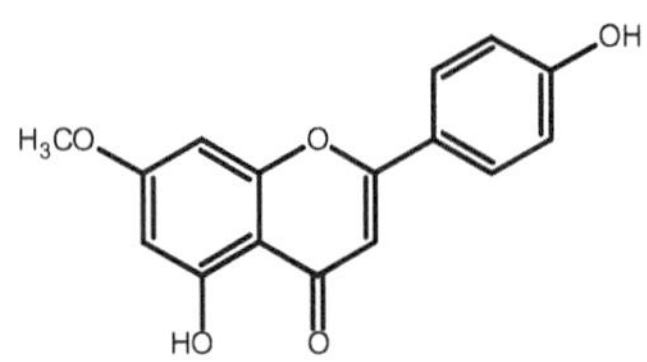

Iso-acacetin

Part B: Chemical profiling and quality control

10. Chromatography analysis

10.1 High-performance thin-layer chromatography (HPTLC) fingerprint analysis

General instrumentation: A CAMAG HPTLC instrument consisting of an automatic TLC sampler (ATS 4), automatic developing chamber (ADC 2), CAMAG TLC Visualiser 2, CAMAG derivatiser and TLC plate heater. *HPTLC plates*: Silica gel glass plates 60 F_{254} (Merck).

10.1.1 Non-volatile fraction analysis

Plant part: Aerial parts, 10% acetone:methanol extract. *Sample application*: Application volume of 2 µL extract (10 mg/mL) and 10 µL standard (1 mg/mL) spotted as 10 mm bands. Plates developed in a 20 × 10 × 4 cm glass twin-trough chamber to a migration distance of 80 mm. *Tank saturation*: 20 min at 15 °C and 40% RH, with 25 mL of mobile phase. *Mobile phase*: Ethyl acetate:water:formic acid (18:1:1, v/v/v). *Derivatisation*: Natural Product reagent (NPR) and polyethylene glycol reagent (PEGR). The plate was heated for 3 min at 100 °C on a TLC plate heater, sprayed with 3 mL of the NPR + PEGR (1:1, v/v) mixture, and then visualised. *Visualisation:* The plate was viewed under 366 nm radiation.

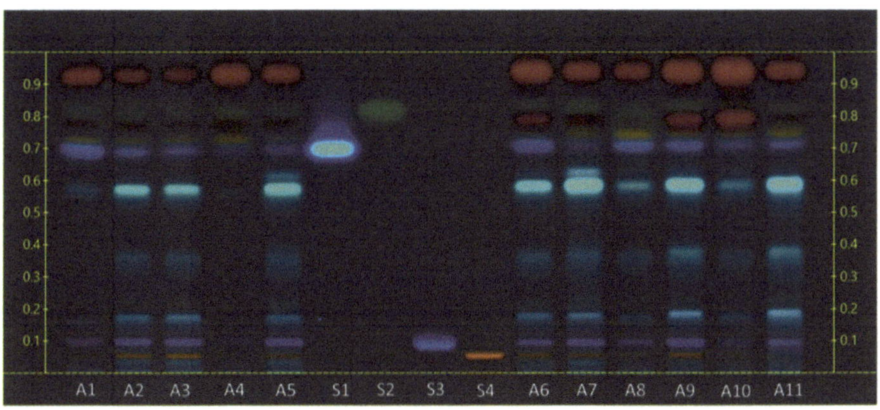

HPTLC plate of *Artemisa afra* extracts from various localities (A1–A5, A6–A11) and the standards (S1–S4). The samples are characterised by a dark blue band for scopoletin (S1) (R_f = 0.70), a yellow-green band for acacetin (S2) (R_f = 0.82), a dark blue band for scopolin (S3) (R_f = 0.10) and an orange band for rutin (S4) (R_f = 0.06).

10.1.2 Essential oil analysis

Plant part: Aerial parts, essential oil. *Sample application*: Application volume of 2 μL essential oil (25 μL/mL in toluene) spotted as 10 mm bands. Plates developed in a 20 × 10 × 4 cm glass twin-trough chamber to a migration distance of 70 mm. *Tank saturation*: 20 min at 15 °C and 40% RH, with 25 mL of mobile phase. *Mobile phase*: Toluene:ethyl acetate (90:10, v/v). *Derivatisation*: *p*-Anisaldehyde. The plate was sprayed with 3 mL of *p*-anisaldehyde reagent and heated on a TLC plate heater at 100 °C until colour developed. *Visualisation:* The plate was viewed under white reflectance light.

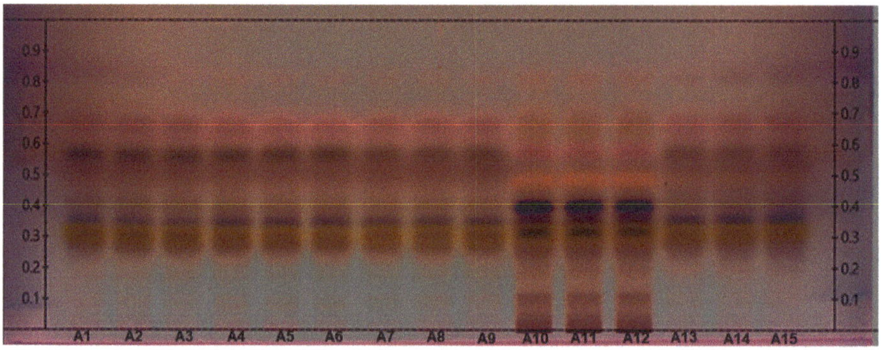

HPTLC plate of *Artemisa afra* essential oils from various localities (A1–A15). The samples are characterised by a yellowish-green band (R_f = 0.31) and a light blue band (R_f = 0.35). Variation was observed with samples A10–A12 showing a distinct dark blue band (R_f = 0.41), orange band (R_f = 0.49) and a pink band (R_f = 0.58) absent in other samples.

10.2 Ultra-performance liquid chromatography (UPLC) analysis

General instrumentation: Waters Acquity Ultra-Performance Liquid Chromatography system with photodiode array (PDA) detector combined with a Xevo G2QToF mass spectrometer (Waters, USA). *Plant part*: Aerial parts, acetone:methanol extract. *Sample application*: Injection volume: 1.0 μL (full-loop injection) at 1 mg/mL. *Column*: Acquity UPLC BEH C_{18} column (150 mm × 2.1 mm, i.d., 1.7 μm particle size, Waters). *Mobile phase*: 0.1% formic acid in water (solvent A) and acetonitrile (solvent B). *Analysis conditions*: Gradient elution at a flow rate of 0.35 mL/min, changing as follows: 80% A: 20% B to 40% A: 60% B in 13.5 min, to 0% A: 100% B within 2 min, keeping for 1 min and back to initial ratio, equilibrating the system for 2.0 min, total run time 18 min. *Mass spectrometry*: ESI^- (negative ionisation mode), N_2 used as desolvation gas, desolvation temperature 350 °C at a flow rate of 500 L/h and source temperature at 100 °C. Capillary and cone voltages, 2500 and 45 V, respectively. Data collected between *m/z* 100 and 1200.

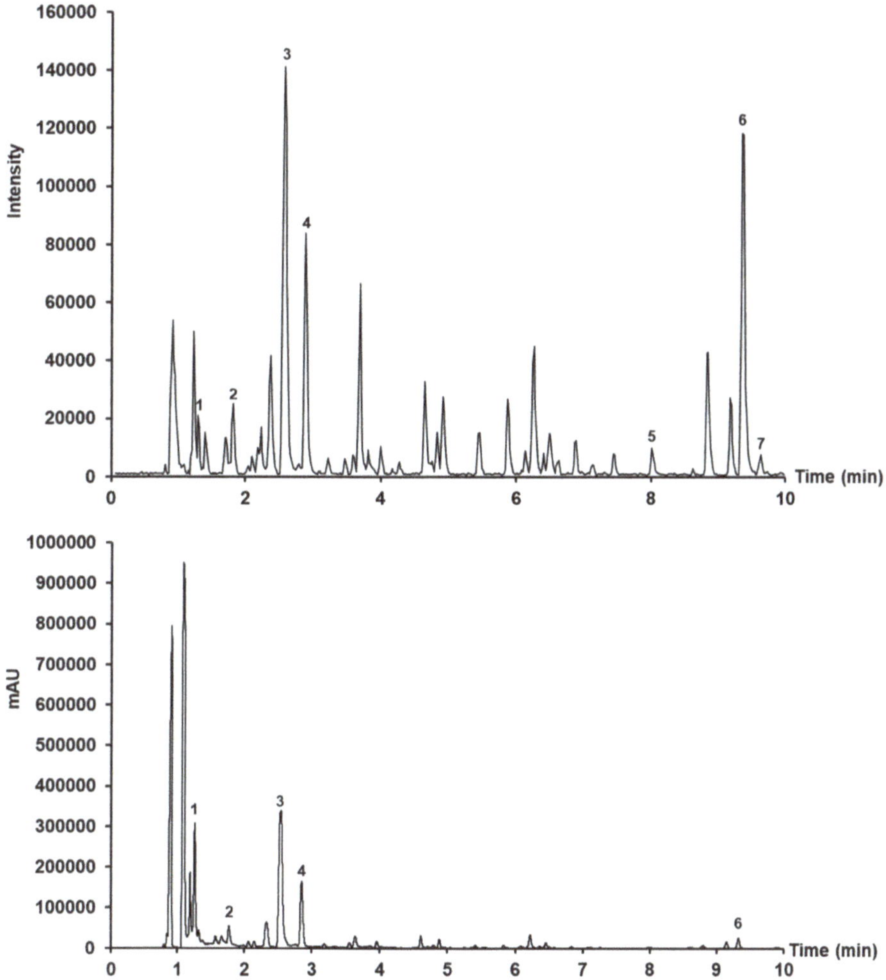

UPLC-ToF-MS ESI$^-$ (upper) and PDA (lower) chromatograms of *Artemisia afra* acetone:methanol extract. [1]=scopolin *m/z* 353.0874, [2]=rutin *m/z* 609.1456, [3]=scopoletin *m/z* 191.0559, [4]=3,5-di-*O*-caffeoylyquinic acid *m/z* 515.1190, [5]=chrysoeriol *m/z* 299.0556, [6]=acacetin *m/z* 283.0605, [7]=isoacacetin *m/z* 283.0607.

10.3 Gas chromatography (GC) analysis

General instrumentation: An Agilent 6860N chromatograph (Agilent Technologies, Hanova, USA) fitted with a flame ionisation detector (FID) and a mass spectrometer. *Plant part*: Aerial parts, essential oil. *Sample application*: Injection volume of 1 µL (split) at 20% (v/v) in hexane, split ratio: 1:200 and inlet temperature 250 °C. *Column*: HP-Innowax, 60 m × 250 µm × 0.25 µm (polyethylene glycol column, Agilent Technologies, Hanova, USA). *Analysis conditions*: Helium carrier gas, flow rate: 1.2 mL/min, pressure: 24.79 psi. Starting oven temperature at 60 °C and then rise to 220 °C at 4 °C/min, holding for 10 min and increased to 240 °C at 1 °C/min. *Mass spectrometry conditions*: Chromatograms obtained on electron impact at 70 eV using an Agilent 5973 mass selective detector, scanning range: *m/z* 35–550 (Agilent Technologies, Hanova, USA). *Identification*: Authentic standards, NIST® and Mass Finder®.

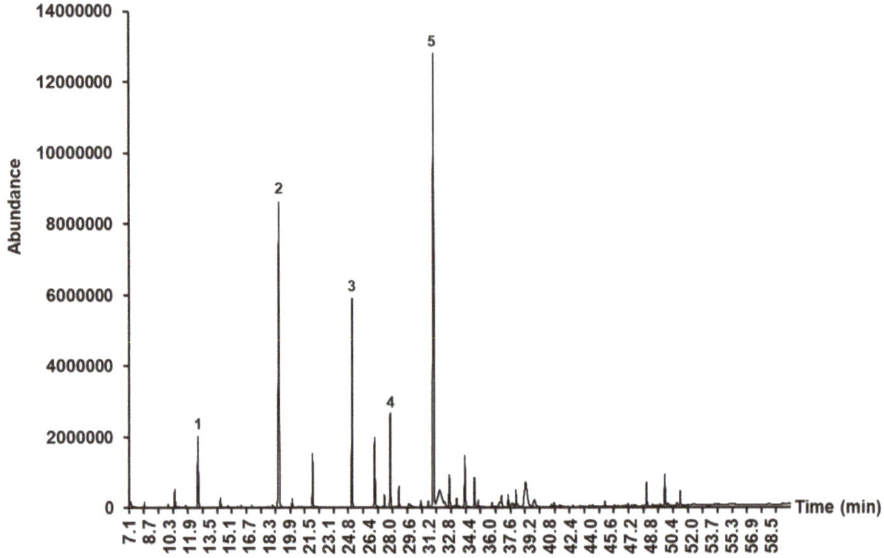

Total ion chromatogram (TIC) of *Artemisia afra* essential oil indicating major compounds. [1] = camphene (R_t 12.60, *m/z* 136.1252), [2] = 1,8-cineole (R_t 19.10, *m/z* 154.1357), [3] = artemisia ketone (R_t 25.05, *m/z* 152.1201), [4] = β-thujone (R_t 28.09, *m/z* 152.1201), [5] = camphor (R_t 31.53, *m/z* 152.1201).

11. Mid-infrared (MIR) spectroscopy analysis

General instrumentation: Alpha-P Bruker spectrometer, mounted with an attenuated total reflectance (ATR) diamond crystal. *Spectral acquisition*: Spectrum obtained in absorbance mode, with a spectral resolution of 4 cm^{-1} over the range 4000–550 cm^{-1} and captured using OPUS 6.5 software.

11.1 Powder analysis

Plant part: Aerial parts. *Sample preparation*: Aerial parts powdered, sieved (<500 μm) and placed directly onto the surface of the diamond crystal.

11.2 Essential oil analysis

Plant part: Aerial parts, essential oil. *Sample preparation*: Hydro-distillation to obtain essential oil, placed directly onto the surface of the diamond crystal.

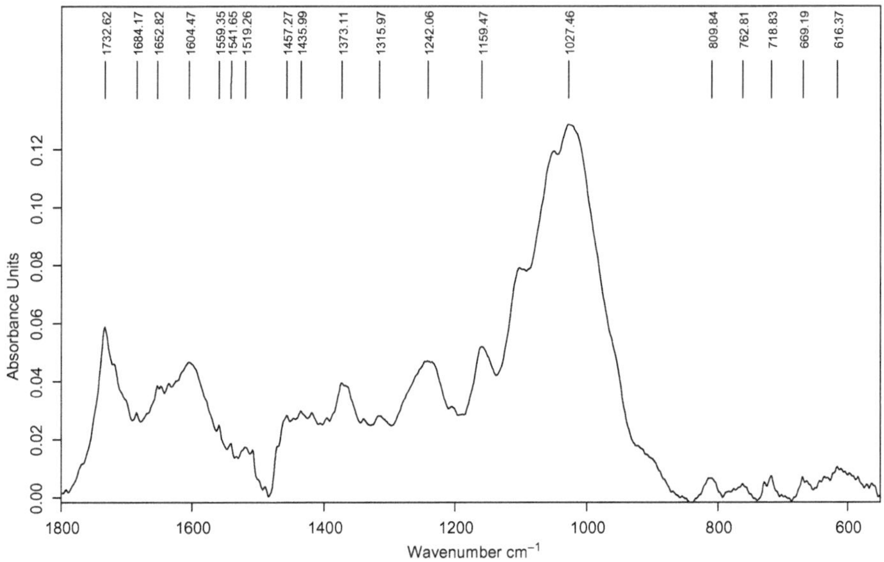

Mid-infrared spectrum of *Artemisia afra* powder displaying the fingerprint region (1800–550 cm^{-1}).

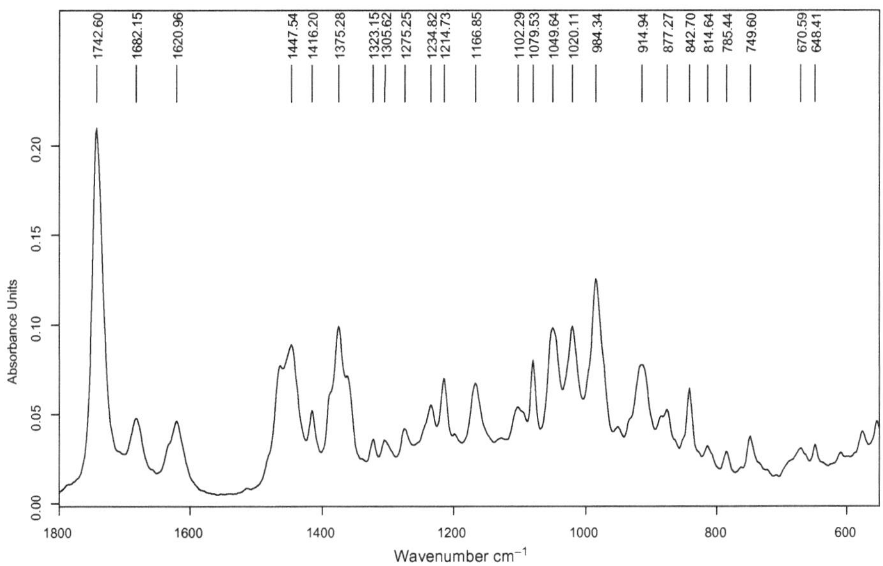

Mid-infrared spectrum of *Artemisia afra* essential oil displaying the fingerprint region (1800–550 cm^{-1}).

References

Adeogun, O.O., Maroyi, A., Afolayan, A.J., 2018. Trop. J. Pharm. Res., 17:519–528.

Afolayan, A.J., Sunmonu, T.O., 2011. Biosci. Biotechnol. Biochem., 75:2083–2086.

Afolayan, A.J., Sunmonu, T.O., 2012. Afr. J. Tradit. Complement. Altern. Med., 10:15–20.

Asekun, O.T., Grierson, D.S., Afolayan, A.J., 2007. J. Essent. Oil Bear. Plants, 10:5–9.

Ashafa, A.O.T., Pitso, T.R., 2014. J. Essent. Oil Bear. Plants, 17:1087–1093.

Avula, B., Wang, Y.-H., Smillie, T.J., Mabusela, W., Vincent, L., Weitz, F., Khan, I.A., 2009. J. AOAC Int., 92:633–644.

Bohlmann, F., Zdero, C., 1972. Phytochemistry, 11:2329–2330.

Braithwaite, M., Van Vuuren, S.F., Viljoen, A.M., 2008. J. Ethnopharmacol., 119:501–506.

Braünlich, P.M., Inngjerdingen, K.T., Inngjerdingen, M., Johnson, Q., Paulsen, B.S., Mabusela, W., 2018. Fitoterapia, 124:182–187.

Burits, M., Asres, K., Bucar, F., 2001. Phytother. Res., 15:103–108.

Buwa, L.V., Afolayan, A.J., 2009. Afr. J. Biotechnol., 8:6683–6687.

Charlson, A.J., 1980. J. Ethnopharmacol., 2:323–335.

Clarkson, C., Maharaj, V.J., Crouch, N.R., Grace, O.M., Pillay, P., Matsabisa, M.G., Bhagwandin, N., Smith, P.J., Folb, P.I., 2004. J. Ethnopharmacol., 92:177–191.

Fouché, G., Cragg, G.M., Pillay, P., Kolesnikova, N., Maharaj, V.J., Senabe, J., 2008. J. Ethnopharmacol., 119:455–461.

Germishuizen, G., Meyer, N.L., Steenkamp, Y., Keith, M., 2006. A Checklist of South African Plants. Southern African Botanical Diversity Network Report No. 41. SABONET, Pretoria, South Africa.

Graven, E.H., Webber, L., Venter, M., Gardner, J.B., 1990. J. Essent. Oil Res., 2:215–220.

Graven, E.H., Dean, S.G., Svoboda, K.P., Mavi, S., Gundidza, M.G., 1992. Flavour Fragr. J., 7:121–123.

Guantai, A.N., Addae-Mensah, I., 1999. Pharm. Biol., 37:351–356.

Hübsch, Z., Van Zyl, R.L., Cock, I.E., Van Vuuren, S.F., 2014. S. Afr. J. Bot., 93:185–197.

Jackson, W.P.U., 1990. Origins and Meanings of Names of South African Plant Genera. UCT Ecolab, Cape Town, South Africa.

Jakupovic, J., Klemeyer, H., Bohlmann, F., Graven, E.H., 1988. Phytochemistry, 27:1129–1133.

Liu, N.Q., Van der Kooy, F., Verpoorte, R., 2009. S. Afr. J. Bot., 75:185–195.

Liu, N.Q., Cao, M., Frédérich, M., Choi, Y.H., Verpoorte, R., Van der Kooy, F., 2010. J. Ethnopharmacol., 128:230–235.

Lubbe, A., Seibert, I., Klimkait, T., Van Der Kooy, F., 2012. J. Ethnopharmacol., 141:854–859.

Mangena, T., Muyima, N.Y.O., 1999. Lett. Appl. Microbiol., 28:291–296.

Masoko, P., Nxumalo, K.M., 2013. Evid. Based Complement. Alternat. Med., Art. No. 586247, https://doi.org/10.1155/2013/586247.

Mbokane, E.M., Moyo, N.A.G., 2018. Aquaculture, 482:197–202.

Mjiqiza, S.J., Syce, J.A., Obikeze, K.C., 2013. J. Ethnopharmacol., 149:648–655.

Molefe, N.I., Tsotetsi, A.M., Ashafa, A.O.T., Thekisoe, O.M.M., 2012. Bangl. J. Pharmacol., 7:157–163.

More, G., Lall, N., Hussein, A., Tshikalange, T.E., 2012. Evid. Based Complement. Alternat. Med., Art. No. 252758, https://doi.org/10.1155/2012/252758.

Moyo, P., Botha, M.E., Nondaba, S., Niemand, J., Maharaj, V.J., Eloff, J.N., Louw, A.I., Birkholtz, L., 2016. J. Ethnopharmacol., 185:235–242.

Mukinda, J.T., Syce, J.A., 2007. J. Ethnopharmacol., 112:138–144.

Mungho, T.C., Tobela, G.E., Olasunkanmi, A.O., Rufaro, S.-R.C., Omowumi, O.A., Oyehan, O.O., Ngwenchi, N.-C.B., 2018. Res. J. Biotechnol., 13:20–25.
Muyima, N.Y.O., Nkata, L., 2005. J. Essent. Oil Bear. Plants, 8:224–232.
Muyima, N.Y.O., Zulu, G., Bhengu, T., Popplewell, D., 2002. Flavour Fragr. J., 17:258–266.
Mwangi, J.W., Achola, K.J., Sinei, K.A., Lwande, W., Laurent, R., 1995. J. Essent. Oil Res., 7:97–99.
Naidoo, V., McGaw, L.J., Bisschop, S.P.R., Duncan, N., Eloff, J.N., 2008. Vet. Parasitol., 153:214–219.
Ntutela, S., Smith, P., Matika, L., Mukinda, J., Arendse, H., Allie, N., Estes, D.M., Mabusela, W., Folb, P., Steyn, L., Johnson, Q., Folk, W.R., Syce, J., Jacobs, M., 2009. Tuberculosis, 89:S33–S40.
Oyedeji, A.O., Afolayan, A.J., Hutchings, A., 2009. Nat. Prod. Commun., 4:849–852.
Rabe, T., Van Staden, J., 1997. J. Ethnopharmacol., 56:81–87.
Roberts, M., 1990. Indigenous Healing Plants. Southern Book Publishers, Halfway House, South Africa.
Rood, B., 1994. Uit die Veldapteek. Tafeberg Publishers, Cape Town, South Africa.
Silbernagel, E., Spreitzer, H., Buchbauer, G., 1990. Monats. Chem. Chem. Mon., 121:433–436.
Spies, L., Koekemoer, T.C., Sowemimo, A.A., Goosen, E.D., Van de Venter, M., 2013. S. Afr. J. Bot., 84:104–109.
Sotenjwa, V.Z., Chen, W., Veale, C.G.L., Anokwuru, C.P., Tankeu, S.Y., Combrinck, S., Kamatou, G.P.P., Viljoen, A.M., 2020. Fitoterapia, 147:104740.
Stafford, G.I., Jäger, A.K., Van Staden, J., 2005. J. Ethnopharmacol., 100:210–215.
Suliman, S., Van Vuuren, S.F., Viljoen, A.M., 2010. S. Afr. J. Bot., 76:655–661.
Sunmonu, T.O., Afolayan, A.J., 2010. Food Chem. Toxicol., 48:1969–1972.
Sunmonu, T.O., Afolayan, A.J., 2012. Pak. J. Nutr., 11:520–525.
Sunmonu, T.O., Afolayan, A.J., 2013. Evid. Based Complement. Alternat. Med., Art. No. 929074, https://doi.org/10.1155/2013/929074.
The Merck Index, 1989. 11th ed. Merck & Co., Inc., Rahway, New Jersey, USA.
Tisserand, R., Balacs, T., 1995. Essential Oil Safety: A Guide for Health Care Professionals. Churchill Livingstone, Edinburgh, Scotland, pp. 199–200.
Treurnicht, F.T., 1997. An Evaluation of the Toxic and Potential Antiviral Effects of some Plants used by South Africans for Medicinal Purposes. M.Sc. dissertation, University of Stellenbosch, Stellenbosch, South Africa.
Vagionas, K., Graikou, K., Chinou, I.B., Runyoro, D., Ngassapa, O., 2007. J. Essent. Oil Res., 19:396–400.
Van Vuuren, S., Muhlarhi, T., 2017. S. Afr. J. Bot., 112:186–192.
Van Wyk, B.E., Van Oudtshoorn, B., Gericke, N., 2009. Medicinal Plants of South Africa, third ed. Briza Publications, Pretoria, South Africa.
Venables, L., Koekemoer, T.C., Van de Venter, M., Goosen, E.D., 2016. S. Afr. J. Bot., 103:216–221.
Viljoen, A.M., Van Vuuren, S.F., Gwebu, T., Demirci, B., Başer, K.H.C., 2006. J. Essent. Oil Res., 18:19–25.
Watt, J.M., Breyer-Brandwijk, M.G., 1962. The Medicinal and Poisonous Plants of Southern and Eastern Africa, second ed. E. & S. Livingstone Ltd, Edinburgh and London, UK.
Worku, T., Rubiolo, P., 1996. J. Essent. Oil Res., 8:355–357.

CHAPTER

Aspalathus linearis

5

Elizabeth Joubert[a], Gerda Fouche[b], Ilze Vermaak[c,d], Nduvho Mulaudzi[c] and Weiyang Chen[c]

[a]*Plant Bioactives Group, Post-Harvest and Agro-Processing Technologies, Agricultural Research Council (Infruitec Nietvoorbij), Stellenbosch, South Africa*

[b]*Chemistry Department, University of Pretoria, Pretoria, South Africa*

[c]*Department of Pharmaceutical Sciences, Tshwane University of Technology, Pretoria, South Africa*

[d]*SAMRC Herbal Drugs Research Unit, Faculty of Science, Tshwane University of Technology, Pretoria, South Africa*

Abstract

Aspalathus linearis (Burm.f) R.Dahlgren, commonly referred to as 'rooibos tea', is the best-known indigenous South African herbal tea. It is considered the success story of indigenous product development and marketing, and it is a prime export product, marketed globally. Rooibos is endemic to the Fynbos Biome and is found in the far southwestern part (Nieuwoudtville) of the Northern Cape Province, but chiefly in the Citrusdal and Clanwilliam regions (Cederberg area) of the Western Cape Province. Rooibos tea is anecdotally consumed to relieve colic, indigestion, heartburn and nausea. It also reduces nervous tension, promotes sound sleep and improves appetite. Rooibos extracts are included as anti-oxidant in a wide range of nutraceutical products. The use of rooibos extract in products for topical application for a range of dermatological issues and in a collection of skin-care products is well-established in South Africa. The 'fermentation' process is important for the development of the characteristic aroma, flavour and colour of the 'traditional' tea product, notable for its red–brown colour. The phytochemistry of rooibos tea has been extensively investigated, especially with regard to the aspalathin (dihydrochalcone) content and that of other major flavonoids, and the quantitative differences between unfermented (green) and fermented rooibos. Much has been documented concerning the anti-oxidant activity of rooibos tea and its role in alleviating oxidative stress. The potential of rooibos, in particular green rooibos extract and aspalathin, in the prevention of metabolic syndrome has been the focus of many studies. Other investigations include antispasmodic, anticancer, bone health and antistress activities. High-performance liquid chromatography (HPLC) with diode array detection (DAD) has been used extensively for the quantification of aspalathin, other major flavonoids and Z-2-(β-D-glucopyranosyloxy)-3-phenylpropenoic acid in rooibos. Other techniques, such as semi-automated high-performance thin-layer chromatography (HPTLC), ultra-performance liquid chromatography coupled to mass spectrometry (UPLC–MS), and mid-infrared (MIR) spectroscopy, were used to determine the chemical profiles of rooibos tea.

The South African Herbal Pharmacopoeia. https://doi.org/10.1016/B978-0-323-99794-2.00001-5

Keywords: *Aspalathus linearis*, Rooibos tea, Fermentation, Aspalathin, Flavonoids, HPLC–DAD, HPTLC, UPLC–MS, MIR spectroscopy

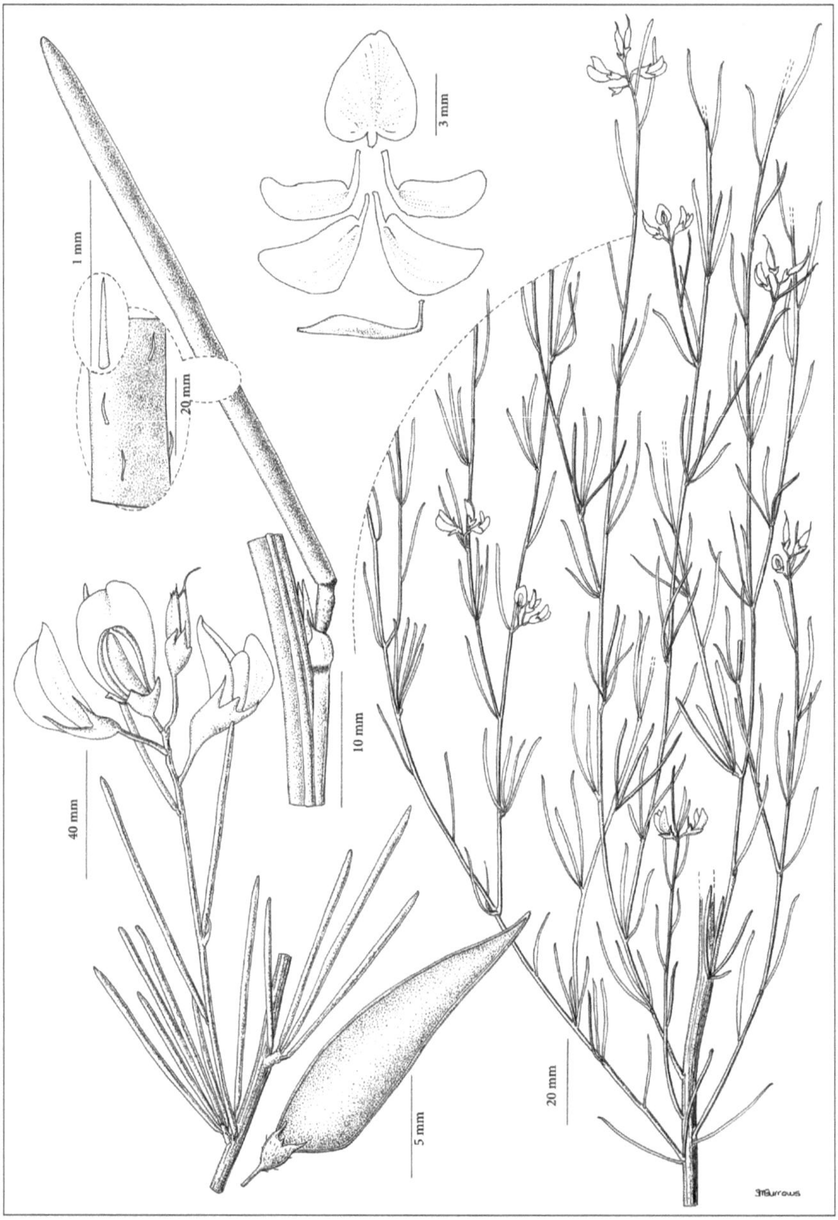

Part A: General overview

1. Synonyms

Aspalathus linearis (Burm.f.) R.Dahlgren subsp. *pinifolia* (Marloth) R.Dahlgren, *Aspalathus cognata* C.Presl, *Aspalathus corymbosa* E.Mey., *Aspalathus tenuifolia* DC., *Borbonia pinifolia* Marloth, *Lebeckia linearis* (Burm.f.) DC., *Psoralea linearis* Burm.f.[a]

2. Common name(s)

Rooibos tea, Red tea, Koopman's tea, bush tea, veld tea; '*rooibostee*', '*bossietee*', '*naalde tee*', '*maktee*', '*spelde tee*', '*swart tee*', '*rooibossie*', '*rooi tee*', '*sprinkaan tee*' (Afrikaans).[a]

3. Conservation status

Least concern.[a]

4. Botany

Aspalathus linearis (Burm.f.) R.Dahlgren, indigenous to the Cape Floristic Region, is one of more than 270 species of the genus *Aspalathus* (Family Fabaceae, Tribe Crotalarieae). Until recently, it was the only reported source of aspalathin, a *C*-glucosyl dihydrochalcone. Stander et al. (2017) determined that *Aspalathus pendula* R.Dahlgren, a closely related species, also contains aspalathin. The genus name *Aspalathus* is derived from '*aspalathos*' (Greek), the name of a scented bush that grew in Greece, and the epithet '*linearis*' (Latin) meaning linear, referring to the leaf shape. *Aspalathus* L. is the largest genus of Fabaceae in South Africa. *Aspalathus linearis* is an erect, highly variable shrub or shrublet up to 2 m high, with green, needle-like leaves (15–60 mm long and up to about 1 mm thick) on straight, slender branches (A). The leaves are without stalks and stipules and may be densely clustered (C). The young branches are often reddish. The small, yellow flowers of the cultivated type appear in spring to early summer (D). They are solitary, or arranged in groups, at the tips of branches. The fruit is a small lance-shaped pod, usually containing one to two hard seeds. The aerial parts of *A. linearis* in the unfermented (unoxidised; known as green rooibos) or fermented (oxidised) forms have commercial value (B) as herbal tea and for the production of extracts. The species is exceptionally polymorphic, with ecotypes differing in morphology and fire survival strategy (reseeding

[a] Red List of South African Plants (http://redlist.sanbi.org).

or resprouting). Seven new species of *Aspalathus* from South Africa were recently described by Stirton and Muasya (2016): *A. eriocephaloides* C.H.Stirt. & Muasya, *A. eustonbrownii* C.H.Stirt. & Muasya and *A. nickhelmei* C.H.Stirt. & Muasya from the Western Cape Province; *A. dahlgrenii* C.H.Stirt. & Muasya and *A. spinifera* C.H.Stirt. & Muasya from KwaZulu Natal Province; and *A. modesta* C.H.Stirt. & Muasya and *A. usnoides* C.H.Stirt. & Muasya from the Eastern Cape Province. New distribution records were added for the rare and little-known species, *A. macrocarpa* Eckl. & Zeyh. and *A. barbigera* R.Dahlgren, and conservation statuses were re-assessed.

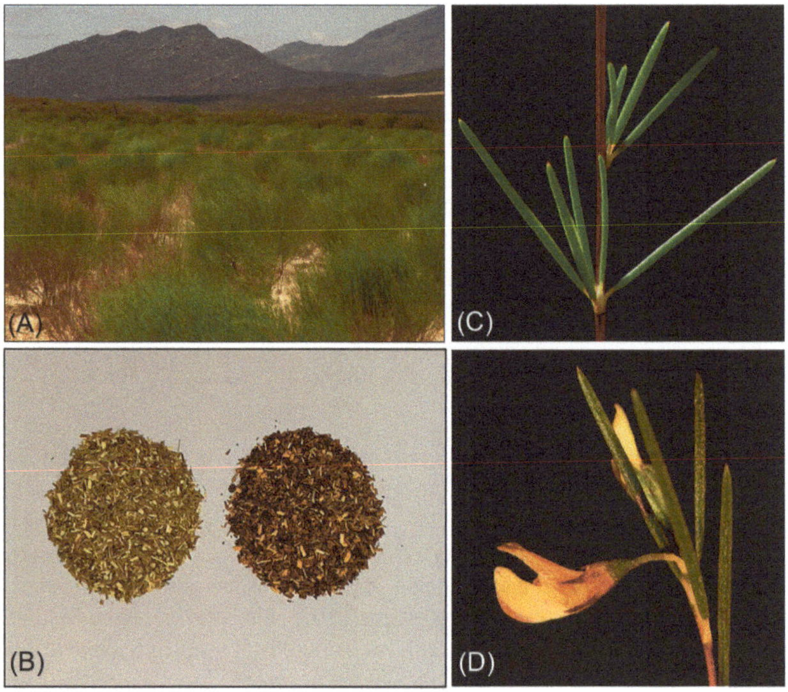

Aspalathus linearis shrub (A) with straight, slender reddish branches (C) and small, yellow flowers (D). Aerial parts are commercialised in unfermented (unoxidised) or fermented (oxidised) forms (B).

5. Geographical distribution

Aspalathus linearis has a narrow geographic distribution and is endemic to the Fynbos Biome of the Cape Floristic Region. It is naturally distributed from about Vanrhynsdorp and Nieuwoudtville in the north, to the Cape Peninsula and the Betty's Bay area in the south (Dahlgren, 1968). This area typically has cold, wet winters, with about 300–350 mm of rain per annum, and a hot and dry summer season. The rooibos plant is naturally found and cultivated in the Northern Cape Province, specifically Nieuwoudtville and the Bokkeveld plateau on the border with the Western Cape Province. This small geographical region provides the ideal environment for the cultivation of rooibos due to its Mediterranean climate and deep, coarse, acidic sandy soils. Temperatures range from 0 °C in the winter months to 45 °C in summer, with an annual rainfall of 200–450 mm. Compared to the Nieuwoudtville area, the Clanwilliam and Citrusdal areas, situated at a lower elevation, have higher average minimum and maximum daily temperatures. Rooibos is a hardy dry land crop and it is often exposed to drought conditions, as no irrigation is applied. The plant survives due to its tap root that extends down 3 m or more into the well-drained, cool and sandy soil.

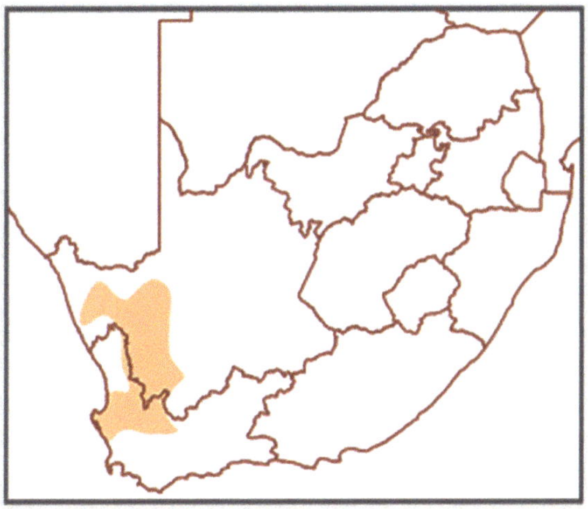

Geographical distribution of *Aspalathus linearis* in South Africa.

6. Ethnopharmacology

The Swedish botanist Carl Thunberg noted the use of *Bordonia cordata* as tea during his travels in the interior of the Cape of Good Hope (1772–75). According to Van Wyk and Gorelik (2017), 'this anecdote is sometimes uncritically cited and erroneously associated with rooibos tea (*A. linearis*)'. Marloth (1917) indicated several sources of wild teas. His entry for rooibos tea reads: 'Rooibos tee, Rooi tee, Naald tee or Koopman's tee, is *Borbonia pinifolia*; a small shrublet of the Olifant's river and Cedarberg mountains. The twigs and leaves are cut up and fermented like the *Cyclopia* plant. A pleasant beverage, especially in hot weather, free from tannin and stimulating ingredients'. He also gave the name 'spelde tee' as a synonym of 'rooi tee', the Afrikaans for 'red tea'. Although several authors have assumed that rooibos tea originated from the local inhabitants of the Cederberg, there are unfortunately no earlier ethnobotanical records, and no Khoi or San vernacular names have ever been recorded. Statements saying that rooibos tea is a traditional drink of Khoi-descended people of the Cederberg and 'poor whites' are correct. However, this tradition could not be traced back further than the last quarter of the 19th century (Van Wyk and Gorelik, 2017). The traditional processing method of rooibos tea was reported to be through beating the material on a flat rock in an area where there is a slight depression. A heavy wooden pole or club, such as a stump of the sand olive (*Dodonaea viscosa*), or a large wooden hammer usually made from wild olive wood (*Olea europaea* subsp. *africana*), was used. It is reported that rooibos is used for the treatment of allergy, stomach cramps, eczema, nappy rash, chest troubles, constipation, heartburn and as an appetite stimulant, while an infusion with '*jantjiebêrend*' is used to treat high blood pressure (Nortje and Van Wyk, 2015). It was the discovery in the 1960s that rooibos tea contributes considerably to calm and convalesce a colicky baby that stimulated interest in rooibos tea as a 'healthy' drink for the modern consumer.

7. Commercialisation

A merchant of Clanwilliam, Benjamin Ginsberg, was the first person to realise the commercial potential and started marketing rooibos as a herbal tea in 1904. He obtained the tea from descendants of the Khoi, who crudely processed it during the warm summer months. Seed selection and improved cultivation and processing started in the 1920s. The agricultural value of rooibos was only recognised in 1930 by a medical practitioner and nature lover, P. Le Fras Nortier of Clanwilliam. His early cultivation experiments, carried out with the help of local farmers, O. Bergh and H. Riordan, laid the foundation for the industry (Joubert and De Beer, 2011). Other farmers in the area started to participate in rooibos production, mainly concentrated in the Clanwilliam area. Since large-scale expansion in later years, due to growing demand, has threatened the biodiversity of the Greater Cederberg Biodiversity Corridor, the South African Rooibos Council, in partnership with CapeNature, formed the Rooibos Biodiversity Initiative (Pretorius, 2007). In the early years, different *Aspalathus* species and ecotypes, naturally occurring in the Cederberg area, were used to produce rooibos tea. For commercial cultivation, only the Rocklands/Nortier variety of rooibos has been selected for use (Wynberg, 2017). The red type is divided into the selected, improved Nortier type, and the Cederberg type (wild growing). Tea is also sometimes made from small quantities of a closely related species, *A. pendula* R.Dahlgren, and several wild types of *A. linearis* (Van Heerden et al., 2003). The grey, black and red–brown types were harvested in the wild, processed, and sold to the Rooibos Tea Control Board until 1966, after which the marketing of the grey and black types was discontinued due to poor quality. A recent assessment of wild types demonstrated morphological (Malgas et al., 2010), genetic (Malgas et al., 2010), chemical (Van Heerden et al., 2003) and ecological (Hawkins et al., 2011) variation. Differences in the phenolic profiles of the wild types can be attributed to genetics, and may be useful in developing regional products such as Wupperthal tea and Heiveld tea. Wild rooibos comprises only a small percentage of annual production (Joubert and De Beer, 2011).

The early years of the industry saw a growing demand, due to a shortage of black tea (*Camellia sinensis*) as a result of the Second World War, followed by the market collapse in the years after the war. Total sales were only 524 tonnes in 1955. When one-channel marketing was abolished on 1 October 1993, total sales had reached in excess of 4000 tonnes. The entry of new marketing companies and access to new markets resulted in strong growth in sales during subsequent years, due to steady growth in the domestic market and expansion of global markets. Organic production of rooibos, as well as the demand for green rooibos, is still small in relation to conventional rooibos (Joubert and De Beer, 2011). Rooibos tea constitutes less than 0.3% of the global tea market, but it represents 10% of the growing herbal tea market, and 30.9% of the South African tea market (Wynberg, 2017). A recent addition of the designation 'Rooibos' to the register of the European Union of Protected Designations of Origin and Protected Geographical Indications not only offers ownership of this particular name to South Africa, but it will ensure that the term will be applicable only to rooibos products.

With the continued growth in the popularity of rooibos, the need to profile the aroma and flavour of rooibos has become essential to ensure effective quality control, exploit niche markets, and support rooibos as a geographical indicator. The characteristic aroma notes of fermented rooibos are 'rooibos-woody', 'fynbos-floral', and 'honey', with 'fruity-sweet', 'caramel', and 'apricot' present in many production batches (Koch et al., 2012; Jolley et al., 2017). At low intensity, the 'hay/dried grass' aroma note is also considered to be part of the characteristic aroma profile of rooibos, but at high intensity, it is detrimental to quality. Steam pasteurisation of fermented rooibos leaves and stems, a processing step introduced in the 1980s to ensure a microbially safe product, changed the sensory profile slightly, i.e. the infusions were slightly less astringent and the intensities of most of the aroma and flavour attributes decreased. 'Green' and 'caramel' notes exhibited the largest reductions in intensity (Koch et al., 2013). Cold-brewing of rooibos has recently gained popularity in Japan. In a study on the effect of the brewing procedure on the sensory profile of rooibos tea, the tea was prepared by infusing the leaves for 8 h in cold water ($<5\,^{\circ}C$) (cold brew), freshly boiled water for 5 min (regular brew), or boiling for 5 min (boiled brew). It was found that the method did not have an effect on the intensities of some of the primary aroma attributes ('rooibos-woody', 'fynbos-floral' and 'honey') of fermented rooibos. The cold-brewed fermented rooibos samples tasted sweeter and less astringent than the regular- and boiled-brewed teas. The impact of the brewing procedure on the sensory profile of green rooibos, dominated by a 'hay/dried grass' aroma, bitter taste and astringency, was greater than for fermented rooibos, but mostly, cold and regular brews had similar aroma attribute intensities (Muller et al., 2020).

The first value addition of rooibos was the use of a fermented rooibos extract in cosmetic care products (Joubert and Schulz, 2006), first sold in the South African market, but later distributed more widely. Published scientific studies dealing with the topical/cosmetic application of rooibos extract are very limited. Changing consumer attitudes towards natural products and their role in health and wellness created a market for other value-added products. This led to the addition of fermented rooibos extract to yogurt, drinking yogurt, bread and other food products. However, the most successful and enduring products are the convenience beverage products, the ready-to-drink (RTD) rooibos iced teas, instant rooibos tea, and 'instant rooibos cappuccino', a formulated ready-to-use powdered product.

8. Pharmacological evaluation

Rooibos flavonoids are implicated, or either confirmed, to play an integral role in the bioactivity and pharmacological effects of rooibos. Of these compounds, aspalathin has been studied in depth to gain insight into the ability of rooibos extracts, in particular green rooibos extracts that contain high levels of the compound, to modulate the metabolic syndrome. In this section, the focus will fall predominantly on extracts. A few studies on compounds will be highlighted. No distinction will be made between hot water extract and infusion when discussing testing performed *in vitro*. Aqueous extracts and infusions were prepared by boiling or steeping of the plant material in hot water. Preparation procedures varied between studies. Japanese studies mostly used much lower solid-to-solvent ratios for the preparation of infusions (Joubert et al., 2008a). If no reference is made to the 'fermentation' (oxidation) status of the plant material (green *vs* fermented), it was not stated in the paper, but it was most likely fermented rooibos. Many studies did not report the phenolic composition of the extracts and infusions.

Several reviews have dealt with studies evaluating the pharmacological potential of rooibos extracts and the flavonoid constituents, some providing an overview of the many studies (McKay and Blumberg, 2007; Joubert et al., 2008a; Chaudhary et al., 2021). Reviews by Marnewick and co-workers concentrated on *in vivo* and *in vitro* anti-oxidant activity and oxidative stress-induced conditions (Marnewick, 2014; Ajuwon et al., 2015). Others focused on cardiovascular disease (CVD) (Smith and Swart, 2018; Windvogel, 2019; Maarman, 2019), cardioprotective effects relating to hyperglycaemia-induced injury (Dludla et al., 2017), metabolic syndrome (Muller et al., 2018; Johnson et al., 2018) and ovarian health (Sirotkin, 2021). Sasaki et al. (2018) made a systematic review and meta-analysis of the beneficial role of rooibos in diabetes mellitus. Bond and Derbyshire (2020) wrote a systematic review of rooibos tea and health, encompassing evidence from the last two decades. The main body of research focused on the role of rooibos in protecting against the detrimental effects of oxidative stress (as this is an underlying cause of many diseases) and in modulating the metabolic syndrome.

8.1 *In vitro* and *ex vivo* studies

8.1.1 Anti-oxidant activity

The general interest and hype around anti-oxidants as 'anti-ageing' phytochemicals in the 1990s occasioned the first studies by Japanese researchers on the ability of fermented rooibos to neutralise reactive oxygen species (ROS) (Yoshikawa et al., 1990;

Ito et al., 1991). Prompted by their findings, the rooibos industry initiated South African research on the anti-oxidant activity of rooibos and compounds. Extracts from green rooibos, prepared for the first time, and specifically to demonstrate the effect of fermentation of the plant material on its anti-oxidant activity (Von Gadow et al., 1997a), were shown to be more effective than extracts from fermented rooibos, an outcome explained by the substantially higher levels of aspalathin and its relative potency (Von Gadow et al., 1997b). These outcomes formed the basis for commercialisation of green rooibos, and patenting of a vacuum drying process for the production of green rooibos. Other studies followed, highlighting the effects of processing of the plant material, the role of aspalathin in the higher anti-oxidant (Standley et al., 2001; Schulz et al., 2003; Joubert et al., 2004) and pro-oxidant (Joubert et al., 2005) activity of green rooibos compared to fermented rooibos, and the anti-oxidant activity of aspalathin in relation to its flavanone and flavone oxidation products (Snijman et al., 2009; Krafczyk et al., 2009a). Xue et al. (2020) made use of the density functional theory to provide insight into the radical scavenging mechanism of aspalathin. A study of a large number of green rooibos samples showed a linear relationship between the total anti-oxidant capacity of their extracts and aspalathin content (Joubert et al., 2008b). Several reviews covered details of the early and other studies on the anti-oxidant activity of rooibos and aspalathin (Joubert and Schulz, 2006; Joubert et al., 2008a; Joubert and De Beer, 2014; Chaudhary et al., 2021). Literature abounds with studies on the anti-oxidant capacity of various plant extracts that include rooibos for comparative purposes.

Of physiological importance is the ability of rooibos to protect against ROS and its effect on anti-oxidant enzymes in a cellular or subcellular environment. Rooibos extract protected human polymorphonuclear leucocytes against superoxide anion and hydroxyl radicals (Yoshikawa et al., 1990). It also protected mouse L5178Y cells against H_2O_2-induced oxidative stress (Ito et al., 1991). Hitomi et al. (1999) made use of rabbit erythrocyte membrane, rat liver microsome and rat liver homogenate to show that rooibos may help to prevent lipid peroxidation of cell membranes. Inhibition of peroxide-induced hemolysis of Japanese quail erythrocytes by rooibos served as a model for its ability to protect biomembranes against oxidative damage (Simon et al., 2000). Hot water and a 75% ethanolic rooibos extract dose-dependently inhibited peroxyl radical-induced DNA strand scission (Lee and Jang, 2004). The viability of Chinese hamster lung fibroblast V79-4 cells subjected to H_2O_2-induced oxidative stress was increased by rooibos extract, a protective effect linked to increased activity of the anti-oxidant enzymes, superoxide dismutase (SOD) and catalase (CAT) (Yoo et al., 2008). Human red blood cells, pretreated with rooibos extract, were less prone to oxidation when exposed to the free radical-generating azo compound, 2,2′-azobis(2-amidinopropane) dihydrochloride (AAPH) (Blasa et al., 2011). Lawal et al. (2019) showed that pretreatment of human umbilical vein endothelial cells (HUVECs) with green and fermented rooibos extracts reduced ROS production caused by air pollutants, i.e. diesel exhaust particles. Other indices of oxidative stress in the particle-exposed HUVECs, i.e. increased thiobarbituric acid reactive substances (TBARS), conjugated diene and carbonyl protein levels, and reduced glutathione redox status (GSH:GSSG), were also modulated by the rooibos extracts. Xiao et al. (2020) concluded that rooibos reduced Fe^{3+}-induced oxidative stress in rat liver homogenates, as evidenced by reduced malondialdehyde (MDA) levels, and increased reduced glutathione (GSH) levels and SOD and CAT activity.

The ROS-scavenging ability of rooibos extract was also investigated in *in vitro* disease models. Rooibos extract reduced ROS levels and increased SOD and CAT activities dose-dependently in hyperglycaemia-induced HUVECs (for diabetes) and HeLa cells (for cancer) (Waisundara and Hoon, 2015). A number of other studies focused on the protective effect of rooibos, aspalathin and another rare rooibos compound, Z-2-(β-D-glucopyranosyloxy)-3-phenylpropenoic acid (PPAG), to counteract oxidative stress relating to hyperglycaemia and diabetes. These studies focused on cardiomyocytes exposed to high glucose concentrations (Dludla et al., 2014, 2016, 2020a,b). Aspalathin protected the β-cell line, Insulinoma IE (INS-1E), against ROS, induced by streptozotocin (STZ) or H_2O_2 (Moens et al., 2020). However, PPAG was ineffective in decreasing superoxide anion radical generation by STZ in the same model (Himpe et al., 2016).

8.1.2 Ameliorative effects on risk factors of metabolic syndrome

A large body of studies, using cell models that address elements related to diabetes, obesity and metabolic syndrome, has been published to date. The metabolic syndrome is a cluster of interrelated pathophysiological features, including insulin resistance, obesity, dyslipidaemia, hyperglycaemia and chronic inflammation that increase the risk for CVD and type 2 diabetes. Two comprehensive reviews have covered the potential of rooibos extracts, in particular green rooibos extract, and the compounds, aspalathin and PPAG (Muller et al., 2018; Johnson et al., 2018). A review by Dludla et al. (2017) focused specifically on the protection of the diabetic heart at risk from hyperglycaemia-induced injury. These reviews also provide insight into mechanisms explaining the effect of rooibos and compounds on glucose and lipid metabolism.

New *in vitro* studies published since, elucidated further the protective role of rooibos extract, aspalathin and PPAG, on risk factors of the metabolic syndrome and the mechanisms involved. Following studies showed that an aspalathin-enriched green rooibos extract (18.4% aspalathin) reversed palmitate-induced insulin resistance in C2C12 skeletal muscle cells and 3T3-L1 adipocytes (as reviewed by Muller et al., 2018). Mazibuko-Mbeje et al. (2019a) reported that the same extract attenuated palmitate-induced insulin resistance in liver (C3A) cells. The extract improved impaired glucose and lipid uptake, reduced lipid accumulation, increased lipolysis, and modulated key genes and proteins involved in insulin resistance. The extract increased phosphatidylinositol-4,5-bisphosphate 3-kinase/protein kinase B (PI3K/AKT) and AMP-activated protein kinase (AMPK) phosphorylation, reversed the palmitate-induced reduction of glucose transporter 2 (GLUT2) expression, and promoted gene expression of proteins linked to fatty acid oxidation (Forkhead box protein O1, FOXO1; and carnitine palmitoyl transferase 1, CPT1). A further study confirmed the role of aspalathin in ameliorating impaired glucose and lipid metabolism in palmitate-induced insulin-resistant C3A cells, evident from improved insulin signalling and mitochondrial bioenergetics (Mazibuko-Mbeje et al., 2019b). The study by Moens et al. (2020) provided mechanistic insight into the role of aspalathin in the protection of INS-1E β-cells from oxidative stress and cell death caused by glucotoxicity. The same study also demonstrated the β-cytoprotective effect of aspalathin against glucotoxicity and oxidative stress-induced apoptosis in isolated primary rat islet β-cells. Oxidative stress is a key factor in β-cell dysfunction and cell death. As a mechanism, they proposed the direct interaction of aspalathin with the stress-sensitive protein and redox sensor, sequestosome-1 (P62) protein. P62 interacts with the NRF2–KEAP1–ARE pathway that induced the expression of NRF2-regulated anti-oxidant enzymes. The aspalathin-treated β-cells showed increased expression of the anti-oxidant target genes, *Hmox1*, NAD(*P*)H quinone dehydrogenase 1 (*Nqo-1*), and superoxide dismutase 1 (*Sod1*).

Dludla et al. (2020b) used H9c2 cardiomyocytes, exposed to high glucose concentrations that induced a state of myocardial substrate inflexibility, to show that fermented rooibos extract improved impaired mitochondrial bioenergetics, and enhanced intracellular GSH and SOD levels and free fatty acid utilisation, with an effectivity similar to metformin. Treatment with the rooibos extracts also increased intracellular coenzyme Q_{10} levels. In a further study, the combination of aspalathin and PPAG to protect H9c2 cardiomyocytes from hyperglycaemia-induced oxidative cardiac damage was investigated (Dludla et al., 2020a). Treatment with this combination improved the impaired myocardial substrate metabolism, maintained the mitochondrial membrane potential (MMP), and showed comparable efficacy to metformin in modulating the hyperglycaemia-induced oxidative stress by reducing ROS levels and increasing NADPH oxidase activity and GSH content. Similar to metformin, the combination treatment of aspalathin and PPAG modulated genes involved in energy metabolism, i.e. it upregulated mRNA expression for glucose transporter 4 (GLUT4), peroxisome proliferator-activated receptor-α (PPARα) and acetyl-CoA carboxylase (ACC). Additionally, the combination treatment was more effective than metformin in ameliorating DNA damage caused by chronic exposure of the cardiomyocytes to a high glucose concentration. Low plasma levels of sex hormone-binding globulin (SHBG) are associated with obesity, metabolic syndrome and non-alcoholic fatty liver disease. Rooibos treatment of HepG2 liver cells increased SHBG production (Laura et al., 2021).

8.1.3 Antimutagenic, anticlastogenic and anticancer activity

An aqueous extract of rooibos suppressed chromosome aberrations in Chinese hamster ovary cells induced by benzo[*a*]pyrene (B(*a*)P) or mitomycin C (MMC) in the presence of rat liver microsomal enzymes (S9). The rooibos extract was also effective in suppressing chromosome aberrations by MMC in the absence of metabolic activation. The clastogen-suppressing effects were demonstrated when cells were exposed to rooibos before and/or after mutagen treatment (Sasaki et al., 1993; Shimoi et al., 1994). A rooibos extract inhibited X-ray-induced oncogenic transformation of C3H10T 1/2 mouse embryo fibroblast cells in a concentration- and time-dependent manner (Komatsu et al., 1994). It also inhibited cell proliferation concentration-dependently in embryonic chick skeletal muscle cells (Lamošová et al., 1997). Aqueous extracts of green and fermented rooibos inhibited mutagenesis induced by the aromatic amide, 2-acetylaminofluorene (2-AAF) and the fungal mycotoxin, aflatoxin B_1 (AFB_1), in the *Salmonella typhimurium* mutagenicity assay, using tester strains TA98 and TA100, in the presence of metabolic activation (Marnewick et al., 2000). The fermented rooibos extract was more effective than the green rooibos extract, but both extracts were less effective in inhibiting mutagenesis induced by the direct-acting mutagens, methyl methanesulphonate, cumolhydroperoxide, and hydrogen peroxide, using TA102, a strain used to detect oxidative mutagens and carcinogens. Two studies investigated the effect of fermentation of rooibos on its antimutagenic potency against 2-AAF in TA98 with metabolic activation. Standley et al. (2001) and Van der Merwe et al. (2006) obtained opposite results. Both studies employed several rooibos samples (6–10) of each type, but the samples were randomly selected and therefore did not originate from the same batch of plant material. This discrepancy could be attributed to natural variation in the chemical composition of the plant material, which confounds the issue.

The antigenotoxic effects of rooibos against 2-AAF and the heterocyclic aromatic amines, 2-amino-1-methyl-6-phenylimidazo [4,5-b]pyridine (PhIP) and 2-amino-3-methylimidazo(4,5-*f*)quinoline (IQ), were determined by Edenharder and co-workers. The inhibitory effect of rooibos varied, showing a stronger inhibitory effect against 2-AAF than PhIP in genetically modified Chinese hamster lung fibroblasts, expressing cytochrome P450 1A2 (CYP1A2) and sulphotransferase 1C1 (SULT1C1) (Edenharder et al., 2002). The antimutagenic effects were attributed to the inhibition of CYP1A2 and SULT1C1. In a subsequent study, genetically engineered V79 Chinese hamster fibroblasts (V79-hCYP1A2-hNAT2*4) were used to demonstrate moderate protection by rooibos against genotoxicity of IQ (Platt et al., 2010).

Aqueous extracts of green and fermented rooibos and a methanol extract of green rooibos were investigated for their ability to suppress mutagenesis induced by the tobacco-specific mutagens, 4-(methylnitrosamino)-1-(3-pyridyl)-1-butanone (NNK) and 4-(methyl nitrosamino)-1-(3-pyridyl)-1-butanol (NNAL), in *Salmonella typhimurium* tester strain TA1535 (in the presence of metabolic activation) (Gelderblom et al., 2017). The methanol extract was more effective than the aqueous extracts in suppressing NNK-induced mutagenesis. NNAL-induced mutagenesis was effectively suppressed by both the methanol and aqueous extracts of green rooibos, with the aqueous extract of fermented rooibos extract being less effective.

Huang and co-workers investigated the potential of an aspalathin-rich green rooibos extract (GRT; 12.8% aspalathin) for the treatment of prostate cancer. The extract exhibited dose-dependent suppression of the proliferation of castration-resistant androgen receptor (AR)-rich LNCaP 104-R1 cells, AR-positive androgen-dependent LNCaP FGC cells and AR-negative PC-3 cells. Inhibition of AKT signalling by the rooibos extract was responsible for suppressing LNCaP 104-R1 cell proliferation (Huang et al., 2019). A follow-up study showed that GRT and aspalathin could suppress the migration and invasion of human castration-resistant prostate cancer cells (CRPC) (LNCaP C4-2B and 22Rv1), partly *via* the inhibition of Yes-associated protein (YAP) signalling (Huang et al., 2020).

8.1.4 Skin treatment

Studies on rooibos relating to skin, focused on protection against skin cancer, stimulation of melanogenesis and enhancement of wound healing. Magcwebeba and co-workers investigated the chemopreventive properties of aqueous and methanolic extracts of green rooibos in skin cells. The methanol extract, with a higher content of aspalathin and other flavonoids, was more active than the aqueous extract in disrupting cell viability of non-malignant normal fibroblast-like skin cells (CRL 7761) and premalignant skin cells (HaCaT), but less active in basal carcinoma malignant skin cells (CRL 7762) (Magcwebeba et al., 2016a). Next, the anti-inflammatory effects of these extracts were investigated in UVB/HaCaT keratinocytes, using the accumulation of intracellular interleukin-1α (icIL-1α) as biomarker (Magcwebeba et al., 2016b). The same skin cell models were used to demonstrate that the rooibos extracts enhanced UVB-induced inhibition of cell viability, proliferation and induction of apoptosis, a process that facilitates the removal of icIL-1α. A differential effect was shown for the methanol extract, targeting premalignant cells; proliferation was inhibited at lower extract concentrations, and apoptosis was induced at higher extract concentrations *via* membrane depolarisation at the higher concentrations (Magcwebeba et al., 2016c). Akinfenwa et al. (2021) demonstrated the role of rooibos dihydrochalcones in the protection of human skin cells against UVB-induced oxidative stress and toxicity.

Organic solvent extracts of green and fermented rooibos were investigated for their ability to inhibit skin pigmentation by assessing the inhibition of tyrosinase (Popoola et al., 2019). Ethanol extracts were more effective than chloroform extracts, with the extracts of green rooibos exhibiting higher enzyme inhibitory activity. Another study focused on the stimulation of melanogenesis by assessing the effect on tyrosinase, the rate-limiting enzyme of this process (Van Staden et al., 2021). An ethanol extract of rooibos, its fractions, and aspalathin all stimulated tyrosinase to varying degrees.

Pringle et al. (2018) used RAW 264.7 cells to determine the potential wound healing effects of aqueous extracts of green and fermented rooibos. The fermented rooibos extract, but not the green rooibos extract, increased nitric oxide (NO) production and levels of cellular inducible nitric oxide synthase (iNOS) and cyclooxygenase-2 (COX-2), enzymes that are characteristic markers for classically activated macrophages. The green rooibos extract reduced COX-2 levels. Both extracts inhibited the cellular production of ROS and apoptotic/necrotic cell death. It was concluded that the pro-inflammatory nature of the fermented rooibos extract may have therapeutic value for the healing of early diabetic wounds, which are characterised by a delayed initial inflammatory phase, whilst wounds associated with excessive inflammation would probably benefit more from treatment using the green rooibos extract.

8.1.5 Immunomodulating effects

Kunishiro et al. (2001) investigated the effect of rooibos on antigen-specific antibody production and cytokine generation in murine splenocytes. Aqueous rooibos extract affected antibody (IgM) production in murine splenocytes treated with the antigen, ovalbumin (OVA), in a concentration-dependent manner, with stimulation at low concentrations (1–100 μg/mL) and suppression at a substantially higher concentration (1000 μg/mL). The same effect was observed for the particulate antigen, sheep red blood cells (SRBC), but the extract had no effect on lipopolysaccharide (LPS)-stimulated splenic B-cells. Rooibos extract also had a concentration-dependent effect on cytokine production. It stimulated interleukin (IL)-2 secretion in OVA-treated splenocytes, while suppressing IL-4 secretion. In a follow-up study by Ichiyama et al. (2007), rooibos extract suppressed IL-2 generation in OVA-treated splenocytes, contradictory to the previous finding, however, anti-OVA IgM augmentation was not affected. The extract suppressed interferon-gamma (IFN-γ) generation, enhanced IL-10 production. It had no effect on IL-4 at low concentrations (10 and 30 μg/mL), but decreased the level of this cytokine at higher concentrations (100 and 300 μg/mL). Fractionation of the crude extract on a macroporous resin, by stepwise elution with increasing methanol concentration (water, 25%, 50%, 75% and 100%), produced five fractions, differing in anti-OVA IgM production. The water fraction (A) increased anti-OVA IgM production at the same level as the whole extract, and enhanced antigen production concentration-dependently. Fractions C and D suppressed anti-OVA IgM production, whilst fractions B and E had no effect on antigen production. Further investigation of fraction A demonstrated a similar effect to the crude extract on the cytokines, IL-2, IL-4, IL-10 and IFN-γ.

Hendricks and Pool (2010) demonstrated that rooibos tea modulated immune function *in vitro*, by exposing stimulated and non-stimulated cultures of whole blood cells to rooibos. The levels of IL-6, IL-10 and INF-γ, biomarkers for inflammation, humoral immunity, and cell-mediated immunity, respectively, were determined. Higher levels of these biomarkers were reported in non-stimulated cells after incubation with rooibos. While secretion of INF-γ was not affected, IL-6 secretion increased, and IL-10 secretion decreased in stimulated whole blood cultures after the addition of rooibos extract (Hendricks and Pool, 2010). Rooibos extract was found to suppress antigen-stimulated degranulation in rat basophilic leukaemia (RBL-2H3) cells (Morishita et al., 2019). Pedretti and Peter (2020) used whole blood from atopic patients *ex vivo* to demonstrate that aqueous extracts of green and fermented rooibos inhibited basophil activation (CD63 upregulation) in a concentration-dependent manner. The fermented rooibos extract displayed a stronger inhibitory effect.

8.1.6 Antispasmodic and bronchodilatory activities

An aqueous extract of rooibos demonstrated an antispasmodic effect by dose-dependent relaxation of contractions of rabbit jejunum, induced by K^+. The extract was less effective at the higher K^+ concentration (25 mM *vs* 80 mM). Organic fractions were more effective than the aqueous extract. The contraction effect was postulated to be the activation of K^+ channel opening and weak Ca^{2+} antagonism (Gilani et al., 2006). The aqueous extract also displayed a bronchodilatory effect by inhibiting contractions of guinea-pig trachea induced by the low K^+ concentration. Similar to the jejunum, the effect was weak at the high K^+ concentration (Khan and Gilani, 2006).

8.1.7 Bone health

Several studies investigated the effect of rooibos on bone health. Nash and Ward (2016) established that an aqueous extract of rooibos enhanced mineralisation, maintained alkaline phosphatase (ALP), increased cellular activity, and reduced cellular toxicity of SaoS-2 osteoblasts. It affected osteoblast inflammatory and bone markers, specific to osteoblast metabolism. The levels of the pro-inflammatory markers, IL-6 and tumour necrosis factor α (TNFα), were reduced, whereas the levels of the bone markers, osteopontin (OPN), sclerostin (SOST), and osteoprotegerin (OPG), were increased, decreased and not affected at day 7 of treatment, respectively. Studies by Coetzee and co-workers (Moosa et al., 2018; Sagar et al., 2020) investigated bone remodelling. Osteoporosis is characterised by overactive osteoclasts and the rate of osteoclastic bone resorption exceeding osteoblastic bone formation, resulting in lower bone mineral density. Their first study investigated the effects of aqueous extracts of green and fermented rooibos on receptor activator of NF-κB ligand (RANKL)-induced osteoclast formation and bone resorption in RAW264.7 murine macrophages (Moosa et al., 2018). The fermented rooibos extract was more effective in inhibiting RANKL-induced osteoclastogenesis and decreasing bone resorption. The fermented rooibos extract decreased the expression of downstream genes important for osteoclast fusion and resorption. The green rooibos extract was less effective in suppressing gene expression. Both extracts attenuated NF-κB activity. The role of aspalathin in bone protection *in vitro*, through reduction of osteoclast activity and promotion of osteoblast formation and function activity, was reported by Sagar et al. (2020). Further insight into the stimulation of bone mineralisation by fermented rooibos extract was provided by the study of McAlpine et al. (2019) in a SaoS-2 osteoblast cell model. Mineralisation increased with increasing concentrations of rooibos extract (0.1–10 μg/mL). Protein expression of nucleotide pyrophosphatase/phosphodiesterase 1 (NPP1), ALP, SOST and OPN changed over the treatment time. After 5 days of mineralisation in the presence of rooibos extract, the expression of ALP and NPP1 remained unchanged, elevated levels of SOST were observed at rooibos concentrations >1 μg/mL, and the differences observed in OPN protein expression after 3 days of mineralisation, disappeared. Munmun et al. (2021) showed that rooibos increased the differentiation of human adult mesenchymal stem cells to osteoblasts.

8.1.8 Male and female reproduction systems

The effect of rooibos on testosterone production was investigated by Opuwari and Monsees (2015). TM3 Leydig cell cultures were treated with extracts of green and fermented rooibos in the presence or absence of human chorionic gonadotropin (hCG). Exposure of the non-stimulated cells to the extracts reduced testosterone production. The effect of the extracts on testosterone production was even greater under hCG stimulation.

Ros-Santaella and Pintus (2017) used semen from boars to show that aqueous extracts of green and fermented rooibos preserved sperm during storage. Indicators were sperm motility, acrosome structure and membrane integrity. The beneficial effects of the extracts were concentration- and time-dependent. Another study by Takalani et al. (2021) used human sperm to demonstrate that an aqueous extract of fermented rooibos did not affect functional sperm parameters (motility, vitality, intracellular ROS and acrosome reaction), but that rooibos reduced the percentage of spermatozoa with fragmented DNA. The effect of rooibos on MMP was concentration-dependent. At a low concentration, the extract reduced the percentage of sperm with intact MMP, whilst the higher concentration restored the percentage of sperm with intact MMP to normal. This was attributed to the anti-oxidant activity of the extract.

Štochmaĉová et al. (2015) used rabbit ovarian fragments to demonstrate that rooibos has a direct effect on ovarian functions and their response to gonadotropins. Treatment with rooibos extract stimulated the release of insulin-like growth factor I (IGF-I) and progesterone, and inhibited the release of testosterone. When the ovarian fragments were treated with a combination of rooibos and the hormonal regulators for reproduction, follicle-stimulating and luteinising hormone (FSH + LH), the presence of rooibos extract induced the suppressive effect of FSH + LH on progesterone release. Rooibos also stimulated the action of FSH + LH on testosterone release and suppressed the response of IGF-I to treatment with FSH + LH. Porcine ovarian granulosa cells were used in a follow-up study to show that rooibos extract inhibited cell proliferation (decreased accumulation of proliferating cell nuclear antigen, PCNA), was pro-apoptotic (increased accumulation of Bcl-2-associated X protein, bax) and suppressed the release of progesterone and leptin (Štochmaĉová et al., 2018). Rooibos extract was able to mitigate the adverse effects of the environmental contaminant, xylene, on ovarian cell function. The extract abrogated the inhibitory effect of xylene on PCNA accumulation, mitigated the suppressive effect of xylene on bax, promoted instead of suppressing the release of progesterone by xylene, and prevented the reduction in estradiol released by xylene. Treatment of the cells with rooibos alone promoted PCNA accumulation and reduced progesterone release, but had no effect on bax accumulation or the release of estradiol (Sirotkin et al., 2021a), contrary to the findings by Štochmaĉová et al. (2018) for PCNA and progesterone. Rooibos extract also modified the effects of benzene, another environmental contaminant, on ovarian cell function. It mitigated the inhibitory effect of benzene on ovarian cell viability and progesterone release, but induced or promoted the suppressing effect of benzene on apoptosis and estradiol release (at high concentration) (Sirotkin et al., 2021b). In the latter study, treatment of ovarian cells with rooibos alone promoted accumulation of PCNA and release of progesterone, but it did not affect cell viability or the levels of bax and estradiol. Both studies used granulosa cells isolated from the ovaries of non-cycling pubertal gilts (Sirotkin et al., 2021a,b). Differences in the effects of rooibos alone were attributed to differences in the initial state of the ovarian cells.

8.1.9 Antiviral and antimicrobial activity

An alkaline extract (1% sodium hydroxide) of rooibos containing polysaccharides, suppressed HIV-induced cytopathicity of HIV (HTLV-III) infected MT-4 cells, but a hot water extract was ineffective. Disaccharides and trisaccharides derived from acid degradation also inhibited HIV-induced cytopathoxicity (Nakano et al., 1997a,b). An aqueous rooibos extract showed inhibition of the rotavirus (Knipping et al., 2012). *In vitro* testing of an alkaline extract of rooibos (1% sodium bicarbonate) and extracts prepared with ethanol, ethyl acetate and *n*-hexane indicated that the alkaline extract was the most potent towards the influenza A virus (Rahmasari et al., 2017). It was also active against several other influenza viruses, including oseltamivir-resistant influenza viruses A and B. The late stages of influenza virus replication were found to be targeted predominantly by the alkaline extract. Idriss et al. (2021) confirmed anti-influenza virus activity for a cold water extract of rooibos. It inhibited the replication of several strains of the virus.

Aqueous extracts of fermented and green rooibos, as well as their ethyl acetate fractions, inhibited the growth of *Escherichia coli* in a concentration-dependent manner (Scheepers, 2001). The aqueous extract of fermented rooibos was more effective than the green rooibos extract (35% decrease), and their ethyl acetate fractions were less effective than the crude extracts. *Escherichia coli* was able to resume growth when the extracts were removed, indicating a bacteriostatic effect. The crude extracts also display inhibitory activity against *Saccharomyces cerevisiae*, *Listeria monocytogenes*, *Bacillus cereus*, *Streptococcus mutans* and *Staphylococcus aureus.* The highest inhibitory activity was achieved towards *S. aureus*, with higher growth inhibition recorded for the fermented rooibos extract. The fermented rooibos extract stimulated the growth of *Zygosaccharomyces rouxii*. Almajano et al. (2008) showed that an aqueous extract of rooibos has some antibacterial activity against *B. cereus* and *Micrococcus luteus* and anticandidal activity towards *Candida albicans.* The extract was inactive towards *Pseudomonas aeruginosa*, *E. coli* and *Lactobacillus acidophilus*. A green rooibos extract stimulated the growth of *Botrytis cinerea*, an important fungal crop pathogen (Coetzee et al., 2008). Kühnast and Braun (2013) investigated the antimicrobial activity of a fermented rooibos extract against lactic acid bacteria (*Lactobacillus* spp., *Carnobacterium* spp., *Leuconostoc carnosum*), food spoilage organisms (*Bacillus* spp., *Brochothrix* spp., *Pseudomonas fluorescens*) and foodborne pathogens (*L. monocytogenes*, *Salmonella enteritidis*). The extract inhibited the growth of *L. monocytogenes* and lactic acid bacteria to some extent, but not that of *Salmonella enteritidis*.

Human et al. (2020) showed that green rooibos extract was more effective against *L. monocytogenes* than towards *E. coli* and *S. aureus* and that the extent of growth inhibition decreased with prolonged exposure to the extract.

Park et al. (2014) evaluated the antimicrobial activity of various combinations of a rooibos infusion, potassium lactate and sodium diacetate towards the growth of *Clostridium perfringens* vegetative cells and spores in ready-to-eat Jokbal (pig's trotters). A combination of rooibos and the two chemicals prevented the growth and spore germination of *C. perfringens* at room temperature. Hübsch et al. (2014) studied the link between the antimicrobial and toxicity effects of aqueous and organic extracts of rooibos combined with seven antibiotics in general use (ciprofloxacin, erythromycin, gentamicin, penicillin G, tetracycline, amphotericin B and nystatin). The most potent activity was recorded for the extracts combined with penicillin G against Gram-positive bacteria. Various combination ratios of these test substances were found to work synergistically against *S. aureus*. Antagonistic action against the Gram-negative bacteria and yeasts was observed for four combinations.

An ethanol extract of rooibos exhibited a minimum inhibitory concentration (MIC) of 125 µg/mL against *Propionibacterium acnes*, a bacterium linked to skin acne (Sharma and Lall, 2014). A rooibos infusion showed antibacterial activity towards a large number of *Helicobacter pylori* strains. Of the 54 *H. pylori* strains tested, 26% and 63% of the strains showed $\geq 8 \times 10^4$ colony forming units (CFU) reduction by rooibos extract (7.5 mg/mL) within 1 and 2 h, respectively (Boyanova, 2014). Ethanol extracts of green and fermented rooibos were not effective in inhibiting the growth of *Mycobacterium tuberculosis* H37Rv (Reid et al., 2020). A collagen-based electrospun scaffold containing an aqueous extract of fermented rooibos was evaluated for potential wound-healing application (Ilomuanya et al., 2020). The extract-loaded scaffold showed antimicrobial activity against *S. aureus*, methicillin-resistant *S. aureus*, *P. aeruginosa* and *E. coli*.

8.1.10 Other effects

Persson et al. (2006) investigated the effect of rooibos extract on angiotensin-converting enzyme (ACE) and NO production in HUVECs for a potential cardioprotective role. The enzyme catalyses the conversion of angiotensin I to angiotensin II, a potent vasoconstrictor, and NO is a vasodilator. Rooibos had no significant effect on ACE activity, but NO production was dose-dependently increased. Following the demonstration that rooibos inhibited ACE *in vivo* (Persson et al., 2010), an enzyme kinetics study was performed that showed rooibos inhibited ACE according to a mixed inhibitor mechanism (Persson, 2012).

Diabetic cardiomyopathy is a disorder of the heart muscle that contributes to cardiovascular deaths in diabetics. An *ex vivo* study by Dludla et al. (2014) provided evidence of the protection offered by rooibos to the diabetic heart. Cardiomyocytes, isolated from the hearts of STZ-induced diabetic rats and exposed to H_2O_2 or an ischaemic solution, showed a decrease in metabolic activity and GSH content with a concomitant increase in apoptosis and intracellular ROS. Pretreatment with an aqueous extract of fermented rooibos was able to combat these effects better than the known anti-oxidant, vitamin E.

Schloms et al. (2012) investigated the effects of rooibos on adrenal steroidogenesis. A methanol extract of green rooibos inhibited P450 17α-hydroxylase/17,20 lyase (CYP17A1) and P450 21-hydroxylase (CYP21A2) in COS-1 cells, and reduced the total steroid level produced under basal conditions and in forskolin-stimulated adrenal H295R cells (to mimic a stress response). Aldosterone and cortisol precursors were significantly reduced. A further study showed that rooibos inhibited 11β-hydroxysteroid dehydrogenase type 1 (11βHSD1), but not 11β-hydroxysteroid dehydrogenase type 2 (11βHSD2), in CHO-K1 cells. This resulted in a significant reduction in the cortisol:cortisone ratio. Rooibos was also effective in reducing the levels of cortisol and corticosterone (CORT) in forskolin-stimulated adrenal H295R cells (Schloms et al., 2014). Rooibos had a greater inhibitory effect on glucocorticoid production (CORT, deoxycorticosterone and 11-dehydroxycorticosterone) in forskolin-stimulated H205R cells than under basal conditions, independent of the presence of cytokines, IL-6 and IL-10 (Smith and Swart, 2016).

'Anti-ageing' has been a mantra used in connection with phenolic anti-oxidants. Hattingh et al. (2019) investigated the anti-ageing properties of rooibos by assessing its ability to modulate age-related decline in preadipocyte function, as relating to mitochondrial dysfunction. An aspalathin-enriched extract of green rooibos was more effective than an aqueous extract of fermented rooibos to preserve the functional capacity of preadipocytes.

8.1.11 Modulation of drug-metabolising enzymes and herb–drug interaction

Abrahams et al. (2019) used primary rat hepatocytes to demonstrate that an aspalathin-enriched green rooibos extract (18.4% aspalathin) had no effect on the expression of genes encoding the xenobiotic-metabolising enzymes, catechol-*O*-methyl transferase (Comt), 17β-hydroxysteroid dehydrogenase 2 (Hsd117β2) and cytochrome P450 2e1 (Cyp2e1). Aspalathin showed a differential effect on gene expression, i.e. *Comt* was upregulated, *Hsd117*β*2* was downregulated, and C*yp2e1* was marginally upregulated.

Given that the pharmacokinetics of a drug might vary when co-administered in the presence of rooibos extract, potential herb–drug interaction of rooibos extracts was investigated with a specific focus on the cytochrome P450 enzymes, CYP2C8, CYP2C9 and CYP3A4, using Vivid® recombinant P450 enzymes (Patel et al., 2016). These P450 enzymes are important in the metabolism of hypoglycaemic drugs (thiazolidinediones and sulphonylureas) and hypocholesterolemic drugs such as atorvastatin. An aqueous extract of fermented rooibos and GRT, the aspalathin-rich extract of green rooibos, were tested for their effects on these enzymes. Both extracts dose- and time-dependently inhibited CYP2C8 and CYP3A4 activity, whilst inhibition of CYP2C9 activity was time-dependent. Fantoukh et al. (2019) showed that a methanol extract of green rooibos inhibited CYP2C9, CYP3A4, CYP2D6, CYP2C19 and CYP1A2, with the strongest effect observed for CYP3A4, followed by CYP2C19. The extract increased pregnane X receptor (PXR) activity in a concentration-dependent manner, indicating the CYP induction potential of the extract through the PXR mechanism. The extract showed no inhibition of *P*-glycoprotein, an efflux transporter in many tissues.

Two *in vitro* studies concentrated on drug-induced toxicity. Aspalathin reverted cardiotoxicity induced by doxorubicin, a chemotherapeutic agent, without decreasing the anticancer efficacy of the drug (Johnson et al., 2017). This was achieved through increased autophagy and decreased expression of p53/mTOR/p62 signalling. Millar et al. (2020) determined that GRT was not effective in modulating atorvastatin-induced toxicity in C3A liver cells.

8.2 *In vivo* studies and clinical trials

Most *in vivo* studies used rodent models to research the beneficial effects of rooibos. Only one study reported the use of a primate model. A limited number of human studies have been undertaken to investigate the potential health-promoting effects of rooibos.

8.2.1 Anti-oxidant properties and oxidative stress

Many studies have dealt with the anti-oxidant properties of rooibos *in vivo* and its ability to modulate oxidative stress, particularly induced in the liver by exposure to a variety of stressors. These have been reviewed by Marnewick and co-workers (Marnewick, 2014; Ajuwon et al., 2015). More animal studies have been published since. This section will focus on human studies. Sauter (2004) demonstrated that a 14-day treatment of 20 volunteers, who received a twice-daily dose of an aspalathin-enriched (15% aspalathin) green rooibos extract (250 mg/tablet) in addition to a restricted flavonoid diet, failed to increase the anti-oxidant status of their blood plasma based on results of the 2,2′-azino-bis(3-ethylbenzothiazoline-6-sulphonic acid) ($ABTS^{\bullet+}$) scavenging and Cu^{2+}-induced low-density lipoprotein (LDL) oxidation test systems. However, a reduction in their plasma anti-oxidant status was observed as measured using the xanthine/xanthine oxidase assay.

Nikolova et al. (2007) used a randomised placebo-controlled intervention (8-week duration) trial of male workers occupationally exposed to lead to demonstrate that drinking rooibos tea improved their anti-oxidant status—reduced elevated SOD and lipid peroxidation-malondialdehyde levels and increased GSH levels. Rooibos drinking had no effect on the lead levels in the blood. In an acute intervention human study with a cross-over design, 15 healthy volunteers drank 500 mL of either water, green rooibos tea or fermented rooibos tea. The total radical-trapping anti-oxidant potential of the plasma of the green rooibos group was 28% higher compared to that of the fermented rooibos group. No changes were observed in their triacylglycerol, cholesterol or uric acid levels (Villaño et al., 2010).

Marnewick et al. (2011) used 40 healthy volunteers, but at risk for CVD, in a 6-week study that entailed drinking six cups of fermented rooibos tea daily. Consumption of rooibos tea reduced serum levels of LDL-cholesterol and triacylglycerol, and reduced oxidative stress by decreasing lipid peroxidation (as measured by conjugated dienes and MDA) and increasing GSH levels and the GSH:GSSG ratio.

8.2.2 Antimutagenic and anticancer effects

Oral gavage of rooibos tea at 1 mL/mouse/day for 4 weeks suppressed induction of chromosome aberrations (formation of micronucleated reticulocytes) by B(*a*)P and MMC (Sasaki et al., 1993). Oral administration of rooibos tea for 28 days (*ad libitum*) also reduced the frequency of γ-ray irradiation (1.5 Gy)-induced micronucleated reticulocytes in mice (Shimoi et al., 1994). In a follow-up study, the frequency of micronucleated reticulocytes in mice was reduced by single gastric intubation (1 mL extract or flavonoid of rooibos) 2 h prior to γ-ray irradiation (Shimoi et al., 1996).

Marnewick et al. (2005) conducted a study on the inhibition of tumour promotion in mouse skin, using a two-stage mouse skin carcinogenesis assay with dimethylbenzantrachene as initiator and 2-*O*-tetradecanoyl-phorbol 13-acetate (TPA) as cancer promoter. Topical application of green and fermented rooibos extracts (ethanol/acetone-soluble fraction of a methanol extract), prior to cancer promotion, reduced the number and size of skin tumours in the Institute of Cancer Research (ICR) mice. The fermented rooibos extract was more effective than the unfermented rooibos extract. Infusions of green and fermented rooibos also displayed chemoprotective effects against cancer promotion in rat liver by a fumonisin B1 (FB1)-diet (Marnewick et al., 2009). Consumption of rooibos (*ad libitum*) by male Fischer rats commenced 1 week after cancer initiation with diethylnitrosamine and continued for 3 weeks. Green rooibos was more effective than fermented rooibos in arresting the proliferation of altered glutathione *S*-transferase Pi ($GSTP^+$) cells.

Sissing et al. (2011) studied the effects of rooibos on oesophageal squamous cell carcinoma, induced in male Fischer F344 rats using methylbenzylnitrosamine (MBM). Following a 5-week treatment with MBM and 1 week after initiation, the rats were treated for 25 weeks with either green or fermented rooibos infusions as their sole drinking fluid. Green rooibos reduced the mean total papilloma size due to the absence of large papillomas ($>10\,mm^3$). The fermented rooibos was less effective in reducing the mean total papilloma size.

Huang et al. (2019) reported that an aspalathin-rich green rooibos extract (GRT) suppressed tumour volume and weight of androgen-independent LNCaP 104-R1-induced xenografts in castrated nude mice. The mice were treated with GRT by gavaging 400 mg/kg body weight (bw) three times a week for 74 days. Inhibition of AKT and YAP signalling by rooibos extract is involved (Huang et al., 2019, 2020).

8.2.3 Modulation of metabolic syndrome

This section highlights new studies on rooibos and aspalathin not covered by the comprehensive reviews of Johnson et al. (2018) and Muller et al. (2018). The results of combination therapy of rooibos or aspalathin with hypoglycaemic and hypolipidaemic drugs are covered.

An aspalathin-rich green rooibos extract (GRT) effectively improved insulin sensitivity in obese insulin-resistant (OBIR) Wistar rats (Mazibuko-Mbeje et al., 2019a). The OBIR rats were maintained on a high-fat, high-sugar diet, and were daily administered with GRT at different doses for 12 weeks. The different doses of GRT (32, 97 and 195 mg/kg bw) were extrapolated from human equivalent consumption of one (32 mg/kg), three (97 mg/kg) and six (195 mg/kg) cups of tea, based on the soluble solid content of a cup of rooibos infusion (~ 230 mg/200 mL) and an average human weight of 70 kg. Vildagliptin, the drug reference control, was administered at a dose of 10 mg/kg bw. The two highest doses reduced blood glucose concentrations after week 4, but after week 12 no effect on blood glucose concentration was observed. Only the highest dose was effective in lowering the plasma insulin concentration and HOMA-IR value, by modulating PI3K/AKT and activated protein kinase (AMPK) pathways. The effect of GRT on gluco-lipidic and oxidative indices was subsequently assessed in high-fat diet-induced diabetic and normal non-human vervet monkeys (*Chlorocebus aethiops*) (Orlando et al., 2019). The diabetic model is characterised by glucose intolerance and increased total cholesterol and LDL levels. The primates were treated thrice daily with a GRT dose (90 mg/kg bw) as part of a 30 g bolus. Treatment lasted for 4 weeks, followed by a 1-month washout period. Supplementation improved all indices in the diabetic primates (intravenous glucose tolerance test, glycaemic area under curve, and total cholesterol, due to a decrease in LDL). The non-diabetic monkeys benefitted from an increase in high-density lipoprotein (HDL) levels. It was concluded that GRT has the potential to counteract hyperglycaemia, oxidative stress and dyslipidaemia, thereby lowering fundamental cardiovascular risk factors associated with diabetes. A histomorphometric study on the hepatoprotective effects of GRT in a diet-induced obese rat model (6-week treatment with 60 mg/kg bw daily) showed that GRT reduced the increased body and liver mass of these obese rats (Layman et al., 2019). The extract was also effective in reducing the percentage, location and type of steatosis, as well as the presence of inflammation and hepatocellular injury. Obesity-induced CVD risk factors in obese male Wistar rats on a high-fat diet for 16 weeks were modulated by a GRT treatment (60 mg/kg bw/day) for the last 6 weeks. The untreated obese rats had increased blood pressure, impaired vasodilation, decreased anti-oxidant enzyme activity, increased MDA levels, attenuated PKB and AMPK expression, and increased phosphorylated eNOS levels (Obasa et al., 2021).

A study using SHBG transgenic mice showed that treatment with rooibos extract increased their SHBG production, suggestive of its role in the antidiabetic and cardiovascular beneficial effects of rooibos (Laura et al., 2021). Dludla et al. (2018) showed that aspalathin (13 and 130 mg/kg bw) used in combination with metformin (150 mg/kg bw) performed better than metformin as a monotherapy in lowering fasting plasma glucose (FPG) levels, homeostatic model assessment-insulin resistance (HOMA-IR) and insulin levels in obese diabetic (*db/db*) mice treated daily through oral gavage for 6 weeks. The results also indicated that long-term treatment with combination therapy might be more effective than short-term treatment. Patel et al. (2021) reported on the co-therapy of GRT with the hypoglycaemic drug, pioglitazone, and hypolipidaemic drug, atorvastatin, on blood glucose and lipid profiles in obese diabetic (*db/db*) mice. The *db/db* mice were treated daily for 5 weeks either with pioglitazone (25 mg/kg bw), atorvastatin (80 mg/kg bw), GRT (100 mg/kg bw), a combination of either drug with GRT or a combination of GRT, pioglitazone and atorvastatin (GPA). Co-therapy of GRT with pioglitazone and atorvastatin, respectively, as well as GPA, lowered their FPG levels. The GRT, pioglitazone and atorvastatin monotherapies had no FPG lowering effect. The GPA combination was not more effective in reducing FPG levels than the co-therapy of GRT and pioglitazone, but it was more effective than atorvastatin in reducing triglyceride levels. The combination of GRT and atorvastatin had no effect on triglyceride levels of the *db/db* mice. The study also demonstrated changes in the expression of genes involved in lipogenesis, cholesterol, fatty acid transport, β-oxidation, and synthesis and storage of fatty acids.

Co-administration of aspalathin (50 mg/kg bw) with atorvastatin (50 mg/kg bw) to Wistar rats affected the pharmacokinetics of this statin (Patel et al., 2019). Aspalathin increased the maximum plasma concentration of atorvastatin and increased the area of the plasma concentration-time curve by 5.8- and 5.9-fold, respectively. The same aspalathin dose co-administered with metformin (150 mg/kg bw) did not affect the plasma concentration of metformin (Patel et al., 2019).

8.2.4 Stress

Plasma from volunteers at risk for CVD, who took part in the human study by Marnewick et al. (2011), showed that daily consumption of six cups of rooibos tea for 6 weeks increased cortisone levels in males, but not in females. Rooibos consumption reduced the cortisol:cortisone ratio in both males and females (Schloms et al., 2014). In Wistar rats, CORT and deoxycorticosterone levels decreased following the consumption of a methanol extract of green rooibos (40 mg/animal, administered twice daily by oral gavage for 10 days). Testosterone and 11-dehydrocorticosterone levels were not affected, whilst the CORT:testosterone ratio was marginally reduced (Schloms et al., 2014). The same rooibos extract and duration of treatment were not effective in reducing elevated CORT and deoxycorticosterone levels in Wistar rats subjected to acute restraint stress for 1 h. This treatment elicited a mild glucocorticoid response (Smith and Swart, 2016). Hong et al. (2014) previously demonstrated that treatment with rooibos attenuated immobilised-induced oxidative stress in rat brain. This included a reduction in increased levels of stress-related metabolites, free fatty acids and 5-hydroxyindoleacetic acid, the primary metabolite of serotonin. For the study, Sprague Dawley rats received rooibos tea as the sole drinking fluid for 4 weeks and they were immobilised for 1 h/day to induce stress.

8.2.5 Male and female reproduction systems

Egg production in Japanese quail (*Coturnix coturnix japonica*) was affected by fermented rooibos tea (drinking fluid or diet-supplementation), depending on their age (Juráni et al., 2008). Rooibos did not increase egg production in young hens, but it reduced the decrease in egg production of aged hens (360-days of age), indicating an extension of the productive period of aged poultry. Another positive outcome was that rooibos increased the body weight of the young hens up to 100-days of age.

Awoniyi et al. (2012) demonstrated that aqueous extracts of green and fermented rooibos increased sperm count and motility in male Wistar rats subjected to oxidative stress, in addition to alleviating the oxidative stress. Oxidative stress was induced by intraperitoneal injection of *t*-butyl hydroperoxide in the last 2 weeks of a 10-week treatment. Fermented and green rooibos tea, consumed as the sole drinking fluid, affected reproduction functions of male Wistar rats, as assessed after a 52-day treatment period (Opuwari and Monsees, 2014). Seminiferous tubules displayed complete spermatogenesis. Tubule diameter and germinal epithelial height were decreased, whilst the epithelial height of epididymis (caput) increased. Green rooibos enhanced sperm concentration, viability and motility. Fermented rooibos also improved sperm vitality, but increased spontaneous acrosome reaction, which may interfere with their fertilisation potential. A study on STZ-induced diabetic Wistar rats showed that a 7-week treatment with fermented rooibos improved the altered testicular and epididymal morphology of the diabetic rats (Omolaoye et al., 2021).

The potential oestrogenic effect of rooibos was investigated on female Wistar rats. The rats were treated with fermented and green rooibos for 21 days (Monsees and Opuwari, 2017). Their hormone levels (FSH and LH) were not affected. Green rooibos increased the relative uterus weight, whilst fermented rooibos decreased the relative ovary weight. Both green and fermented rooibos slightly increased the endometrium thickness, whereas the myometrium thickness remained unchanged.

8.2.6 Cardioprotective properties

A human randomised, three-phase, cross-over study with 17 healthy volunteers, consuming a single oral dose of 400 mL rooibos tea, indicated inhibited ACE activity of the ACE II genotype, 60 min after intake. The treatment had no effect on the NO concentration. These results suggest that rooibos tea may have cardiovascular effects through inhibition of ACE activity (Persson et al., 2010). Green and fermented rooibos were evaluated for their cardioprotective effects against ischaemia/reperfusion injury in male Wistar rats (Pantsi et al., 2011). The treatments improved aortic output recovery after reperfusion and affected the level of the pro-apoptotic proteins during reperfusion. Both fermented and green rooibos decreased the level of cleaved poly (ADP-ribose) polymerase, but they had opposite effects on caspase-3 activation (decreased by fermented rooibos; increased by green rooibos). The human study involving 40 healthy volunteers at risk for CVD, conducted by Marnewick et al. (2011), showed that consumption of six cups of fermented rooibos tea for 6 weeks improved their lipid profiles (decreased serum LDL-cholesterol and triacylglycerol levels; increased HDL-cholesterol levels), in addition to decreased lipid peroxidation, and increased GSH levels and GSH:GSSH ratio (Section 8.2.1). Serum iron, ferritin, transferrin, TIBC and Fe saturation levels of the study participants were not affected (Marnewick et al., 2013).

Smit et al. (2022) confirmed the therapeutic potential of GRT to prevent ischaemia/reperfusion injury in CVD-compromised rats. A 6-week GRT treatment (60 mg/rat/day) lowered their pre-ischaemic heart rate, reduced infarct size, and improved heart function pre- and post-ischaemia in male Wistar rats on a high-calorie diet. The study also provided insight into the mechanisms involved. HIV-infected populations receiving antiretroviral therapy (ART) have an increased risk of CVD. Webster et al. (2019) investigated whether rooibos could ameliorate harmful cardiovascular side effects induced by ART. Rats receiving ART (efavirenz, emtricitabine, tenofovir) for 9 weeks were co-treated with rooibos (as sole drinking fluid). Rooibos treatment reduced total serum cholesterol levels, but not when combined with ART. *Ex vivo*, hearts exposed to ischaemia-reperfusion injury had increased infarct sizes compared to the controls. This was not observed for the co-treatment of ART and rooibos. The co-treatment also improved aortic relaxation, which was reduced with ART treatment.

8.2.7 Anti-allergic and immunomodulatory properties

Ingestion and topical application of rooibos tea on type I skin allergic reaction failed to demonstrate an anti-allergic effect in volunteers with symptoms of allergic disease (asthma or hay fever). The use of antihistamines was discontinued 1 week before the study (Hesseling and Joubert, 1982). The study monitored the skin response after a skin prick test using 16 common allergens. Seven volunteers consumed large quantities of fermented rooibos tea (500 mL three times a day for 1 week) prior to testing. In addition, a rooibos poultice (500 g in 500 mL water) was also applied to one arm 15 min before the skin prick test.

Kunishiro et al. (2001) investigated the effects of rooibos extract on antigen-specific antibody production and cytokine generation in immunosuppressed rats. Female Wistar/ST rats, pretreated with rooibos extract for 1 week, were injected intraperitoneally with OVA. The immunosuppressor, cyclosporin A, was administered intravenously 24 h before the OVA challenge. Rooibos largely countered the reduction in OVA-specific antibody production (IgM) by cyclosporin A. Ingestion of a column fraction (fraction A; Section 8.1.5) of an aqueous extract of rooibos by OVA-immunised mice, increased the serum anti-OVA IgM level. Rooibos tea was ingested *ad libitum* by BALB/c mice, starting 1 week before their first immunisation with OVA and aluminium hydroxide as adjuvant (twice with a 2-week interval), and continued for 5 weeks (Ichiyama et al., 2007).

8.2.8 Brain

Magnetic resonance images of the brains of 24-month-old Wistar female rats, treated with rooibos tea for 21 months, were similar to that of 5-week-old rats. The brains of 24-month-old rats not receiving rooibos treatment, showed a decrease in signal intensity in the cerebral cortex, hippocampus and cerebellum. Additionally, chronic rooibos tea administration prevented age-related accumulation of lipid peroxides in several regions of the rat brain (Inanami et al., 1995). Akinrinmade et al. (2017) investigated the effects of long-term consumption of fermented rooibos on ischaemia/reperfusion (I/aR)-induced brain injury in adult male Wistar rats. Rooibos tea was administered *ad libitum* to the animals for 7 weeks prior to induction of ischaemic injury followed by reperfusion. Rooibos tea reduced brain oedema and neuronal apoptosis, but it did not attenuate blood–brain barrier damage following cerebral ischaemia. Other effects of rooibos on the brain were reduced lipid peroxidation levels, increased total anti-oxidant capacity and improved neurobehavioural outcomes, when compared with untreated animals. Pyrzanowska et al. (2019) evaluated possible behavioural and neurochemical effects of long-term oral administration (12 weeks) of fermented rooibos infusions to adult male Sprague–Dawley rats. Rooibos consumption improved their long-term spatial memory and increased the levels of striatal dopamine and its metabolite, 3-methoxytyramine.

8.2.9 Tear and saliva secretion

Extreme dryness of the eyes and mouth affects the quality of life. Two studies showed that rooibos extract stimulates tear and saliva secretion in mice and humans. The active ingredient was identified as eriodictyol-6-*C*-β-D-glucoside, an oxidation product of aspalathin (Nishimachi et al., 2019; Arakaki et al., 2019). This flavanone stimulated exocrine glands *via* the M3 muscarinic acetylcholine receptor. Yuyama et al. (2020) confirmed the absorption and distribution of eriodictyol-6-*C*-β-D-glucoside to exocrine glands after oral administration in mice.

8.2.10 Cosmetics

Despite the widespread use of rooibos in a variety of cosmetic products, scientific studies related to cosmetics are limited. Rooibos tea extract has been commercialised in Tealine® (Cosmetochem, Switzerland) and was developed into a stable cosmetic gel (0.15%). It showed greater reduction of wrinkles (9.9%) in a 28-day randomised, single-blind study of 20 volunteers than *Gingko* extract (Flavonoids complex SC®, Cosmetochem), having the same flavonoid content (Kanlayavattanakul and Lourith, 2015). According to Glynn (2010), the topical application of a herbal mixture, containing green rooibos extract, alleviates male pattern baldness. A US patent application deals with the protective effect of rooibos extract against hair colour loss (Joppe et al., 2009).

8.2.11 Other effects

Shindo and Kato (1991) demonstrated that drinking rooibos tea could decrease the incidence of herpes simplex and the itching sensation in patients with atopic dermatitis. Rooibos also seems to have a beneficial effect on inflammatory disease with infiltration of polymorphonuclear leucocytes, steroid-induced dermatitis, and photosensitivity as a result of UV irradiation. Hydrogels loaded with green or fermented rooibos extract improved the healing of a surgical wound on the back skin of Swiss albino mice. The topical application of the hydrogel loaded with green rooibos extract was more effective and shortened the time for complete wound closure from 14 to 10 days (Elegbede et al., 2020).

A human study was carried out to determine if rooibos tea has a deleterious effect on iron absorption. It was reported that Fe absorption was not affected by a single serving of 200 mL rooibos (40 mL milk and 20 sugar added). The participants in the study were 30 males, aged between 21 and 34 years (Hesseling et al., 1979). Another study by Breet et al. (2005) showed that a twice daily intake of rooibos tea (200 mL with milk and sugar added) by 175 children over a 16-week period did not affect their iron status (serum ferritin, transferrin, total iron-binding capacity and transferrin saturation).

Khan and Gilani (2006) reported that rooibos tea dose-dependently reduced the arterial blood pressure of rats under anaesthesia. Hypouricaemic effects of an aspalathin-rich fraction (21.4%) of green rooibos and aspalathin were demonstrated in hypouricaemic mice. Both extract and aspalathin suppressed increased plasma uric acid levels in a dose-dependent manner (Kondo et al., 2013). The suppressed plasma uric acid level was attributed to their xanthine oxidase (XOD)-inhibitory activity. A preliminary human study showed that drinking rooibos tea did not reduce the physiochemical and peroxidative risk factors of calcium oxalate renal stone formation. The limited number of volunteers ($n=8$), the short duration of treatment (30 days) and the dosage may have resulted in the apparent lack of effect (Rodgers et al., 2016). Rooibos consumption, three times daily for 30 days, reduced urinary levels of the bone resorption marker, C-terminal telopeptide of type I collagen, in humans with osteopenia (Munmun et al., 2021). Green rooibos and aspalathin, administered *ad libitum* through the diet (0.2% or 0.04%, respectively) enhanced the physical endurance of mice in a swimming test (Watanabe et al., 2014). This was evident after 2 and 4 weeks on the supplemented diet. The livers and muscles of these mice, after 30 min swimming at the end of the 5-week experimental period, showed higher glycogen levels than the control group. Utter et al. (2010) reported that drinking rooibos tea was not more effective than water in promoting rehydration in athletes.

8.2.12 Herb–drug interaction and gene expression of xenobiotic-metabolising enzymes

Consumption of rooibos affected drug-metabolising enzymes. Aqueous extracts of green and fermented rooibos, provided as sole drinking fluids, enhanced cytosolic glutathione *S*-transferase α levels in the livers of male Fischer 344 rats after 10 weeks

(Marnewick et al., 2003). The expression of CYP2C11 was lowered in rats drinking a rooibos infusion for 3 days (Jang et al., 2004). Rooibos also increased the expression and activity of CYP3A, a key enzyme in the metabolism of a large number of therapeutic drugs, in the intestine (Matsuda et al., 2007). Rooibos also affected gene expression in the liver and kidneys of rats administered a diet supplemented with an aspalathin-enriched green rooibos extract (GRE) for 28 days (Abrahams et al., 2019). In the liver, GRE upregulated genes encoding aldehyde dehydrogenase, glucose phosphate isomerase and cytochrome P450, whilst 17β-hydroxysteroid dehydrogenase 2 (Hsd17β2) was downregulated. In the kidneys, GRE upregulated genes encoding the phase II xenobiotic metabolism enzymes, glutathione-*S*-transferase mμ and microsomal glutathione-*S*-transferase, whilst downregulating genes encoding the ATP binding cassette transporter, cytochrome P450, gamma glutamyltransferase 1 and *N*-acetyltransferase 1.

8.2.13 Bioavailability studies

Several studies demonstrated the bioavailability of aspalathin and other rooibos flavonoids and the identification of metabolites (reviewed by Muller et al., 2018). Of importance is that aspalathin can be absorbed by the intestine as a *C*-glucoside, as well as being cleaved into an aglycone and a sugar moiety.

8.2.14 Non-therapeutic uses

The use of fermented rooibos as a potential meat preservative against lipid oxidation has been investigated for several meat products, i.e. ostrich and rabbit meat patties (Cullere et al., 2013, 2019) and '*droëwors*' produced from the meats of ostrich, blesbok, springbok and fallow deer (Hoffman et al., 2014; Jones et al., 2015a,b). Rooibos was not successful to inhibit or delay lipid peroxidation in all products, but it showed potential as a flavour enhancer (Jones et al., 2015a,b). '*Droëwors*' is a traditional South African dried sausage product. Rooibos is sometimes used in cooking for its flavour. Its use as an antimicrobial in meat preservation is discussed in Section 8.1.9.

8.3 Safety

The historical and modern use of rooibos as a beverage for everyday consumption has led to a general assumption of its safety, as no reports of toxicity for its routine use as herbal tea have been documented. Although no toxicological studies have been conducted, a number of studies have addressed aspects of the safety and toxicity of rooibos. Chronic consumption of aqueous extracts of unfermented and fermented rooibos by rats for a 10-week period did not cause any adverse effects on the liver or kidney. In addition, serum iron and cholesterol levels were also not significantly altered (Marnewick et al., 2003). Three case reports of possible hepatotoxic effects of rooibos tea have been published (Sinisalo et al., 2010; Engels et al., 2013; Reddy et al., 2016). The Perishable Products Export Control Board of South Africa certifies that rooibos tea meets standards of quality with respect to bacteria and impurities. The detection of pyrrolizidine alkaloids in various teas, including rooibos tea, destined for the European market, has resulted in the screening of rooibos. Van Wyk et al. (2017) showed that the weed, *Senecio angustifolius*, is the major source of pyrrolizidine alkaloid contamination of rooibos tea.

9. Phytochemistry

9.1 Volatile constituents

Habu et al. (1985) identified 26 ketones, 19 aldehydes, 16 alcohols, 12 esters, nine hydrocarbons, seven phenols, four acids, three ethers and three miscellaneous compounds in the vacuum steam-distilled volatile fraction of fermented rooibos tea, using gas chromatography coupled to mass spectrometry (GS–MS). When extracted with heptane, the major compounds were guaiacol, 6-methyl-3,5-heptadien-2-one, damascenone, geranylacetone, β-phenylethyl alcohol and 6-methyl-5-hepten-2-one. Headspace analysis yielded 218 positive or tentative identifications, including 47 alcohols, 41 ketones, 39 aldehydes, 27 hydrocarbons, 24 esters, 13 ethers, seven phenols, six acids and 14 miscellaneous compounds. Kawakami et al. (1993) compared the volatile fraction of fermented rooibos, brewed for 10 min and then extracted using dichloromethane, to that obtained by steam distillation and extraction (SDE) of the plant material, using GC–MS. The dichloromethane extract yielded 50 compounds, including high levels of 2-phenylethanol, guaiacol and methylethylmaleimide, and lactones such as 2-methoxy-2-buten-4-olide, dihydroactinidiolide, and 4-butanolide. This aroma fraction had a strong resemblance to that of rooibos tea itself. The SDE sample consisted of 123 components, including acetic acid, β-damascenone, geranylacetone, guaiacol, hexanoic acid, 3-methylbutanoic acid, 2-phenylethanol and 6,10,14-trimethylpentadecanone, but mostly lacked lactones. Song et al. (2021) employed SDE and steam distillation under reduced pressure (DRP; for analysing thermally unstable volatiles) to obtain the volatile fraction of fermented rooibos tea. From the 50 volatile compounds identified using GC–MS, the SDE and DRP fractions delivered 26 and 25 aroma-active compounds, respectively. A shelf-life study on a ready-to-use green rooibos iced tea powder, containing the extract microencapsulated with inulin and mixed with xylitol and citric acid, demonstrated that the aroma profile of the product changed from a predominantly green, vegetal character to an aroma more reminiscent of fermented rooibos (Human et al., 2021a). By using headspace and GC-MS analysis, the presence of a large number of compounds, of which 37 compounds were identified, were demonstrated in the powder after reconstitution to beverage strength. Semiquantitative analysis showed that the concentrations of 31 identified compounds increased (e.g. limonene and geranyl acetone) or decreased (e.g. linalool) during the 1-month accelerated storage. The change in aroma profile was attributed to a decrease in the concentration of 2-hexenal, (*Z*)-2-heptenal, (*E*)-2-octenal, (*E*)-2-nonenal, (*E,Z*)-2,6-nonadienal and (*E*)-2-decenal, associated with 'green-like' aromas, rather than an increase in fruity and sweet aroma-impact compounds.

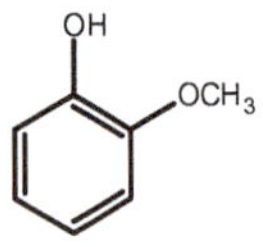
Guaiacol

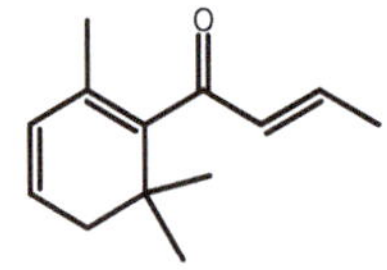
Damascenone

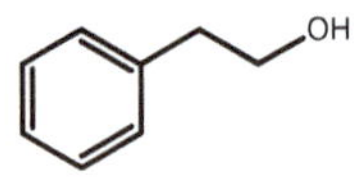
2-Phenylethanol

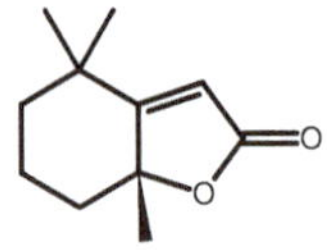
Dihydroactinidiolide

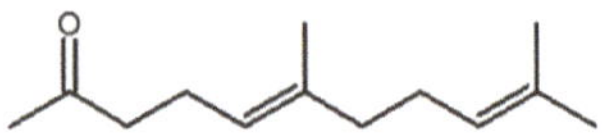
Geranylacetone

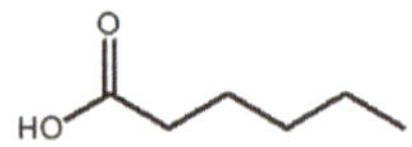
Hexanoic acid

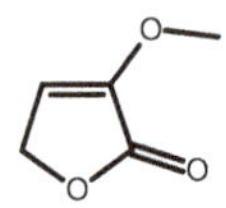
2-Methoxy-2-buten-4-olide

9.2 Non-volatile constituents

Rooibos tea contains less tannins than black tea (*Camellia sinensis*) and it does not contain caffeine, as recently confirmed using a highly specific method with a limit of detection (LOD) of 0.2 μg/L (Stander et al., 2019). Information on the tannin structures found in rooibos is sparse, but the dimer, procyanidin B3, the trimer, bis-fisetinidol-(4β,6:4β,8)-catechin, and a pentamer have been reported in a tannin fraction (Ferreira et al., 1995). Two unique phenolic compounds found in rooibos are a cyclic dihydrochalcone, aspalalinin (Shimamura et al., 2006) and linearthin, a dihydrochalcone containing a *C*-fructofuranoside unit (Akinfenwa et al., 2021). The dihydrochalcone *C*-glucoside, aspalathin, only occurs in rooibos and *A. pendula*. Another rare dihydrochalcone *C*-glucoside present in rooibos is nothofagin. The presence of the *C*-5′-hexosyl derivative of aspalathin was demonstrated by Beelders et al. (2012a) and its structure was later confirmed to be a *C*-5′-glucosyl derivative, 3-hydroxyphloretin-3′,5′-di-*C*-glucoside, when the same compound was isolated from *Cyclopia subternata* (Human et al., 2021b). Rooibos contains many other major phenolic compounds: the flavones such as vitexin and isovitexin, orientin and isoorientin, as well as luteolin, luteolin-7-*O*-glucoside and chrysoeriol; flavanones including dihydro-orientin, dihydro-isoorientin and hemiphlorin; and the flavonols rutin, quercetin, isoquercitrin and hyperoside (Ferreira et al., 1995; Shimamura et al., 2006). Coumarins such as esculin and esculetin, the flavonol quercetin-3-*O*-robinobioside, phenolic acids, lignans, flavone diglycosides, (+)-catechin, and a phenylpyruvic acid glycoside, PPAG, have also been identified (Marais et al., 1996; Shimamura et al., 2006).

Van Heerden et al. (2003) demonstrated qualitative and quantitative differences in wild-type rooibos populations and provenances. Aspalathin was absent in some wild rooibos populations, whereas other flavonoids, including orientin, isoorientin and rutin, were present as the major phenolic compounds. *Aspalathus pendula*, which is rarely used to make rooibos tea and is closely related to *A. linearis*, was reported to have rutin as the main compound (Van Heerden et al., 2003). Stander et al. (2017)

noted no diagnostically different discontinuities between the species. Aspalathin was also detected in *A. pendula* for the first time by Stander et al. (2017). Northern resprouters from Gifberg and Nieuwoudtville contained higher PPAG levels, whilst populations from Wupperthal and surrounding areas contained the dihydrochalcones, phloridzin and a sieboldin analogue, both reported in rooibos for the first time.

Analysis of green and fermented rooibos extracts is challenging due to the complex nature of the samples. Rooibos extracts contain many phenolic compounds that cannot be separated and identified using a single chromatographic technique, within a reasonable run time. Beelders et al. (2012b) used a systematic approach to optimise the reversed phase-liquid chromatographic separation (RP-LC) of 15 major phenolic compounds in rooibos tea. Thirteen additional phenolic compounds, including a new luteolin-6-*C*-pentoside-8-*C*-hexoside and the novel *C*-5′-hexosyl derivative of aspalathin reported for the first time, were detected in rooibos infusions using mass spectrometric (MS) and tandem MS methods. To achieve separation and tentative identification of a larger number of compounds, two-dimensional (2D) separation was first employed by Beelders et al. (2012a). Phenolic compounds were separated according to polarity by hydrophilic interaction chromatography (HILIC) in the first dimension, whilst reversed-phase liquid chromatography (RP-LC) provided separation according to hydrophobicity in the second dimension. Both off-line and online modes were investigated. Using the HILIC × RP-LC method, large qualitative differences in the phenolic composition of green and fermented rooibos could be established (Beelders et al., 2012a). Walters et al. (2017a) employed an off-line 2D method comprising normal phase high-performance countercurrent chromatography (NP-HPCCC) as the first dimension and RP ultra-high-performance liquid chromatography (RP-UHPLC) as the second dimension. The large polarity range of the HPCCC gradient separation allowed phenolic compounds, including relatively polar flavonoid di-*C*-glycosides and less polar mono- and di-*O*-glycosides, to be spread across the retention space. This 2D method resulted in the efficient separation of rooibos phenolic compounds with a high degree (~80%) of orthogonality, within a 17-h total analysis time. The qualitative analysis of both fermented and green rooibos extracts allowed for the separation and tentative identification of 39 compounds, 18 of which were reported for the first time in rooibos. Hesperidin (flavanone), scolymoside (flavone) and phloretin-3′,5′-di-*C*-glucoside (dihydrochalcone), previously reported in *Cyclopia* spp. (honeybush), were identified for the first time in rooibos by comparison with authentic reference standards (Walters et al., 2017a).

Rooibos tea is available in two forms, fermented (oxidised) and unfermented (unoxidised; green). The fermentation process results in major chemical changes, especially with regard to its phenolic composition. Most notable is the oxidation of aspalathin to isoorientin and orientin *via* its flavanone analogues (Marais et al., 2000). Krafczyk and Glomb (2008) elucidated the oxidation mechanism, which includes the conversion of dihydro-isoorientin ((*R*)- and (*S*)-eriodictyol-6-*C*-glucoside) to isoorientin. However, dihydro-orientin ((*R*)- and (*S*)-eriodictyol-8-*C*-glucoside), forming in lesser quantities, does not oxidise directly to orientin as demonstrated for dihydro-isoorientin and its flavone, isoorientin. Orientin forms irreversibly from isoorientin. It undergoes the opening of its vinyl ester structure to form a chalcone intermediate that is then converted to orientin. Furthermore, three colourless aspalathin dimers, two coloured compounds with dibenzofuran skeletons and brown high molecular compounds form as a result of aspalathin oxidation (Krafczyk et al., 2009b; Heinrich et al., 2012).

The green rooibos plant contains high levels of aspalathin (2.5%–4.5%) with lower levels of orientin, isoorientin and nothofagin (<0.5%) (De Beer et al., 2017). The nothofagin and aspalathin content of green rooibos exhibited seasonal variation, with the highest levels occurring in mid-spring to early summer (De Beer et al., 2017). Other factors affecting the aspalathin content include plant-to-plant variation due to plant propagation from open-pollinated seeds (Joubert and De Beer, 2011), and leaf-to-stem ratio (De Beer et al., 2017). In contrast, fermented plant material contains much lower levels of aspalathin (<1%) and nothofagin (<0.5%), with orientin and isoorientin levels around 0.5% (Joubert and De Beer, 2014). The PPAG content of green and fermented rooibos plant material is similar (Joubert et al., 2013). Walters et al. (2017b) quantified the major phenolic compounds in green and fermented plant material, originating from the same batches. This allowed a direct comparison of the effect of fermentation. Changes to the phenolic composition during fermentation included a substantial decrease in dihydrochalcone content, a moderate to small decrease in flavonol content, and an increase in the content of eriodictyol-glucopyranoside isomers, due to the oxidative conversion of aspalathin. In a follow-up study, the phenolic composition of rooibos plant material was monitored over 6 h during laboratory-scale simulated fermentation at various temperatures (37–50 °C) (De Beer et al., 2019). The degradation of aspalathin and nothofagin and the formation of eriodictyol-glucoside isomers were modelled using the fraction conversion model, based on first-order reaction kinetics. Changes in other compounds were not extensive enough to allow kinetic modelling. The data obtained in this study support the postulation that endogenous enzymes in rooibos participate in the oxidation of aspalathin and that the process does not solely involve chemical oxidation.

The HPLC–DAD method developed by Beelders et al. (2012b) was applied for the analysis of 'cup-of-tea' infusions of a large sample set ($n = 114$) of fermented rooibos, representing three production years (2009, 2010 and 2011) and four quality grades (A, B, C and D) (Joubert et al., 2012). The major phenolic constituents of the infusions were isoorientin and orientin (>10 mg/L), with quercetin-3-*O*-robinobioside, PPAG and aspalathin present at >5 mg/L. Isovitexin, vitexin and hyperoside were present at <3 mg/L, and rutin, ferulic acid and isoquercitrin at <2 mg/L. Nothofagin was present at much lower concentrations (<1 mg/L) than aspalathin. Only traces of luteolin-7-*O*-glucoside and the aglycones, quercetin, luteolin and chrysoeriol, were detected. On average, rooibos of a higher quality grade contained higher concentrations of all phenolic compounds, except PPAG and ferulic acid.

Steam pasteurisation is performed on fermented rooibos postproduction to ensure microbial safety. This processing step decreases the aspalathin concentration of infusions significantly (Koch et al., 2013). None of the other phenolic compounds quantified were affected by steam pasteurisation. De Beer et al. (2015) developed a high-performance countercurrent chromatography (HPCCC) method to isolate the valuable bioactive compounds, aspalathin and nothofagin. In addition, a rapid 16 min HPLC–DAD method was developed and validated to quantify aspalathin, nothofagin, isoorientin and orientin, the four major compounds. The pH was shown to have an effect on the stability of aspalathin in solution, with 91% remaining after 29 h at pH 3, compared to 45% remaining after 29 h at a pH of 7. Semipreparative HPLC yielded high purity aspalathin (99%) and nothofagin (100%) from HPCCC fractions. It was noted that acidification of the HPCCC solvent system prevents the degradation of the selected analytes.

Joubert et al. (2016) embarked on a study to determine whether the production area affects the phenolic composition of rooibos infusions. This is relevant to climate change, as production in the western areas of South Africa could become less suitable, necessitating production at a higher elevation. A large sample set ($n = 209$) comprising different grades of unpasteurised, fermented rooibos samples was obtained over a period of three production years (2011–13) from two major rooibos processing and marketing companies, located in the Western Cape and Northern Cape provinces, respectively. Hot water infusions at 'cup-of-tea' strength (as prepared for grading) were analysed to quantify the content of 10 flavonoid glycosides, PPAG and ferulic acid. Principal component analysis (PCA) of the data showed no clear grouping of samples according to the production area, although samples from the Western Cape Province contained slightly, but significantly, more aspalathin and nothofagin. Discriminant analysis showed grouping according to year, but not production area.

Vibrational spectroscopic techniques have been investigated for rapid quality control. Manley et al. (2006) developed near-infrared (NIR) spectroscopy calibration models for the quantification of the aspalathin and nothofagin content of green rooibos. The models were suitable for screening the plant material, however, the transmission NIR calibration model for the prediction of the aspalathin concentration (0.3–51 mg/L) in dilute, aqueous extracts did not give acceptable results. Hyperspectral imaging (HSI) was investigated as a potential rapid quality control method by Djokam et al. (2017). Using the sisuChema shortwave-infrared (SWIR) hyperspectral pushbroom imaging system, images of rooibos, buchu, honeybush and cancerbush 'raw' plant materials and intact tea bags were acquired (920–2514 nm) and chemometric data analysis was performed on the images. The PCA scores plot revealed a clear separation between the plant materials. Partial least-squares discriminant analysis (PLS-DA) models were developed and subsequently successfully used to predict the raw material constituents, and accurately determine the relative proportions of blends. Ultra-high-performance liquid chromatography coupled to mass spectrometry (UHPLC–MS) was used to confirm the results. This method showed the possible non-destructive application of HSI in the industry, as the intact teabag could be analysed.

Dihydrochalcones

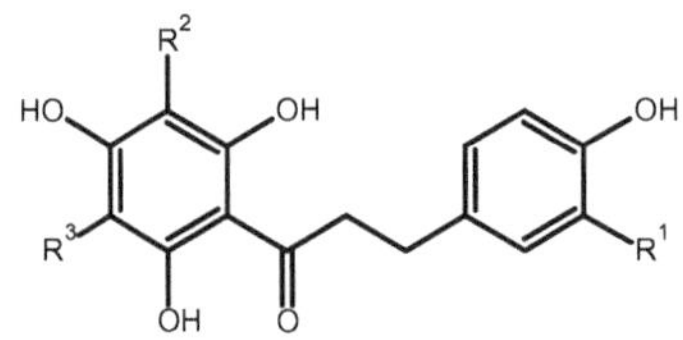

Aspalathin: R^1=OH; R^2=H; R^3=β-D-glucopyranosyl
Nothofagin: R^1, R^2=H; R^3=β-D-glucopyranosyl

Flavones

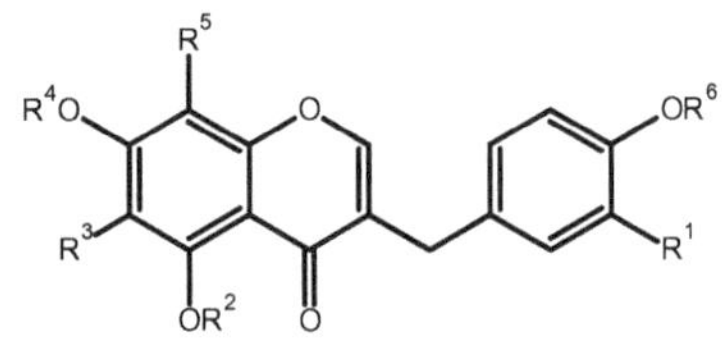

Orientin: R^1=OH; R^2, R^3, R^4, R^6=H; R^5=β-D-glucopyranosyl
Isoorientin: R^1=OH; R^2, R^4, R^5, R^6=H; R^3=β-D-glucopyranosyl
Vitexin: R^1, R^2, R^4, R^3, R^6=H; R^5=β-D-glucopyranosyl
Isovitexin: R^1, R^2, R^4, R^5, R^6=H; R^3=β-D-glucopyranosyl
Luteolin: R^1=OH; R^2, R^3, R^5, R^4=H
Chrysoeriol: R^1=OCH_3; R^2, R^3, R^5, R^4=H
Luteolin-7-*O*-glucopyranoside: R^1=OH; R^2, R^4, R^5, R^6=H; R^4=β-D-glucopyranosyl

Flavanones

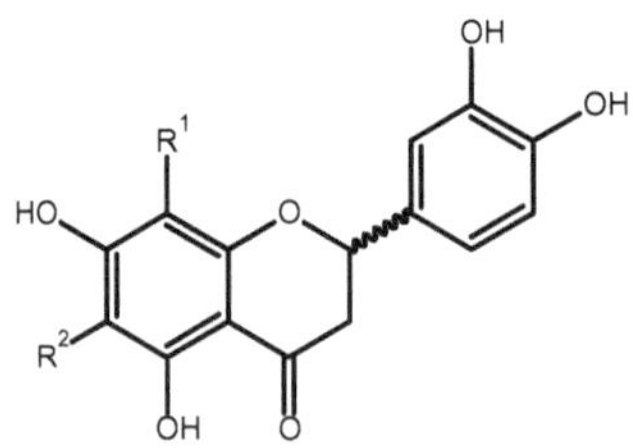

(*S*)/(*R*)-Eriodictyol-6-*C*-glucopyranoside: R^1=H, R^2=β-D-glucopyranosyl
(*S*)/(*R*)-Eriodictyol-8-*C*-glucopyranoside: R^1=β-D-glucopyranosyl, R^2=H

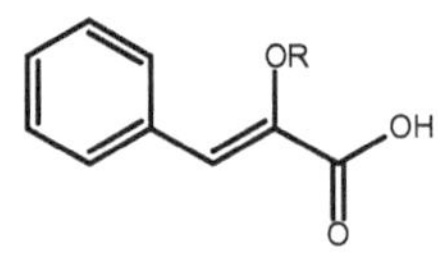

Z-2-(β-D-Glucopyranosyloxy)-3-phenylpropenoic acid (PPAG): R=β-D-glucopyranosyl

Flavonols

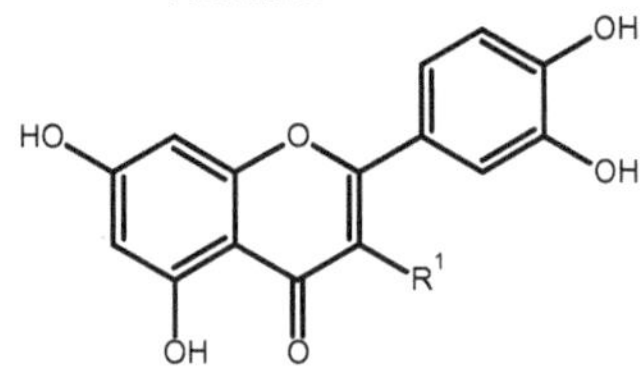

Hyperoside: R^1=*O*-β-D-galactopyranosyl
Isoquercitrin: R^1=*O*-β-D-glucopyranosyl
Rutin: R^1=*O*-α-L-rhamnopyranosyl-(1→6)-β-D-glucopyranosyl
Quercetin-3-*O*-robinobioside: R^1=*O*-α-L-rhamnopyranosyl-(1→6)-β-D-galactopyranosyl

Part B: Chemical profiling and quality control

10. Chromatography analysis

10.1 High-performance thin-layer chromatography (HPTLC) fingerprint analysis

General instrumentation: CAMAG HPTLC instrument consists of an automatic TLC sampler (ATS 4), automatic developing chamber (ADC 2), CAMAG TLC visualiser 2, CAMAG derivatiser, and TLC plate heater. *HPTLC plates:* Silica gel glass plates 60 F_{254} (Merck). *Plant part:* Aerial parts, methanol extract. *Sample application:*

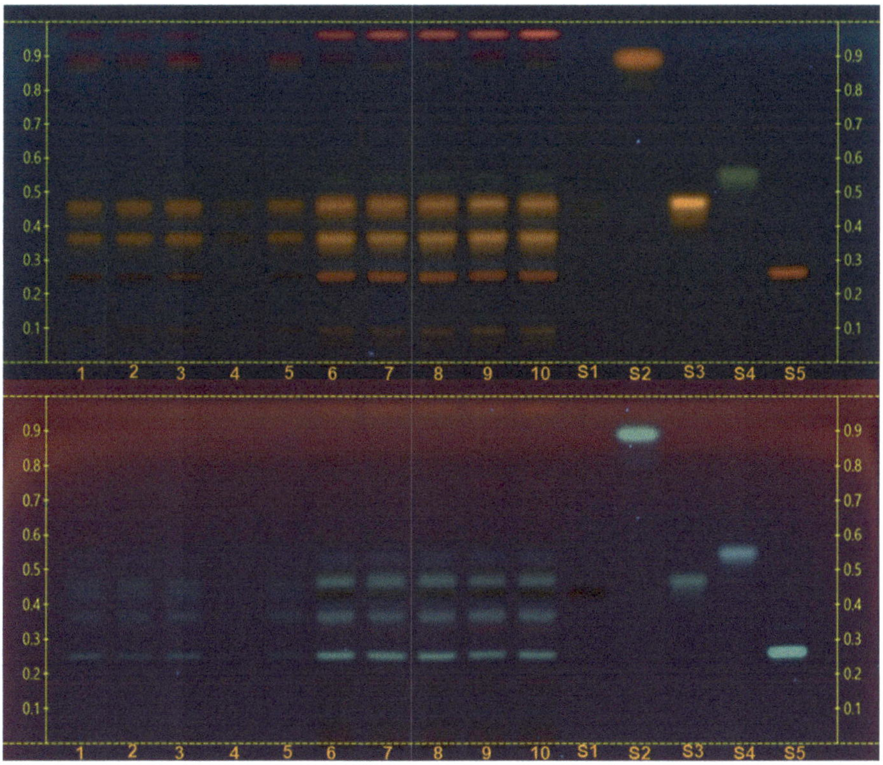

HPTLC plates of *Aspalathus linearis* methanol extracts (fermented 1–5, unfermented 6–10) and the standards (S1–S5) were viewed under 366 nm radiation and derivatised with NP reagent (top) and anisaldehyde (bottom). The samples are characterised by a brown band for aspalathin (S1) (R_f=0.44) (bottom plate), an orange band for quercetin (S2) (R_f=0.88), a yellow band for orientin (S3) (R_f=0.48), a green band for vitexin (S4) (R_f=0.56) and an orange band for rutin (S5) (R_f=0.27).

Application volume of 2 µL methanol extract (100 mg/mL) and standards (1 mg/mL) spotted as 10 mm bands. Plates were developed in a 20 × 10 × 4 cm glass twin-trough chamber to a migration distance of 70 mm. *Tank saturation:* 20 min at 15 °C and 33% RH, with 25 mL of the mobile phase. *Mobile phase:* Ethyl acetate:water:formic acid (16:1:1 v/v/v). *Derivatisation:* Reagent A, Natural Product reagent (NP) (1 g 2-aminoethyl diphenylborinate + 100 mL methanol) and polyethylene glycol (PEG) (5 g polyethylene glycol + 100 mL 96% ethanol). The plate was heated for 3 min at 100 °C and sprayed with 3 mL of NP+PEG (1:1 v/v). Reagent B, *p*-anisaldehyde reagent (85 mL methanol + 10 mL acetic acid + 5 mL sulphuric acid + 0.5 mL *p*-anisaldehyde). The plate was sprayed with 3 mL of anisaldehyde reagent, followed by heating the plate for 3 min at 100 °C and then visualised. *Visualisation:* The plate was viewed under 366 nm radiation.

10.2 Ultra-performance liquid chromatography (UPLC) analysis

General Instrumentation: Waters Acquity Ultra-Performance liquid chromatography system with photodiode array (PDA) detector combined with Xevo G2QToF mass spectrometer (Waters, United States). *Plant part:* Aerial parts, methanol extract. *Sample application:* Injection volume of 1.0 µL (full-loop injection) at 1 mg/mL concentration. *Column:* Acquity UPLC BEH C_{18} column (150 mm × 2.1 mm i.d., 1.7 µm particle size, Waters). *Mobile phase:* 0.1% formic acid in water (solvent A) and acetonitrile (solvent B). *Analysis conditions:* Gradient elution at a flow rate of 0.3 mL/min, initially 90% A: 10% B to 75% A: 25% B in 8 min, to 50% A: 50% B in 2 min, keeping for 0.5 min and back to initial ratio in 0.2 min, equilibrating the system for 1.3 min, total run time 12 min. *Mass spectrometry:* ESI^+ (positive ionisation mode), N_2 used as desolvation gas at a flow rate of 500 L/h, desolvation temperature 350 °C, and source temperature at 100 °C. Capillary and cone voltages, 3000 and 40 V, respectively. Data were collected between *m/z* 100 and 1200.

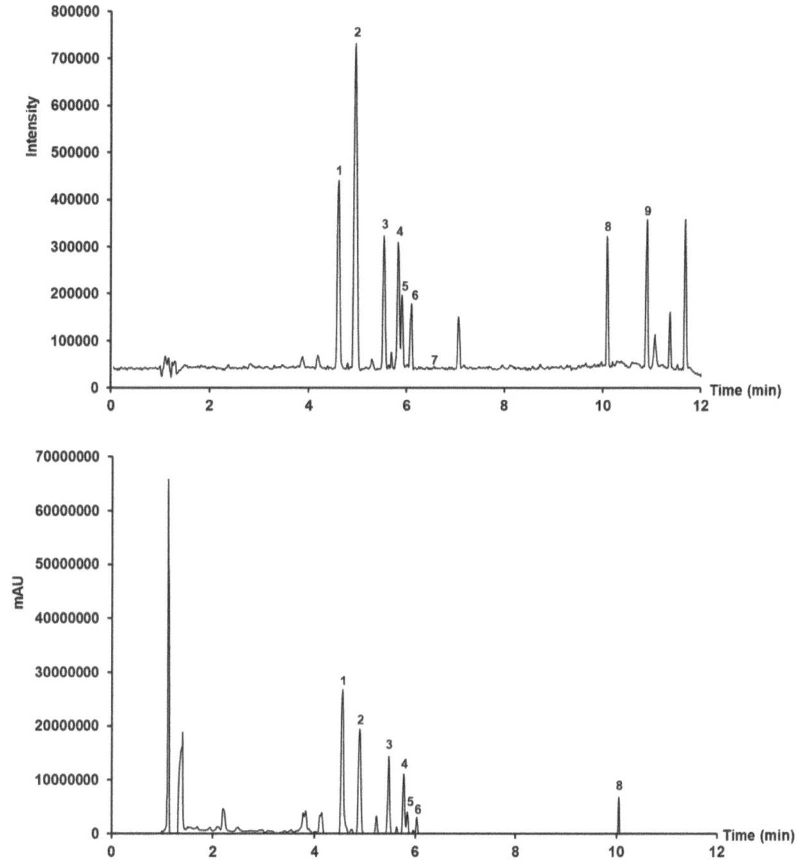

UPLC–ToF–MS ESI$^+$ (upper) and PDA (lower) chromatograms of *Aspalathus linearis* methanol extract. [1] = isoorientin *m/z* 449.1083, [2] = orientin *m/z* 449.1097, [3] = aspalathin *m/z* 453.1417, [4] = isovitexin *m/z* 433.1138, [5] = hyperoside *m/z* 465.1033, [6] = isoquercitrin *m/z* 465.1040, [7] = luteolin-7-*O*-glucoside *m/z* 449.1076, [8] = luteolin *m/z* 287.0562, [9] = chrysoeriol *m/z* 301.0714.

11. Mid-infrared (MIR) spectroscopy analysis

General instrumentation: Alpha-P Bruker spectrometer, mounted with an attenuated total reflectance (ATR) diamond crystal. *Spectral acquisition:* Spectra obtained in absorbance mode, with a spectral resolution of 4 cm^{-1} over the range 4000–550 cm^{-1} and captured using OPUS 6.5 software. *Plant part:* Aerial parts. *Sample preparation:* Samples were powdered and sieved (<500 μm) and placed directly onto the surface of the crystal.

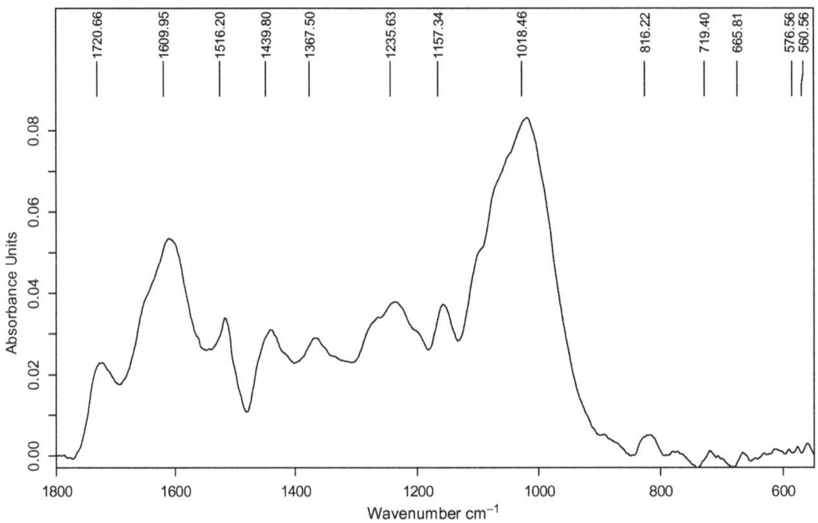

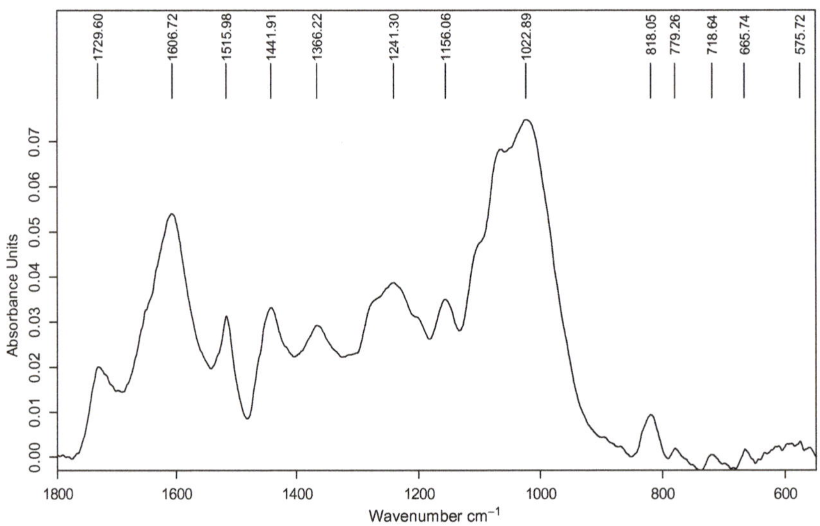

Mid-infrared spectra of fermented (*upper*) and unfermented (*lower*) *Aspalathus linearis* powder displaying the fingerprint region (1800–550 cm^{-1}).

References

Abrahams, S., Samodien, S., Lilly, M., Joubert, E., Gelderblom, W., 2019. Planta Med., 85:6–13.

Ajuwon, O., Marnewick, J., Davids, L., 2015. Rooibos (*Aspalathus linearis*) and its major flavonoids—potential against oxidative stress-induced conditions. In: Gowder, S.J.T. (Ed.), Basic Principles and Clinical Significance of Oxidative Stress. IntechOpen, London, UK, https://doi.org/10.5772/61614.

Akinfenwa, A.O., Abdul, N.S., Marnewick, J.L., Hussein, A.A., 2021. Plants, 10, Art. No. 1936, https://doi.org/10.3390/plants10091936.

Akinrinmade, O., Omoruyi, S., Dietrich, D., Ekpo, O., 2017. Acta Neurobiol. Exp., 77:94–105.

Almajano, M.P., Carbo, R., Jimenez, J.A.L., Gordon, M.H., 2008. Food Chem., 108:55–63.

Arakaki, R., Ushio, A., Kisoda, S., Sato, M., Nakamura, Y., Yuyama, K., Tateyama, R., Morishita, S., Monoi, N., Kudo, Y., Ishimaru, N., 2019. J. Oral Biosci., 61:179–182.

Awoniyi, D.O., Aboua, Y.G., Marnewick, J., Brooks, N., 2012. Phytother. Res., 26:1231–1239.

Beelders, T., Kalili, K.M., Joubert, E., De Beer, D., De Villiers, A., 2012a. J. Sep. Sci., 35:1808–1820.

Beelders, T., Sigge, G.O., Joubert, E., De Beer, D., De Villiers, A., 2012b. J. Chromatogr. A, 1219:128–139.

Blasa, M., Angelino, D., Gennari, L., Ninfali, P., 2011. Food Chem., 125:685–691.

Bond, T., Derbyshire, E., 2020. Nutr. Food Technol. Open Access, 6, https://doi.org/10.16966/2470-6086.166.

Boyanova, L., 2014. World J. Microbiol. Biotechnol., 30:1633–1637.

Breet, P., Kruger, H.S., Jerling, J.C., Oosthuizen, W., 2005. Nutr. Res., 25:983–994.

Chaudhary, S.K., Sandasi, M., Makolo, F., Van Heerden, F.R., Viljoen, A.M., 2021. Phytochem. Rev., Art. No. 09741-9.

Coetzee, G., Marx, I.J., Pengilly, M., Bushula, V.S., Joubert, E., Bloom, M., 2008. S. Afr. J. Enol. Vitic., 29:33–38.

Cullere, M., Hoffman, L.C., Dalle Zotte, A., 2013. Meat Sci., 95:72–77.

Cullere, M., Tasoniero, G., Secci, G., Parisi, G., Smit, P., Hoffman, L.C., Dalle Zotte, A., 2019. LWT - Food Sci. Technol., 108:31–38.

Dahlgren, R., 1968. Revision of the genus *Aspalathus*. Bot. Notiser, 12:195–197.

De Beer, D., Malherbe, C.J., Beelders, T., Willenburg, E.L., Brand, D.J., Joubert, E., 2015. J. Chromatogr. A, 1381:29–36.

De Beer, D., Miller, N., Joubert, E., 2017. S. Afr. J. Bot., 110:138–143.

De Beer, D., Tobin, J., Walczak, B., Van der Rijst, M., Joubert, E., 2019. Food Res. Int., 121:185–196.

Djokam, M., Sandasi, M., Chen, W., Viljoen, A., Vermaak, I., 2017. Appl. Sci., 7, Art. No. 268, https://doi.org/10.3390/app7030268.

Dludla, P.V., Muller, C.J.F., Louw, J., Joubert, E., Salie, R., Opoku, A.R., Johnson, R., 2014. Phytomedicine, 21:595–601.

Dludla, P.V., Muller, C.J.F., Joubert, E., Louw, J., Gabuza, K.B., Huisamen, B., Essop, M.F., Johnson, R., 2016. Planta Med., 82:1468–1474.

Dludla, P.V., Joubert, E., Muller, C.J.F., Louw, J., Johnson, R., 2017. Nutr. Metab., 14, Art. No. 45, https://doi.org/10.1186/s12986-017-0200-8.

Dludla, P.V., Gabuza, K.B., Muller, C.J.F., Joubert, E., Louw, J., Johnson, R., 2018. Physiol. Res., 67:813–818.

Dludla, P.V., Muller, C.J.F., Louw, J., Mazibuko-Mbeje, S.E., Tiano, L., Silvestri, S., Orlando, P., Marcheggiani, F., Cirilli, I., Chellan, N., Ghoor, S., Nkambule, B.B., Essop, M.F., Huisamen, B., Johnson, R., 2020a. Nutrients, 12, Art. No. 1151, https://doi.org/10.3390/nu12041151.

Dludla, P.V., Johnson, R., Mazibuko-Mbeje, S.E., Muller, C.J.F., Louw, J., Joubert, E., Orlando, P., Silvestri, S., Chellan, N., Nkambule, B.B., Essop, M.F., Tiano, L., 2020b. S. Afr. J. Bot., 131:143–150.

Edenharder, R., Sager, J.W., Glatt, H., Muckel, E., Platt, K.L., 2002. Mutat. Res., 521:57–72.

Elegbede, R.D., Ilomuanya, M.O., Sowemimo, A.A., Nneji, A., Joubert, E., De Beer, D., Koekemoer, T., Van de Venter, M., 2020. Wound Med., 29, Art. No. 100186, https://doi.org/10.1016/j.wndm.2020.100186.

Engels, M., Wang, C., Matoso, A., Maidan, E., Wands, J., 2013. ACG Case Rep. J., 1:58–60.

Fantoukh, O.I., Dale, O.R., Parveen, A., Hawwal, M.F., Ali, Z., Manda, V.K., Khan, S.I., Chittiboyina, A.G., Viljoen, A., Khan, I.A., 2019. J. Agric. Food Chem., 67:4967–4975.

Ferreira, D., Marais, C., Steenkamp, J.A., Joubert, E., 1995. Rooibos tea as a likely health food supplement. In: Proceedings of Recent Development of Technologies on Fundamental Foods for Health. Korean Society of Food Science and Technology, Seoul, Korea, pp. 73–88.

Gelderblom, W.C.A., Joubert, E., Gamieldien, K., Sissing, L., Malherbe, C.J., Maritz, G., 2017. S. Afr. J. Bot., 110:194–200.

Gilani, A.H., Khan, A.-U., Ghayur, M.N., Ali, S.F., Herzig, J.W., 2006. Basic Clin. Pharmacol. Toxicol., 99:65–373.

Glynn, K.M., 2010. From *In-Vitro* to *In-Vivo*: Corporate Development and Efficacy of a Topical Hair Growth Agent Derived From Natural Extracts. Masters dissertation, Grand Valley State University, Michigan, USA.

Habu, T., Flath, R.A., Mon, T.R., Morton, J.F., 1985. J. Agric. Food Chem., 33:249–254.

Hattingh, A.C., Van de Venter, M., Koekemoer, T.C., 2019. J. Funct. Foods, 55:184–192.

Hawkins, H.-J., Malgas, R., Biénabe, E., 2011. S. Afr. J. Bot., 77:360–370.

Heinrich, T., Willenberg, I., Glomb, M.A., 2012. J. Agric. Food Chem., 60:5221–5228.

Hendricks, R., Pool, E.J., 2010. J. Immunoass. Immunochem., 31:169–180.

Hesseling, P.B., Joubert, J.R., 1982. S. Afr. Med. J., 62:1037–1038.

Hesseling, P.B., Klopper, J.F., Van Heerden, P.D.R., 1979. S. Afr. Med. J., 55:631–632.

Himpe, E., Cunha, D.A., Song, I., Bugliani, M., Marchetti, P., Cnop, M., Bouwens, L., 2016. PLoS One, 11, Art. No. e0157604, https://doi.org/10.1371/journal.pone.0157604.

Hitomi, E., Tamura, S., Tsurumoto, Y., Tsuda, T., Nakano, M., 1999. Nippon Shokuhin Kagaku Kogaku Kaishi, 46:779–785.

Hoffman, L.C., Jones, M., Muller, N., Joubert, E., Sadie, A., 2014. Meat Sci., 96:1289–1296.

Hong, I.-S., Lee, H.-Y., Kim, H.-P., 2014. PLoS One, 9, Art. No. e87061, https://doi.org/10.1371/journal.pone.0087061.

Huang, S.-H., Tseng, J.-C., Lin, C.-Y., Kuo, Y.-Y., Wang, B.-J., Kao, Y.-H., Muller, C.J.F., Joubert, E., Chuu, C.-P., 2019. Phytomedicine, 64, Art. No. 153068, https://doi.org/10.1016/j.phymed.2019.153068.

Huang, S.-H., Kao, Y.-H., Muller, C.J.F., Joubert, E., Chuu, C.-P., 2020. Phytomedicine, 69, Art. No. 153210, https://doi.org/10.1016/j.phymed.2020.153210.

Hübsch, Z., Van Vuuren, S.F., Van Zyl, R.L., 2014. S. Afr. J. Bot., 93:148–156.

Human, C., De Beer, D., Aucamp, M., Marx, I.J., Malherbe, C.J., Viljoen-Bloom, M., Van der Rijst, M., Joubert, E., 2020. LWT - Food Sci. Technol., 117, Art. No. 108653, https://doi.org/10.1016/j.lwt.2019.108653.

Human, C., De Beer, D., Muller, M., Van der Rijst, M., Aucamp, M., Tredoux, A., De Villiers, A., Joubert, E., 2021a. Molecules, 26, Art. No. 5260, https://doi.org/10.3390/molecules26175260.

Human, C., Danton, O., De Beer, D., Maruyama, T., Alexander, A., Malherbe, C., Hamburger, M., Joubert, E., 2021b. Food Chem., 351, Art. No. 129273, https://doi.org/10.1016/j.foodchem.2021.

Ichiyama, K., Tai, A., Yamamoto, I., 2007. Biosci. Biotechnol. Biochem., 71:598–602.

Idriss, M.T., Abdelgadir, A.A., Nour, A.H., 2021. Trop. J. Nat. Prod. Res., 5:686–691.

Inanami, O., Asanuma, T., Inukai, N., Jin, T., Shimokawa, S., Kasai, N., Nakano, M., Sato, F., Kuwabara, M., 1995. Neurosci. Lett., 196:85–88.

Ilomuanya, M.O., Adebona, A.C., Wang, W., Sowemimo, A., Eziegbo, C.L., Silva, B.O., Adeosun, S.O., Joubert, E., De Beer, D., 2020. SN Appl. Sci., 2, Art. No. 881, https://doi.org/10.1007/s42452-020-2701-8.

Ito, A., Shinohara, K., Kator, K., 1991. Protective action of rooibos tea (*Aspalathus linearis*) extracts against inactivation of L5178Y cells by H_2O_2. In: Proceedings of the International Symposium on Tea Science, The Organizing Committee of ISTS, Shizuoka, Japan, pp. 381–384.

Jang, E.H., Park, Y.C., Chung, W.G., 2004. Food Chem. Toxicol., 42:1749–1756.

Johnson, R., Shabalala, S., Louw, J., Kappo, A., Muller, C., 2017. Molecules, 22, Art. No. 1589, https://doi.org/10.3390/molecules22101589.

Johnson, R., De Beer, D., Dludla, P., Ferreira, D., Muller, C., Joubert, E., 2018. Planta Med., 84:568–583.

Jolley, B., Van der Rijst, M., Joubert, E., Muller, M., 2017. S. Afr. J. Bot., 110:161–166.

Jones, M., Hoffman, L.C., Muller, M., 2015a. Meat Sci., 103:54–60.

Jones, M., Hoffman, L.C., Muller, M., 2015b. S. Afr. J. Sci., 111 (11/12), Art. No. 014-0347, https://doi.org/10.17159/sajs.2015/20140347.

Joppe, H., Hermann, M., Wiedemann, J., 2009. Use of Rooibos Extract for the Protection of Hair Colour. U.S. Patent Application No. US 2009/0104298 A1.

Joubert, E., De Beer, D., 2011. S. Afr. J. Bot., 77:869–886.

Joubert, E., Winterton, P., Britz, T.J., Ferreira, D., 2004. Food Res. Int., 37:133–138.

Joubert, E., Winterton, P., Britz, T.J., Gelderblom, W.C.A., 2005. J. Agric. Food Chem., 53:10260–10267.

Joubert, E., Schulz, H., 2006. J. Appl. Bot. Food Qual., 80:138–144.

Joubert, E., Gelderblom, W.C.A., Louw, A., De Beer, D., 2008a. J. Ethnopharmacol., 119:376–412.

Joubert, E., Manley, M., Botha, M., 2008b. Phytochem. Anal., 19:169–178.

Joubert, E., Beelders, T., De Beer, D., Malherbe, C.J., De Villiers, A., Sigge, G.O., 2012. J. Agric. Food Chem., 60:9171–9179.

Joubert, E., De Beer, D., Malherbe, C.J., Muller, N., Bonnet, S.L., Van der Westhuizen, J.H., Ferreira, D., 2013. Food Chem., 136:1078–1085.

Joubert, E., De Beer, D., 2014. Antioxidants of rooibos beverages: role of plant composition and processing, In: Preedy, V. (Ed.), Processing and Impact on Antioxidants in Beverages. Academic Press, San Diego, USA, pp. 131–144.

Joubert, E., Jolley, B., Koch, I.S., Muller, M., Van der Rijst, M., De Beer, D., 2016. S. Afr. J. Bot., 103:162–169.

Juráni, M., Lamošsová, D., MáčAjová, M., Košťál, L., Joubert, E., Greksák, M., 2008. Br. Poult. Sci., 49:55–64.

Kanlayavattanakul, M., Lourith, N., 2015. J. Cosmet. Laser Ther., 17:343–352.

Kawakami, M., Kobayashi, A., Kator, K., 1993. J. Agric. Food Chem., 41:633–636.
Khan, A., Gilani, A.H., 2006. Eur. J. Nutr., 45:463–469.
Knipping, K., Garssen, J., Vant Land, B., 2012. Virol. J., 9, Art. No. 137, https://doi.org/10.1186/1743-422X-9-137.
Koch, I.S., Muller, M., Joubert, E., Van der Rijst, M., Næs, T., 2012. Food Res. Int., 46:217–228.
Koch, I.S., Muller, N., De Beer, D., Næs, T., Joubert, E., 2013. Food Res. Int., 53:704–712.
Komatsu, K., Kator, K., Mitsuda, Y., Mine, M., Okumura, Y., 1994. Cancer Lett., 77:33–38.
Kondo, M., Hirano, Y., Nishio, M., Furuya, Y., Nakamura, H., Watanabe, T., 2013. J. Food Sci., 78:H1935–H1939.
Kühnast, K., Braun, P.G., 2013. Arch. Leb., 64:24–30.
Kunishiro, K., Tai, A., Yamamoto, I., 2001. Biosci. Biotechnol. Biochem., 65:2137–2145.
Krafczyk, N., Glomb, M.A., 2008. J. Agric. Food Chem., 56:3368–3376.
Krafczyk, N., Woyand, F., Glomb, M.A., 2009a. Mol. Nutr. Food Res., 53:635–642.
Krafczyk, N., Heinrich, T., Porzel, A., Glomb, M.A., 2009b. J. Agric. Food Chem., 57:6838–6843.
Lamošová, D., Juráni, M., Greksák, M., Nakano, M., Vaneková, M., 1997. Comp. Biochem. Physiol. C Pharmacol. Toxicol. Endocrinol., 116:39–45.
Laura, B.K., Pheiffer, C., Fuertes, R.L., Ramos, P.L., Hernandez, C., Simo., Martinez, D., 2021. Endocr. Abstr., Art. No. EP88880, https://www.endocrine-abstracts.org/ea/0073/ea0073ep88.
Lawal, A.O., Davids, L.M., Marnewick, J.L., 2019. Phytomedicine, 59, Art. No. 152898, https://doi.org/10.1016/j.phymed.2019.152898.
Layman, J.I., Pereira, D.L., Chellan, N., Huisamen, B., Kotzé, S.H., 2019. Acta Histochem., 121:646–656.
Lee, E.-J., Jang, H.-D., 2004. Biofactors, 21:285–292.
Maarman, G.J., 2019. S. Afr. J. Sci., 115:8–11.
Magcwebeba, T.U., Riedel, S., Swanevelder, S., Swart, P., De Beer, D., Joubert, E., Gelderblom, W.C.A., 2016a. J. Pharm. Pharmacol., 68:1440–1453.
Magcwebeba, T., Swart, P., Swanevelder, S., Joubert, E., Gelderblom, W., 2016b. Molecules, 21, Art. No. 1323, https://doi.org/10.3390/molecules21101323.
Magcwebeba, T., Swart, P., Swanevelder, S., Joubert, E., Gelderblom, W.C.A., 2016c. Molecules, 21, Art. No. 1622, https://doi.org/10.3390/molecules21121622.
Malgas, R.R., Potts, A.J., Oettlé, N.M., Koelle, B., Todd, S.W., Verboom, G.A., Hoffman, M.T., 2010. S. Afr. J. Bot., 76:72–81.
Manley, M., Joubert, E., Botha, M., 2006. J. Near Infrared Spectrosc., 14:213–222.
Marais, C., Steenkamp, J.A., Ferreira, D., 1996. Tetrahedron Lett., 37:5763–5764.
Marais, C., Janse van Rensburg, W., Ferreira, D., Steenkamp, J.A., 2000. Phytochemistry, 55:43–49.
Marloth, R., 1917. Dictionary of Common Names of South African Plants. The Speciality Press, Cape Town, South Africa.
Marnewick, J.L., Gelderblom, W.C.A., Joubert, E., 2000. Mutat. Res., 471:157–166.
Marnewick, J.L., Joubert, E., Swart, P., Van der Westhuizen, F., Gelderblom, W.C., 2003. J. Agric. Food Chem., 51:8113–8119.
Marnewick, J.L., Joubert, E., Joseph, S., Swanevelder, S., Swart, P., Gelderblom, W.C.A., 2005. Cancer Lett., 224:193–202.
Marnewick, J.L., Van der Westhuizen, F.H., Joubert, E., Swanevelder, S., Swart, P., Gelderblom, W.C.A., 2009. Food Chem. Toxicol., 47:220–229.

Marnewick, J.L., Rautenbach, F., Venter, I., Neethling, H., Blackhurst, D.M., Wolmarans, P., Macharia, M., 2011. J. Ethnopharmacol., 133:46–52.
Marnewick, J.L., Venter, I., Rautenbach, F., Neethling, H., Kotze, M., 2013. ACS Symp. Ser., 1127:103–114.
Marnewick, J.L., 2014. Antioxidant properties of rooibos (*Aspalathus linearis*)—*in vitro* and *in vivo* evidence. In: Laher, I. (Ed.), Systems Biology of Free Radicals and Antioxidants. Springer Berlin, Heidelberg, Germany, pp. 4083–4108.
Matsuda, K., Nishimura, Y., Kurata, N., Iwase, M., Yasuhara, H., 2007. J. Pharmacol. Sci., 103:214–221.
Mazibuko-Mbeje, S.E., Dludla, P.V., Roux, C., Johnson, R., Ghoor, S., Joubert, E., Louw, J., Opoku, A.R., Muller, C.J.F., 2019a. Int. J. Mol. Sci., 20, Art. No. 633, https://doi.org/10.3390/ijms20030633.
Mazibuko-Mbeje, S.E., Dludla, P.V., Johnson, R., Joubert, E., Louw, J., Ziqubu, K., Tiano, L., Silvestri, S., Orlando, P., Opoku, A.R., Muller, C.J.F., 2019b. PLoS One, 14, Art. No. e0216172, https://doi.org/10.1371/journal.pone.0216172.
McAlpine, M.D., Gittings, W., MacNeil, A.J., Ward, W.E., 2019. Beverages, 5, Art. No. 69, https://doi.org/10.3390/beverages5040069.
McKay, D.L., Blumberg, J.B., 2007. Phytother. Res., 21:1–16.
Millar, D.A., Bowles, S., Windvogel, S.L., Louw, J., Muller, C.J.F., 2020. J. Cell. Physiol., 235:9487–9496.
Moens, C., Bensellam, M., Himpe, E., Muller, C.J.F., Jonas, J., Bouwens, L., 2020. Mol. Nutr. Food Res., 64, Art. No. 1901009, https://doi.org/10.1002/mnfr.201901009.
Monsees, T.K., Opuwari, C.S., 2017. S. Afr. J. Bot., 110:208–215.
Moosa, S., Kasonga, A.E., Deepak, V., Marais, S., Magoshi, I.B., Bester, M.J., Kruger, M.C., Coetzee, M., 2018. Food Funct., 9:3301–3312.
Morishita, Y., Ikeda, K., Matsuno, H., Ito, H., Tai, A., 2019. Nat. Prod. Res., 33:1472–1476.
Muller, C.J.F., Malherbe, C.J., Chellan, N., Yagasaki, K., Miura, Y., Joubert, E., 2018. Crit. Rev. Food Sci. Nutr., 58:227–246.
Muller, M., De Beer, D., Truzzi, C., Annibaldi, A., Carloni, P., Girolametti, F., Damiani, E., Joubert, E., 2020. LWT - Food Sci. Technol., 132, Art. No. 109919, https://doi.org/10.1016/j.lwt.2020.109919.
Munmun, F., Linden, A., Hanlon, H., Enderby, H., Witt-Enderby, P., 2021. Melatonin Res., 4:270–298.
Nakano, M., Itoh, Y., Mizuno, T., Nakashima, H., 1997a. Biosci. Biotechnol. Biochem., 61:267–271.
Nakano, M., Nakashima, H., Itoh, Y., 1997b. Leukemia, 11 (Suppl. 3):28–130.
Nash, L.A., Ward, W.E., 2016. Food Funct., 7:1166–1175.
Nikolova, V., Petrova, S., Petkova, V., Pavlova, A., Georgieva, T., 2007. Toxicol. Lett., 172:120–121.
Nishimachi, S., Iwai, T., Nakamura, Y., Yuyama-Masuda, K., Tsutsui, T., Monoi, N., Uchiyama, A., Nakamura, S., 2019. Funct. Foods, 55:248–254.
Nortje, J.M., Van Wyk, B.-E., 2015. J. Ethnopharmacol., 171:205–222.
Obasa, Z., Van Vuuren, M.A., Huisamen, B., Windvogel, S.L., 2021. Cardiovasc. J. Afr., 32:33–43.
Omolaoye, T.S., Windvogel, S., Du Plessis, S.S., 2021. Asian Pacific J. Reprod., 10:11–20.
Opuwari, C.S., Monsees, T.K., 2014. Andrologia, 46:867–877.
Opuwari, C.S., Monsees, T.K., 2015. Andrologia, 47:52–58.

Orlando, P., Chellan, N., Louw, J., Tiano, L., Cirilli, I., Dludla, P., Joubert, E., Muller, C.J.F., 2019. Molecules, 24, Art. No. 1713, https://doi.org/10.3390/molecules24091713.

Pantsi, W.G., Marnewick, J.L., Esterhuyse, A.J., Rautenbach, F., Van Rooyen, J., 2011. Phytomedicine, 18:1220–1228.

Park, H.J., Park, K.-C., Yoon, K.S., 2014. J. Food Sci., 79:M2507–M2515.

Patel, O., Muller, C., Joubert, E., Louw, J., Rosenkranz, B., Awortwe, C., 2016. Molecules, 21, Art. No. 1515, https://doi.org/10.3390/molecules21111515.

Patel, O., Muller, C.J.F., Joubert, E., Rosenkranz, B., Taylor, M.J.C., Louw, J., Awortwe, C., 2019. Front. Pharmacol., 10, Art. No. 1243, https://doi.org/10.3389/fphar.2019.01243.

Patel, O., Muller, C.J.F., Joubert, E., Rosenkranz, B., Louw, J., Awortwe, C., 2021. PLoS One, 16, Art. No. e0251069, https://doi.org/10.1371/journal.pone.0251069.

Pedretti, S., Peter, J., 2020. J. Ethnopharmacol., 252, Art. No. 112353, https://doi.org/10.1016/j.jep.2019.112353.

Persson, I.A.-L., Josefsson, M., Persson, K., Andersson, R.G.G., 2006. J. Pharm. Pharmacol., 58:1139–1144.

Persson, I.A.-L., Persson, K., Hägg, S., Andersson, R.G.G., 2010. Public Health Nutr., 13:730–737.

Persson, I.A., 2012. Phytother. Res., 26:517–521.

Platt, K.L., Edenharder, R., Aderhold, S., Muckel, E., Glatt, H., 2010. Mutat. Res., 703:90–98.

Popoola, O., Adedara, T., Ajao, A., Akinrinlola, M., Olasanmi, A., 2019. Biomed. J. Sci. Tech. Res., 20:15195–15202.

Pretorius, G., 2007. Rooibos Biodiversity Initiative (RBI). Biodiversity Best Practice Guidelines for the Sustainable Production of Rooibos. Natura Libra Environmental Consultants CC, Malmesbury, South Africa.

Pringle, N.A., Koekemoer, T.C., Holzer, A., Young, C., Venables, L., Van de Venter, M., 2018. Planta Med., 84:645–652.

Pyrzanowska, J., Fecka, I., Mirowska-Guzel, D., Joniec-Maciejak, I., Blecharz-Klin, K., Piechal, A., Wojnar, E., Widy-Tyszkiewicz, E., 2019. J. Ethnopharmacol., 238, Art. No. 111881, https://doi.org/10.1016/j.jep.2019.

Rahmasari, R., Haruyama, T., Charyasriwong, S., Nishida, T., Kobayashi, N., 2017. Nat. Prod. Commun., 12:599–602.

Reddy, S., Mishra, P., Qureshi, S., Nair, S., Straker, T., 2016. J. Clin. Anesth., 35:96–98.

Reid, A., Oosthuizen, C.B., Lall, N., 2020. S. Afr. J. Bot., 128:257–263.

Rodgers, A., Mokoena, M., Durbach, I., Lazarus, J., de Jager, S., Ackermann, H., Breytenbach, I., Okada, A., Usami, M., Hirose, Y., Ando, R., Yasui, T., Kohri, K., 2016. Urolithiasis, 44:299–310.

Ros-Santaella, J.L., Pintus, E., 2017. PLoS One, 12, Art. No. e0183682, https://doi.org/10.1371/journal.pone.0183682.

Sagar, T., Kasonga, A., Baschant, U., Rauner, M., Moosa, S., Marais, S., Kruger, M., Coetzee, M., 2020. J. Funct. Foods, 64, Art. No. 103616.

Sasaki, Y.F., Yamada, H., Shimoi, K., Kator, K., Kinae, N., 1993. Mutat. Res. Fundam. Mol. Mech. Mutagen., 286:221–232.

Sasaki, M., Nishida, N., Shimada, M., 2018. Molecules, 23, Art. No. 839, https://doi.org/10.3390/molecules23040839.

Sauter, W., 2004. Vergleich Antioxidativer Eigenschaften von Extrakten aus *Camellia sinensis*, *Rosmarinus officinalis*, *Cyclopia genistoides*, *Cyclopia sessiliflora* und *Aspalathus linearis*. PhD dissertation, Technischen Universität München, Weihenstephan, Germany.

Scheepers, S., 2001. Anti-Microbial Activity of Rooibos Tea (*Aspalathus linearis*) on Food Spoilage Organisms and Potential Pathogens. MSc (Food Science) thesis, Stellenbosch University, Stellenbosch, South Africa.
Schloms, L., Storbeck, K.-H., Swart, P., Gelderblom, W.C.A., Swart, A.C., 2012. J. Steroid Biochem. Mol. Biol., 128:128–138.
Schloms, L., Smith, C., Storbeck, K.-H., Marnewick, J.L., Swart, P., Swart, A.C., 2014. Mol. Nutr. Food Res., 58:537–549.
Schulz, H., Joubert, E., Schütze, W., 2003. Eur. Food Res. Technol., 216:539–543.
Sharma, R., Lall, N., 2014. S. Afr. J. Sci., 110 (11–12), Art. No. 8, https://doi.org/10.1590/sajs.2014/20130293.
Shimamura, N., Miyase, T., Umehara, K., Warashina, T., Fujii, S., 2006. Biol. Pharm. Bull., 29:1271–1274.
Shimoi, K., Hokabe, Y., Sasaki, Y.F., Yamada, H., Kator, K., Kinae, N., 1994. ACS Symp. Ser., 547:106–113.
Shimoi, K., Masuda, S., Shen, B., Furugori, M., Kinae, N., 1996. Mutat. Res., 350:153–161.
Shindo, Y., Kato, K., 1991. Effect of rooibos tea on some dermatological diseases. In: Proceedings of the International Symposium on Tea Science, The Organizing Committee of ISTS, Shizuoka, Japan, pp. 385–389.
Simon, M., Horovská, L., Greksák, M., Dušinský, R., Nakano, M., 2000. Gen. Physiol. Biophys., 19:365–371.
Sinisalo, M., Enkovaara, A.L., Kivistö, K.T., 2010. Eur. J. Clin. Pharmacol., 66:427–428.
Sirotkin, A.V., 2021. J. Anim. Physiol. Anim. Nutr., https://doi.org/10.1111/jpa.13624.
Sirotkin, A.V., Macejková, M., Tarko, A., Fabova, Z., Alwasel, S., Harrath, A.H., 2021a. Environ. Sci. Pollut. Res., 28:7431–7439.
Sirotkin, A.V., Macejková, M., Tarko, A., Fabova, Z., Alrezaki, A., Alwasel, S., Harrath, A.H., 2021b. Environ. Sci. Pollut. Res., 28:3434–3444.
Sissing, L., Marnewick, J., De Kock, M., Swanevelder, S., Joubert, E., Gelderblom, W., 2011. Nutr. Cancer, 63:600–610.
Smit, S.E., Manirafasha, C., Marais, E., Johnson, R., Huisamen, B., 2022. Planta Med., 88:62–78.
Smith, C., Swart, A.C., 2016. J. Funct. Foods, 27:42–54.
Smith, C., Swart, A., 2018. Food Funct., 9:5041–5058.
Snijman, P.W., Joubert, E., Ferreira, D., Li, X.-C., Ding, Y., Green, I.R., Gelderblom, W.C.A., 2009. J. Agric. Food Chem., 57:6678–6684.
Song, N., Kim, M.K., Lee, K., Jang, H.W., 2021. Food Res. Int., 141, Art. No. 109942, https://doi.org/10.1016/j.foodres.2020.109942.
Stander, M., Van Wyk, B., Taylor, M.J.C., Long, H.S., 2017. J. Agric. Food Chem., 65:10270–10281.
Stander, M.A., Joubert, E., De Beer, D., 2019. J. Food Compos. Anal., 76:39–43.
Standley, L., Winterton, P., Marnewick, J.L., Gelderblom, W.C.A., Joubert, E., Britz, T.J., 2001. J. Agric. Food Chem., 49:114–117.
Stirton, C.H., Muasya, A.M., 2016. S. Afr. J. Bot., 104:35–46.
Štochmačová, A., Kádasi, A., Vlčková, R., Sopková, D., Nltray, J., Nltrayová, S., Slrotkin, A.V., 2015. Biologia, 70:1424–1428.
Štochmačová, A., Kádasi, A., Alexa, R., Bauer, M., Harrath, A.H., Sirotkin, A.V., 2018. J. Anim. Physiol. Anim. Nutr., 102:e550–e557.
Takalani, N.B., Adefolaju, G.A., Henkel, R., Opuwari, C.S., 2021. Andrologia, 53, Art. No. e14114, https://doi.org/10.1111/and.14114.

Utter, A.C., Quindry, J.C., Emerenziani, G.P., Valiente, J.S., 2010. Res. Sports Med., 18:85–89.
Van der Merwe, J.D., Joubert, E., Richards, E.S., Manley, M., Snijman, P.W., Marnewick, J.L., Gelderblom, W.C.A., 2006. Mutat. Res., 611:42–53.
Van Heerden, F.R., Van Wyk, B.-E., Viljoen, A.M., Steenkamp, P.A., 2003. Biochem. Syst. Ecol., 31:885–895.
Van Staden, A.B., Oosthuizen, C.B., Lall, N., 2021. Sci. Rep., 11, Art. No. 7020, https://doi.org/10.1038/s41598-021-86410-z.
Van Wyk, B.-E., Gorelik, B., 2017. S. Afr. J. Bot., 110:18–38.
Van Wyk, B.-E., Stander, M.A., Long, H.S., 2017. S. Afr. J. Bot., 110:124–131.
Villaño, D., Pecorari, M., Testa, M.F., Raguzzini, A., Stalmach, A., Crozier, A., Tubili, C., Serafini, M., 2010. Food Chem., 123:679–683.
Von Gadow, A., Joubert, E., Hansmann, C.F., 1997a. Food Chem., 60:73–77.
Von Gadow, A., Joubert, E., Hansmann, C.F., 1997b. J. Agric. Food Chem., 45:632–638.
Waisundara, V.Y., Hoon, L.Y., 2015. J. Tradit. Complement. Med., 5:174–178.
Walters, N.A., De Villiers, A., Joubert, E., De Beer, D., 2017a. J. Chromatogr. A, 1490:102–114.
Walters, N.A., De Villiers, A., Joubert, E., De Beer, D., 2017b. J. Food Compos. Anal., 55:20–29.
Watanabe, N., Hara, Y., Sakuda, S., Mori, Y., Furuya, Y., Watanabe, T., 2014. Food Nutr. Sci., 5:127–131.
Webster, I., Imperial, E.G., Westcott, C., Strijdom, H., 2019. Cardiovasc. J. Afr., 30:95–102.
Windvogel, S., 2019. Rooibos (*Aspalathus linearis*) and honeybush (*Cyclopia* spp.): from bush teas to potential therapy for cardiovascular disease. In: Hueda, M.C. (Ed.), Nutraceuticals—Past, Present and Future. IntechOpen, London, UK, https://doi.org/10.5772/intechopen.86410.
Wynberg, R., 2017. S. Afr. J. Bot., 110:39–51.
Xiao, X., Erukainure, O.L., Sanni, O., Koorbanally, N.A., Islam, M.S., 2020. J. Food Sci. Technol., 57:4345–4354.
Xue, Y., Liu, Y., Xie, Y., Cong, C., Wang, G., An, L., Teng, Y., Chen, M., Zhang, L., 2020. Phytochemistry, 179, Art. No. 112393, https://doi.org/10.1016/j.phytochem.2020.112393.
Yoo, K.M., Lee, C.H., Lee, H., Moon, B., Lee, C.Y., 2008. Food Chem., 106:929–936.
Yoshikawa, T., Naito, Y., Oyamada, H., Ueda, S., Tanigawa, T., Takemura, T., Sugino, S., Kondo, M., 1990. Scavenging effect of *Aspalathus linearis* (rooibos tea) on active oxygen species. In: Emerit, I., Packer, L., Auclair, C. (Eds.), Antioxidants in Therapy and Preventative Medicine. Plenum Press, New York, USA, pp. 171–174.
Yuyama, K., Nakamura, Y., Tateyama, R., Arakaki, R., Tsutsui, T., Ishimaru, N., 2020. J. Chromatogr. B, 1137, Art. No. 121881, https://doi.org/10.1016/j.jchromb.2019.121881.

CHAPTER

Athrixia phylicoides

6

Lefa Lerotholi, Weiyang Chen and Sandra Combrinck

Department of Pharmaceutical Sciences, Tshwane University of Technology, Pretoria, South Africa

Abstract

Athrixia phylicoides DC. (Asteraceae), known as bush tea, is a leafy shrub that grows abundantly in South Africa and its neighbouring countries, including Lesotho and Swaziland. The plant is recognised as one of South Africa's indigenous teas, since infusions of the aerial parts are enjoyed as a beverage. Several indigenous groups prepare decoctions, infusions and pastes from various parts of the plant to treat an array of ailments, including infections, pain, inflammation, and conditions of dermatological, gastrointestinal, genito-urinary, cardiovascular and endocrine origin. In vitro studies have indicated that A. phylicoides has antidiabetic effects, and suggest that bush tea is safe to consume, but clinical trials to confirm this are lacking. Although bush tea has not been commercialised and is only informally traded, ongoing fundamental research coupled with models derived from successfully commercialised local herbal teas revealed potential for the development of bush tea products. Leaves and twigs of A. phylicoides from several natural populations were extracted using methanol: water (1:1). The chemical profiles of the extracts were established using semi-automated high-performance thin-layer chromatography (HPTLC) and ultra-performance liquid chromatography coupled with mass spectrometry (UPLC–MS). Compounds identified as chemical markers for the species were visible on derivatised HPTLC plates (viewed under 366 nm radiation) and on the UPLC–MS chromatograms.

Keywords: *Athrixia phylicoides*, Bush tea, Flavonoids, Chlorogenic acid, 3-*O*-dimethyldigicitrin, Hydroxy-6,7,8,3′,4′,5′-hexamethoxyflavon-3-ol, HPTLC, UPLC–MS, MIR spectroscopy

The South African Herbal Pharmacopoeia. https://doi.org/10.1016/B978-0-323-99794-2.00014-3

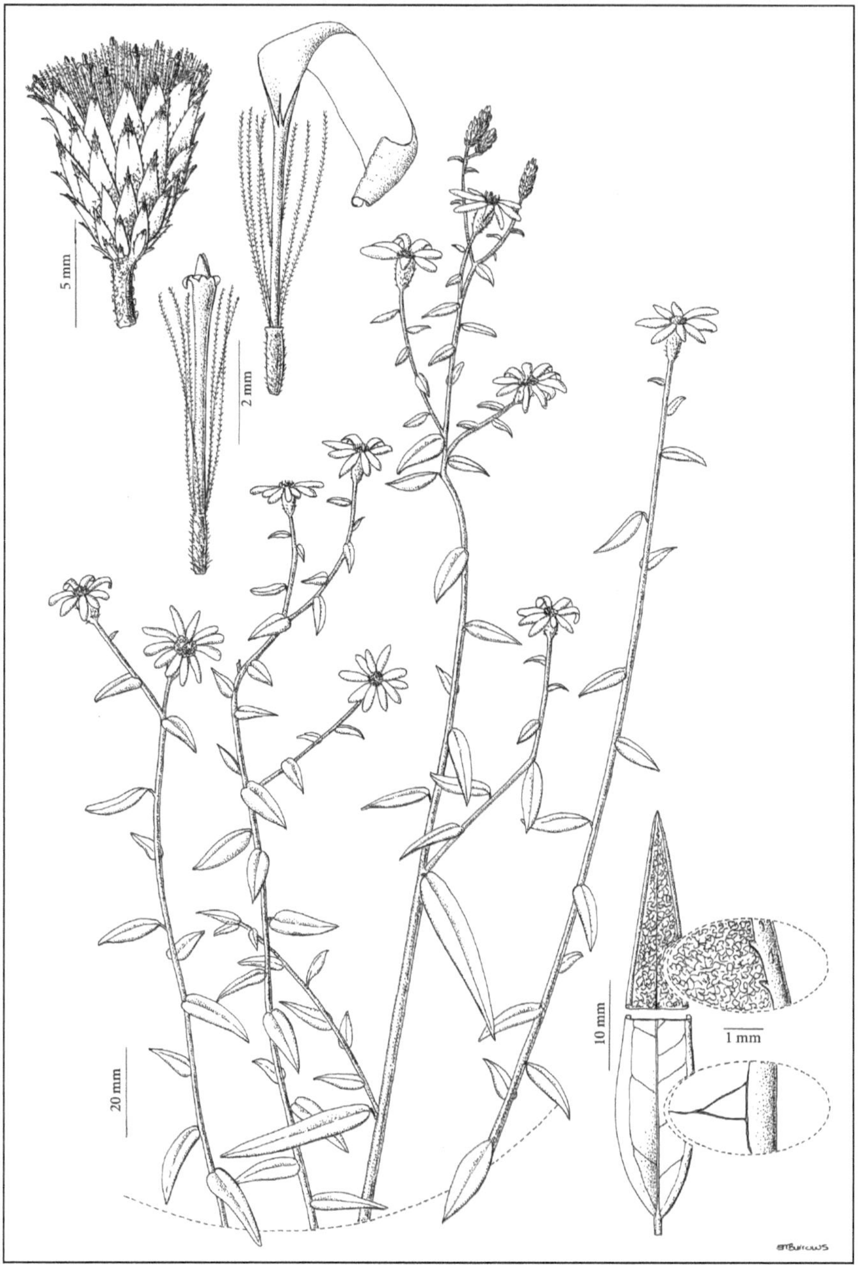
5 mm
2 mm
20 mm
10 mm
1 mm

Part A: General overview

1. Synonyms

No synonyms recorded.

2. Common name(s)

Bushman's tea, bush tea, Zulu tea (English), '*Boesmanstee*' (Afrikaans), '*icholo-cholo', 'itshelo', 'mohlahlaishi*' (Sepedi), '*mutshatshaila*' (Tshivenda), '*luphephe-tse*' (siSwati), '*sephomolo*' (Sesotho), '*umtshanelo*', '*icholocholo*', or '*itshelo*' (isiZulu).[a]

3. Conservation status

Least concern.[a]

4. Botany

Athrixia phylicoides is a member of the family Asteraceae (daisy family) and is classified under the tribe Inucleae and subtribe Athrixiinae. The shrub reaches a height of approximately 1 m. Leafy stems occur throughout, and appear white and fluffy. These stems are gathered and bundled by locals for domestic and medicinal use. The alternate leaves are aromatic, fine, linear, about 30 × 10 mm in size, and are sometimes radical and sessile (A). The adaxial leaf surfaces are shiny and dark green, while the undersides appear grey-white and smooth. The hairy leaf bases are often decurrent, lanceolate, and frequently display revolute margins. Flowers with mauve ray florets and yellow disc florets adorn the shrub throughout the year (B), but are most prolific between March and May. Flower heads are sessile, terminal and axillary towards the ends of the branches. The Greek word '*thrix*', meaning hair, is the origin of the genus name *Athrixia* and refers to the leaves, while the specific epithet *phylicoides* indicates its similarity to the genus *Phylica*, from the family Rhamnaceae (Mbambezeli, 2005). The leaves are harvested, dried (C) and used for various medicinal purposes.

[a] Red List of South African Plants (http://redlist.sanbi.org).

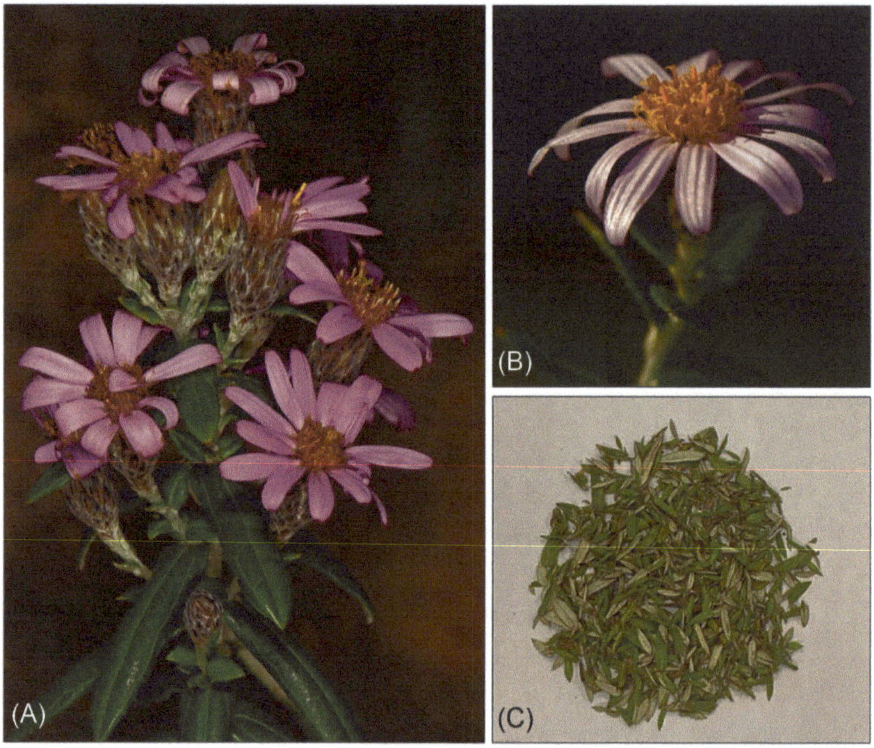

Athrixia phylicoides shrub (A) with purple flowers at the end of the branch (B) and small, dark green leaves with a hairy leaf base (C).

5. Geographical distribution

Athrixia phylicoides is widely distributed throughout the northern and eastern parts of South Africa, extending from the Limpopo and Mpumalanga provinces to the KwaZulu-Natal and Eastern Cape provinces. The plant also occurs in neighbouring Swaziland (Eswatini) and Lesotho (Germishuizen et al., 2006). It is prevalent in bushveld, rocky and sloping grassland and forests. The plant is adapted to altitudes from 600 to 2000 m above sea level. Flowering depends on the prevailing environmental conditions. The shrub prefers loamy soil and direct sunlight, with sufficient space for branching. It is found in the Drakensberg Mountains, but also grows abundantly along the coast.

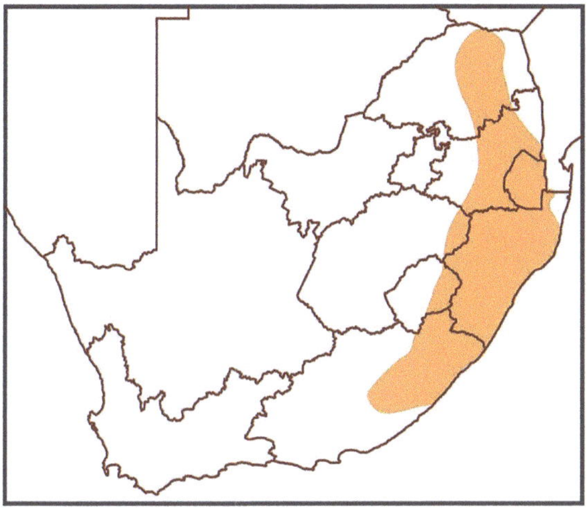

Geographical distribution of *Athrixia phylicoides* in South Africa.

6. Ethnopharmacology

A wide range of disorders, including skin conditions (Hutchings et al., 1996; Rampedi and Olivier, 2005), heart problems, diabetes, diarrhoea and vomiting, are treated using *A. phylicoides*. The herbal remedy is also used as an anthelmintic, cough remedy and a purgative (Watt and Breyer-Brandwijk, 1962). Various ethnic groups in South Africa use different parts of *A. phylicoides* for medicinal and other domestic purposes (Van Wyk and Gericke, 2000). The aerial parts of the plant are collected for use as a beverage. The gathered material is tied together and the bundles suspended from the rafters of the roof to protect them from moisture. A decoction is prepared by boiling a handful of leaves and twigs in water for a few minutes. After straining, the tea is enjoyed as a relaxing, caffeine-free refreshment (Rampedi and Olivier, 2005). The leaves are chewed by the Sotho and Xhosa people to relieve colds, coughs and throat infections (Mbambezeli, 2005), while the Venda use extracts from soaked roots and leaves as an aphrodisiac (Van Wyk and Gericke, 2000) and as an anthelmintic (Mbambezeli, 2005). Since this concoction is believed to arouse sexual desire, bachelors are discouraged from taking the root infusions (Hutchings et al., 1996; Rakuombo, 2007). The popular use of the plant as a beverage (Rampedi and Olivier, 2005; McGaw et al., 2013) suggests that it is has commercial potential. The traditional use of *Athrixia* for cleansing the womb, kidneys and veins, and to purify blood, indicates its detoxifying effect. Infusions are taken to treat leg wounds, influenza and stomach ache (Rakuombo, 2007), as well as for treating infected wounds and cuts, boils and headaches (Joubert et al., 2008). It is also applied for skin cleansing and as a lotion to combat acne and to alleviate skin rashes. Decoctions are gargled to treat laryngitis. Decoctions and infusions prepared from leaves and twigs are widely used by rural people to treat diabetes, hypertension, poor blood circulation and heart problems, vomiting and diarrhoea (Rampedi and Olivier, 2005), while decoctions of the root are used as a purgative (Watt and Breyer-Brandwijk, 1962). The Sotho people use leaf decoctions to soothe painful feet. The leaves are masticated to remedy sore throats, probably associated with inflammation of the pharynx (Watt and Breyer-Brandwijk, 1962). One of the most common uses of *A. phylicoides* is making brooms, by stripping the leaves from long branches and then binding the ends together to form the broom handle (Van Wyk and Gericke, 2000; Rampedi and Olivier, 2005).

7. Commercialisation

The informal trade in tea and brooms in the Gauteng Province is the only commercial activity involving *A. phylicoides* (Rampedi and Olivier, 2005). However, a survey among rural and urban communities in the northern parts of South Africa indicated interest in commercial *A. phylicoides* products, stemming from generations of use of the plant by rural communities. Traders from Gauteng hire labourers in the area of Wolkberg, a mountainous part of Limpopo, to harvest *A. phylicoides* (Rampedi and Olivier, 2005). In autumn, large quantities of the material destined for making brooms to be sold by hawkers on the streets of the city, are transported to Gauteng. This practice is unsustainable and threatens the bush tea populations along the lower parts of Wolkberg. In many cases, the entire plant is uprooted and is unable to recover. The local villagers, who are careful to pick only a few branches from each plant, find that bush tea is becoming unavailable, with flourishing populations occurring further from habitation. A shift away from broom-making to high-end products in the beverage sector will add value and generate considerably more income. Such activities, if developed sustainably, could contribute to the economic growth of rural regions of South Africa and promote employment opportunities (Rampedi and Olivier, 2005; Joubert et al., 2008).

Several researchers (Rampedi and Olivier, 2005; Chellan et al., 2008) have directly or indirectly contributed towards commercialisation through their research. There is general consensus that bush tea must compete strongly with rooibos and honeybush teas with respect to its medicinal properties, or serve to complement them, if it is to take its rightful place (Lehlohonolo et al., 2013). Bush tea can be mass cultivated more easily than rooibos and honeybush teas, which are restricted to specific habitats (Joubert et al., 2008). Propagation and cultivation should enhance the consistency and quality of the tea, in addition to improving the sustainability of the species. A number of studies have been conducted on various aspects of *A. phylicoides* to assist in its development as a commercial herbal beverage (Joubert et al., 2008; McGaw et al., 2013). Various propagation techniques were investigated by Maudu et al. (2012), who compared the quality of cultivated and wild plants prepared from new growth, whole plant or older plant parts. For cultivated plants, new growth and whole plant propagation yielded better tea quality, as reflected by the polyphenol, tannin and anti-oxidant content, than the older leaves. However, new and older growths of wild-harvested plants contained similar concentrations of total polyphenols and anti-oxidants. Araya (2005) studied the effects of different propagation techniques on cuttings and seed germination. Variables included the cutting position, growth medium, season (spring, summer, autumn or winter), the application of plant hormones at different concentrations, the survival of transplants and effects of light and temperature. The conditions yielding the best vegetative growth and survival were established and can be implemented by future developers of the tea. The trade in *A. phylicoides* through informal markets and as brooms (Rampedi and Olivier, 2005) has little economic impact. Bush tea is a well-known beverage amongst various ethnic groups in South Africa and should be a popular addition to the caffeine-free and healthy alternative beverage sector. South African indigenous teas have built up a good reputation, and a new entrant may be welcomed internationally (Lerotholi et al., 2017).

8. Pharmacological evaluation

8.1 *In vitro* studies

8.1.1 Anti-oxidant activity

The anti-oxidant activity of an infusion, a decoction, and aqueous and ethanolic extracts of *A. phylicoides* was determined by McGaw et al. (2007). The infusion, decoction and cold water extract (at concentrations of 0.5, 1 and 2 mg/mL) exhibited good free-radical-scavenging ability when tested using the Trolox Equivalent Anti-oxidant Capacity (TEAC) assay. The decoction displayed better anti-oxidant activity than rooibos tea, which was explained by the lower phenolic content of rooibos extract compared to that of bush tea. Although several compounds with anti-oxidant activity were detected using a thin-layer chromatography (TLC)-based bioassay, specific compounds were not identified. In a study conducted by Mavundza et al. (2010), the anti-oxidant activity of three compounds isolated from *A. phylicoides*, namely 5-hydroxy-6,7,8,3′,4′,5′-hexamethoxyflavon-3-ol, 3-*O*-demethyldigicitrin and quercetin, was compared to that of the crude ethanol extract using the 2,2-diphenyl-1-picryl-hydrazyl-hydrate (DPPH)-spectrophotometric assay. The extract at concentrations from 3.9 to 500 μg/mL displayed concentration-dependent radical scavenging activity with a half maximal effective concentration (EC_{50}) of 10.64 ± 0.08 μg/mL. The radical scavenging ability of quercetin was the best of the three pure compounds tested, with 3-*O*-demethyldigicitrin displaying the poorest activity. The anti-oxidant activity of an aqueous extract of *A. phylicoides* was determined by De Beer et al. (2011) using an assortment of free-radical-scavenging assays, namely the azino-*bis*(3-ethylbenzothiazoline-6-sulphonic acid) (ABTS) ($ABTS^{\bullet +}$), DPPH•, and oxygen radical absorption capacity (ORAC) scavenging assays. The ferric reducing anti-oxidant power (FRAP), iron-chelating activity, inhibition of lipid peroxidation and linoleic acid emulsion oxidation were also determined. The results obtained after testing both polar and aqueous extracts indicated that bush tea is an excellent source of anti-oxidants. In addition, compared to the hot aqueous extract of rooibos tea, the same extract of bush tea displayed higher anti-oxidant activity. However, the DPPH• scavenging activity and reducing potential of the extract were lower than those of the corresponding extract from unfermented rooibos. *Athrixia* inhibited the peroxidation of microsomes to a larger degree than unfermented rooibos. It was also reported that the ORAC and $ABTS^{\bullet +}$ scavenging activities were comparable to the activities of fermented rooibos extracts, but the iron-chelation activity of *A. phylicoides* was higher than those of the corresponding extracts prepared from honeybush and rooibos. The limitation of the mentioned studies of McGaw et al. (2007) and De Beer et al. (2011) is that they did not take chemical variation within *A. phylicoides* into account, since only a few samples were used. However, their studies substantiated the anti-oxidant activity of bush tea and indicated that the activity is on par with that of other indigenous herbal teas. A study to link the soaking (fermentation) conditions of bush tea to the anti-oxidant activity was conducted by Negukhula et al. (2011). They found that the combination of bush tea and black tea resulted in a significant reduction in the anti-oxidant activity. However, an increase in the fermentation temperature to 90 °C for 3 min led to an increase in the activity of the tea combination. Mavundza et al. (2010) demonstrated the role of three compounds in *A. phylicoides* in the anti-oxidant activity, but earlier research by McGaw et al. (2007) had indicated that many compounds with anti-oxidant activity are present in the plant. Some of these compounds could potentially be used to reflect the quality of plant material for tea production.

8.1.2 Antimicrobial activity

The microdilution technique was used by Tshivhandekano et al. (2014) to determine the antimicrobial activity of ethanol extracts of *A. phylicoides* against a number of human pathogens. The minimum inhibitory concentrations (MICs) ranged from 1.56 to 12.50 mg/mL, while the minimum microbicidal concentrations (MMCs) ranged from 0.78 to 12.50 mg/mL, indicating poor activity and variation in susceptibility of the organisms. Padayachee (2011) also reported variation in the antimicrobial activity of the methanol extract and essential oil against a diverse range of human pathogens. A compound that was highly active against *Staphylococcus aureus* (MIC 19.5 µg/mL) was isolated and identified as 4-hydroxyphenylpropyl coumarate, previously isolated and reported as *p*-hydroxyphenylpropan-3-ol-coumarate by Bohlmann and Zdero (1977), from *A. phylicoides*. The activity worth noting obtained for the pure compounds suggested that the crude extract contained only low concentrations of the active compounds, since the activity was poor. The antimicrobial activities of *A. phylicoides* and several other plant species, with popular traditional use to combat skin conditions, were evaluated by Mabona et al. (2013). Recorded MICs ≥1 mg/mL reflected poor activity for both dichloromethane/methanol and water extracts. The influence of different methods of drying (sun, freeze, shade and oven drying) on the antimicrobial activities of *A. phylicoides*, revealed that drying, regardless of the method, had no effect (Mudau and Ngezimana, 2014). Their results merely confirmed the poor activity reported by others, since MICs of 6.3 mg/mL were determined for all the Gram-negative organisms, and 3.1 mg/mL and higher were recorded for the Gram-positive bacteria. The antibacterial and antifungal activities of extracts (10 mg/mL) prepared from dried, ground, aerial parts of bush tea using organic solvents of different polarities and water, were mildly active towards *Escherichia coli*, but inactive towards *Pseudomonas aeruginosa* (McGaw et al., 2013). Growth inhibition of *Cryptococcus neoformans*, *Enterococcus faecalis* and *S. aureus*, as well as the fungus *Candida albicans*, was recorded, following exposure to the diethyl ether, dichloromethane/methanol, ethyl acetate and ethanol extracts.

The organic extracts contained more compounds with antimicrobial activity than the water extract. Seven compounds with antibacterial or antifungal activity were detected, but could not be identified, in the organic extracts. Many of the traditional uses of *A. phylicoides* indicate that the plant has antimicrobial activity; yet, the overall activity reported by numerous researchers does not substantiate this assumption. It is possible that other chemotypes with better antimicrobial activity exist. It is also possible that extracts of the plant interfere with communication of bacteria, rather than through inducing physical damage to the organism (Lerotholi et al., 2017). Assays that allow the identification of compounds with antiquorum sensing activities should be used to investigate this possibility.

8.1.3 Antidiabetic activity

The potential antidiabetic properties of chlorogenic acid, present in *A. phylicoides*, was revealed by its ability to upregulate glucose transporter 4 (GLUT4) and elevate the expression of the peroxisome proliferator-activated receptor gamma ($PPAR_{\gamma}$) gene (Prabhakar and Doble, 2009). The *in vitro* antidiabetic effects of hot water extracts prepared from the aerial parts of *A. phylicoides* at three concentrations (0.025, 0.050, 0.10 μg/μL) were determined by Chellan et al. (2012) in three cell lines C2C12 (ATCC CRL-1772), Chang (ATCC CCL-13) and 3T3-L1 (ATCC CL-173). The extract induced an increase in cellular glucose uptake and metabolism in all three cell types. No effect was observed on the rate of conversion in 3T3-L1 cells, but there was a significant increase in the oxidation of ^{14}C-glucose to $^{14}CO_2$ by C2C12 and Chang myocytes. The amount of glycogen stored in Chang cells increased significantly at all three concentrations tested, but the glycogen content of C2C12 myocytes remained unchanged. These results imply that metabolic disorders associated with type 2 diabetes and obesity can be mitigated by hot water extracts of the plant, which accelerate the metabolism of glucose in insulin-responsive tissues. The ability of *A. phylicoides* to modulate the effects of diabetes and obesity was attributed to the presence of the phenolic acids, 1,3-di-caffeoylquinic acid and chlorogenic acid, and other hydroxycinnamic acid derivatives (Joubert et al., 2012). However, these researchers warned that the results of metabolic studies involving cancer cells, such as Chang cells, must be further substantiated, since processes such as glucose utilisation and storage may be very specific and not indicative of metabolic processes in normal cells.

8.1.4 Other activities

The *in vitro* antiplasmodial activity of the methanol extract and essential oil of *A. phylicoides* against a chloroquine-resistant *Plasmodium falciparum* (FCR-3) strain was investigated by Padayachee (2011), using the titrated hypoxanthine-incorporated assay. Poor activity ($IC_{50}=83.49\pm5.48$ μg/mL) was reported for the methanol extract, but the essential oil was strongly active ($IC_{50}=1.006\pm0.060$ μg/mL) towards the chloroquine-resistant parasite, although the activity was substantially poorer than that of quinine, the positive control (0.034 ± 0.002 μg/mL). Kleynhans et al. (2017) determined the antityrosinase activity and the antibacterial activity of ethanol leaf extracts against *Propionibacterium acnes*, in an attempt to find cosmetic applications for *A. phylicoides*. However, the extracts were inactive towards the bacterium. Nine prominent phenolic compounds were identified in the aqueous extract of *A. phylicoides* (Bowles et al., 2017). The intestinal transport of these compounds across a fully differentiated Caco-2 cell monolayer was investigated, to predict their bioavailability and to identify metabolite formation. Significant amounts of three of the nine compounds (protocatechuic acid, caffeic acid and *p*-coumaric acid) were transported across the Caco-2 monolayer, as reflected by P_{app} values of 4.52×10^{-6} cm/s, 4.35×10^{-6} cm/s and 2.3×10^{-5} cm/s, respectively. *p*-Coumaric acid was predicted to have the highest bioavailability of the compounds evaluated (Bowles et al., 2017). The anti-inflammatory activity of the essential oil and methanol extract of *A. phylicoides* was assessed by Padayachee (2011), using an *in vitro* assay. The activity of the essential oil (IC_{50} 25.68 µg/mL) was poorer than that of nordihydroguaiaretic acid (IC_{50} 5.0 µg/mL), used as the positive control. However, the methanol extract was completely inactive, even at the highest concentration tested ($IC_{50} > 100$ µg/mL), suggesting that the water extracts used traditionally would not have anti-inflammatory activity, unless it involved action *via* a different pathway.

8.2 *In vivo* studies

The effects of prolonged intake of high doses of aqueous *A. phylicoides* extract on a daily basis by mature Wistar rats (3-month-old) were determined (Chellan et al., 2008). Dried extract at 30, 90 or 180 mg/kg/body weight/day was administered over a 3-month period. At the end of the period, blood and tissues were analysed. Serum creatinine, alkaline phosphatase and urea levels were normal for all groups. Histopathology indicated that the liver, kidney and gastrointestinal tract were not affected. An increase in urine production in the groups receiving 90 and 180 mg/kg, compared to the untreated controls, indicated that the extract has mild diuretic properties. No morbidity or mortality was recorded throughout the study, supporting claims that the tea is safe to consume.

8.3 Safety

A preliminary toxicological evaluation of a decoction and infusion, together with water and ethanol extracts of *A. phylicoides*, was done in the Vero monkey kidney cell line by McGaw et al. (2007). The absence of cytotoxicity of the plant extracts, tested over the concentration range 1–1000 µg/mL, was affirmed by half-maximal lethal dose (LD_{50}) values of above 1000 µg/mL for the aqueous extract and 252 µg/mL for the ethanol extract. The ethanol and aqueous extracts at concentrations of 0.1 to 5 mg/mL also failed to induce mortality in the brine shrimp larval assay. The high half-maximal lethal concentration (LC_{50}) values, which were above 1000 µg/mL, and 394 µg/mL for the aqueous and ethanol extracts, respectively, confirmed the absence of toxicity. Two *A. phylicoides* samples were also screened by these researchers for the presence of pyrrolizidine alkaloids, highly toxic compounds produced by some members of the Asteraceae family (Wiedenfeld, 2011). These carcinogenic, hepatotoxic and genotoxic compounds (Fu et al., 2004) could not be detected. The toxicity of infusions of ground aerial parts of *A. phylicoides* at concentrations of 0.025, 0.05 and 0.1 µg/µL were tested in the MTT (3-(4,5-dimethylthiazol-2-yl)-2,5-diphenyltetrazolium bromide) cytotoxicity assay (Chellan et al., 2012). No inhibition of mitochondrial activity or reduction in Chang cell viability was reported, indicating that the extracts were not cytotoxic. Mavundza et al. (2010) investigated the cytotoxicity of the ethanol extract (3.13–400 μg/mL), and that of four pure compounds (1.56 to 200 μg/mL) isolated from *A. phylicoides*. The ethanol extract was reported to be non-toxic (IC_{50} = 107.8 ± 0.13 μg/mL), while quercetin displayed only a small degree of toxicity (IC_{50} = 81.38 ± 0.33 μg/mL). 3-*O*-Demethyldigicitrin (IC_{50} = 28.92 ± 0.12 μg/mL) and 5-hydroxy-6,7,8,3′,4′,5′-hexamethoxyflavon-3-ol (IC_{50} = 27.91 ± 0.18 μg/mL) were the most toxic of the compounds tested. Following the review of literature on *A. phylicoides*, Lerotholi et al. (2017) concluded that since there were no reported detrimental effects towards cells, experimental animals, or humans, through its traditional use as a beverage or medicine, the plant is probably non-toxic or has very low undocumented toxicity.

9. Phytochemistry

9.1 Volatile constituents

Several volatile organic compounds have been identified from *A. phylicoides*. Germacrene D, linoleic acid and *p*-hydroxyphenylpropan-3-ol-coumarate were reported from the leaves by Bohlmann and Zdero (1977). Padayachee (2011) also identified germacrene D as a major constituent of the essential oils isolated, using hydrodistillation (0.47% yield) from seven samples of *A. phylicoides*. Other major compounds (>10%) identified in the volatile oil, using gas chromatography–mass spectrometry (GC–MS) analysis, were α-pinene, β-pinene, myrcene, β-caryophyllene, spathulenol and caryophyllene oxide.

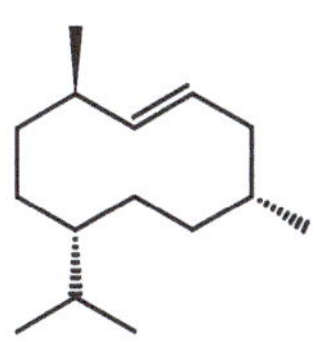
Germacrene D

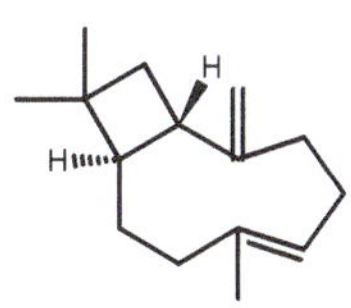
β-Caryophyllene

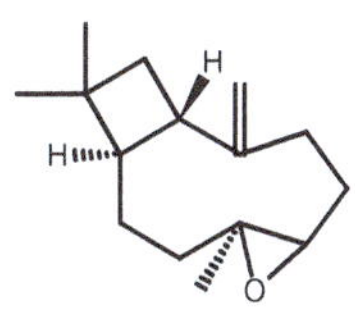
Caryophyllene oxide

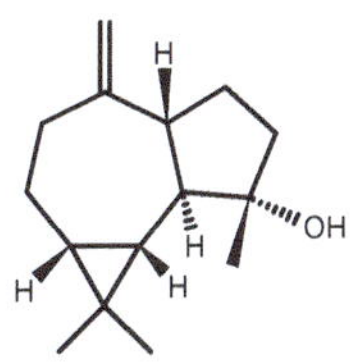
Spathulenol

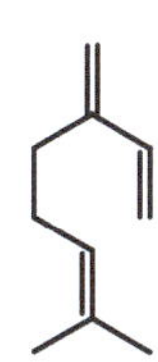
Myrcene

9.2 Non-volatile constituents

Bush tea is rich in flavonoids and tannins, compounds that are frequently used as indicators of herbal tea quality. The flavonoid, 5-hydroxy-6,7,8,3′,4′,5′-hexamethoxyflavon-3-ol, was isolated by Mashimbye et al. (2006) from an acetone extract of the green leaves. Mavundza et al. (2010) isolated several flavonoids, namely 5,6,7,8,3′,4′-hexamethoxyflavone-3-ol, quercetin and 3-*O*-dimethyldigicitrin, from an ethanolic extract of aerial plant parts. 6-Hydroxyluteolin-7-*O*-β-glucoside, a strong anti-oxidant, was isolated from an aqueous extract of twigs and leaves using high-performance countercurrent chromatography (HPCCC), combined with semi-preparative high-performance liquid chromatography (HPLC) (De Beer et al., 2011). Chlorogenic acid, 1,3-dicaffeoylquinic acid and dicaffeoylquinic acids (3,4-dicaffeoylquinic acid and 3,5-dicaffeoylquinic acid), which are hydroxycinnamic acid derivatives, in addition to 6-hydroxyluteolin-7-*O*-β-glucoside and quercetagetin-7-*O*-β-glucoside, were identified using mass spectral and ultraviolet–visible spectroscopy data. A study on the influence of temperature and time during fermentation on the chemical composition of *A. phylicoides* indicated that the total polyphenolic content was increased by high fermentation temperature, while there was a slight decrease in the tannin content (Hlahla et al., 2010). The concentrations of total polyphenols and tannins were enhanced significantly when the duration of fermentation was increased. Sensory evaluation of the tea would enable the optimum fermentation time to be selected, since the tannin content affects the taste of the tea. The total phenolic and tannin contents of leaves of *A. phylicoides* were reported as 6.41 mg/100 g and 0.34 mg/100 g, respectively (Tshivhandekano et al., 2014). The nutritional value of *A. phylicoides* was investigated by Olivier et al. (2012). They reported that the plant material contained 13% non-structural carbohydrates, 8% proteins, 2.5% fatty acids, low concentrations of tannins, vitamins B1, B2, C and E, and minerals (aluminium, calcium, copper, fluoride, iron, magnesium, manganese, phosphorus, potassium, sodium, sulphur and zinc). Bush tea was found to be richer in most minerals than the popular indigenous herbal teas, rooibos and honeybush.

The phenolic compounds in a hot aqueous extract of *A. phylicoides* were determined using HPLC with diode array detection (DAD) (Chellan et al., 2012). Compound identities were verified by ultra-performance liquid chromatography coupled to mass spectroscopy (UPLC–MS) analysis. The aqueous extract contained 5-hydroxy-6,7,8,3′,4′,5′-hexamethoxyflavon-3-ol, in addition to hydroxybenzoic acid, protocatechuic acid, hydroxycinnamic acid, caffeic acid, and the chlorogenic acid isomers, neochlorogenic and cryptochlorogenic acids. Both De Beer et al. (2011) and Chellan et al. (2012) reported the presence of 6-hydroxyluteolin-7-*O*-β-glucoside and quercetagetin-7-*O*-glucoside in *A. phylicoides*. High-temperature liquid chromatography and fast centrifugal partition chromatography were used to isolate compounds from a methanol extract of bush tea (Reichelt et al., 2012). Two dicaffeoyl quinic acids, 3′-*O*-methylcalycopterin, one coumaric acid ester and four polymethoxylated flavones, together with quercetin-3′-*O*-glucoside and a methoxylated quercetin derivative, were isolated and identified. Several compounds with antimicrobial activity were identified by McGaw et al. (2013) using HPLC, and TLC bioautography as a guide. Quercetin, caffeic acid, inositol, kaempferol, apigenin, hymenoxin and oleanolic acid were identified as active compounds. Several studies have been conducted to investigate the chemical variation within classes of compounds (hydrolysable or condensed tannins, or phenolic compounds) in *A. phylicoides*. The degree of variation of specific compounds or complete chemical profiles has received less attention (Lehlohonolo et al., 2012). Variation in the chemical composition of bush tea was attributed to the influence of season, altitude and edaphic factors. Lehlohonolo et al. (2012) conducted a study of wild-harvested bush tea to establish the link between environmental factors and the phenolic composition. Samples were sourced from localities exposed to different climates and edaphic factors and at different altitudes. Plants growing at high altitudes (944–1410 m above sea level) contained significantly higher concentrations of soluble phenolic compounds. The tannin content, however, was not influenced by altitude. Surprisingly, the total anti-oxidant content of samples from different altitudes did not differ significantly. The results also indicated that the total polyphenol, total tannin and total anti-oxidant contents were not influenced by rainfall, temperature, soil macroelements, or the pH of the soil.

The effects of different drying methods, namely sun, freeze, shade and oven drying on total polyphenol content, tannins, total anti-oxidants and phytochemical content of bush tea, were evaluated (Mudau and Ngezimana, 2014). The chemical composition of the plant material was significantly affected by drying. Freeze- and shade-drying had the least effect on the total phenolic content, with values as high as 8.34 mg/100 g reported, compared to less than 6.50 mg/100 g in sun- and oven-dried samples. The chemical variation within *A. phylicoides* was investigated extensively by Lerotholi et al. (2018). The chemical profiles of 48 samples from 12 locations in South Africa were obtained using ultra-performance liquid chromatography time-of-flight mass spectrometry (UPLC-ToF-MS). Chemometric analysis of the aligned data using hierarchical cluster analysis (HCA), indicated two groups that could be distinguished based on their chemical compositions. Five marker compounds, identified through visual inspection and with the aid of a constructed discriminant analysis model, were evident on the chromatograms. Three hydroxy methoxyflavones and a coumarate were identified after targeted isolation of the marker compounds. Using the isolated compounds as reference standards, a UPLC method with photodiode array (PDA) detection was developed and validated for the determination of the marker compounds. The concentrations of all the markers were found to be higher in samples clustered in one group, than in samples from the second group. It was speculated that these chemical differences resulted from differences in the environmental conditions to which the wild-harvested plants had been exposed. The identification of these marker compounds is important for the quality control of *A. phylicoides*, an important element of sustainable commercialisation. A comparative phytochemical study incorporating bush tea, rooibos and honeybush tea was conducted by Malongane et al. (2018). Nuclear magnetic resonance (NMR) spectroscopy and high-resolution liquid chromatography-mass spectrometry (HRLC-MS) were used to determine differences between the teas by comparing signals and peak area intensities. The concentrations of lignans, including justicidin A, justicidin B and diphylin, were higher in bush tea than in the other teas investigated.

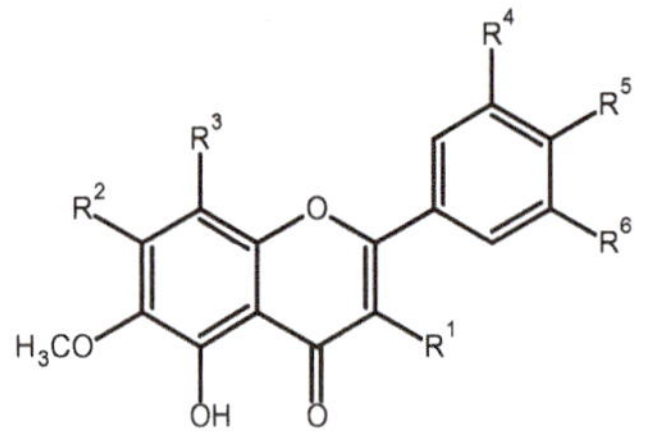

5-Hydroxy-6,7,8,3′,4′,5′-hexamethoxyflavon-3-ol: R^1=OH; R^2, R^3, R^4, R^5, R^6=OCH_3
3-*O*-Dimethyldigicitrin: R^1, R^4=OH; R^2, R^3, R^5, R^6=OCH_3
3′-*O*-Methylcalycopterin: R^5=OH; R^1, R^2, R^3, R^4=OCH_3; R^6=H
5,7-Dihydroxy-3,6,8,3′,4′,5′-hexamethoxyflavone: R^2=OH; R^2, R^3, R^4, R^5, R^6=OCH_3
5,7,3′-Trihydroxy-3,6,8,4′,5′-pentamethoxyflavone: R^2, R^4=OH; R^1, R^3, R^5, R^6=OCH_3
5,7,4′-Trihydroxy-3,6,3′-trimethoxyflavone: R^2, R^5=OH; R^1, R^6=OCH_3; R^4, R^3=H

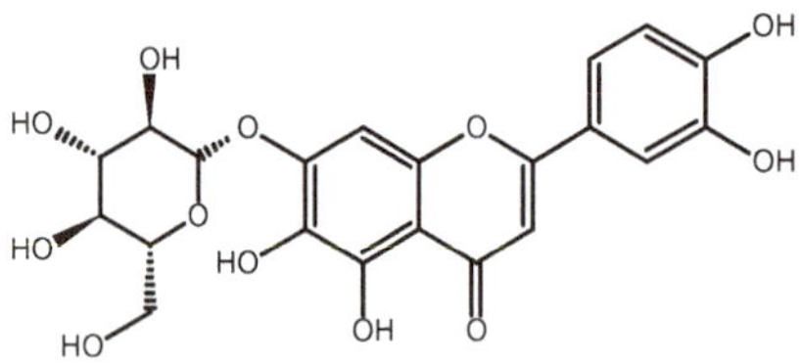

6-Hydroxyluteolin-7-*O*-β-glucoside

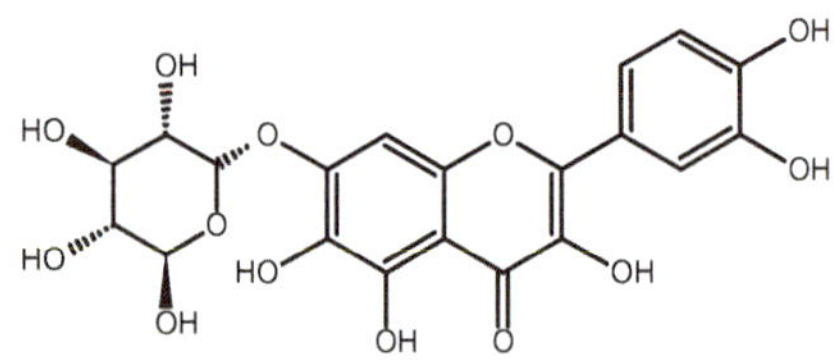

Quercetagetin-7-*O*-β-glucoside

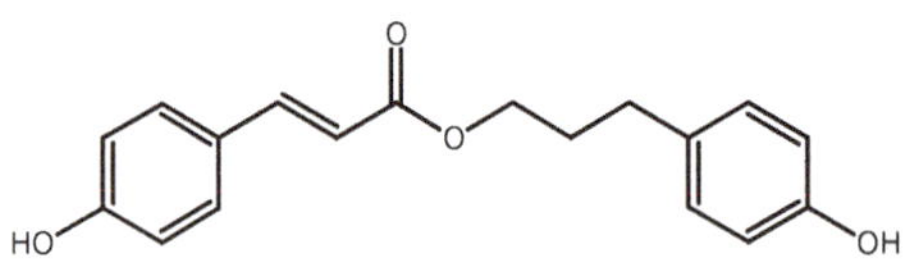

p-Hydroxyphenylpropan-3-ol-coumarate

Part B: Chemical profiling and quality control

10. Chromatography analysis

10.1 High-performance thin-layer chromatography (HPTLC) fingerprint analysis

General instrumentation: A CAMAG HPTLC instrument consisting of an automatic TLC sampler (ATS 4), automatic developing chamber (ADC 2), CAMAG TLC Visualizer 2, CAMAG derivatiser and TLC plate heater. *HPTLC plates:* Silica gel glass plates 60 F_{254} (Merck). *Plant part:* Leaves and twigs, methanol extract. *Sample application:* Application volume of 2 μL methanol extract (100 mg/mL) spotted as 10 mm bands. Plates developed in a 20×10×4 cm glass twin-trough chamber to a migration distance of 70 mm. *Tank saturation:* 20 min at 15 °C and 33% RH, with

25 mL of mobile phase. *Mobile phase:* Ethyl acetate: water: formic acid (12:1:1, v/v/v). *Derivatisation:* Natural Product reagent and polyethylene glycol reagent mixture. The plate was heated for 3 min at 100 °C on a TLC plate heater, sprayed with 3 mL of the derivatisation mixture and then visualised. *Visualisation:* The plate was viewed under 366 nm radiation.

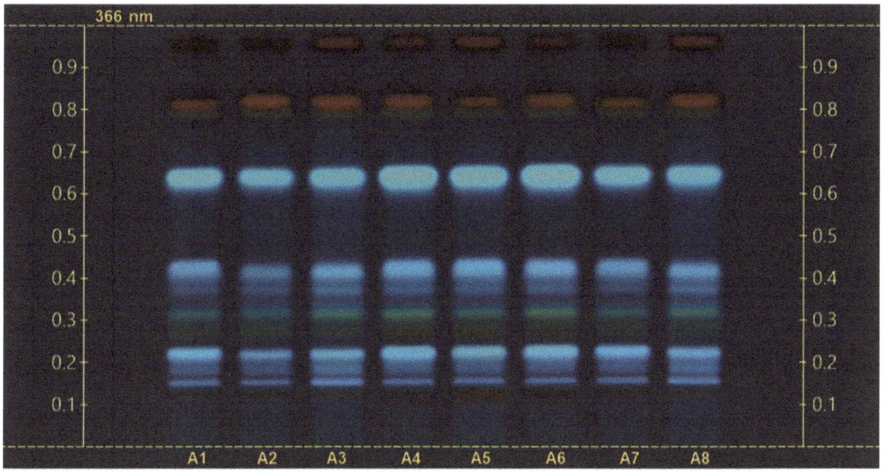

HPTLC plate of *Athrixia phylicoides* methanol extracts (n=8) (A1–A8). The samples are characterised by a light blue band for 5,7,5′-trihydroxy-3,6,8,3′,4′-pentamethoxyflavone (*m/z* 419) (R_f=0.43) and another for 5,7-dihydroxy-3,6,8,3′,4′,5′-hexamethoxyflavone (*m/z* 433) at R_f=0.65.

10.2 Ultra-performance liquid chromatography (UPLC) analysis

General instrumentation: Waters Acquity Ultra-Performance Liquid Chromatography system with photodiode array (PDA) detector combined with a Xevo G2QToF mass spectrometer (Waters, USA). *Plant part:* Leaves and twigs, methanol: water (1:1) extract. *Sample application:* Injection volume: 2.0 μL (full-loop injection) at 1 mg/mL. *Column:* Acquity UPLC BEH C_{18} column (150 mm × 2.1 mm, i.d., 1.7 μm particle size, Waters). *Mobile phase:* 0.1% formic acid in water (solvent A) and acetonitrile (solvent B). *Analysis conditions:* Gradient elution at a flow rate of 0.3 mL/min, changing as follows: 90% A: 10% B, changed to 50% A: 50% B in 11 min, to 10% A: 90% B in 4 min, held for 1 min, back to initial ratio in 1 min, equilibrating for 1 min, total run time of 18 min. *Mass spectrometry*: ESI^- (negative ionisation mode), N_2 used as desolvation gas, desolvation temperature 350 °C at a flow rate of 500 L/h and a source temperature at 100 °C. Capillary and cone voltages, 2500 and 45 V, respectively. Data collected between *m/z* 100 and 1200.

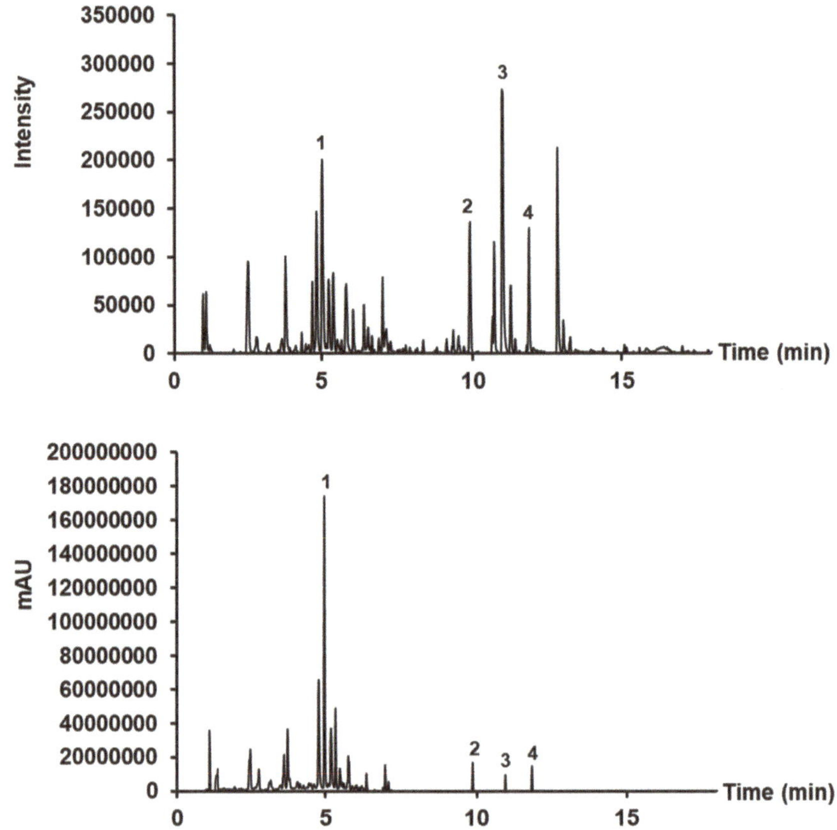

UPLC-ToF-MS ESI⁻ (upper) and PDA (lower) chromatograms of *A. phylicoides* methanol: water (1:1) extract. [1]=chlorogenic acid *m/z* 353.0872, [2]=3-*O*-dimethyldigicitrin *m/z* 419.0978, [3]=*p*-hydroxyphenylpropan-3-ol-coumarate *m/z* 297.113, [4]=5-hydroxy-6,7,8,3′,4′,5′-hexamethoxyflavon-3-ol *m/z* 433.1132.

11. Mid-infrared (MIR) spectroscopy analysis

General instrumentation: Alpha-P Bruker spectrometer, mounted with an attenuated total reflectance (ATR) diamond crystal. *Spectral acquisition:* Spectrum obtained in absorbance mode, with a spectral resolution of 4 cm^{-1} over the range 4000–550 cm^{-1} and captured using OPUS 6.5 software. *Plant part:* Aerial parts. *Sample preparation:* Leaves and twigs powdered, sieved (<500 µm) and placed directly onto the surface of the diamond crystal.

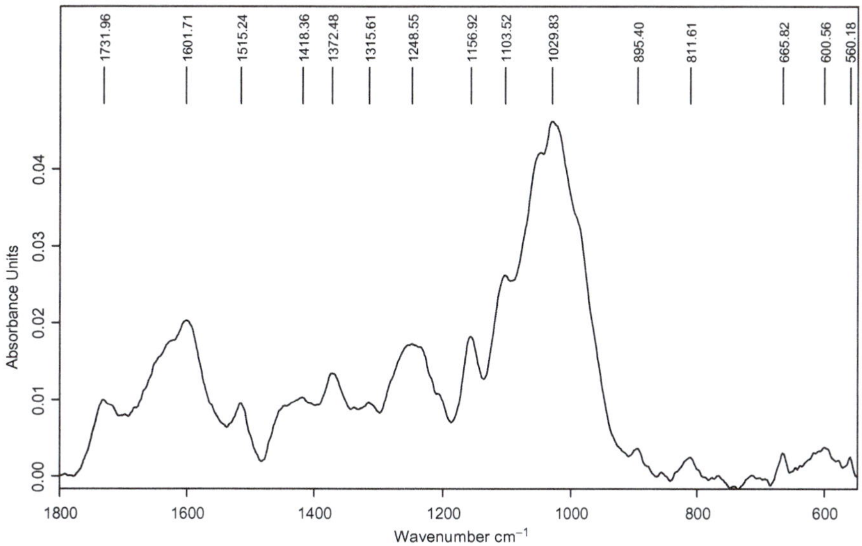

Mid-infrared spectrum of *Athrixia phylicoides* powder displaying the fingerprint region (1800–550 cm^{-1}).

References

Araya, H.T., 2005. Seed Germination and Vegetative Propagation of Bush Tea (*Athrixia phylicoides*). MSc dissertation, University of Pretoria, Pretoria, South Africa.

Bohlmann, F., Zdero, C., 1977. Phytochemistry, 16:1773–1776.

Bowles, S.L., Ntamo, Y., Malherbe, C.J., Kappo, A.M.P., Louw, J., Muller, C.J.F., 2017. J. Ethnopharmacol., 200:45–50.

Chellan, N., De Beer, D., Muller, C., Joubert, E., Louw, J., 2008. Hum. Exp. Toxicol., 2:819–825.

Chellan, N., Muller, C.J.F., De Beer, D., Joubert, E., Page, B.J., Louw, J., 2012. Phytomedicine, 19:730–736.

De Beer, D., Joubert, E., Malherbe, C.J., Brand, D.J., 2011. J. Chromatogr. A, 1218:6179–6186.

Fu, P.P., Xia, Q., Lin, G., Chou, M.W., 2004. Drug Metab. Rev., 36:1–55.

Germishuizen, G., Meyer, N.L., Steenkamp, Y., Keith, M. (Eds.), 2006. A Checklist of South African Plants. Southern African Biodiversity Network Report No. 41, SABONET, Pretoria.

Hlahla, L.N., Mudau, F.N., Mariga, I.K., 2010. J. Med. Plant Res., 4:824–829.

Hutchings, A., Scott, A.H., Lewis, G., Cunningham, A., 1996. Zulu Medicinal Plants: An Inventory. University of Natal Press, Pietermaritzburg, South Africa.

Joubert, E., Gelderblom, W.C.A., Louw, A., De Beer, D., 2008. J. Ethnopharmacol., 119:376–412.

Joubert, E., Muller, C.J.F., De Beer, D., Johnson, R., Chellan, N., Louw, J., 2012. The potential role of phenolic acids in tea and herbal teas in modulating effects of obesity and diabetes. In: Phenolic Acids: Composition, Application and Health Benefits. Nova Science Publishers Inc., New York, USA.

Kleynhans, R., Singh, S., Kishore, N., Lall, N., 2017. S. Afr. J. Bot., 112:319–321.

Lehlohonolo, N., Mudau, F.N., Mariga, I.K., 2012. J. Med. Plant Res., 6:1662–1666.
Lehlohonolo, N., Irvine, K.M., Ngezimana, W., Mudau, F.N., 2013. Esci. J. Crop Prod., 2:37–43.
Lerotholi, L., Chaudhary, S.K., Combrinck, S., Viljoen, A., 2017. S. Afr. J. Bot., 110:4–17.
Lerotholi, L.J., Chaudhary, S.K., Chen, W., Veale, C.G.L., Combrinck, S., Viljoen, A.M., 2018. Planta Med., 84:902–912.
Mabona, U., Viljoen, A., Shikanga, E., Marston, A., Van Vuuren, S., 2013. J. Ethnopharmacol., 148:45–55.
Malongane, F., McGaw, L.J., Nyoni, H., Mudau, F.N., 2018. Food Chem., 257:90–100.
Mashimbye, M.J., Mudau, F.N., Soundy, P., Van Ree, T., 2006. S. Afr. J. Chem., 59:1–2.
Maudu, M.E., Mudau, F.N., Mariga, I.K., 2012. Int. J. Agric. Biol., 14:552–556.
Mavundza, E.J., Tshikalange, T.E., Lall, N., Mudau, F.N., Hussein, A.A., 2010. J. Med. Plant Res., 4:2584–2587.
Mbambezeli, G., 2005. Distribution and habitat of *Athrixia phylicoides*. Available from: https//www.plantzafrica.com.
McGaw, L.J., Steenkamp, V., Eloff, J.N., 2007. J. Ethnopharmacol., 110:16–22.
McGaw, L.J., Bagla, V.P., Steenkamp, P.A., Fouché, G., Olivier, J., Eloff, J.N., Myer, M.S., 2013. BMC Complement. Altern. Med., 13:356–367.
Mudau, F.N., Ngezimana, W., 2014. Int. J. Agric. Biol., 16:1011–1014.
Negukhula, S., Mudau, F.N., Mariga, I.K., Liphadzi, K.B., 2011. Indian J. Hortic., 68:91–95.
Olivier, J., Symington, E.A., Jonker, C.Z., Rampedi, I.T., Van Eeden, T.S., 2012. S. Afr. J. Sci., 108:623–629.
Padayachee, K., 2011. The Phytochemistry and Biological Activities of *Athrixia phylicoides*. MSc in Medicine dissertation, University of the Witwatersrand, Johannesburg, South Africa.
Prabhakar, P.K., Doble, M., 2009. Phytomedicine, 16:1119–1126.
Rakuombo, Z.J., 2007. Indigenous Knowledge of Bush Tea (*Athrixia phylicoides*) and Effects of Fertigation Frequency and Growing Medium on Plant Growth. M. Inst. Agrar. dissertation, University of Pretoria, Pretoria, South Africa.
Rampedi, I., Olivier, J., 2005. Acta Academica, 37:165–183.
Reichelt, K.V., Hoffmann-Lücke, P., Hartmann, B., Weber, B., Ley, T.P., Krammer, G.E., Swanepoel, K.M., Engel, K.H., 2012. S. Afr. J. Bot., 83:1–8.
Tshivhandekano, I., Ntushelo, K., Ngezimana, W., Tshikalange, T.E., Mudau, F.N., 2014. Asian Pac. J. Trop. Med., 7:448–453.
Van Wyk, B.E., Gericke, N., 2000. People's Plants. A Guide to Useful Plants of South Africa, first ed. Briza Publications, Pretoria, South Africa.
Watt, J.M., Breyer-Brandwijk, M.G., 1962. The Medicinal and Poisonous Plants of Southern and Eastern Africa, second ed. E. & S. Livingstone Ltd, Edinburgh and London, UK.
Wiedenfeld, H., 2011. Food Addit. Contam., Part A, 28:282–292.

CHAPTER

Cyclopia genistoides 7

Elizabeth Joubert[a], Nduvho Mulaudzi[b], Weiyang Chen[b], Ilze Vermaak[b,c] and Sandra Combrinck[b]

[a]*Plant Bioactives Group, Post-Harvest and Agro-Processing Technologies, Agricultural Research Council (Infruitec Nietvoorbij), Stellenbosch, South Africa*

[b]*Department of Pharmaceutical Sciences, Tshwane University of Technology, Pretoria, South Africa*

[c]*SAMRC Herbal Drugs Research Unit, Faculty of Science, Tshwane University of Technology, Pretoria, South Africa*

Abstract

Cyclopia genistoides (L.) R.Br (Fabaceae), commonly referred to as 'honeybush tea', is one of 23 Cyclopia species endemic to South Africa. The natural habitat of this small fynbos shrub is restricted to very small areas in the Western Cape Province, spanning from the West Coast to Mossel Bay on the Southern Cape coast. Honeybush tea is mostly enjoyed as a hot beverage of the 'fermented' product. 'Fermentation' refers to the high-temperature oxidation process essential for the development of the sought-after sweet, floral aroma and flavour, and brown colour. Traditional medicinal uses include use as an expectorant in pulmonary tuberculosis, chronic catarrh, and a restorative with astringent properties. 'Caspa Cyclopia Tea' was the first branded product to appear on the market in the 1960s. The development of a formal industry in the 1990s gave rise to different branded honeybush products, and the production of extracts. Several studies investigating the anti-oxidant, anticancer, antidiabetic, anti-obesity, antimicrobial, anti-inflammatory and immunomodulating activities have been documented for different Cyclopia species (fermented and unfermented). Quality control protocols based on the chromatographic profiling of methanol extracts were developed using a semi-automated high-performance thin-layer chromatography (HPTLC) system. The HPTLC profiles of the extracts viewed under 366 nm radiation after derivatisation with vanillin-sulphuric acid reagent revealed the presence of mangiferin, isomangiferin and hesperidin in all samples, compounds ubiquitous to all Cyclopia species. Their presence in the methanol extracts was confirmed by ultra-performance liquid chromatography coupled to mass spectrometry (UPLC–MS).

Keywords: *Cyclopia genistoides*, Honeybush tea, Fermentation, HPTLC, UPLC–MS, MIR spectroscopy, Mangiferin, Isomangiferin, Hesperidin

The South African Herbal Pharmacopoeia. https://doi.org/10.1016/B978-0-323-99794-2.00020-9

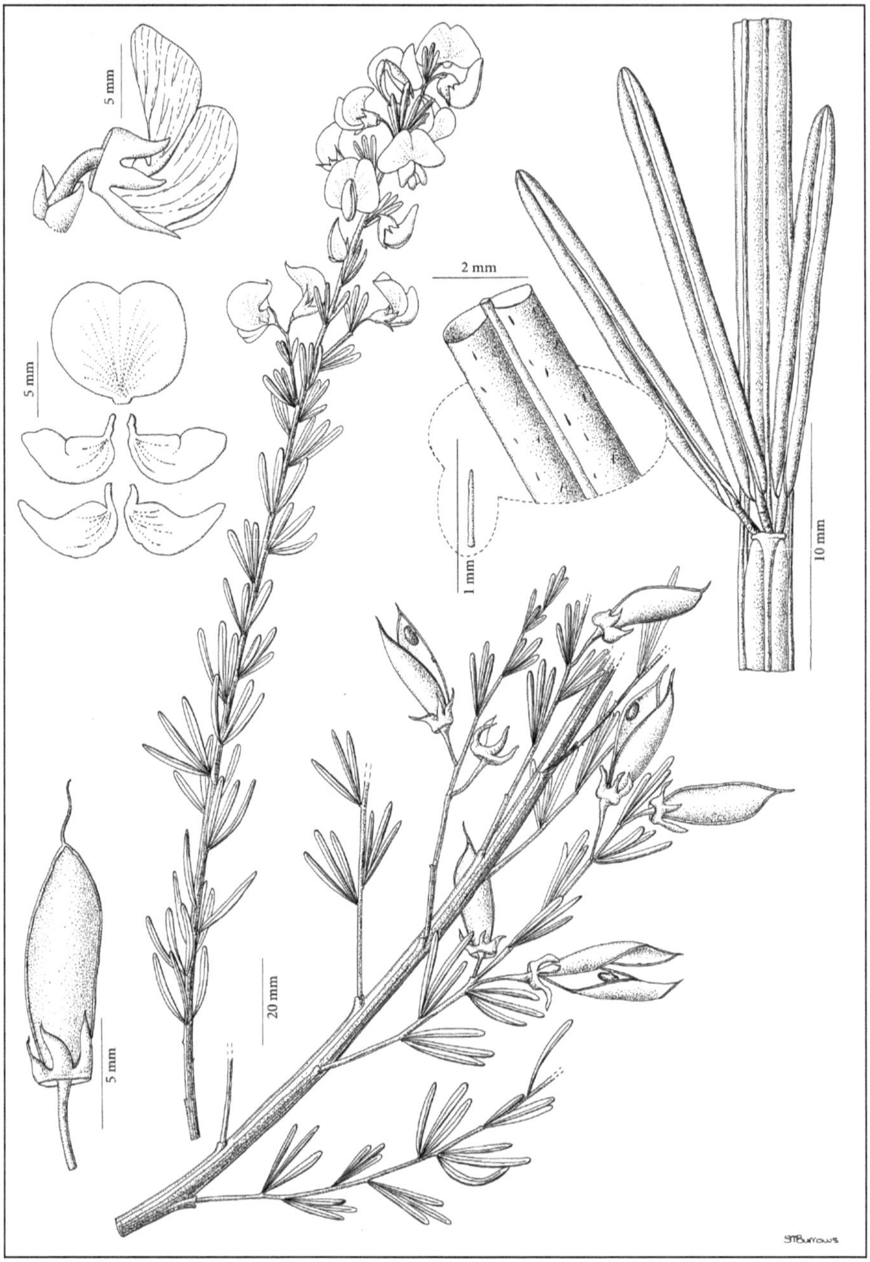
5 mm
5 mm
2 mm
1 mm
10 mm
20 mm
5 mm
SMBurrows

Part A: General overview

1. Synonyms

Cyclopia galioides E.Mey., *Cyclopia genistoides* (L.) R.Br. var. *heterophylla* (Eckl. & Zeyh.) Harv., *C. genistoides* (L.) R.Br. var. *genistoides*, *C. genistoides* (L.) R.Br. var. *teretifolia* (Eckl. & Zeyh.) Kies, *C. genistoides* (L.) R.Br. var. *linearifolia* Eckl. & Zeyh., *Cyclopia teretifolia* Eckl. & Zeyh., *Cyclopia heterophylla* Eckl. & Zeyh., *Ibbetsonia genistoides* Sims, *Galega genistoides* (L.) Thunb., *Sophora genistoides* L., *Podalyria genistoides* (L.) Willd.[a]

2. Common name(s)

Honeybush tea, Cape tea, Boer tea, bush tea, honey tea (English); '*honingtee*', (German); '*heuningbos*', '*heuningtee*', '*heuningbostee*', '*boertee*', '*boss(ies)tee*', '*potbergtee*' (Afrikaans) (Van Wyk and Gorelick, 2017).

3. Conservation status

Near threatened.[a]

4. Botany

The genus *Cyclopia* belongs to the leguminous family Fabaceae and is a member of the tribe Podalrieae. The genus *Cyclopia* is endemic to South Africa and comprises 23 species (Schutte, 1997). *Cyclopia genistoides* (L) R.Br. is a small, multibranched, woody shrub that is easy to miss when not in flower. This typical fynbos shrub with needle-like leaves and yellowish to brown stems, sprouts from a lignotuber and grows to about 1 m in height (C). The name '*Cyclopia*' is derived from the Greek word 'cyclops' meaning 'round-eyed', which refers to the circle-shaped depression or sunken area in the base of the calyx, where the pedicel is attached to the yellow flower (A). Another typical feature of *Cyclopia* species is the trifoliate arrangement of the leaves along the branches (B). Most *Cyclopia* species flower in spring (September–October) when the shrub of *C. genistoides* displays bright yellow, sweetly scented, pea-shaped flowers (A). The seeds are formed in small pods and as they ripen, the coat hardens, the pod turns brown, dries and splits open (SANBI, 2000). The aerial parts are harvested, processed and dried into a popular herbal tea (D).

[a] Red List of South African Plants (http://redlist.sanbi.org).

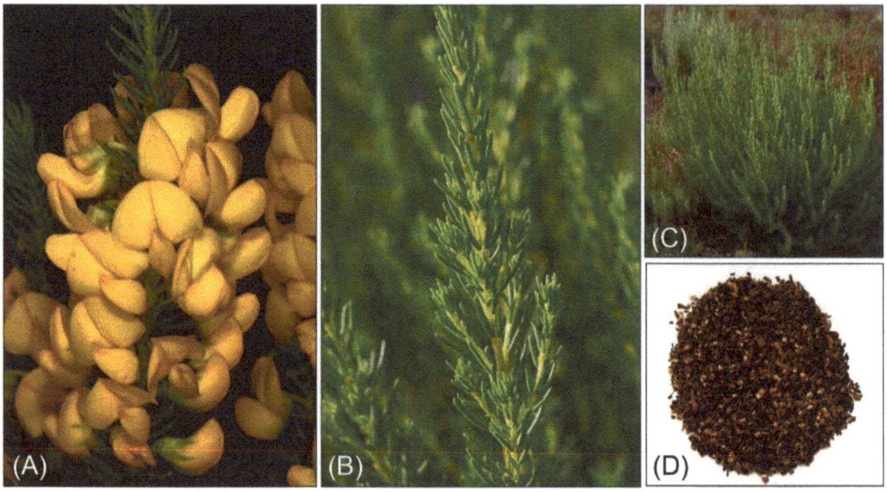

Cyclopia genistoides shrub with bright yellow flowers (A) and needle-like leaves on yellow stems (B). The small shrub is multibranched (C) and the dried aerial parts (D) are of commercial importance.

5. Geographical distribution

All *Cyclopia* species occur in the fynbos region, extending from the Cederberg Mountains, eastwards to Port Elizabeth (Gqeberha) and southwards to the Cape Peninsula. The plants are restricted to very small areas with very specific habitats that include marshlands, high mountain peaks and shale bands. In the mountainous areas, populations of *Cyclopia* are found on the wetter, cooler southern slopes.

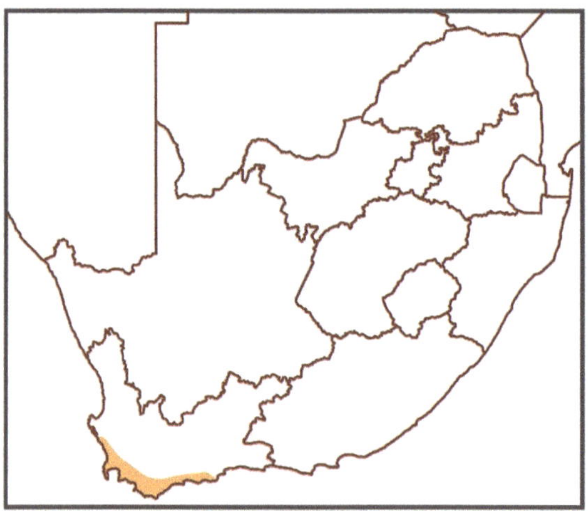

Geographical distribution of *Cyclopia genistoides* in South Africa.

Cyclopia genistoides grows naturally in sandy, coastal areas from the West Coast to Mossel Bay in the Southern Cape (SANBI, 2000).

6. Ethnopharmacology

The use of *Cyclopia* species, specifically pertaining to their use as herbal teas, was well documented in the Cape Province of South Africa during the 19th and early 20th centuries (Van Wyk and Gorelik, 2017). This popular herbal tea, known as 'honeybush tea', was recorded for the first time by Bowie (1829) as 'a decoction of this shrub is much used by the Colonists as a restorative'. *Cyclopia genistoides* was the first of the *Cyclopia* species to be used as a substitute for tea. Early documented medicinal uses of *C. genistoides* include its use as an expectorant in pulmonary tuberculosis, chronic catarrh, and as a restorative with astringent properties (Ecklon and Zeyher, 1836; Pappe, 1868). Tea made from *C. genistoides* is still known locally as honeybush tea or honey tea ('*heuningbostee*', '*heuningtee*'), although internationally it was referred to as Boer tea or Cape tea. Marloth (1925), reported that honeybush was described as wholesome by many colonists, who valued the plant as a stomachic that aids weak digestion, without producing any serious heart stimulation. Infusions of honeybush were noted to stimulate the appetite (Watt and Breyer-Brandwijk, 1962). Anecdotal evidence suggests that it soothes colic in babies, stimulates milk production in breast-feeding women (Rood, 1994), and alleviates nausea and heartburn (Van Wyk et al., 1997).

7. Commercialisation

The first branded product, 'Caspa Cyclopia Tea', appeared on the South African market in the 1960s with the involvement of Mr B. Ginsberg, considered the pioneer of rooibos marketing (Joubert et al., 2011). Other companies that followed were Goldberger Trading in East London and International Foods in Johannesburg. The possibility of exporting *Cyclopia* was investigated by one farmer, but the production was too low to meet the estimated demand. Despite these early marketing efforts, honeybush tea remained an insignificant tea until researchers of the Agricultural Research Council (ARC) and the South African National Biodiversity Institute (SANBI) made a concerted effort from the early 1990s to realise its commercialisation through research and technical support. This gave rise to the establishment of processing facilities in the Western Cape and Eastern Cape provinces to produce the traditional 'fermented' (oxidised) product. One of the facilities focusses largely on the processing of *C. genistoides*. Green honeybush gained the interest of the industry in 2000 as an alternative mangiferin-containing tea product, and the preferred raw material for production of extracts for the nutraceutical, food and cosmetic markets. A patented process was filed for vacuum drying to produce green honeybush tea (De Beer and Joubert, 2002), but this technology was not used on a commercial scale.

A formal breeding programme was developed by the ARC in 1999 to develop improved genetic material for sustainable production. *Cyclopia subternata* and *C. genistoides* plants with vigorous growth were selected from different farms for propagation. The long-term goal of the ARC is to release selected clones to achieve increased biomass yield, while retaining quality based on the sensory profile of the tea and phenolic composition of the plant material (Bester et al., 2016). The commercialisation strategy is based on the development of small, medium and microenterprises (SMMEs) to propagate and distribute improved genetic material (Bester, 2013). The SMME model includes the development of rural communities through job creation and alleviation of poverty.

Most of the tea produced by the industry (95%) is still exported and sold in bulk to international clients. However, it is recognised that it is in the interest of the industry to shift from bulk supply to packaged products ready for the retail market. With the involvement of the major rooibos tea marketing companies, the presence of honeybush in supermarkets has become more commonplace in recent years. Mixtures of fermented *Cyclopia* species are sold as different branded honeybush products. Some up-market farm stalls and speciality shops sell smaller brands that contain only one *Cyclopia* species. Other products available in supermarkets consist of mixtures of rooibos and honeybush, usually with a small percentage of honeybush. A small quantity of the tea, including *C. genistoides*, is sold as green honeybush tea (Joubert et al., 2011).

Cyclopia is one of the few South African plants to have transitioned from regional use to a commercial product, sold in local and global markets. Major markets of *Cyclopia* are the Netherlands, Germany and the United Kingdom (McGregor, 2017). Other international markets include those of countries in the Americas, Far East, Eastern Europe and Africa. Despite the slow pace of commercialisation over the last 100 years, honeybush is likely to become an important export herbal tea/product as new markets and products are developed. Small quantities of *Cyclopia* extract are produced for use in supplements, cosmetics, toiletries and food products. Although the demand for honeybush tea has escalated, commercialisation of *Cyclopia* remains underdeveloped. Joubert and co-workers have contributed to the understanding of the chemical constituents and variation within different *Cyclopia* species (Van Wyk and Gorelik, 2017). Sophisticated procedures and quality control criteria have been developed to provide scientific support for the commercialisation of *Cyclopia* species (Joubert et al., 2019).

To cater for the demand, wild-harvesting of *Cyclopia* species, primarily *C. intermedia*, occurs in the mountainous areas of the fynbos region of South Africa, and still continues to be a major part of the plant material supply (McGregor, 2017). Approximately 200 ha of mostly *C. subternata, C. genistoides* and *C. longifolia* are currently under cultivation. These activities are spread over the fynbos area, from the Langkloof and Tsitsikamma in the Eastern Cape to Overberg in the Western Cape Province. Studies on harvesting practices are limited, but summer harvesting is recommended when high levels of phenolic compounds such as mangiferin, are required in the leaves (Joubert et al., 2014; Mabizela et al., 2020). A study conducted in non-irrigated commercial plantations of *C. subternata* and *C. genistoides* found that harvest date affected the production, growth and quality of the tea. Furthermore, *C. genistoides* harvested annually did not recover to the height of unharvested plants (North et al., 2017). When harvested in February, the regrowth of *C. genistoides* was found to be the fastest with the highest dry mass yield; in September, harvests of the growth flush resulted in the highest mangiferin content and sieve quality (i.e. fraction used as herbal tea). It was also noted that, for the fermented product, the total polyphenol content and hot-water-soluble solids of its 'cup-of-tea' infusion increased with years of harvest, while the mangiferin content of unfermented *C. genistoides* plant material increased with years of harvest. *Cyclopia subternata* plant material harvested during August and September recovered the fastest in height, while the May and August harvests delivered the highest fresh mass yield. Harvesting during August delivered processed tea containing less of the coarse fraction (with a higher stem content) than a February, September or May harvest, but significantly more of the finer processed tea (with a higher leaf content). Annual harvesting is encouraged, but harvesting should not take place during the flowering season (August to September), as the flowers add very little to the final product yield and do not add value to the product. Annually, an estimated production of 10.4 or 8.5 tons/ha of *C. subternata* and *C. genistoides* (fresh plant material) can be achieved based on 10,000 bushes/ha (North et al., 2017).

The bulk of the annual harvest is processed as fermented honeybush tea. The fermentation process is actually a high-temperature oxidation process. Heating of the plant material is required to develop the sweet, characteristic aroma and flavour, and brown leaf and infusion colour. Traditional practice was to heat the plant material in an oven (Hofmeyer and Phillips, 1922) or to place the shredded plant material in a heap for spontaneous heating (Marloth 1909) followed by sun-drying. Remnants of baking ovens, originating from the 1890s, were found in the Garcia Pass near Riversdale in the Southern Cape (Joubert et al., 2011). Modern practice makes use of oxidation ovens, varying in design between factories, but basically employing external heat to reach temperatures in excess of 60 °C. The high temperature is not only critical for development of the sought-after sensory properties, but also to ensure good microbial quality (Du Toit et al., 1999). An increase in oxidation temperature shortens the time to form the sought-after sensory profile. The primary aroma and flavour attributes of fermented honeybush tea are similar for all *Cyclopia* species, but some attributes are more prominent in the fermented product of some species and can be manipulated by oxidation conditions (Joubert et al., 2019). The high temperature and oxidative conditions of the fermentation step cause both qualitative and quantitative changes in the phenolic composition of honeybush tea. Most of the major phenolic compounds of *C. genistoides* are degraded, producing not only an extract with a lower phenolic concentration, but also a lower yield (Beelders et al., 2015).

Retention of high levels of phenolic compounds in green honeybush makes it the preferred plant material for the production of nutraceutical extracts, particularly mangiferin-rich extracts (Joubert et al., 2003; Miller et al., 2020a). By applying a short steam treatment (60 s or longer), the freshly shredded leaves and stems of *C. maculata* (Alexander et al., 2017) and *C. longifolia* (Alexander et al., 2018) developed fruity aroma attributes, while the intensities of the vegetal, green notes of the green honeybush were reduced. The short steam treatment had no detrimental impact on the content of the phenolic compounds or the green leaf colour. Some production batches of green *C. genistoides* and *C. longifolia* may produce a bitter-tasting tea, partly attributed to a high mangiferin content (Alexander et al., 2021).

8. Pharmacological evaluation

8.1 *In vitro and ex vivo* studies

8.1.1 Anti-oxidant activity

Several assays had been used to assess the effect of fermentation on the radical scavenging activity of extracts of several *Cyclopia* species. The superoxide radical ($O_2^{\bullet-}$) scavenging activity of aqueous extracts prepared from *Cyclopia* species (*C. genistoides, C. sessiflora, C. maculata, C. subternata* and *C. intermedia*) was investigated in a β-NADH/phenazine methosulphate (PMS) system (Hubbe and Joubert, 2000). Scavenging activities of the extracts were significantly lower following fermentation of the plant material. The extracts of fermented *C. maculata* and *C. intermedia* had the lowest total polyphenolic content. They also had the weakest $O_2^{\bullet-}$ scavenging activity (EC_{50} 238.2 and 249.3 μg/mL, respectively). The same study showed that fermentation also reduced the 2,2-diphenyl-1-picrylhydrazyl radical (DPPH) scavenging activity of the extracts. Another study, using radical scavenging (2,2-azino-bis-(3-ethylbenzothiazoline-6-sulphonate)) radical cation ($ABTS^{\bullet+}$), ferric ion reduction, and inhibition of Fe^{2+}-induced microsomal lipid peroxidation as criteria for the assessment of *in vitro* anti-oxidant activity of the aqueous extracts of these *Cyclopia* species, confirmed the same trend as found for $O_2^{\bullet-}$ scavenging activity. The only exception was *C. genistoides*, i.e. fermentation did not affect the ability of the extract to inhibit lipid peroxidation (Joubert et al., 2008). Fermentation of *C. genistoides* also did not affect the total anti-oxidant capacity of aqueous extracts assessed using the oxygen radical absorbance capacity (ORAC) assay, i.e. 4460 ± 423 vs 4406 ± 463 μmoL Trolox equivalents/g extract of unfermented and fermented plant material, respectively, despite qualitative and quantitative changes in the phenolic profile of the extracts (Beelders et al., 2015).

8.1.2 Antimutagenic effects

Aqueous extracts of fermented and unfermented *C. intermedia* reduced 2-acetylaminofluorene (2-AAF)-induced and aflatoxin B1 (AFB1)-induced mutagenesis in *Salmonella typhimurium* strains TA98 and TA100, respectively, in the presence of metabolic activation (S9 liver homogenate) (Marnewick et al., 2000). Fermentation decreased the inhibitory effect of the extracts. The extracts displayed weak inhibition of mutagenesis induced by direct-acting mutagens, methyl methanesulphonate, hydrogen peroxide and cumol hydroperoxide. A follow-up study confirmed these findings for aqueous extracts of *C. intermedia* (fermented and unfermented) on 2-AAF- and AFB1-induced mutagenesis in these tester strains (Van der Merwe et al., 2006). Investigation of other *Cyclopia* species demonstrated that fermentation of *C. genistoides* enhanced its antimutagenic effect against 2-AAF-induced mutagenesis, reduced that of *C. sessiliflora*, and had no effect on *C. subternata* (Van der Merwe et al., 2006). An *ex vivo* study demonstrated that the cytosolic liver fraction of male Fischer rats treated for 10 weeks with the aqueous extract of unfermented *C. intermedia* offered protection against both 2-AAF- and AFB1-induced mutagenesis in *S. typhimurium* (Marnewick et al., 2004). The extract from fermented *C. intermedia* was effective against AFB1-induced mutagenesis in strain TA100, but only marginally effective against 2-AAF-induced mutagenesis in strain TA98. The microsomal liver fraction of rats consuming the extract of unfermented *C. intermedia* reduced AFB1-induced mutagenicity, but none of the extracts were effective in decreasing 2-AAF-induced mutagenicity. *Cyclopia intermedia* extracts demonstrated a protective effect against tobacco-specific mutagens, 4-(methylnitrosamino)-1-(3-pyridyl)-1-butanone (NNK) and 4-(methylnitroamino)-1-(3-pyridyl)-1-butanol (NNAL), tested in the *S. typhimurium* strain TA1535 in the presence of metabolic activation (S9) (Gelderblom et al., 2017). Fermentation of the plant material reduced the protective effect of *C. intermedia* extract against NNK, but not against NNAL.

8.1.3 Phyto-oestrogenic and chemopreventive activities

Methanol and water extracts of *C. subternata, C. genistoides, C. intermedia* and *C. sessiliflora* (both unfermented and fermented) were found to displace tritiated estradiol E_2(^3H-E_2) from human estrogen receptors (ER), ERα and ERβ, using a competitive whole-cell ER binding assay. The human ERα and ERβ were transiently transfected into COS-1 cells (Verhoog et al., 2007a). The extent of binding of the extracts to ERα and ERβ differed between *Cyclopia* species, the type of extract and the batch of plant material (harvesting). *Cyclopia subternata* and *C. genistoides* were more effective than *C. intermedia* and *C. sessiliflora,* with the methanol extracts of the unfermented plant material generally displaying greater activity. Some extracts showed significant binding to ERα or ERβ, or both ER isoforms. Further investigation of methanol extracts of another three *C. genistoides* harvestings (P104, P105 and P122) (Verhoog et al., 2007b) confirmed the variation in binding, with only one harvesting, P104, binding to both ER isoforms. The methanol extracts transactivated the oestrogen response element promoter reporter construct in COS-1 cells *via* human ERβ, but not *via* ERα, despite binding to both subtypes (Verhoog et al., 2007a). The extracts of P105 and P104 were able to induce proliferation of ERα- and ERβ-positive MCF-7 BUS cells, but they antagonised E_2-induced MCF-7 BUS cell proliferation. Given that the extracts also induced proliferation of oestrogen-insensitive MDA-MB-231 breast cancer cells, the results suggested that the extracts are able to induce both ER-dependent and ER-independent cell proliferation. In addition, the methanol extracts displaced E_2 from the sex hormone-binding globulin (SHBG).

Mfenyana et al. (2008) benchmarked sequential methanol (SM6Met) and ethyl acetate extracts of unfermented *C. subternata* against four commercial phyto-oestrogenic nutraceuticals. The *Cyclopia* extracts had comparable efficacy and potency to the commercial products. SM6Met and the methanol extract of P104 (*C. genistoides*) and aqueous extracts (preparation as for a cup-of-tea infusion) of the same batches of plant material were evaluated for ER subtype-specific antagonism and agonism, in both transrepression and transactivation (Visser et al., 2013). For transactivation, all extracts displayed ERβ agonism and ERα antagonism when ER subtypes were expressed separately; however, when co-expressed, only agonism was observed. By contrast, for transrepression P104 displayed agonism, both when the subtypes were expressed separately and when co-expressed. SM6Met displayed antagonism when subtypes were expressed separately, and agonism when co-expressed. The breast cancer cell proliferation assays indicated that extracts antagonised cell proliferation in the presence of oestrogen at lower concentrations than required for proliferation. Fractionation of SM6Met showed separation of its desirable oestrogenic activities, namely ERα antagonism, ERβ agonism, and antagonism of E2-induced breast cancer cell proliferation, into different fractions (Mortimer et al., 2015).

The pro-apoptotic and antiproliferative activities of aqueous and methanol extracts of unfermented *C. intermedia* and *C. subternata* in skin cells were evaluated using spontaneously immortalised keratinocytes (HaCaT), non-malignant normal fibroblast-like skin cells (CRL 7761) and basal carcinoma cell line (CRL 7762) skin cells (Magcwebeba et al., 2016a). The aqueous extracts of the *Cyclopia* species inhibited proliferation and induced pro-apoptotic caspase-3 activity in the skin cells. By contrast, the methanol extracts offered less protection against cell proliferation. The methanol extract of *C. intermedia* did not exhibit pro-apoptotic activity in all three cell types, while the methanol extract of *C. subternata* was not effective in inducing caspase-3-activity in normal and cancer cells. Roza et al. (2017) showed that the extract fractions of *C. genistoides* (fermented and unfermented) inhibited the growth of two human cancerous cell lines, A2780 and T47D cells (isolated from ovarian and breast carcinoma, respectively), using the MTT ((3-[4,5-dimethylthiazol-2-yl]-2,5 diphenyl tetrazolium bromide) assay.

8.1.4 Anti-obesity activities

A few studies investigated the anti-obesity properties of *Cyclopia* extracts, using 3T3-L1 adipocytes as an *in vitro* model of obesity. Dudhia et al. (2013) reported that aqueous extracts of fermented and unfermented *C. maculata* and unfermented *C. subternata* inhibited adipocyte differentiation, reduced intracellular triglyceride and lipid accumulation, and inhibited the expression of peroxisome proliferator-activated receptor gamma isoform 2, a key regulator of adipogenesis. Differentiation of 3T3-L1 preadipocytes with the extract of fermented *C. maculata* increased adiponectin secretion, while all the extracts increased leptin secretion. A follow-up study on the same extracts showed that lipolysis was stimulated by all the extracts, but mostly by the extract of fermented *C. maculata.* The increased lipolysis was accompanied by increased expression of hormone-sensitive lipase and perilipin (Pheiffer et al., 2013). Jack et al. (2017) expanded the study of the anti-obesity effects of *Cyclopia* species to include *C. intermedia*, using 40% aqueous methanol for extraction followed by partitioning into two fractions, organic and aqueous. The extracts and their organic fractions decreased the lipid content of 3T3-L1 adipocytes. Investigation of the organic fraction of *C. intermedia* confirmed a decrease in lipid accumulation in 3T3-L1 adipocytes by regulating lipid metabolism [increased mRNA expression of human hormone-sensitive lipase (*HSL*)] and energy homeostasis (increasing mRNA expression of *SIRT1*, *UCP3* and *PPARγ*). Further investigation of the organic fraction of *C. intermedia* demonstrated that its fractionation did not increase the ability to enhance gene expression within a single fraction, i.e. fractions F1 and F2 displayed increased mRNA expression of *HSL*, while F1 and F4 displayed increased *UCP3* expression (Jack et al., 2018).

8.1.5 Antidiabetic activities

Co-exposure of rat islet tumour RIN-5F cells to streptozotocin (STZ), a β-cell-specific cytotoxin, and unfermented *C. maculata* extract (also used by Dudhia et al., 2013, in his study on 3T3-L1 cells) demonstrated that the extract improved cell viability as measured by cellular ATP content, comparable to *N*-acetyl cysteine, an anti-oxidant, and the positive control (Chellan et al., 2014). Aqueous extracts of a large number of batches of unfermented *C. subternata* enhanced glucose uptake in C2C12 myocytes to a varying degree (Schulze et al., 2016). *Cyclopia genistoides* extracts from different batches of plant material, prepared with 40% aqueous ethanol, showed mammalian α-glucosidase inhibitory activity (Bosman et al., 2017). Subsequent preparation of a xanthone-enriched fraction of the extract enhanced inhibition of α-glucosidase activity relative to the extract (Miller et al., 2020b). The potential for dose reduction of acarbose through synergism was demonstrated for combinations of the drug with the xanthone-enriched fraction at the 50% and 75% effect levels, based on the combination index.

8.1.6 Anti-inflammatory activity

The modulatory activity of aqueous and methanol extracts of unfermented *C. intermedia* and *C. subternata* against intracellular interleukin-1α (icIL-1α) accumulation as biomarker was investigated in a UVB/HaCaT keratinocyte model (Magcwebeba et al., 2016b). The aqueous extract of *C. intermedia* facilitated the inhibition of icIL-1α production that strongly correlated with the reduction in cell viability and the induction of caspase-3-activity, implying a mechanism involving apoptosis. The methanol extracts of both *Cyclopia* species enhanced icIL-1α accumulation, suggesting a pro-inflammatory effect associated with a reduction in UVB-induced apoptosis, without adversely affecting cell viability.

8.1.7 Immunomodulating activity

Ethanol: water (40%, v/v) and aqueous extracts, prepared from unfermented *C. subternata*, *C. genistoides* and *C. maculata*, were evaluated for immune-regulating activity using mesenteric lymph node cells and murine splenocytes (Murakami et al., 2018). The 40% aqueous ethanol extracts of *C. subternata* and *C. genistoides* enhanced production of the cytokines, IL-4, IFN-γ, IL-10 and IL-17A, by ovalbumin-stimulated splenocytes and enhanced IFN-γ production in mesenteric lymph node cells, also stimulated with ovalbumin. The extracts increased the ratio of $CD4^+CD25^+Foxp3^+$ Treg cells to total $CD4^+$cells, indicating induction of $Foxp3^+$ Treg cells. A low extract dose induced Treg cells in allergen-stimulated cells, while a high dose activated T cells, suggesting that dose will play an important role in the immune-suppressing or enhancing effect of honeybush.

8.1.8 Other activities

An aqueous extract of fermented *C. intermedia* inhibited anti-osteoclastogenic activity, i.e. receptor activator of NF-κB ligand (RANKL)-induced osteoclast formation and decreased bone resorption in RAW264.7 murine macrophages (Visagie et al., 2015). The extract decreased the expression of crucial resorption genes, tartrate-resistant acid phosphatase (*TRAP*), matrix metalloproteinase-9 (*MMP-9*) and cathepsin K. Agapouda et al. (2020) investigated the effects of *Cyclopia* extracts on neuronal cells and specifically on their mitochondrial function. Pretreatment of human neuroblastoma SH-SY5Y cells with the aqueous extract of unfermented *C. subternata*, and to a lesser extent those of unfermented *C. genistoides* and *C. longifolia*, exhibited a protective effect by rescuing bioenergetics and mitochondrial deficits under H_2O_2-induced oxidative stress. Ros-Santaella et al. (2020) assessed the effect of an aqueous *C. intermedia* extract on boar sperm parameters under induced oxidative stress (Fe^{2+}/ascorbate) and during storage (5 days at 17 °C) without oxidative stress. During exposure to oxidative conditions, the extract improved sperm motility and kinetic parameters, preserved the plasma membrane integrity, and reduced lipid peroxidation in the samples. The positive effects of the extract on the sperm parameters (motility, kinetics, acrosome integrity and mitochondrial activity) were observed from 48 h until 120 h storage. The dichloromethane layers of methanol extracts of unfermented and fermented *C. genistoides* exhibited inhibition of xanthine oxidase activity (Roza et al., 2016). Weak antimicrobial activity was reported against *Streptococcus pyogenes* for a chloroform extract of unfermented *C. intermedia* (Dube et al., 2017). The same study showed weak inhibition of *Staphylococcus aureus* and *Candida albicans* by aqueous and methanol extracts of both fermented and unfermented *C. intermedia*.

8.2 *In vivo* studies and clinical trials

8.2.1 Modulation of hepatic drug-metabolising enzymes

Aqueous extracts of *C. intermedia* (fermented and unfermented), given as the sole drinking fluid to male Fischer rats for 10 weeks, increased the activity of cytosolic glutathione S-transferase α. Microsomal UDP-glucuronyl transferase activity was slightly increased by the extract of unfermented *C. intermedia* (Marnewick et al., 2003).

8.2.2 Anti-oxidant effects and modulation of oxidative stress

The study by Marnewick et al. (2003) also showed that the aqueous extracts of *C. intermedia* (fermented and unfermented) affected no change in hepatic anti-oxidative capacity, measured using the ORAC assay. The extracts reduced oxidised glutathione (GSSG) levels in the liver compared to the water control, but reduced glutathione (GSH) levels were not significantly affected, resulting in higher GSH/GSSG ratios, especially for the extract of unfermented *C. intermedia*. In another study by Van der Merwe et al. (2017), male Fischer rats fed polyphenol-enriched extracts of unfermented *C. genistoides* and *C. subternata* (2.5 g/kg) for 28 and 90 days, respectively, increased glutathione reductase activity in the liver significantly after 28 days. In addition, the *C. subternata* extract decreased the hepatic GSH content significantly after 90 days, resulting in a marked, but not significant, decrease in the GSH/GSSG ratio. Both extracts altered the expression of anti-oxidant defence-related genes and oxidative stress after 28 days to varying degrees. Seven genes were affected by both extracts; namely, the anti-oxidant-related genes: kinesin family member 9 (*Kif9*) and serine (or cysteine) peptidase inhibitor clade B member 1b (*Serpinb1b*) were downregulated, while prostaglandin-endoperoxide synthase 1 (*Ptgs1*) was up-regulated; genes involved in ROS metabolism: thioredoxin-interacting protein (*Txnip*) and xeroderma pigmentosum complementation group A (*Xpa*) were down- and up-regulated, respectively; and oxygen transporter-related genes: Fanconi anaemia, complementation group C (*Fancc*) and vimentin (*Vim*) were both up-regulated. Furthermore, the *C. subternata* extract up-regulated expression of other genes involved in ROS metabolism: NADPH oxidase organiser 1 (*Noxo1*), superoxide dismutase 1 (*Sod1*), and the oxidative stress responsive gene, aminoadipate-semialdehyde synthase (*Aass*). The *C. genistoides* extract up-regulated other genes involved in ROS metabolism, namely NAD(*P*)H dehydrogenase, quinone 1 (*Nqo1*), thyroid peroxidase (*Tpo*), nudix (nucleoside diphosphate linked moiety X)-type motif 15 (*Nudt1*), and proteasome (prosome, macropain) subunit beta type 5 (*Psmb5*).

8.2.3 Anti-obesity activities

A daily 28-day treatment of obese leptin receptor-deficient ($Lepr^{db/db}$) mice by oral gavage with 70 and 352 mg/kg body weight (bw) of an organic fraction of unfermented *C. intermedia* decreased body weight gain by 14% and 21%, respectively (Jack et al., 2017). Treatment had no effect on water intake or food consumption, nor did it affect the oral glucose tolerance of the mice as determined on day 27 of treatment.

8.2.4 Antidiabetic activities

Following studies for patent application (PCT/EP2008/052863) in 2008, the antidiabetic potential of an aqueous extract of unfermented *C. intermedia* was assessed in STZ and obese insulin-resistant male Wistar rats (Muller et al., 2011). An acute dose of the extract reduced the plasma glucose concentration of the STZ-induced diabetic rats over a 6 h period. The obese, insulin-resistant rats, on a high sugar and fat diet, were treated with different doses for 3 months. The average intake of the extract varied from 77 to 531 mg/kg bw. The treatment, irrespective of dose, reduced their hyperglycaemic fasting blood glucose concentrations to normal levels. The treatment also reduced total plasma cholesterol concentrations and decreased average α-cell size, and the α-cell size-to-β-cell size ratio. Chellan et al. (2014) pretreated male Wistar rats for 15 days with an aqueous extract of unfermented *C. maculata* (30 and 300 mg/kg bw) before injection with STZ. The treatment continued for a further 6 days (21 days in total). Pretreatment decreased the percentage of diabetic rats following an STZ injection. The high extract dose significantly reduced the fasting plasma glucose levels and both doses were effective in improving glucose tolerance compared to the STZ controls. Other changes caused by the extract were a reduction in the total serum triglyceride levels, the glucose-to-insulin ratio and plasma nitrate levels, and an increase in the β-cell area to total islet area, and β-cell proliferation. An aqueous extract of unfermented *C. subternata* that was effective in increasing glucose uptake in C2C12 myocytes was shown to improve glycaemic control of STZ-induced diabetic male Wistar rats after acute administration of the extract, dosed at 600 mg/kg bw, but not at 30 and 300 mg/kg bw (Schulze et al., 2016). An aqueous extract of fermented *C. intermedia,* dosed in the drinking water of STZ-induced diabetic male Wistar rats, decreased their elevated fasting plasma glucose levels. Histological evaluation of the testis and caudal epididymis following treatment, showed that disruptions in their morphology in the diabetic animal were mildly ameliorated by the extract (Omolaoye and Du Plessis, 2021).

8.2.5 UVB skin-protective effects

Fermented and unfermented *C. intermedia* were investigated for their photoprotective effect (Petrova et al., 2011). Ethanol extracts of defatted plant material were prepared as 1% (w/v) solutions in ethanol: acetone (1:1, v/v) and applied to the dorsal skin of SKH-1 mice before short UVB exposure (180 mJ/cm^2). The treatment was repeated daily for 10 days. The extracts reduced signs of sunburn, such as peeling, erythema, and hardening of the skin, and also significantly reduced epidermal hyperplasia and oedema and reduced the expression of cyclo-oxygenase-2 (COX-2), GADD45, ornithine decarboxylase (ODC), and OGG1/2, caused by UVB exposure. The extract of fermented *C. intermedia* was more effective than the extract of unfermented *C. intermedia* in reducing lipid peroxidation, and protected against the UV-induced depletion of superoxide dismutase and catalase in the skin.

8.2.6 Phyto-oestrogenic and chemopreventive activities

Given the ability of unfermented *C. subternata* extracts (SM6Met and aqueous) to induce weak proliferation in the absence of oestrogen and to antagonise oestrogen-induced proliferation of MCF-7BUS human breast cancer cell line (Visser et al., 2013), further investigation entailed treatment of immature female Wistar rats with the extracts. The rats were treated daily with oestrogen, SM6Met, or the aqueous extract of *C. subternata* by oral gavage for 30 consecutive days. The extracts, unlike oestrogen, did not increase uterine weight, and SM6Met antagonised oestrogen-induced uterine growth, suggesting that the extract behaves as an anti-oestrogen in the uterus. Other *in vivo* studies on SM6Met were conducted to evaluate its effects on breast cancer (Visser et al., 2016; Oyenihi et al., 2018). In a study focussing on cancer promotion and targeted primary chemoprevention in an *N*-methyl-*N*-nitrosourea (NMU)-induced rat mammary gland carcinogenesis model, SM6Met decreased palpable tumour frequency, mass and volume, and increased tumour latency (by 7 days) and tumour-free survival (by 42 days) in Sprague–Dawley rats. SM6Met was administered daily *via* the diet aiming at 200 mg/kg bw. The study was terminated after 219 days (Visser et al., 2016). Oyenihi et al. (2018) showed that SM6Met decreased LA-induced mammary tumours in female Sprague–Dawley rats comparable to the standard-of-care drug, tamoxifen. SM6Met was administered daily for 28 days, starting 14 days prior to tumour induction. All four doses of SM6Met (100, 200, 300 and 500 mg/kg bw) reduced tumour volume relative to the vehicle.

The modulating effect of the ethanol/acetone-soluble fraction of methanol extracts of *C. intermedia* (unfermented and fermented) on tumour promotion was demonstrated in a two-stage mouse-skin carcinogenesis model (Marnewick et al., 2005). The mice were treated with a single topical application of 7,12-dimethylbenz[*a*]anthracene (DMBA) as tumour initiator, followed by the *C. intermedia* fraction, 30 min prior to application of the cancer promoter, 12-*O*-tetradecanoylphorbol-13-acetate (TPA). Both fractions were effective in suppressing skin tumour promotion by TPA with the fraction of unfermented *C. intermedia* being the more effective. Not only did the fractions reduce the tumour volume and the mean number of tumours per mouse, but tumour development was also delayed.

Ingestion of the aqueous extracts of *C. intermedia* (fermented and unfermented) protected against fumonisin B1 (FB1)-induced cancer promotion in diethyl nitrosamine-initiated rat liver carcinogenesis (Marnewick et al., 2009). The extracts were fed to male Fischer rats *ad libitum* for 1 week after a single dose of the initiator, until completion of the experiment after 6 weeks. Cancer promotion commenced 3 weeks after cancer initiation by giving the FB1-containing diet for 21 days. The extracts marginally reduced foci of different sizes, except for a significant reduction in the number of foci sized 21–30 µm by the extract of unfermented *C. intermedia*. Foci of this size group constituted approximately 20% of the total number of foci in the positive control group. The aqueous extracts of *C. intermedia* also modulated methylbenzylnitrosamine (MBN)-induced oesophageal squamous cell carcinogenesis in male Fischer rats, by reducing the size and number of papillomas (Sissing et al., 2011).

8.2.7 Anti-allergic properties

The immune-regulating activity of 40% aqueous ethanol extracts of unfermented *C. subternata* and *C. genistoides*, which was demonstrated *in vitro* (Murakami et al., 2018), was confirmed *in vivo* (Yoshida et al., 2020). Ovalbumin-specific T-cell receptor transgenic DO11.10 mice were treated with the extracts, dissolved in their drinking water (1 mg/mL), and after 2 days, the mice received a diet containing 20% ovalbumin that was continued for 5 days. The extracts enhanced both Th1- and Th2-type antibody production in the sera and generation of Treg cells in the spleen. The Treg cells isolated from mice treated with *C. subternata* extract were selected for further investigation. These cells display regulatory activity, i.e. inhibition of the production of both Th1- (IFN-γ) and Th2- (IL-4) type cytokines in co-culture with naïve splenocytes. The Treg cells of the treated mice also produced IL-10 at comparable levels to naïve Treg cells.

8.3 Safety

No toxicity or adverse effects related to the consumption of honeybush tea have been documented. Polyphenol-enriched extracts of unfermented *C. genistoides* and *C. subternata,* given to male Fischer rats as part of the diet (2.5 g/kg feed) for 28 and 90 days, respectively, had no effect on body weight gain and kidney or liver weight. The *C. subternata* extract had a marked effect on serum iron (reduced), serum alkaline phosphatase levels (increased), and total serum bilirubin (increased) (Van der Merwe et al., 2017). Further studies on the potential adverse effects are required, in view of the potentially detrimental effects of chronic ingestion of exogenous anti-oxidants at high doses on cellular homeostasis (Van der Merwe et al., 2017). Another consideration is potential herb-drug interaction given the enhanced activity of cytosolic glutathione S-transferase alpha and microsomal UDP-glucuronosyl transferase of rats fed *C. intermedia* extracts (Marnewick et al., 2003). Microbial safety received attention from Du Toit et al. (1999). Five endospore-forming *Bacillus* species, namely *B. badius, B. brevis, B. subtilis, B. stearothermophilus* and *B. pumilus*, and two thermophilic moulds, *Humicola lanuginosa* and *H. grisea* var. *thermoida*, were isolated from the plant material. These microbial contaminants can be eliminated during fermentation of the plant materials by employing temperatures >60 °C.

9. Phytochemistry

9.1 Volatile constituents

The first investigation of the volatile organic compounds (VOCs) of *Cyclopia* entailed headspace analysis of fermented and unfermented *C. genistoides*, using gas chromatography with mass spectrometry (GC–MS) detection (Le Roux et al., 2008). Fermentation of the plant material resulted in quantitative differences, with terpenoids comprising the major compounds of the fermented plant material, and unsaturated and saturated alcohols, methyl ketones and aldehydes those of unfermented plant material. 6-Methyl-5-hepten-2-one, the major constituent of unfermented plant material, is associated with the following reported aroma description: 'pungent-herbaceous, oily-green with grassy fresh green fruity notes'. Linalool, the major aroma constituent identified in fermented *C. genistoides,* is described as 'floral woody and refreshing'. Other compounds with a sweet aroma are geraniol, (*E*)-β-damascenone and 10-*epi*-γ-eudesmol. Unsaturated and saturated C_5–C_{18} aldehydes present in the flowers of *C. genistoides* may have a detrimental effect on the flavour of the tea (Le Roux et al., 2006). A study of the VOCs of fermented *C. subternata* entailed GC–MS and GC-olfactometry (GC-O) (Le Roux et al., 2012). A total of 183 compounds, the majority of which were terpenoids (103), were identified and 37 of these compounds were determined by GC-O to be odour-active. (*R*/*S*)-Linalool, (*E*)-β-damascenone, (*E*)-β-damascone, (*E*)-β-ionone, geraniol and (7*E*)-megastigma-5,7,9-trien-4-one were identified with the highest flavour dilution factors (DF ≥ 512). Compounds exhibiting honeybush-like odours identified by GC-O assessors included (6*E*,8*E*)-megastigma-4,6,8-trien-3-one, (6*E*,8*Z*)-megastigma-4,6,8-trien-3-one, (7*E*)-megastigma-5,7,9-trien-4-one, 10-epi-γ-eudesmol, epi-α-cadinol and epi-α-muurolol. Analysis using GC-O of a sample of fermented *C. maculata* with a distinct cinnamon-like aroma resulted in the identification of only one compound, namely eugenol, with its sweet, spicy and clove-like aroma that could contribute to this aroma note (Theron et al., 2014). Subsequent analysis of the VOCs of the infusions of a set of 15 samples, five each of fermented *C. maculata* (including the sample with the prominent cinnamon-like note), *C. genistoides* and *C. subternata* by GC × GC-FID analysis, resulted in the identification of 84 compounds, of which 5-methylfurfural and butyl benzoate were identified for the first time in *Cyclopia*. Most compounds were common to all three species, with differences primarily in their relative amounts. Principal component analysis of the GC and descriptive sensory data showed that the identification of compounds responsible for differentiation between these *Cyclopia* species according to sensory attributes was not possible (Ntlhokwe et al., 2017). The volatile compounds from infusions were also determined by using two-dimensional gas chromatography coupled to time-of-flight mass spectrometry (GC × GC-ToF-MS). Using reference standards, 101 of a total of 287 compounds were identified, while the remainder were tentatively identified using retention index (RI) and mass spectral data (Ntlhokwe et al., 2018). Some of the compounds were unique to each of the *Cyclopia* species, but the majority of the compounds identified were common to all three species, although differences in their relative abundances were observed. (*E*)-Cinnamaldehyde was tentatively identified in *C. maculata* samples, pointing to the likely contribution of this compound to the cinnamon-like note. Compounds likely to contribute to honey and caramel notes were benzene acetaldehyde and maltol (3-hydroxy-2-methylpyrone).

9.2 Non-volatile constituents

The absence of caffeine in honeybush herbal teas, including *C. genistoides*, reported previously, was confirmed using a highly specific analytical method with a low detection limit (0.2 μg/L) (Stander et al., 2019a). The methylated inositol, pinitol, was isolated from *C. intermedia* and identified by nuclear magnetic resonance (NMR) spectroscopy (Ferreira et al., 1998). The presence of pinitol at ca. 40 mg/g in 40% aqueous ethanol extracts of unfermented *C. genistoides* and *C. subternata* was determined using GC–MS analysis (Yoshida et al., 2020). *Cyclopia subternata* (unfermented) and *C. intermedia* (fermented) were comprehensively studied in terms of their polyphenol composition by Ferreira et al. (1998) and Kamara et al. (2003, 2004). Xanthones (mangiferin and isomangiferin), flavones (5-deoxyluteolin, luteolin, diosmetin and scolymoside), flavanones (eriodictyol, hesperetin, eriocitrin, naringenin, naringenin-5-*O*-β-D-glucopyranoside, narirutin, eriodictyol-7-*O*-β-D-glucopyranoside and eriodictyol-5-*O*-β-D-glucopyranoside), isoflavones (formononetin-diglucoside, formononetin, afrormosin, wistin, calycosin, pseudobaptigenin, orobol, isosakuranetin and fujikinetin), coumestans (flemmichapparin, medicagol and sophoracoumestan), flavonols (kaempferol glucoside derivatives) and others (*p*-coumaric acid, epigallocatechin gallate, tyrosol, tyrosol derivatives and pinitol) were identified after isolation and NMR analysis of the acylated compounds. Subsequently, Kokotkiewicz et al. (2012) isolated three compounds from unfermented *C. subternata* extract and identified them using NMR spectroscopy as phloretin-3′,5′-di-*C*-β-D-glucopyranoside (dihydrochalcone), iriflophenone-3-*C*-β-D-glucopyranoside (benzophenone) and isorhoifolin (flavone). The same group also isolated and identified (using NMR) a number of compounds from unfermented and fermented *C. genistoides*, namely mangiferin, isomangiferin, iriflophenone-3-*C*-β-D-glucopyranoside, maclurin-3-*C*-β-D-glucopyranoside, hesperidin and luteolin (Kokotkiewicz et al., 2013).

A comprehensive analysis of the aqueous extracts of unfermented *C. genistoides* conducted by Beelders et al. (2014b) employing LC–MS, identified two aromatic amino acids (tyrosine and phenylalanine), two flavones (vicenin-2 and diosmin) and two glycosylated flavanones (eriocitrin and narirutin). The dihydrochalcone, phloretin-3′,5′-di-*C*-β-D-glucopyranoside, was also tentatively identified. Beelders et al. (2014a) subsequently isolated and identified (NMR) iriflophenone-3-*C*-β-D-glucopyranoside-4-*O*-β-D-glucopyranoside from the aqueous extract of unfermented *C. genistoides*. Both iriflophenone glucosides, and in some cases the maclurin glucoside, were subsequently identified (LC–MS) in *C. maculata* (Schulze et al., 2014), *C. subternata* (Schulze et al., 2015), *C. longifolia* (Schulze et al., 2015), *C. intermedia* (Jack et al., 2017) and *C. pubescens* (Walters et al., 2019, 2021). Additionally, mangiferin, isomangiferin, vicenin-2, eriocitrin, hesperidin, scolymoside and phloretin-3′,5′-di-*C*-β-D-glucopyranoside were identified (LC–MS) in unfermented *C. maculata* water extracts (Schulze et al., 2014). The hydroxybenzoic acid, protocatechuic acid, was identified in a fraction from a methanol extract of unfermented *C. subternata* (Mortimer et al., 2015). Two aromatic amino acids (tyrosine and phenylalanine), two xanthones (mangiferin and isomangiferin), four flavones (vicenin-2, scolymoside, isorhoifolin and luteolin-7-O-β-D-glucopyranoside) and three flavanones (eriocitrin, narirutin and hesperidin) were identified in fermented *C. longifolia*, using LC–MS, while the dihydrochalcone, phloretin-3′,5′-di-*C*-β-D-glucopyranoside, was tentatively identified (Schulze et al., 2015). Fractionation of the stems and leaves of *C. genistoides* yielded two pterocarpans, (6a*R*,11a*R*)-(−)-maackiain and (6a*R*,11a*R*)-(−)-2-methoxymaackiain, the flavanones, hesperetin and liquiritigenin, as well as 4-hydroxybenzaldehyde, piceol, and the flavone, diosmetin (Roza et al., 2016).

Genistein, isoliquiritigenin, naringenin, helichrysin B, luteolin and 5,7,3′,5′-tetrahydroxyflavanone were isolated through bioassay-guided fractionation of *C. genistoides* extracts (Roza et al., 2017). To date, the flavanone neoponcirin has only been identified (LC–MS) in *C. intermedia* extracts and infusions (Jack et al., 2017; Stander et al., 2019b). De Beer et al. (2021) showed it is either not present or below detectable levels in some batches of *C. intermedia* plant material. Danton et al. (2018) reported the isolation of a naringenin derivative from unfermented *C. genistoides*, identified as (2*S*)-naringenin-5-*O*-neohesperidoside, which epimerises to (2*R*)-naringenin-5-*O*-neohesperidoside, when heated. These two flavanones were also identified in *C. intermedia* infusions and *C. pubescens* extracts (Walters et al., 2019, 2021; De Beer et al., 2021). Stander et al. (2019b) (tentatively) identified (LC–MS) citric acid, psidic acid and butein in leaves from several *Cyclopia* species. Recently, Human et al. (2021) isolated and identified (using NMR) the dihydrochalcone, 3-hydroxyphloretin-3′,5′-di-*C*-β-D-glucopyranoside, from an extract of unfermented *C. subternata*. Walters et al. (2019, 2021) investigated the phenolic composition of unfermented *C. pubescens*, identifying mangiferin, isomangiferin, vicenin-2, narirutin, hesperidin, eriodictyol, *R*-neoeriocitrin, 3,4-dihydroxybenzoic acid-3-*O*-α-L-arabinopyranoside, *Z*-4-hydroxycinnamic acid-4-*O*-β-D-glucopyranoside and 4-(4′-hydroxy-3′-methoxyphenyl-4′-*O*-β-D-glucopyranosyl)-2-butanone. Several polyphenols, identified in other *Cyclopia* species, namely mangiferin, isomangiferin, hesperidin, eriocitrin, iriflophenone-3-*C*-β-D-glucopyranoside, *p*-coumaric acid, scolymoside and phloretin-3′,5′-di-*C*-β-D-glucopyranoside, were also detected in *C. sessiliflora* by LC–MS (De Beer and Joubert, 2010), although the identity of all the compounds was not known at that time.

The major phenolic compounds identified in all the species to date are the flavanone, hesperidin, and the xanthones, mangiferin and isomangiferin. Fermented *C. genistoides* and *C. longifolia* infusions contain substantially more mangiferin and isomangiferin than the other species, although the intraspecies variability is high (Joubert et al., 2019; Alexander et al., 2021; De Beer et al., 2021). Fermented *C. genistoides* infusions also contain high levels of iriflophenone-3-*C*-β-D-glucopyranoside-4-*O*-β-D-glucopyranoside. Fermentation of *C. genistoides* reduces the mangiferin (≈61%), isomangiferin (≈41%) and iriflophenone-3-*C*-β-D-glucopyranoside (≈66%) concentrations in the infusions, while iriflophenone-3-*C*-β-D-glucopyranoside-4-*O*-β-D-glucopyranoside is not affected (Alexander et al., 2021). Hesperidin is present in higher levels in the stems of *C. subternata* and *C. maculata*, while the leaves have higher levels of the xanthones (De Beer et al., 2012; Du Preez et al., 2016). The phenolic composition of extracts is affected by extraction conditions, such as extraction solvent, temperature and time. For instance, extraction with water favours iriflophenone-3-*C*-β-D-glucopyranoside-4-*O*-β-D-glucopyranoside, while extraction with aqueous ethanol mixtures leads to extracts with a higher mangiferin and isomangiferin content (Bosman et al., 2017).

Joubert et al. (2003) reported that *C. genistoides* Overberg type contained less hesperidin and more mangiferin than the West Coast type, with no differences observed in the isomangiferin content. Another study showed that the mangiferin, isomangiferin and iriflophenone-3-*C*-β-D-glucopyranoside content of *C. genistoides* leaves varied according to the harvesting period, with the highest content during summer (Joubert et al., 2014). Genotypic variation in the individual compound content was demonstrated for *C. genistoides* (Bosman et al., 2017) and *C. subternata* (Mabizela et al., 2020).

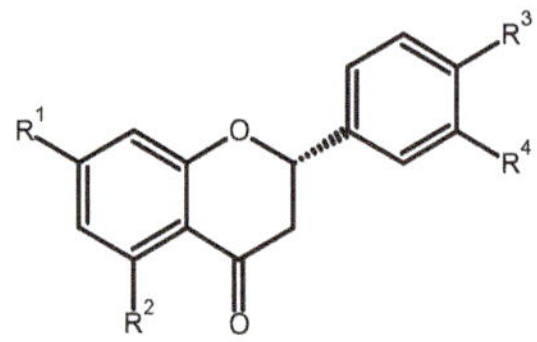

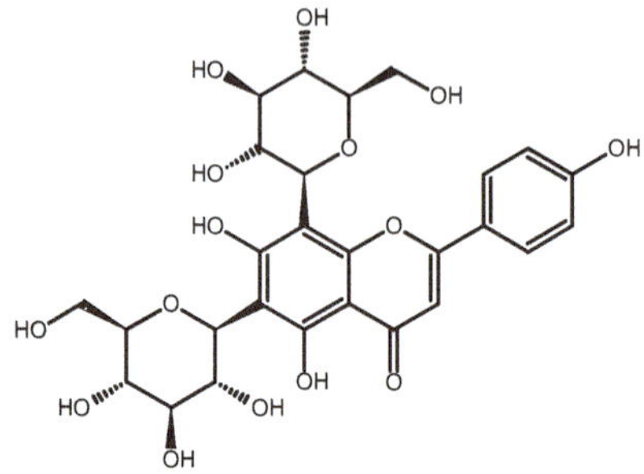

Vicenin-2

Eriocitrin: R¹=*O*-rutinosyl, R², R³, R⁴=OH

Narirutin: R¹=*O*-rutinosyl, R², R³=OH, R⁴=H

Hesperidin: R¹=*O*-rutinosyl, R³=OCH_3, R², R⁴=OH

(2R/S)-naringenin-5-*O*-neohesperidoside: R¹, R³=OH, R²=*O*-neohesperidosyl, R⁴ = H

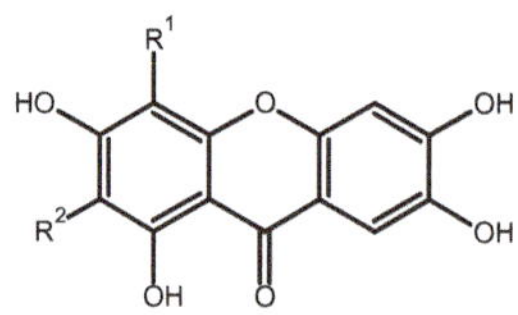

Mangiferin: R¹=H, R²= 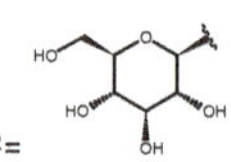

Isomangiferin: R²=H, R¹= 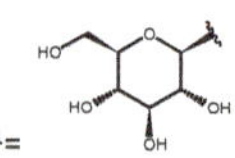

Part B: Chemical profiling and quality control

10. Chromatography analysis

10.1 High-performance thin-layer chromatography (HPTLC) fingerprint analysis

General instrumentation: A CAMAG HPTLC instrument consisting of an automatic TLC sampler (ATS 4), automatic developing chamber (ADC 2), CAMAG TLC Visualizer 2, CAMAG derivatiser and TLC plate heater. *HPTLC plates:* Silica gel glass plates 60F_{254} (Merck). *Plant part:* Aerial parts, methanol extract. *Sample application:* Application volume of 2 μL methanol extract (100 mg/mL) and standards (1 mg/mL) spotted as 15 mm bands. Plates developed in a 20×10×4 cm glass twin-trough chamber to a migration distance of 85 mm. *Tank saturation:* 20 min at 25 °C and 47% RH, with 25 mL of mobile phase. *Mobile phase:* Ethyl acetate: formic acid:

water: acetic acid: methanol (80:10:10:10:5, v/v/v/v/v). *Derivatisation:* Vanillin-sulphuric acid reagent. The plate is sprayed with 3 mL of vanillin reagent, followed by heating for 3 min at 100 °C. *Visualisation:* The plate was viewed under 366 nm radiation after development, and under white light after derivatisation, using the CAMAG TLC Visualizer.

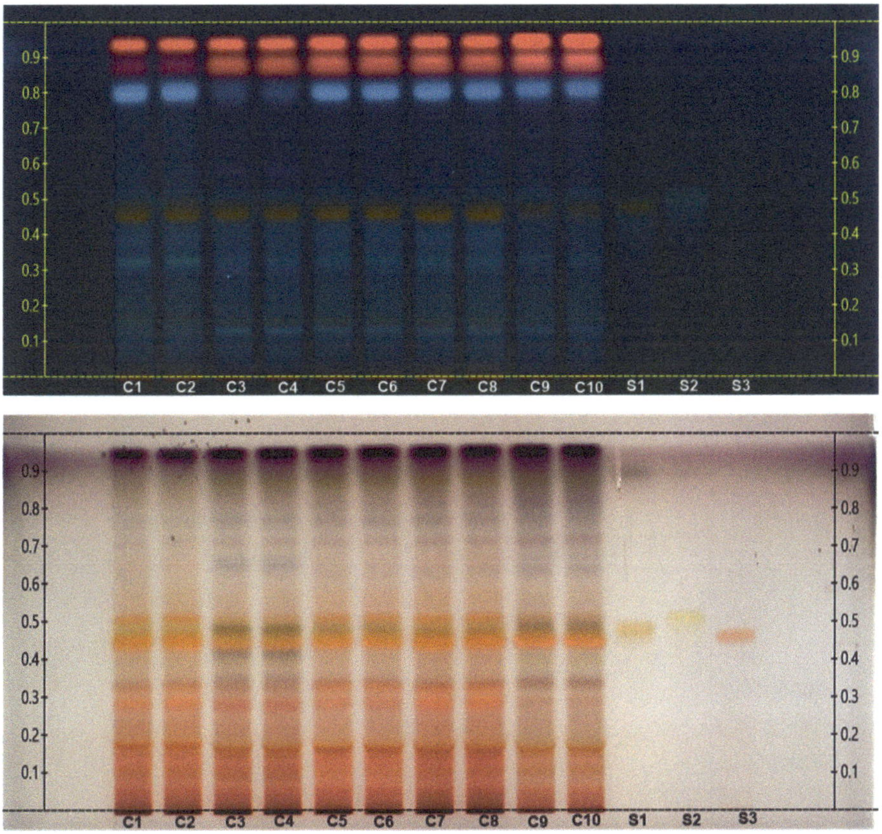

HPTLC plate of *Cyclopia genistoides* methanol extracts ($n=10$) (C1–C10) and the standards mangiferin (S1) ($R_f=0.49$), isomangiferin (S2) ($R_f=0.50$) and hesperidin (S3) ($R_f=0.48$) viewed under 366 nm radiation (upper) and under white light (lower).

10.2 Ultra-performance liquid chromatography (UPLC) analysis

General instrumentation: Waters Acquity Ultra-Performance Liquid Chromatography system with photodiode array (PDA) detector combined with a Xevo G2QToF mass spectrometer (Waters, USA). *Plant part:* Aerial parts, methanol extract. *Sample application:* Injection volume: 1.0 µL (full-loop injection) at 1 mg/mL. *Column:* Acquity UPLC

BEH C18 column (150 mm × 2.1 mm, i.d., 1.7 μm particle size, Waters). *Mobile phase:* 0.1% formic acid in water (solvent A) and acetonitrile (solvent B). *Analysis conditions:* Gradient elution at a flow rate of 0.3 mL/min, changing as follows: 95% A: 5% B to 75% A: 25% B in 5 min, to 50% A: 50% B in 1 min, to 20% A: 80% B in 1 min, keeping for 1.5 min and back to the initial ratio in 0.5 min, equilibrating the system for 3 min, total run time 12 min. *Mass spectrometry*: ESI⁻ (negative ionisation mode), N_2 used as desolvation gas at a flow rate of 500 L/h, desolvation temperature 350 °C, and source temperature at 100 °C. Capillary and cone voltages, 3500 and 55 V, respectively. Data collected between *m/z* 100 and 1200.

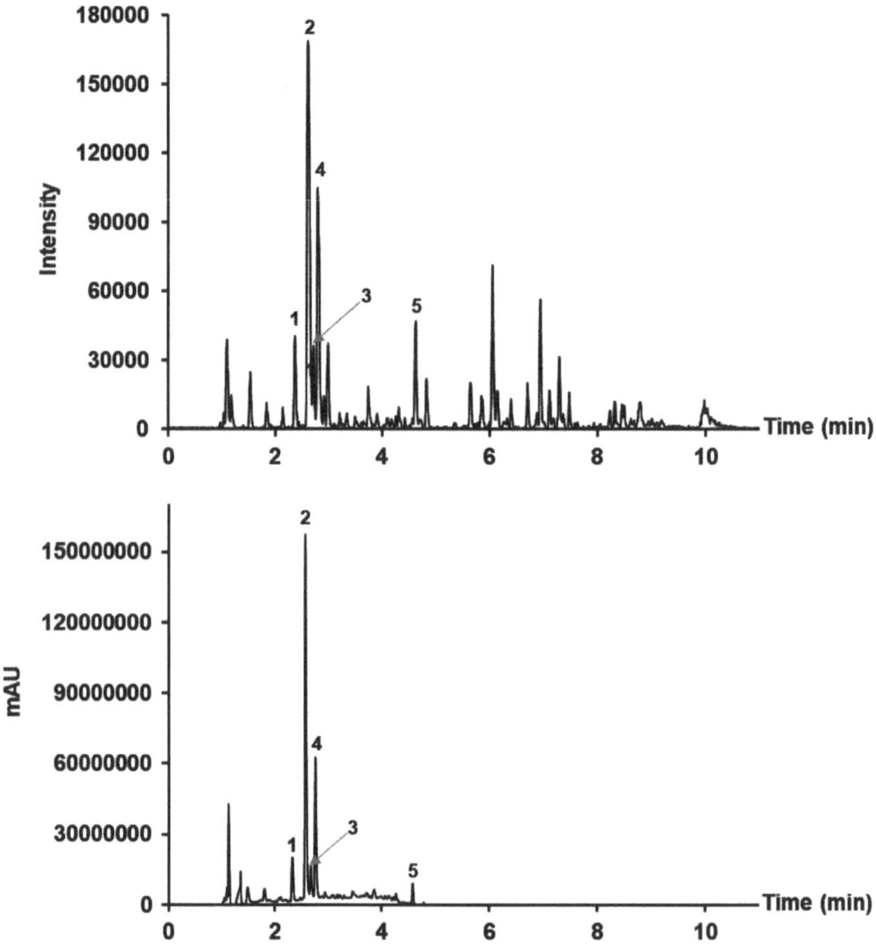

UPLC-ToF-MS ESI⁻ (upper) and PDA (200–400 nm) (lower) chromatograms of *Cyclopia genistoides* methanol extract. [1] = iriflophenone-3-*C*-glucoside *m/z* 407.0948, [2] = mangiferin *m/z* 421.0820, [3] = vicenin-2 *m/z* 593.1508, [4] = isomangiferin *m/z* 421.0807, [5] = hesperidin *m/z* 609.1793.

11. Mid-infrared (MIR) spectroscopy analysis

General instrumentation: Alpha-P Bruker spectrometer, mounted with an attenuated total reflectance (ATR) diamond crystal. *Spectral acquisition:* Spectrum obtained in absorbance mode, with a spectral resolution of 4 cm^{-1} over the range 4000–550 cm^{-1} and captured using OPUS 6.5 software. *Plant part:* Aerial parts. *Sample preparation:* Aerial parts powdered, sieved (< 500 μm) and placed directly onto the surface of the diamond crystal.

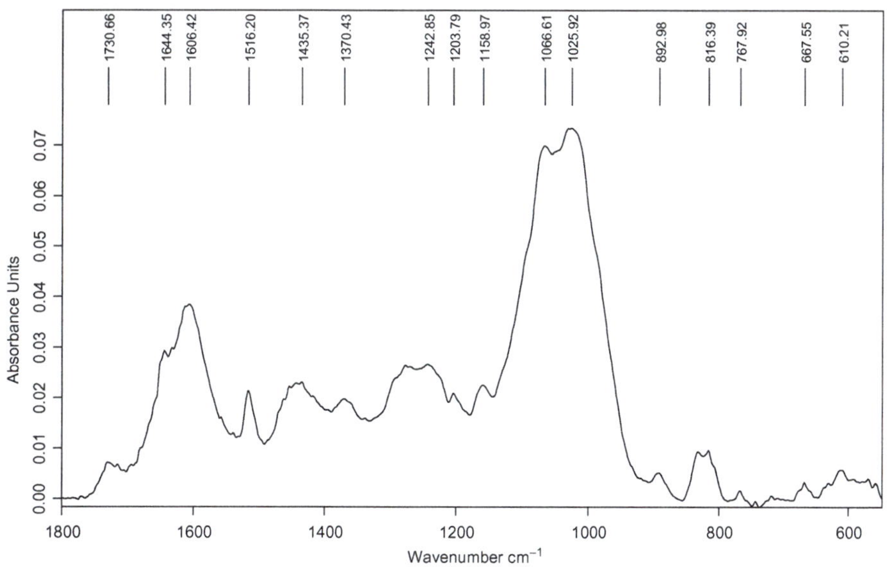

Mid-infrared spectrum of *Cyclopia genistoides* displaying the fingerprint region (1800–550 cm^{-1}).

References

Agapouda, A., Butterweck, V., Hamburger, M., De Beer, D., Joubert, E., Eckert, A., 2020. Oxid. Med. Cell. Longev., 2020, Art. No. 1948602, https://doi.org/10.1155/2020/1948602.

Alexander, L., De Beer, D., Muller, M., Van der Rijst, M., Joubert, E., 2017. LWT - Food Sci. Technol., 82:49–57.

Alexander, L., De Beer, D., Muller, M., Van der Rijst, M., Joubert, E., 2018. S. Afr. J. Bot., 114:316–322.

Alexander, L., Moelich, E.I., De Beer, D., Muller, M., Walczak, B., Joubert, E., 2021. LWT - Food Sci. Technol., 139, Art. No. 110608, https://doi.org/10.1016/j.lwt.2020.110608.

Beelders, T., Brand, D.J., De Beer, D., Malherbe, C.J., Mazibuko, S.E., Muller, C.J.F., Joubert, E., 2014a. J. Nat. Prod., 77:2694–2699.

Beelders, T., De Beer, D., Stander, M.A., Joubert, E., 2014b. Molecules, 19:11760–11790.

Beelders, T., De Beer, D., Joubert, E., 2015. J. Agric. Food Chem., 63:5518–5527.

Bester, C., 2013. Acta Hortic., 1007:889–894.

Bester, C., Joubert, M.E., Joubert, E., 2016. Acta Hortic., 1127:15–22.

Bosman, S.C., De Beer, D., Beelders, T., Willenberg, E.L., Malherbe, C.J., Walczak, B., Joubert, E., 2017. J. Funct. Foods, 33:21–31.

Bowie, J., 1829. S. Afr. Quart. J., 1:27–36.

Chellan, N., Joubert, E., Strijdom, H., Roux, C., Louw, J., Muller, C.J.F., 2014. Planta Med., 80:622–629.

Danton, O., Alexander, L., Hunlun, C., De Beer, D., Hamburger, M., Joubert, E., 2018. J. Nat. Prod., 81:2743–2749.

De Beer, S.W., Joubert, E., 2002. Preparation of Tea-like Beverages. SA Patent No. 2002/2802.

De Beer, D., Joubert, E., 2010. J. Food Compos. Anal., 23:289–297.

De Beer, D., Schulze, A., Joubert, E., De Villiers, A., Malherbe, C., Stander, M., 2012. Molecules, 17:14602–14624.

De Beer, D., Du Preez, B.V.P., Joubert, E., 2021. J. Food Compos. Anal., 104, Art. No. 104154, https://doi.org/10.1016/j.jfca.2021.104154.

Du Preez, B.V.P., De Beer, D., Joubert, E., 2016. Ind. Crop. Prod., 87:132–141.

Du Toit, J., Joubert, E., Britz, T.J., 1999. J. Sci. Food Agric., 79:2040–2044.

Dube, P., Meyer, S., Marnewick, J.L., 2017. S. Afr. J. Bot., 110:184–193.

Dudhia, Z., Louw, J., Muller, C., Joubert, E., De Beer, D., Kinnear, C., Pheiffer, C., 2013. Phytomedicine, 20:401–408.

Ecklon, C.F., Zeyher, K.L.P., 1836. Enumeration Plantarum Africae Australis Extratropicae 2. Perthes and Besser, Hamburg, Germany.

Ferreira, D., Kamara, B.I., Brandt, E.V., Joubert, E., 1998. J. Agr. Food Chem., 46:3406–4310.

Gelderblom, W.C.A., Joubert, E., Gamieldien, K., Sissing, L., Malherbe, C.J., Maritz, G., 2017. S. Afr. J. Bot., 110:194–200.

Hofmeyer, J., Phillips, E.P., 1922. Vent. Bothalia, 1:105–109.

Hubbe, M.E., Joubert, E., 2000. *In vitro* superoxide anion radical scavenging ability of honeybush tea (*Cyclopia*). In: Johnson, I.T., Fenwick, G.R. (Eds.), Dietary Anticarcinogens and Antimutagens—Chemical and Biological Aspects. The Royal Society of Chemistry, Cambridge, UK, pp. 242–244.

Human, C., Danton, O., De Beer, D., Maruyama, T., Alexander, L., Malherbe, C., Hamburger, M., Joubert, E., 2021. Food Chem., 351, Art. No. 129273, https://doi.org/10.1016/j.foodchem.2021.129273.

Jack, B.U., Malherbe, C.J., Huisamen, B., Gabuza, K., Mazibuko-Mbeje, S., Schulze, A.E., Joubert, E., Muller, C.J.F., Louw, J., Pheiffer, C., 2017. S. Afr. J. Bot., 110:216–229.

Jack, B.U., Malherbe, C.J., Willenburg, E.L., De Beer, D., Huisamen, B., Joubert, E., Muller, C.J.F., Louw, J., Pheiffer, C., 2018. Planta Med., 84:100–110.

Joubert, E., Otto, F., Grüner, S., Weinreich, B., 2003. Eur. Food Res. Technol., 216:270–273.

Joubert, E., Richards, E.S., Van der Merwe, J.D., De Beer, D., Manley, M., Gelderblom, W.C.A., 2008. J. Agr. Food Chem., 56:954–963.

Joubert, E., Joubert, M.E., Bester, C., De Beer, D., De Lange, J.H., 2011. S. Afr. J. Bot., 77:887–907.

Joubert, E., De Beer, D., Hernández, I., Munné-Bosch, S., 2014. Ind. Crops Prod., 56:74–82.

Joubert, E., De Beer, D., Malherbe, C.J.M., Muller, M., Louw, A., Gelderblom, W.C.A., 2019. S. Afr. J. Bot., 127:58–79.

Kamara, B.I., Brandt, E.V., Ferreira, D., Joubert, E., 2003. J. Agr. Food Chem., 51:3874–3879.

Kamara, B.I., Brand, D.J., Brandt, E.V., Joubert, E., 2004. J. Agr. Food Chem., 52:5391–5395.

Kokotkiewicz, A., Luczkiewicz, M., Sowinski, P., Glod, D., Gorynski, K., Bucinski, A., 2012. Food Chem., 133:1373–1382.

Kokotkiewicz, A., Luczkiewicz, M., Pawlowska, J., Luczkiewicz, P., Sowinski, P., Witkowski, J., Bryl, E., Bucinski, A., 2013. Fitoterapia, 90:199–208.

Le Roux, M., Cronje, J.C., Burger, B.V., Joubert, E., 2006. Chemical characterization of the aroma of honeybush, *Cyclopia genistoides*. Poster presented at the 29th International Symposium on Capillary Chromatography, 29 May–2 June 2006, Riva del Garda, Italy, poster no. P28.

Le Roux, M., Cronje, J.C., Joubert, E., Burger, B.V., 2008. S. Afr. J. Bot., 74:139–143.

Le Roux, M., Cronje, J.C., Burger, B.V., Joubert, E., 2012. J. Agr. Food Chem., 60:2657–2664.

Mabizela, G., Muller, M., De Beer, D., Van Der Rijst, M., Slabbert, M.M., Joubert, E., Bester, C., 2020. S. Afr. J. Bot., 132:491–501.

Magcwebeba, T.U., Swart, P., Swanevelder, S., Joubert, E., Gelderblom, W.C.A., 2016a. Molecules, 21, Art. No. 1622, https://doi.org/10.3390/molecules21121622.

Magcwebeba, T., Swart, P., Swanevelder, S., Joubert, E., Gelderblom, W., 2016b. Molecules, 21, Art. No. 1323, https://doi.org/10.3390/molecules21101323.

Marloth, R., 1909. Agric. J., 35:634–638.

Marloth, R., 1925. The Flora of South Africa with Synoptical Tables of the Genera of the Higher Plants. Darter Bros & Co., Cape Town, South Africa, pp. 69–72.

Marnewick, J.L., Gelderblom, W.C.A., Joubert, E., 2000. Mutat. Res., 471:157–166.

Marnewick, J.L., Joubert, E., Swart, P., Van Der Westhuizen, F., Gelderblom, W.C., 2003. J. Agric. Food Chem., 51:8113–8119.

Marnewick, J.L., Batenburg, W., Swart, P., Joubert, E., Swanevelder, S., Gelderblom, W.C.A., 2004. Mutat. Res., 558:145–154.

Marnewick, J.L., Joubert, E., Joseph, S., Swanevelder, S., Swart, P., Gelderblom, W.C.A., 2005. Cancer Lett., 224:193–202.

Marnewick, J.L., Van der Westhuizen, F.H., Joubert, E., Swanevelder, S., Swart, P., Gelderblom, W.C.A., 2009. Food Chem. Toxicol., 47:220–229.

McGregor, G.K., 2017. An overview of the honeybush industry. Department of Environmental Affairs and Development Planning, Cape Town, South Africa.

Mfenyana, C., De Beer, D., Joubert, E., Louw, A., 2008. J. Steroid Biochem. Mol. Biol., 112:74–86.

Miller, N., Malherbe, C.J., Joubert, E., 2020a. Sep. Purif. Technol., 237, Art. No. 116465, https://doi.org/10.1016/j.seppur.2019.116465.

Miller, N., Malherbe, C.J., Joubert, E., 2020b. Food Funct., 11:6476–6486.

Mortimer, M., Visser, K., De Beer, D., Joubert, E., Louw, A., 2015. PLoS One, 10, Art. No. e0132950, https://doi.org/10.1371/journal.pone.0132950.

Muller, C.J.F., Joubert, E., Gabuza, K., De Beer, D., Fey, S.J., Louw, J., 2011. Assessment of the antidiabetic potential of an aqueous extract of honeybush (*Cyclopia intermedia*) in streptozotocin and obese insulin resistant Wistar rats. In: Rasooli, I. (Ed.), Phytochemicals—Bioactivities and Impact on Health. InTech, Rijeka, Croatia, pp. 313–332.

Murakami, S., Miura, Y., Hattori, M., Matsuda, H., Malherbe, C.J., Muller, C.J.F., Joubert, E., Yoshida, T., 2018. Planta Med., 84:311–319.

North, M.S., Joubert, E., De Beer, D., De Kock, K., Joubert, M.E., 2017. S. Afr. J. Bot., 110:132–137.

Ntlhokwe, G., Tredoux, A.G.J., Gorecki, T., Edwards, M., Vestner, J., Muller, M., Erasmus, L., Joubert, E., Cronje, J.C., De Villers, A., 2017. Anal. Bioanal. Chem., 409:4127–4138.

Ntlhokwe, G., Muller, M., Joubert, E., Tredoux, A.G.J., De Villiers, A., 2018. J. Chromatogr. A, 1536:137–150.

Omolaoye, T., Du Plessis, S., 2021. Asian Pacific J. Reprod., 10:176–186.

Oyenihi, O.R., Krygsman, A., Verhoog, N., De Beer, D., Saayman, M.J., Mouton, T.M., Louw, A., 2018. Front. Pharmacol., 9, Art. No. 650, https://doi.org/10.3389/fphar.2018.00650.

Pappe, C.W.L., 1868. Florae Capensis Medicae Prodromus, or, an Enumeration of South African Indigenous Plants, Used as Remedies by the Colonists of the Cape of Good Hope. Third Edition: with Corrections and Numerous Additions. W. Britain, Cape Town, South Africa

Petrova, A., Davids, L.M., Rautenbach, F., Marnewick, J.L., 2011. J. Photochem. Photobiol. B, 103:126–139.

Pheiffer, C., Dudhia, Z., Louw, J., Muller, C., Joubert, E., 2013. Phytomedicine, 20, 1168–1171.

Rood, B., 1994. Uit die Veldapteek. Tafelberg-Uitgewers Bpk, Cape Town, South Africa, p. 51.

Ros-Santaella, J.L., Kadlec, M., Pintus, E., 2020. Animals, 10, Art. No. 463, https://doi.org/10.3390/ani10030463.

Roza, O., Martins, A., Hohmann, J., Lai, W.-C., Eloff, J., Chang, F.-R., Csupor, D., 2016. Planta Med., 82:1274–1278.

Roza, O., Lai, W.-C., ZupkÇü, I., Hohmann, J., Jedlinszki, N., Chang, F.-R., Csupor, D., Eloff, J.N., 2017. S. Afr. J. Bot., 110:201–207.

SANBI, South African National Biodiversity Institute, 2000. Liesl van der Walt. Available from: http://pza.sanbi.org/cyclopia-genistoides.

Schulze, A.E., De Beer, D., De Villiers, A., Manley, M., Joubert, E., 2014. J. Agric. Food Chem., 62:10542–10551.

Schulze, A.E., Beelders, T., Koch, I.S., Erasmus, L.M., De Beer, D., Joubert, E., 2015. J. Food Compos. Anal., 44:139–148.

Schulze, A.E., De Beer, D., Mazibuko, S.E., Muller, C.J.F., Roux, C., Willenburg, E.L., Nyunaï, N., Louw, J., Manley, M., Joubert, E., 2016. Anal. Bioanal. Chem., 408, 639–649.

Schutte, A.L., 1997. Edinb. J. Bot., 54:125–170.

Sissing, L., Marnewick, J., De Kock, M., Swanevelder, S., Joubert, E., Gelderblom, W., 2011. Nutr. Cancer, 63:600–610.

Stander, M.A., Joubert, E., De Beer, D., 2019a. J. Food Compos. Anal., 76:39–43.

Stander, M.A., Redelinghuys, H., Masike, K., Long, H., Van Wyk, B.-E., 2019b. Molecules, 24, Art. No. 2352, https://doi.org/10.3390/molecules24132352.

Theron, K.A., Muller, M., Van der Rijst, M., Cronje, J.C., Le Roux, M., Joubert, E., 2014. Food Res. Int., 66:12–22.

Van der Merwe, J.D., Joubert, E., Richards, E.S., Manley, M., Snijman, P.W., Marnewick, J.L., Gelderblom, W.C.A., 2006. Mutat. Res., 611:42–53.

Van der Merwe, J.D., De Beer, D., Swanevelder, S., Joubert, E., Gelderblom, W.C.A., 2017. S. Afr. J. Bot., 110:230–239.

Van Wyk, B.-E., Gorelik, B., 2017. S. Afr. J. Bot., 110:18–38.

Van Wyk, B.-E., Van Oudtshoorn, B., Gericke, N., 1997. Medicinal Plants of South Africa. Briza Publications, Pretoria, South Africa, p. 290.

Verhoog, N.J.D., Joubert, E., Louw, A., 2007a. S. Afr. J. Sci., 103:13–21.

Verhoog, N.J.D., Joubert, E., Louw, A., 2007b. J. Agr. Food Chem., 55:4371–4381.

Visagie, A., Kasonga, A., Deepak, V., Moosa, S., Marais, S., Kruger, M.C., Coetzee, M., 2015. Int. J. Environ. Res. Public Health, 12:13779–13793.

Visser, K., Mortimer, M., Louw, A., 2013. PLoS One, 8, Art. No. e79223, https://doi.org/10.1371/journal.pone.0079223.

Visser, K., Zierau, O., Macejová, D., Goerl, F., Muders, M., Baretton, G.B., Vollmer, G., Louw, A., 2016. J. Steroid Biochem. Mol. Biol., 163:129–135.

Walters, N.A., De Beer, D., De Villiers, A., Walczak, B., Joubert, E., 2019. J. Food Compos. Anal., 78:129–137.

Walters, N.A., Beer, D., Villiers, A., Danton, O., Hamburger, M., Joubert, E., 2021. Phytochem. Anal., 32:347–361.

Watt, J.M., Breyer-Brandwijk, M.G., 1962. The Medicinal and Poisonous Plants of Southern and Eastern Africa, second ed. E. & S. Livingstone Ltd, Edinburgh and London, UK.

Yoshida, T., Malherbe, C.J., Okon, K., Miura, Y., Hattori, M., Matsuda, H., Muller, C.J.F., Joubert, E., 2020. J. Funct. Foods, 64, Art. No. 103704, https://doi.org/10.1016/j.jff.2019.103704.

CHAPTER

Eriocephalus punctulatus 8

Maxleene Sandasi[a,b], Guy Kamatou[a], Nduvho Mulaudzi[a] and Gerda Fouche[c]

[a]*Department of Pharmaceutical Sciences, Tshwane University of Technology, Pretoria, South Africa*

[b]*SAMRC Herbal Drugs Research Unit, Faculty of Science, Tshwane University of Technology, Pretoria, South Africa*

[c]*Chemistry Department, University of Pretoria, Pretoria, South Africa*

Abstract

Eriocephalus punctulatus DC. (Asteraceae), commonly known as Cape chamomile, is a highly aromatic, woody, evergreen shrub characterised by a fluffy 'white head' when fruiting. The species is endemic to South Africa, with a restricted distribution to parts of the Northern and Western Cape provinces. The aerial parts of the plant are used to treat fever, skin diseases and respiratory and gastro-intestinal disorders. Cape chamomile is well known for its characteristic deep-blue essential oil, which has several applications in aromatherapy, perfumery and cosmetics that have led to the development of commercial plantations. The in vitro biological activities of the plant include antibacterial, antifungal, anti-oxidant, anti-inflammatory and acetylcholinesterase effects. Herein, a comprehensive, up-to-date literature review of the medicinal plant is documented. Chemical profiles of E. punctulatus essential oils from various locations were obtained, using a semi-automated high-performance thin-layer chromatography (HPTLC) system and gas chromatography coupled to mass spectrometry (GC–MS). The HPTLC profiles viewed under white light reflectance, after derivatisation with an anisaldehyde reagent, revealed a consistent chemical profile characterised by various bands. Isobutyl isobutyrate, iso-amyl butyrate, isobutyl angelate, 2-methyl-1-butyl angelate and pogostol were identified in the hydrodistilled essential oil using GC–MS.

Keywords: *Eriocephalus punctulatus*, Cape chamomile, Essential oil, HPTLC, GC–MS, MIR spectroscopy, Isobutyl isobutyrate, Isobutyl angelate, 2-Methyl-1-butyl angelate, Pogostol

The South African Herbal Pharmacopoeia. https://doi.org/10.1016/B978-0-323-99794-2.00023-4

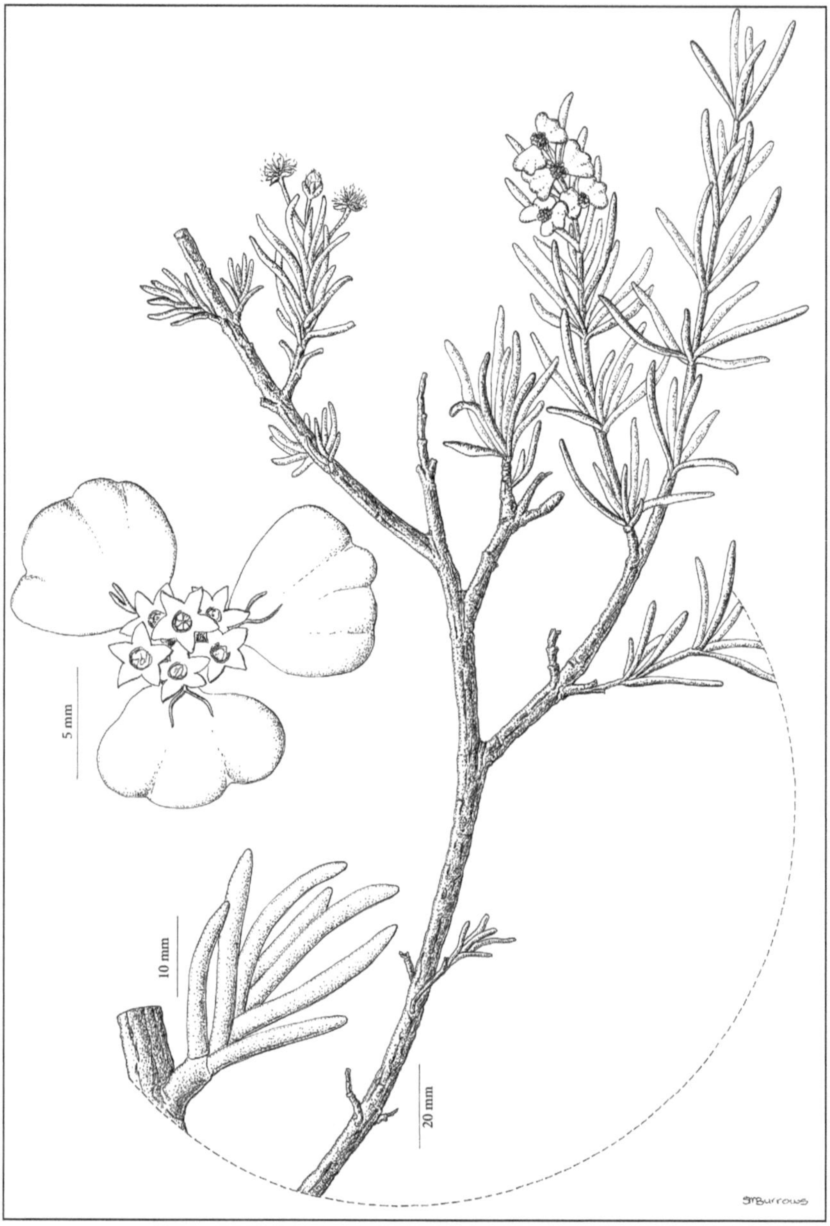
5 mm
10 mm
20 mm

Part A: General overview

1. Synonyms

Eriocephalus punctulatus var. *pedicellaris* (DC.) Harv., *Eriocephalus punctulatus* var. *brevifolius* DC., *Eriocephalus punctulatus* var. *tenuifolius* (DC.) Harv.[a]

2. Common name(s)

Cape chamomile (English); '*boegoekapok*', '*boegoekapokbossie*', '*kapokbos*' (Afrikaans).[b]

3. Conservation status

Least concern.[b]

4. Botany

The genus *Eriocephalus* derives its name from two Greek words '*erion*' and '*kephale*' meaning wool and head, respectively. 'Wool head' is characteristic of the white fluffy fruiting heads that generally give the appearance of cotton balls and snow cover over the plants. *Eriocephalus punctulatus* is a woody, evergreen shrub of up to 1.3 m in height with a vertical stem that branches (A and D). The leaves are small, mostly opposite, but alternate on flowering shoots with felty indumentum to glabrescent. The tiny flowers bear white ray florets (B) and flowering occurs between May and October, reaching a peak from July to September (SANBI, 2012). Hydro-distillation of the aerial parts yields a characteristic bright blue oil known as Cape chamomile oil (C) (Van Wyk et al., 1997). The species can be distinguished from its close taxonomically *Euklastaxon tenuifolius*, mainly by leaf size and characteristics, and the fact that *E. punctulatus* is hardly browsed, whereas *E. tenuifolius* is heavily browsed (Müller et al., 2001).

[a] World Flora Online (http://www.worldfloraonline.org).
[b] The Red List of South African Plants (http://redlist.sanbi.org).

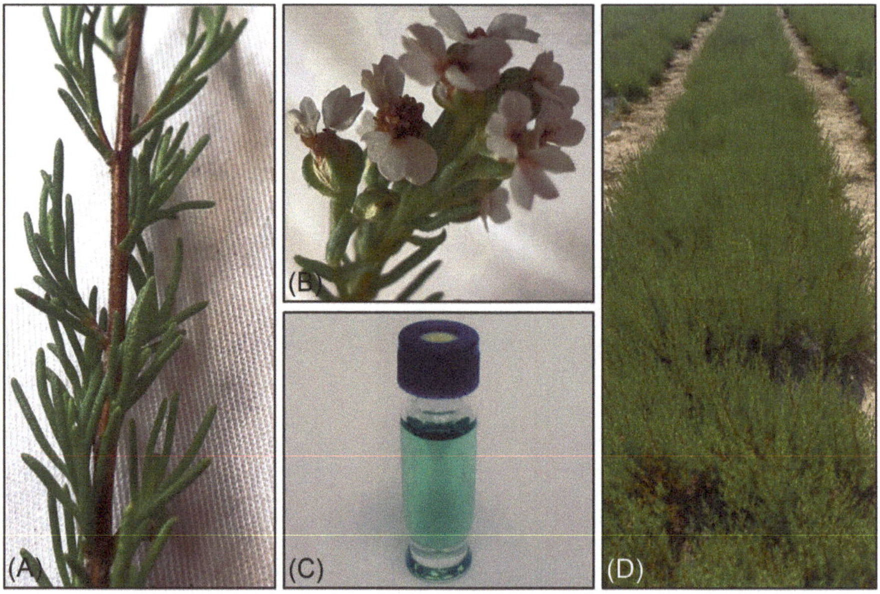

Eriocephalus punctulatus has a woody stem that bears small, opposite leaves (A) and white flowers (B). A characteristic light blue essential oil (C) is isolated from the aerial parts of the evergreen shrub (D).

5. Geographical distribution

Eriocephalus punctulatus is endemic to South Africa and is mostly restricted to the greater Cape floristic region. Its distribution extends from Springbok and

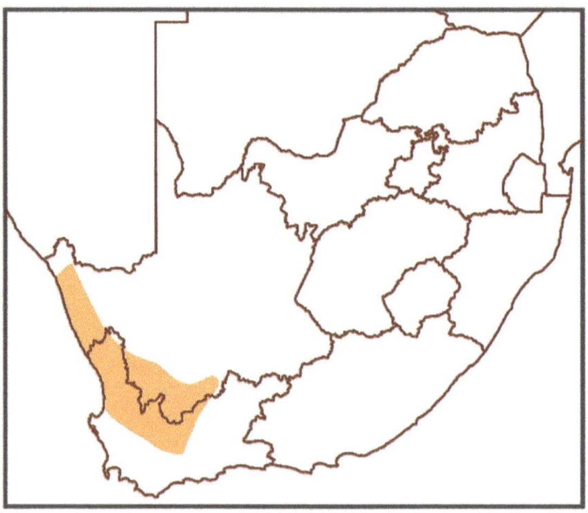

Geographical distribution of *Eriocephalus punctulatus* in South Africa.

Nieuwoudtville in the Northern Cape to the western parts (the Roggeveld and Wittenberg mountains) of the Western Cape Province. The species occurs mostly in high-lying mountainous areas, approximately 300 m above sea level, on the coast, inland, or on plains, and in the desert (Müller et al., 2001).

6. Ethnopharmacology

Eriocephalus species have been used as a traditional remedy for the relief of gastro-intestinal, respiratory and skin disorders. *Eriocephalus punctulatus* is reported for the treatment of stomach ailments (Mierendorff et al., 2003; Njenga and Viljoen, 2006), while the Griqua and the Nama use this plant and other *Eriocephalus* species as diuretics and diaphoretics (Watt and Breyer-Brandwijk, 1962; Van Wyk et al., 1997). The Southern Sotho of South Africa utilise the plant as a fumigant in combination with *Metalasia muricata*, to disinfect huts following sickness or death.[c] A closely related species, *E. africanus*, has diverse medicinal applications that include the treatment of respiratory, gastro-intestinal, gynaecological and skin disorders, as well as stress and depression (Van Wyk and Gericke, 2000; Njenga and Viljoen, 2006). Both plants produce fragrant oils that are used as ingredients of perfumes and cosmetics (Njenga and Viljoen, 2006), while *E. africanus* is also used as a culinary herb as an alternative to rosemary.

7. Commercialisation

The strong aromatic odour, characteristic of the genus, is the result of high concentrations of terpenes. The essential oil of *E. punctulatus* (Cape chamomile) has a characteristic bright blue colour that is attributed to the presence of azulenic compounds formed from the decomposition of pro-azulenes during distillation (Van Wyk et al., 1997). Cape chamomile oil is considered the ‘fourth chamomile’ after German, Roman and Moroccan chamomiles (Watt and Breyer-Brandwijk, 1962; Van Wyk et al., 1997; Van Wyk and Gericke, 2000), and it bears a fruity fragrance similar to Roman chamomile. The oil has been widely used in the perfumery and cosmetics industries since the early 1970s and is an ingredient of the popular cosmetic range ‘Sea-sational products’. The therapeutic properties of Cape chamomile include anti-inflammatory, analgesic, soothing, anti-allergenic, antidepressant and antiseptic, which render the oil useful for skin care and aromatherapy.[d] The potential for use as a flavour enhancer has been mentioned, based on the low taste threshold value of the oil.

While it is generally accepted that the botanical origin of Cape chamomile is *E. punctulatus*[e] (Mierendorff et al., 2003), doubts have been expressed due to certain morphological similarities shared with *E. tenuifolius* (Müller et al., 2001).

[c] http://www.africasgarden.com.
[d] http://www.gnp.co.za/essential oils/chamomile
[e] http://www.aromaceuticals.com.

Furthermore, there are reports that the parent material used in commercial cultivation is originally from Lesotho (personal communication between Graven and Viljoen, 2004). *Eriocephalus punctulatus* does not occur in Lesotho; however, its close taxonomically *E. tenuifolius* does, which has prompted further research. Sandasi et al. (2011) reported similarities in the chemical profiles of commercial Cape chamomile oil to *E. tenuifolius*, based on gas chromatography–mass spectrometry (GC–MS) and vibrational spectroscopy data. The results deepen the controversy of *E. punctulatus* being the commercial species from which Cape chamomile oil is derived. Commercial plantations of *E. punctulatus* have been developed as a result of successful propagation of plant material with favourable chemical and organoleptic properties by The Grassroots Natural Products Company.[d]

8. Pharmacological evaluation

8.1 *In vitro* studies

8.1.1 Antibacterial and antifungal activity

The antimicrobial properties of various *Eriocephalus* species have been investigated. Njenga (2005) evaluated the antimicrobial activity of *E. punctulatus* essential oils and extracts against a range of pathogens. The results indicated good activity of the oil towards *Cryptococcus neoformans*, *Candida albicans*, *Bacillus cereus* and *Bacillus subtilis*. Antimicrobial actions against *Staphylococcus aureus*, *Klebsiella pneumoniae* and *Escherichia coli* were recorded as moderate to low. In addition, the crude extracts also displayed good activity against *C. neoformans* and *B. cereus*, as well as moderate to low activity towards the remainder of the pathogens. Hexane and methanol leaf extracts of *E. tenuifolius* exhibited antibacterial activity against the Gram-positive *B. subtilis* and *S. aureus* (Shale et al., 2004). Storage of the leaf material under various conditions revealed that storage over 3 months at 10 °C, at room temperature, and outdoors, resulted in an increase in antibacterial action. However, storage for longer than 3 months caused a gradual decrease in activity, although some inhibitory activity was still observed after 12 months for the methanol extracts (Shale et al., 2004). Behiry et al. (2019) reported good antimicrobial activity of *E. africanus* oil against plant pathogens that include *Agrobacterium tumefaciens*, *Dickeya solani*, *Erwinia amylovora*, *Pseudomonas cichorii* and *Serratia plymuthica*. The most susceptible pathogen was *D. solani* with a zone inhibition of 18.33 mm and a minimum inhibitory concentration (MIC) of 100 μg/mL.

8.1.2 Anti-oxidant and anti-inflammatory activity

The *in vitro* anti-inflammatory activity of *E. tenuifolius* was investigated for water, methanol and hexane extracts, using the cyclooxygenase-1 (COX-1) assay (Shale et al., 2004). Aqueous extracts exhibited lower activity (COX-1 <20%) compared to methanol and hexane extracts (COX-1 >80%), while the activity of hexane extracts remained high even after 12 months storage of leaf material at 10 °C, room temperature, and outdoors (Shale et al., 2004). The methanol extracts however, lost activity after storage of leaf material for longer than 3 months and after being exposed to higher storage temperatures. *Eriocephalus* species have been reported to exhibit moderate anti-oxidant activity when tested using the 2,2-diphenyl-1-picrylhydrazyl (DPPH) radical scavenging method (Njenga and Viljoen, 2006). The acetone extracts of 22 *Eriocephalus* species exhibited moderate activity with IC_{50} values ranging between 21.5 µg/mL (*E. punctulatus*) and 79 µg/mL. The essential oils did not display anti-oxidant activity even at the highest concentration tested. The presence of 5-lipoxygenase (5-LOX) enzyme inhibitors was detected, with IC_{50} values ranging from 19 µg/mL (*E. africanus*) to 98.9 µg/mL (*E. purpureus*).

8.1.3 Acetylcholinesterase activity

Preliminary thin layer chromatography (TLC) screening of *E. punctulatus* oil indicated the presence of acetylcholinesterase enzyme inhibitors (Njenga, 2005). In a study by Seo et al. (2014), essential oil constituents of tested oils from plants belonging to the Asteraceae family exhibited acetylcholinesterase inhibition activity, with IC_{50} values ranging from 0.03 to 0.67 mg/mL for compounds that included α-pinene, limonene and β-phellandrene.

8.2 *In vivo* studies and clinical trials

There is a need for *in vivo* animal studies and clinical trials to confirm the reported *in vitro* biological activities and potential toxic effects of *E. punctulatus* and other *Eriocephalus* species that are used in traditional medicine systems. Seo et al. (2014) investigated the toxic effects of essential oils from plants belonging to the Asteraceae family towards the Japanese termite *Reticulitermes speratus*. *Eriocephalus punctulatus*, in addition to the essential oils of *Chamaemelum nobile*, *Santolina chamaecyparissus* and *Ormenis multicaulis*, displayed good fumigant activity after 2 days of treatment, and the activity was concentration- and exposure time-dependent.

8.3 Safety

Safety and toxicity information on the plant is scarce. There is a need for research to investigate the acute, chronic, organ and reproductive toxicity/safety, amongst others, of *E. punctulatus* extracts, essential oils and isolated compounds.

9. Phytochemistry

Hydro-distillation of the aerial parts of *E. punctulatus* yields a characteristic blue essential oil that is commonly known as Cape chamomile. The essential oil profile of Cape chamomile has been extensively studied and various classes of compounds have been identified. Similar to other *Eriocephalus* species, *E. punctulatus* essential oil is reported to contain α- and β-pinene, yomogi alcohol, *ρ*-cymene, 1,8-cineole, camphor, 4-terpineol, spathulenol, caryophyllene oxide, α-copaene and β-caryophyllene (Njenga, 2005). Lall and Kishore (2014) identified 2-methylbutyl isobutyrate and 2-methylpropyl isobutyrate, in addition to the above-mentioned profile. In another study, Mierendorff et al. (2003) identified 50 aliphatic esters in the oil accounting for more than 50% of the composition. The compounds occurring in large amounts in this class were identified as 2-methylbutyl-2-methylpropanoate (21.2%), 2-methylbutyl-2-methylbutanoate (5.6%), 2-methylpropyl-2-methylpropanoate (5.3%) and 7-methyl-2-octylacetate (4.5%). Linalyl acetate (4.4%) and α-pinene (1.9%) were prominent in the terpenoid fraction, which accounted for about 37% of the total composition. Accounting for less than 10% were artedouglasia oxides A-D that occurred in the higher boiling fraction, davanones, and laciniata furanones, together with oxygenated sesquiterpenes (Mierendorff et al., 2003). In a study investigating the differences between *E. punctulatus* and *E. tenuifolius* essential oils from South Africa, GC–MS analysis revealed both qualitative and quantitative differences between the oils, with *E. punctulatus* oil displaying high levels of 1,8-cineole, piperitone, yomogi alcohol and pogostol (Sandasi et al., 2011). Multivariate data analysis revealed compositional differences between the two species based on both GC–MS and vibrational spectroscopy techniques. The results of both techniques also indicated that the commercial Cape chamomile oil profiled displayed a similar profile to *E. tenuifolius* oil and not to that of *E. punctulatus*. A study that profiled essential oils from other *Eriocephalus* species from Namibia identified camphor, estafiatin, ivangustin, linalyl acetate, nerolidol, squalene, quercetin, parthenolide, costic acid derivatives, a seco-eudesmane diketone and a chrysanthemol derivative. The species profiled include *E. africanus*, *E. ambiguus*, *E. ericoides*, *E. kingesii*, *E. giessii*, *E. merxmuelleri*, *E. pauperrimus* and *E. scariosus* (Zdero et al., 1987). Davies-Coleman et al. (1992) isolated and confirmed the presence of two bitter compounds, 8-isobutyloxycumambrin-B and cumambrin-A, together with L-2-*O*-methylchiroinositol, in *E. punctulatus*.

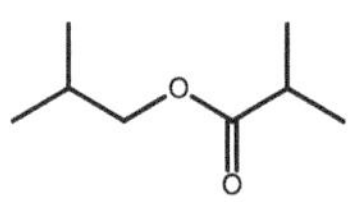

Isobutyl isobutyrate

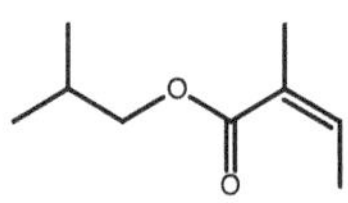

Isobutyl angelate

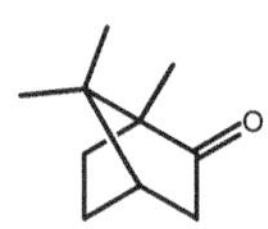

Camphor

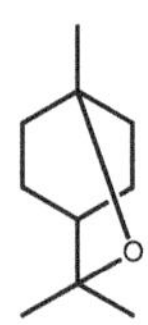

1,8-Cineole

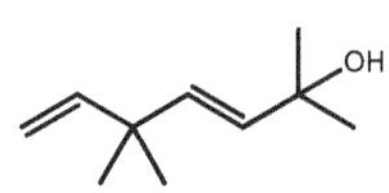

2-Methyl-1-butyl angelate

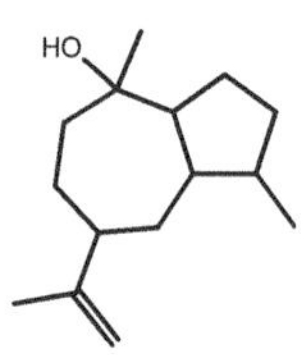

Pogostol

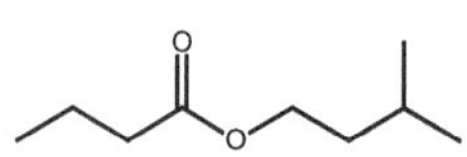

Iso-amyl butyrate

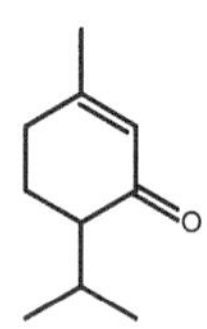

Piperitone

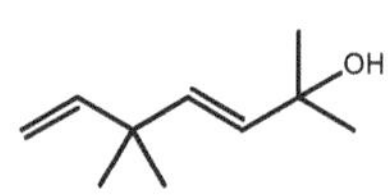

Yomogi alcohol

Part B: Chemical profiling and quality control

10. Chromatography analysis

10.1 High-performance thin-layer chromatography (HPTLC) fingerprint analysis

General instrumentation: A CAMAG HPTLC instrument consisting of an automatic TLC sampler (ATS 4), automatic developing chamber (ADC 2), CAMAG TLC Visualizer 2, CAMAG derivatiser, and TLC plate heater. *HPTLC plates*: Silica gel glass plates 60 F_{254} (Merck). *Plant part*: Aerial parts, essential oil. *Sample application*: Application volume of 2 μL essential oil (25 μL/mL in toluene) spotted as 10 mm bands. Plates developed in a 20×10×4 cm glass twin-trough chamber to a migration distance of 70 mm. *Tank saturation*: 20 min at 15 °C and 33% RH, with 25 mL of mobile phase. *Mobile phase*: Toluene:ethyl acetate (95:5, v/v). *Derivatisation*: *p*-Anisaldehyde sulphuric acid reagent. The plate was sprayed with 3 mL of the reagent, heated for 3 min at 100 °C on a TLC plate heater, and visualised. *Visualisation*: The plate was viewed under white light reflectance.

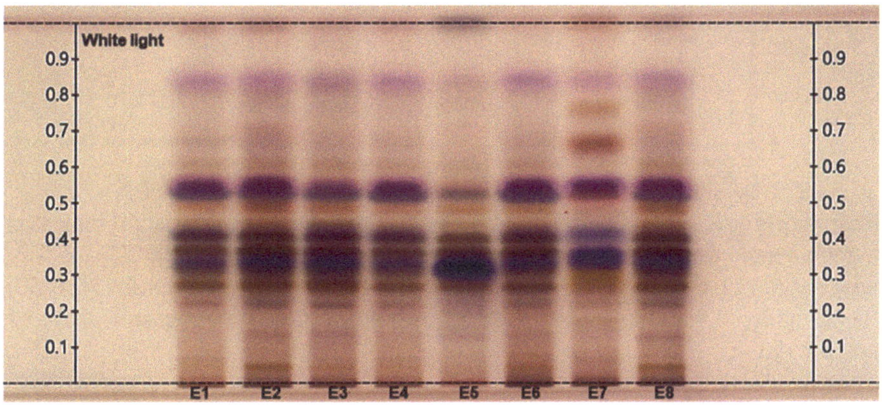

HPTLC plate of *Eriocephalus punctulatus* essential oil ($n=8$) (E1–E8), characterised by dark blue bands ($R_f=0.33$; 0.41), brown band ($R_f=0.36$), light brown band ($R_f=0.50$) and purple bands ($R_f=0.55$; 0.85).

10.2 Gas chromatography (GC) analysis

General instrumentation: An Agilent 6860 N chromatograph (Agilent Technologies, Hanova, USA) fitted with a flame ionisation detector and a mass spectrometer. *Column*: HP-Innowax, 60 m×250 μm×0.25 μm (polyethylene glycol column, Agilent Technologies, Hanova, USA). *Plant part*: Aerial parts, essential oil. *Sample application*: Injection volume of 1 μL (split) at 20% (v/v) in hexane. *Analysis conditions*: Inlet temperature 250 °C, split ratio: 1:200, helium carrier gas, flow rate: 1.2 mL/min, pressure: 24.79 psi. Starting oven temperature at 60 °C, and then rise to 220 °C at 4 °C/min, holding for 10 min and increased to 240 °C at 1 °C/min. *Mass spectrometry conditions*: Chromatograms obtained on electron impact at 70 eV using an Agilent 5973 mass selective detector, scanning range: m/z 35 to 550 (Agilent Technologies, Hanova, USA). *Identification*: Authentic standards, NIST®, Mass Finder®.

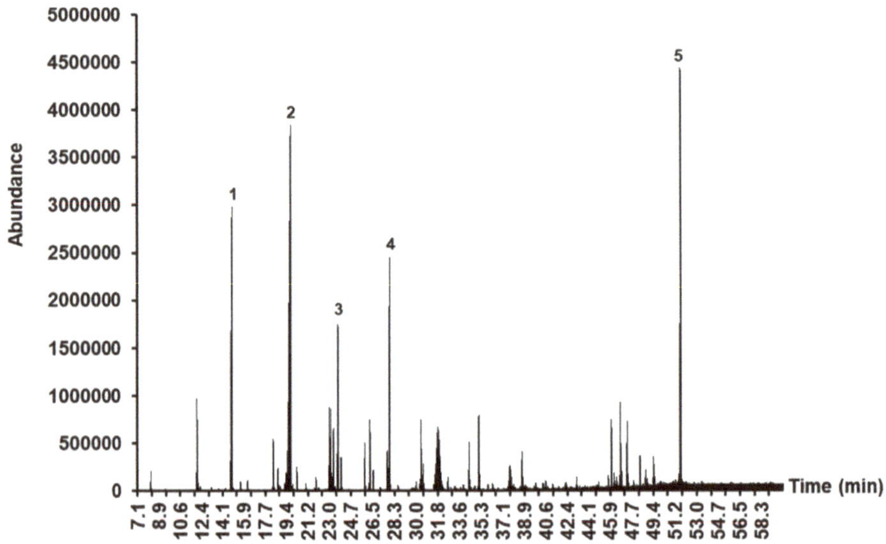

Total ion chromatograms (TIC) of *Eriocephalus punctulatus* essential oil indicating major compounds. [1] = isobutyl isobutyrate (R_t 14.89, m/z 144.1150), [2] = iso-amyl butyrate (R_t 19.64, m/z 158.1308), [3] = isobutyl angelate (R_t 23.68, m/z 156.1150), [4] = 2-methyl-1-butyl angelate (R_t 27.84, m/z 170.1306), [5] = pogostol (R_t 51.61, m/z 222.1983).

11. Mid-infrared (MIR) spectroscopy analysis

General instrumentation: Alpha-P Bruker spectrometer, mounted with an attenuated total reflectance (ATR) diamond crystal. *Spectral acquisition*: Spectrum obtained in absorbance mode, with a spectral resolution of 4 cm^{-1} over the range 4000–550 cm^{-1} and captured using OPUS 6.5 software. *Plant part*: Aerial parts, essential oil. *Sample preparation*: Aerial parts, hydro-distillation to obtain essential oil, placed directly onto the surface of the diamond crystal.

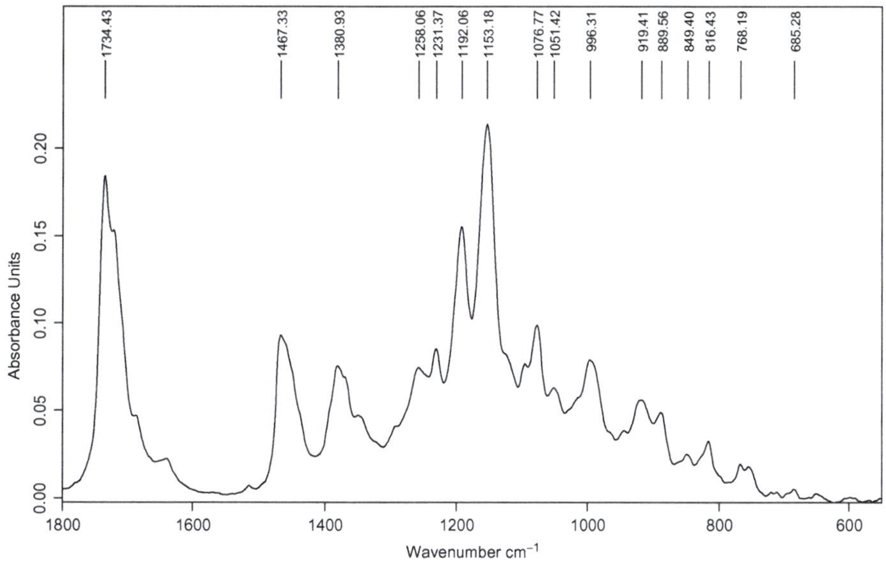

Mid-infrared spectrum of *Eriocephalus punctulatus* essential oil displaying the fingerprint region (1800–550 cm^{-1}).

References

Behiry, S.I., EL-Hefny, M., Salem, M.Z.M., 2019. Nat. Prod. Res., 34:3394–3398.

Davies-Coleman, M.T., English, R.B., Rivett, D.E.A., 1992. Phytochemistry, 31:2165–2167.

Lall, N., Kishore, N., 2014. J. Ethnopharmacol., 153:61–84.

Mierendorff, H.G., Stahl-Biskup, E., Posthumus, M.A., Van Beek, T.A., 2003. Flavour Fragr. J., 18:510–514.

Müller, M.A.N., Herman, P.P.J., Kolberg, H.H., 2001. Flora of Southern Africa, Asteraceae. National Botanical Institute, Pretoria, South Africa.

Njenga, E.W., 2005. The Chemotaxonomy, Phylogeny and Biological Activity of the Genus *Eriocephalus* L. (Asteraceae). PhD thesis, University of the Witwatersrand, Johannesburg, South Africa.

Njenga, E.W., Viljoen, A.M., 2006. S. Afr. J. Bot., 72:637–641.

SANBI, South African National Biodiversity Institute, 2012. Bronwynne Busch and Anthony R. Magee. Compton Herbarium, Kirstenbosch National Botanical Garden, Cape Town, South Africa. Available from: http://pza.sanbi.org/eriocephalus.

Sandasi, M., Kamatou, G.P.P., Viljoen, A.M., 2011. Biochem. Syst. Ecol., 39:328–338.

Seo, S.-M., Kim, J., Kang, J., Koh, S.-H., Ahn, Y.-J., Kang, K.-S., Park, I.-K., 2014. Pestic. Biochem. Physiol., 113:55–61.

Shale, T.L., Stirk, W.A., Van Staden, J., 2004. S. Afr. J. Bot., 70:602–610.

Van Wyk, B.E., Gericke, N., 2000. People's Plants: A Guide to Useful Plants of Southern Africa, first ed. Briza Publications, Pretoria, South Africa.
Van Wyk, B.E., Van Oudtshoorn, B., Gericke, N., 1997. Medicinal Plants of South Africa, first ed. Briza Publications, Pretoria, South Africa.
Watt, J.M., Breyer-Brandwijk, M.G., 1962. The Medicinal and Poisonous Plants of Southern and Eastern Africa, second ed. E. & S. Livingstone Ltd, Edinburgh and London, UK.
Zdero, C., Bohlmann, F., Muller, M., 1987. Phytochemistry, 26:2763–2775.

CHAPTER

Harpagophytum procumbens 9

Nontobeko Mncwangi[a], Weiyang Chen[a], Nduvho Mulaudzi[a], Ilze Vermaak[a,b] and Alvaro Viljoen[a,b]

[a]*Department of Pharmaceutical Sciences, Tshwane University of Technology, Pretoria, South Africa*

[b]*SAMRC Herbal Drugs Research Unit, Faculty of Science, Tshwane University of Technology, Pretoria, South Africa*

Abstract

Harpagophytum procumbens (Burch.) DC. ex Meisn. is an important traditional medicine that grows in the Kalahari region of southern Africa, where it is taken as a general health tonic and anti-inflammatory to treat arthritis, rheumatism, pain, sprains, fever, ulcers and boils. Iridoid glycosides and phenyl derivatives have been the focus of phytochemical investigations, and the biological activity has been ascribed to iridoid glycosides, which are common in nature and are known to have anti-inflammatory activity. Additionally, H. procumbens has been shown to have analgesic, anti-oxidant, antidiabetic, anti-epileptic, antimicrobial and antimalarial activities. The main exporter of this highly commercialised plant is Namibia. The high demand for health products based on this plant has led to overharvesting, raising concerns about sustainability, as the secondary root tubers are utilised commercially, and the whole plant is often destroyed during harvesting. Methods are being assessed to promote sustainable harvesting and propagation of the species. Harpagophytum procumbens is commonly adulterated by its close taxonomic ally H. zeyheri, and this affects the quality of the raw material. Methods such as semi-automated high-performance thin-layer chromatography (HPTLC), ultra-performance liquid chromatography coupled to mass spectrometry (UPLC–MS), and mid-infrared (MIR) spectroscopy have been investigated as quality control methods to profile the non-volatile constituents in H. procumbens raw material. The marker compound harpagoside in the non-volatile fraction was detected in both HPTLC and UPLC–MS analyses.

Keywords: *Harpagophytum procumbens*, *Harpagophytum zeyheri*, Devil's Claw, Anti-inflammatory, HPTLC, UPLC–MS, MIR spectroscopy, Harpagoside, Iridoids, Phenylpropanoid glycosides

The South African Herbal Pharmacopoeia. https://doi.org/10.1016/B978-0-323-99794-2.00007-6

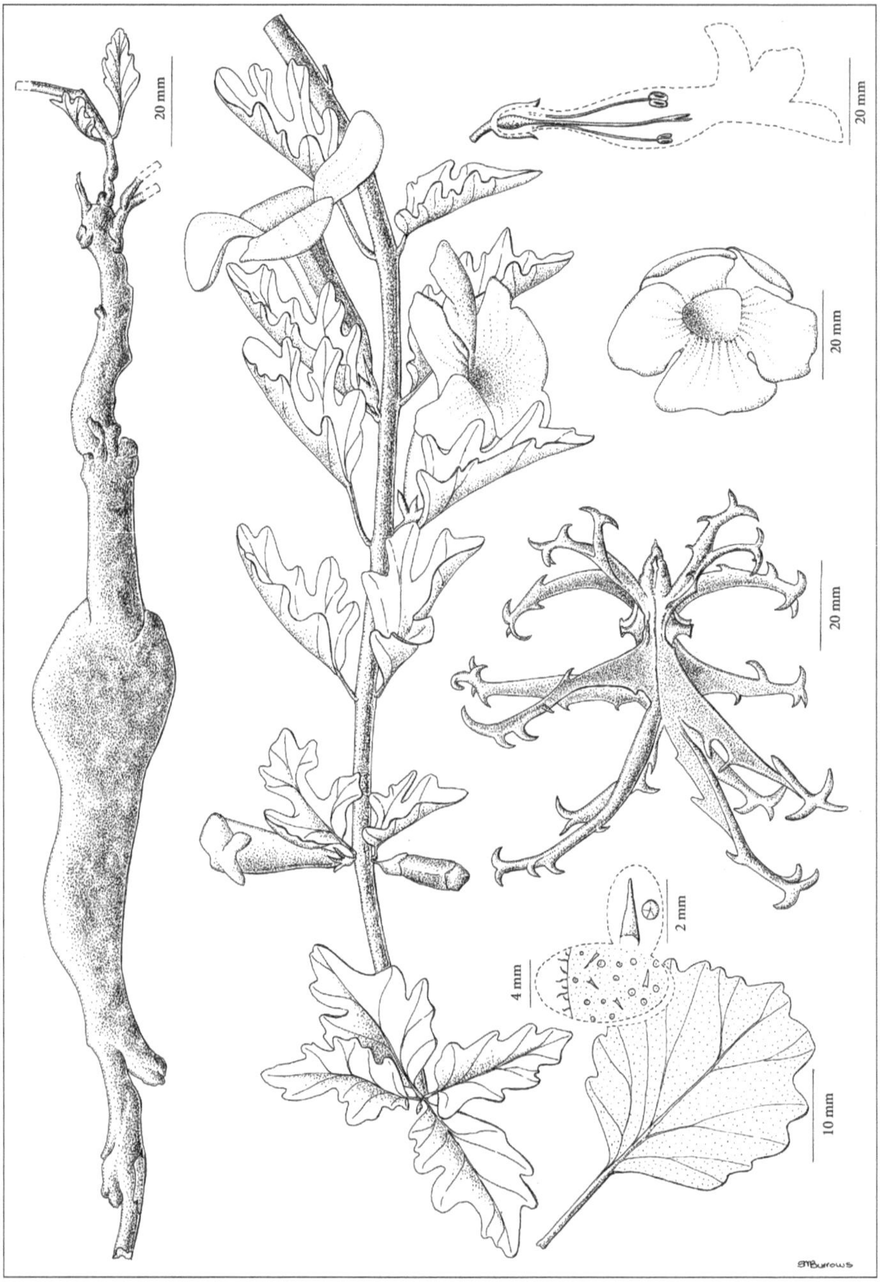
20 mm
20 mm
20 mm
20 mm
2 mm
4 mm
10 mm

Part A: General overview

1. Synonyms

Harpagophytum procumbens subsp. *procumbens, Harpagophytum procumbens* var. *sublobatum* (Engl.) Stapf.[a]

2. Common names

Devil's Claw, harpago, grapple plant, wool- and woodspider (English); '*duiwelsklou*', '*bobbejaandubbeltjie*', '*kloudoring*', '*veldspinnakop*' (Afrikaans); '*teufelskralle*' (German).

3. Conservation status

Least concern.[b]

4. Botany

Harpagophytum procumbens (Pedaliaceae) is a weedy, perennial tuberous plant with creeping annual stems that can reach a length of up to 2 m, spreading from a central thick, fleshy, tuberous taproot. The blue-green leaves are usually divided into several lobes in an irregular manner. The tubular flowers are a deep mauve-pink, with a yellow and white throat (A). The flowers and leaves are visible only during the active growing season, when the climatic conditions are favourable (Wynberg, 2004). Flowers open only for a single day and are pollinated by bees (Von Willert and Sanders, 2004). The aboveground stems emerge after the first rains, but die back during dry spells and in the winter. The fruits are characterised by long protrusions covered with sharp, grapple-like hooks, and two straight thorns on the upper surface; from there comes the colloquial name of the genus *Harpagophytum*, Devil's Claw (B). Seed dispersal occurs when the fruit becomes tangled in the wool, tails or feet of animals, and the seeds are later released and germinated in sandy soils (Ernst et al., 1988). This seed dispersal method is related to the origin of the name Devil's Claw, which illustrates the frantic movements of animals when they try to get rid of the fruit trapped in their hooves (Moatti et al., 1983). The secondary tubers grow up to 2 m deep and are 4–25 cm in length, with a diameter of up to 6 cm (C) (Van Wyk et al., 1997). The tubers are harvested and dried (D) before export or use.

[a] World Flora Online (http://www.worldfloraonline.org).
[b] Redlist of South African Plants (http://redlist.sanbi.org).

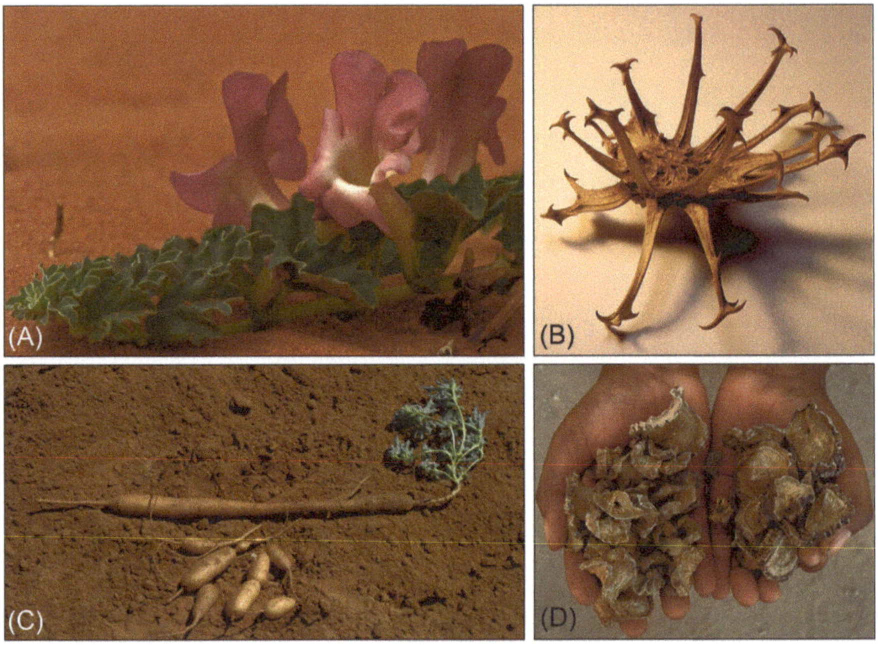

Harpagophytum procumbens is a tuberous creeping plant with blue-green leaves and deep purple-pink flowers (A), spiny fruiting bodies (B), and secondary tubers (C) that are processed by drying (D).

5. Geographical distribution

Harpagophytum procumbens occurs in regions between 15° and 30° latitude in southern Africa (Namibia, Botswana, South Africa, Angola, and to a lesser extent, Zambia, Zimbabwe and Mozambique) (Ihlenfeldt and Hartmann, 1970). The plant typically grows in the red sandy soils of the Kalahari Desert, in areas with low annual rainfall (160–500 mm/year). The formation of secondary root tubers that can store water is the key to the plant's ability to survive long, very dry spells. These tubers branch off horizontally from the main taproot. The amount of rainfall dictates the abundance of the species and how visible it is. It prefers areas where there is less than 25% grass cover and not more than 20% herb and woody vegetation cover. The plant is prevalent in overgrazed areas that are open and where the soil is hard and trampled, as well as on road verges, firebreaks and the slopes of dunes (Hachfeld and Schippmann, 2002).

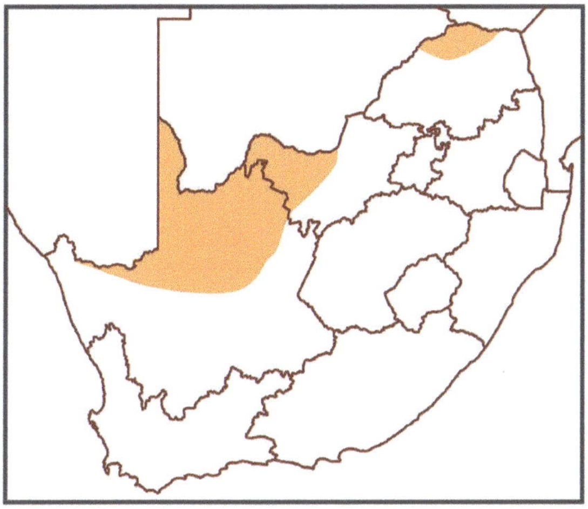

Geographical distribution of *Harpagophytum procumbens* in South Africa.

6. Ethnopharmacology

Harpogophytum procumbens is best known as a remedy to treat inflammation-related conditions. Traditionally, it is prepared in the form of infusions or decoctions to reduce arthritis and pain. However, it is also a trusted medicine to treat dyspepsia, fever, blood diseases, urinary tract infections, postpartum pain, sprains, sores, ulcers and boils (Watt and Breyer-Brandwijk, 1962). Daily intake of *H. procumbens* results in a mild laxative effect. Taken in small amounts, the extract is used to relieve menstrual cramps, while large amounts stimulate the expulsion of a retained placenta after childbirth. The dry, powdered root is applied to wounds, or mixed with animal fat or even Vaseline® and applied to wounds and burns to accelerate healing (Watt and Breyer-Brandwijk, 1962; Van Wyk and Gericke, 2000). Pregnant women ingest about 250 mg of the dry, powdered tuber up to three times daily, to relieve pain. After delivery of the baby, treatment is continued using a reduced dose. An ointment prepared from the fresh root is rubbed into the abdomen of women to ease delivery. It is also applied to the skin to alleviate sores, ulcers, boils and cancerous growths (Watt and Breyer-Brandwijk, 1962).

The secondary tubers are taken as a decoction, or chewed, by the Topnaar people of Namibia to relieve stomach and postpartum pains. They place a needle or a button in the soil above the plant to 'buy the tubers from the earth', before digging them out (Van den Eynden et al., 1992). Patients with high fever are treated by administering a tuber infusion, which is also taken as a bitter tonic, and for the treatment of unspecified 'blood diseases'. Infusions are also taken orally to relieve rheumatism and to treat ailments affecting the liver, kidney, pancreas and stomach (Von Koenen, 1996). A combination of dried *H. procumbens* secondary tuber and *Clerodendrum uncinatum* roots are burnt on a clay shard and the smoke is directed onto the back of a person suffering from back pain. An ointment, prepared by mixing the finely ground ash with fat, is then massaged into the back. A hot water infusion of the two plants is sometimes used as an enema (Von Koenen, 1996). *Harpagophytum procumbens* is the preferred treatment of the Molapo community of South Africa, for menstrual cramps. Although other plants are mostly used, this community sometimes administers Devil's Claw orally, immediately after childbirth, to hasten the expulsion of a retained placenta. However, pregnant women from this community avoid using *H. procumbens*, since they associate the plant with abortion or stillbirth. However, it is used to induce labour, if there is a delayed onset of labour, and is also administered to ease labour pains (Mncwangi et al., 2012).

7. Commercialisation

According to Stewart and Cole (2005), the tubers of *H. procumbens* were first studied in the 1950s by B. Zorn at the University of Jena, Germany. Although initially exported to Germany in small volumes, the large-scale export of the tubers started in 1962 (Raimondo et al., 2003). By 2001, *H. procumbens* was recognised as the third most-frequently used medicinal plant in Germany. Sales increased by 113% between 1999 and 2000, and by another 59% between 2000 and 2001 (Strobach and Cole, 2007). However, since 2002, the sales of Devil's Claw have declined. Several reasons have been proposed for the decrease in demand and these include (i) concerns regarding the sustainability of wild-harvesting of the plant, which were triggered by the proposed listing in April 2000 of *H. procumbens* in Appendix II by the Convention of International Trade in Endangered Species (CITES). In view of this, manufacturers and marketers may have moved their focus to other alternative anti-arthritic products, such as glucosamine. (ii) Prior to 2004, Kathe et al. (2003) reported that 57 pharmaceutical products from the species were marketed by 46 different companies with a value of approximately €30 million in Germany alone. However, a number of natural products, including *H. procumbens*, were removed from the German Medical Aid list in 2004 (Strobach and Cole, 2007). The implication was that medical insurance would no longer cover the cost of prescriptions for these products. The result was a 50% reduction in the sales of herbal medicines in Germany over a 6-month period. (iii) The introduction and enforcement of the Traditional Herbal Medicines Products Directive 2004/24/EC, aimed at streamlining the regulation of medicines in Europe, influenced the production of herbal products. This directive was issued by the European Parliament and by the Council of Europe and came into force in April 2011. It stipulated that all herbal medicines marketed in the EU are regulated and must comply with stringent quality control procedures. The expense involved to become compliant with the regulations forced smaller companies to reduce the range of products that they sell. (iv) The economic downturn experienced globally towards the end of 2008 may have contributed to a reduction in the sales of *H. procumbens*. The national income in Namibia from *H. procumbens* exports in 2009 was estimated at approximately €1.06 million or N$12.16 million. This was of considerably lower value when compared to the figures representing the annual retail sales of *H. procumbens* products worldwide (Ridgway and Krugmann, 2011).

Harvesting of Devil's Claw is done in three ways: traditional wild-harvesting where the sustainability of the tubers is considered; controlled/organised harvesting requiring a permit and harvesters are trained to ensure sustainability; and commercial cultivation where cultivation and harvesting take place on farms (Grote, 2003). Organised harvesters that practice sustainable harvesting and/or are certified as delivering organic raw materials, earn only about 2% of the retail market value. However, according to Ridgway and Krugmann (2011), informal harvesters may receive far less than 1%, while exporters earn approximately 4% of the retail market value. They were convinced that the uneven playing field, exacerbated by open access to the resource and the poverty of the harvesters, contribute to some of the problems faced by the industry. These include overharvesting and the use of harvesting methods that threaten the sustainability of the plant. Several patents related to *H. procumbens* have been filed. One application describes the use of plant extracts, including that of *H. procumbens*, to treat pain, inflammation and/or reduced mobility associated with diseases such as arthritis and osteoarthritis (Rabovsky et al., 2011). Various formulations of pure compounds from the plant, including harpagoside and paeoniflorin, were patented by Shikhman (2010) for the treatment of inflammation, pain, conditions related to arthritis and chronic rheumatic diseases, as well as muscle spasms and headache.

Namibia is the main producer and exporter of Devil's Claw, with 85%–99% of total raw material exports sourced from this country (Stewart and Cole, 2005). Smaller amounts originate from South Africa and Botswana. Europe is the dominant importer of harvested dried roots (Raimondo et al., 2003). Harvesting and trade of the plant for commercial purposes started in Namibia as far back as 1962 when dried tubers were exported by Harpago Pty Ltd. to Erwin Hagen Naturheilmittel GmbH, a German company (Stewart and Cole, 2005). The peak of the global annual market (900 metric tons) was reached in 2002. Exports vary in volume from year to year and seasonally, since demand is inconsistent and may be influenced by stockpiling by overseas companies and erratic sales. Products based on Devil's Claw are readily available in shops marketing natural and wellness products and can be purchased on the internet. Such products are regulated and must be registered in France and Germany as Herbal Medicine or as Food Supplements in the United Kingdom, Netherlands, the United States and the Far East (Cole, 2003). The current European Scientific Cooperative on Phytotherapy (ESCOP, 2003) monograph indicates *H. procumbens* formulations for symptomatic treatment of backache, arthritis and dyspepsia, and to stimulate appetite. In Europe, tea blends containing *H. procumbens* are available and the ground raw material is processed as an ingredient of capsules, tablets, liquid extracts, topical ointments and infusions.

8. Pharmacological evaluation

8.1 *In vitro* studies

8.1.1 Anti-arthritis and anti-inflammatory properties

Kundu et al. (2005) reported that the methanol extract of *H. procumbens* caused inhibition of 12-*O*-tetradecanoylphorbol-13-acetate (TPA)-induced cyclo-oxygenase-2 (COX-2) expression in mouse skin. Extracts of the secondary tubers reportedly inhibited the *in vitro* production of metalloproteinases in human chondrocytes, which are induced by interleukin (IL) (Schulze-Tanzil et al., 2004), and suppressed the expression of COX-2 and inducible nitric oxide (iNOS), which are stimulated by lipopolysaccharide (LPS), in a fibroblast cell line L929 (Jang et al., 2003). The ability of *H. procumbens* to suppress TPA-induced COX-2 expression in human breast epithelial cells (MCF10A) was reported (Na et al., 2004), as well as the inhibition of the release of cytokines (tumour necrosis factor (TNF)-α, IL-6, IL-1β) and prostaglandin induced by LPS (Berthod et al., 2009). Fiebich et al. (2001) showed that the anti-inflammatory activity of *H. procumbens* was related to the inhibition of TNF-α synthesis in primary monocytes stimulated with LPS. The ability of *H. procumbens* to reduce pain and inflammation resulting from rheumatoid arthritis and osteoarthritis is thought to be associated with its efficacy in blocking the production of mediators of inflammation, such as prostaglandin E_2 (PGE2) (Aberham et al., 2007).

An ethanol extract of Devil's Claw tubers was evaluated simultaneously with several of the main extract constituents, namely acteoside (verbascoside), harpagoside, harpagide and 8-*p*-coumaroylharpagide, for their inhibitory effect towards COX-2 expression in excised porcine skin (Abdelouahab and Heard, 2008). The Western blot and immunocytochemical assays indicated good activity for the extract. Exposure of the skin to harpagoside and 8-*p*-coumaroylharpagide reduced COX-2 expression more than exposure to acteoside, 6h after application. However, an increase in COX-2 expression resulted from exposure to harpagide. The researchers found that the ratios of the four major active compounds determined the efficacy of *H. procumbens.* The anti-inflammatory effect of topically applied *H. procumbens* was investigated in the deeper skin layers (Ouitas and Heard, 2009). Freshly excised porcine skin mounted on Franz-type diffusion cells was exposed to an ethanol extract of powdered *H. procumbens* tuber. The liquid in the receptor compartment was analysed after 24h and found to contain harpagoside (0.8 μmol/mL), harpagide (25 μmol/mL), verbascoside (1.8 μmol/mL) and 8-*O*-*p*-coumaroyl-harpagide (0.003 μmol/mL). Freshly excised skin membranes were subsequently exposed to the receptor fluid for 6h. Using immunocytochemistry and Western blotting, the skin was analysed to determine the expression of the three major enzymes involved in the inflammatory factors, namely COX-2 and its product PGE-2, lipoxygenase (5-LOX) and iNOS. The receptor fluid inhibited the expression of COX-2 and its product PGE-2 when applied to the skin, but the effect on 5-LOX and iNOS was insignificant when compared to the controls. The results suggest that transcutaneous delivery of *H. procumbens* may be an effective route to treat inflammation caused by arthritis, which manifests in deeper tissues.

The inhibitory activity of 10 iridoid glycosides isolated from *H. procumbens* tubers was investigated in RAW 264.7 macrophages (Qi et al., 2006a). Chemiluminescence detection revealed that only 8-*O*-*p*-coumaroylharpagide displayed strong activity (IC_{50} 32.4 mM). Concentration-dependent inhibition of nitrite formation (80%) in renal mesangial cells was induced by harpagoside at concentrations ranging from 0.3 to 1 mg/mL (Kaszkin et al., 2004). This activity was associated with the inhibition of iNOS expression at the level of its transcriptional activation. This study suggested that the activity of the extract is higher than that of pure harpagoside. The anti-inflammatory mode of action of the compound was investigated in human HepG2 hepatocarcinoma and RAW 264.7 macrophages (Huang et al., 2006). Harpagoside at 200 mM was reported to suppress LPS-induced mRNA levels and protein expression of COX-2 and iNOS in HepG2 cells. The compound also reduced the release of NO from LPS-stimulated cells, dose-dependently, with an IC_{50} value of 39.8 mM reported. The mode of action determined *in vitro* was found to correspond to that reported for the crude extract. It was also reported (Loew et al., 2001) that the inhibition of biosynthesis of some cysteinyl leukotrienes and thromboxane B2 in Ca2þ ionophore A23187-stimulated human whole blood by *H. procumbens*, was dependent on the harpogoside concentration of the extracts. It was postulated that harpagoside is converted by plasma constituents into a more active form.

The inhibitory activities of fractions isolated from *H. procumbens* towards COX-1 and COX-2 and on NO production were investigated using an LPS-stimulated human whole blood assay (Anauate et al., 2010). The harpagoside concentrations of the fractions, obtained using flash chromatography, were determined. Platelet thromboxane B2 production in blood clotting and PGE-2 production was used to quantify COX-1 and COX-2 activity, respectively. The Griess reaction was used to establish the total NO_2^-/NO_3^- concentration. The fraction containing the highest harpagoside concentration inhibited COX-1 and COX-2 (37.2% and 29.5%, respectively) the most and suppressed NO production (66%). Notably, the fraction rich in iridoids increased COX-2 activity, without affecting NO production or COX-1 activity. In contrast, the cinnamic acid-rich fraction only suppressed NO production by 67%. These results demonstrated that the effect of Devil's Claw on these enzyme activities can be attributed to the harpagoside fraction. In a separate study (Ebrahim and Uebel, 2011), a methanol extract of *H. procumbens* was tested, together with harpagoside and harpagide, as direct inhibitors of COX-2. Direct inhibition of COX-2 was reported for the extract. Harpagoside and harpagide at a concentration equivalent to that in the extract (3% and 1%, respectively) caused only 1.5% and 13% inhibition. Devil's Claw is a popular herbal medicine for treating inflammatory conditions and bone degeneration. The effects of a herbal product Pascoe®-Agil, comprising 60% (v/v) ethanolic Devil's Claw extract, on the production and release of important pro-inflammatory mediators in LPS-stimulated human monocytes were determined by Fiebich et al. (2012). They also investigated the intracellular signalling pathways involved in inflammation. The extract suppressed TNF-α and interleukin (IL)-6, IL-1β and PGE_2 in a dose-dependent manner, in addition to inhibiting the expression of TNF-α and IL-6 mRNA in human monocytes and COX-2 in RAW 264.7 cells. The LPS-stimulated AP-1-mediated gene transcription activity and binding to the AP-1 response elements were also reduced by the extract. However, it did not influence the binding of nuclear factor-kB, induced by LPS, in RAW 264.7 cells. Neither did it affect LPS-induced degradation of IķBα or LPS-induced activation of mitogen-activated protein kinases (MAPK), p38MAPK and JNK in human monocytes. The findings indicate that the standardised extract may be involved in blocking the AP-1 pathway, thereby inhibiting the induction of pro-inflammatory gene expression.

The cytotoxicity and effect of a *H. procumbens* extract, metabolically activated with rat liver S9 mix, on the release of pro-inflammatory cytokines were investigated in LPS-stimulated monocytic THP-1 cells (Hostanska et al., 2014). The release of TNF-α, IL-6 and IL-8 was inhibited by the extract at concentrations shown to be non-cytotoxic (50–250 μg/mL). Metabolic activation of the extract did not influence the cytotoxicity or change its inhibitory effect. However, greater inhibition of TNF-α was reported in the case of the metabolically activated extract (EC_{50} 49 ± 3.5 μg/mL) compared to the extract alone (EC_{50} 116 ± 8.2 μg/mL). Although metabolic activation of the extract reduced the concentrations of harpagoside and derivatives of caffeic acid, no effect was noted on cytokine production.

A study to elucidate the mechanism of harpagoside and harpagide inhibition of COX-2 was conducted by Rahimi et al. (2016). The focus was to establish the drug-likeness and pharmacokinetic characteristics of these natural anti-inflammatory and anti-analgesic compounds. The interaction of both compounds with COX-2 was simulated through molecular docking, with binding energies of −9.13 and −5.53 kcal/mol predicted for harpagoside and harpagide, respectively. Furthermore, stable interactions within the active site of COX-2 were reflected by 7 and 10 hydrogen bonds for the compounds, respectively. Harpagoside and harpagide can be considered moderate G protein-coupled receptor ligands, nuclear receptor-, protease- and enzyme inhibitors, according to the bio-activity scores obtained. Harpagide can also be classified as an ion channel modulator. Both compounds can act as highly selective COX-2 inhibitors (Rahimi et al., 2016). The effects of these two compounds on TNF-α-secretion in undifferentiated and phorbol myristate acetate (PMA)-differentiated THP-1 cells, under inflammatory conditions, were investigated (Schopohl et al., 2016). Their activity towards cellular migration into inflamed tissue was also studied. A decrease in TNFα-secretion in the differentiated cells was induced by both iridoids, while undifferentiated cells remained largely unaffected. Both compounds enhanced mRNA-expression in undifferentiated cells of specific proteins that play a role in leukocyte transmigration. High levels of TNF-α and ICAM-1 mRNA-expression in particular, were recorded after 3 h of exposure, and the enhanced expression was maintained for up to 48 h. L-Selectin and PSGL-1 were strongly induced after 48 h of stimulation. The study found that the immunomodulatory activity of the two iridoids is related to their ability to stimulate the migration of cells into inflamed tissue, thereby promoting the innate anti-inflammatory function of the resident macrophages.

The *in vitro* efficacy of *H. procumbens* in suppressing the production of inflammatory cytokines induced by LPS was demonstrated by Inaba et al. (2010). The ability of harpagoside to inhibit interleukin (IL)-6 production in primary human osteoarthritis chondrocytes, challenged with IL-1β, was consistently observed (Haseeb et al., 2017). Excessive oxidative stress is a hallmark of inflammatory bowel diseases (IBDs), especially ulcerative colitis. The potential protective effects of Devil's Claw in IBDs were evaluated in a preliminary preclinical study. Locatelli et al. (2017) demonstrated the protective effect of a Devil's Claw water extract in isolated LPS-challenged rat colon (Menghini et al., 2018). The concentrations of several markers of inflammation and oxidative stress were suppressed, these included prostanoids, cytokines and serotonin. These findings support the application of the herbal drug in the treatment of ulcerative colitis. A study (Chung et al., 2018) was initiated using LPS-induced RAW 264.7 cells, to investigate the activities of Shinbaro3, which is clinically used to treat arthritis in Korea. The formulation contains hydrolysed roots of *H. procumbens*. Shinbaro3 suppressed the production of NO generation in the cells in a dose-dependent manner. It also dose-dependently downregulated mRNA and protein expression of inflammatory mediators. Three potential mechanisms illuminating the role of Shinbaro3 in RAW 264.7 cells were proposed, namely: (1) suppression of the extracellular signal-regulated kinase 1 and 2 (ERK1/2), stress-activated protein kinase (SAPK)/c-Jun N-terminal protein kinase (JNK), and p38 mitogen-activated protein kinase (MAPK) pathways; (2) inhibition of IκB kinase-*α*/*β* (IKK-*α*/*β*) phosphorylation and nuclear factor-kappa B (NF-κB) subunits in the NF-κB pathway that play a role in MyD88-dependent signaling; and (3) downregulation of IFN-*β* mRNA expression through inhibition of interferon regulatory factor 3 (IRF3) and Janus-activated kinase 1 (JAK1)/signal transducer and activator of transcription 1 (STAT1) phosphorylation, which is associated with TRIF-dependent signaling. Shinbaro3 displayed anti-inflammatory activity in RAW 264.7 macrophage cells stimulated with LPS *via* modulation of the TLR4/MyD88 pathways (Chung et al., 2018).

8.1.2 Antimicrobial and anti-oxidant activity

An extract of *H. procumbens* prepared using supercritical carbon dioxide, yielded a minimum inhibitory concentration (MIC) of 100 μg/mL against *Candida krusei* (Weckesser et al., 2007). Pure harpagoside alone was not effective in the screening. The researchers suggested the existence of synergy between the biologically active constituents. Several researchers have investigated the anti-oxidant activity of Devil's Claw. Betancor-Fernandez et al. (2003) used the Trolox equivalent anti-oxidant capacity (TEAC) assay and reported that the *H. procumbens* extract tested contained active water-soluble anti-oxidants. However, harpagoside did not contribute significantly to the anti-oxidant effects. An IC_{50} value of 19.84 ± 0.13 mg/L was reported for a methanol extract of Devil's Claw (Frum and Viljoen, 2006), reflecting moderate activity in the DPPH (2,2-diphenyl-1-picrylhydrazyl) radical scavenging assay. The extract prepared from secondary tubers and a commercial tincture displayed effective anti-oxidant activity as demonstrated through DPPH radical-scavenging, inhibition of nitrite in LPS-stimulated RAW 264.7 macrophages, and dose-dependent suppression of *N*-formyl-methionyl-leucyl-phenylalanine (fMLP) and acetic acid-induced neutrophil myeloperoxidase (MPO) (Grant et al., 2009).

The most active anti-oxidants derived from *H. procumbens* were found to be β-OH-verbascoside in the DPPH superoxide radical scavenging assay and leucosceptoside A in the oxygen radical anti-oxidant capacity (ORAC) assay (Georgiev et al., 2010). A pilot study conducted by Mazila et al. (2016) was focused on determining the anti-oxidant activity, and the total phenols and main metabolite content of several *Harpagophytum* species. The ability of the selected plants to suppress a respiratory burst of reactive oxygen species (ROS) produced by PMA-challenged human neutrophils, opsonised *Staphylococcus aureus* and *Fusobacterium nucleatum,* was also investigated. A new clone of *H. procumbens* showed the highest degree of anti-oxidative capacity of the specimens tested. Three *Harpagophytum* species were reported to inhibit inflammation induced by PMA when compared to the phosphate-buffered saline (PBS) control. A hybrid of *H. procumbens* and *H. zeyheri* had a pro-inflammatory effect on the response of neutrophils to *F. nucleatum* when compared to the vehicle control treatment (Muzila et al., 2016). Lall et al. (2019) evaluated the biological activities of 25 extracts prepared from 16 plant families in a battery of assays. Besides testing their antityrosinase, anti-oxidant and cytotoxic activities, the anti-acne potential of the extracts was evaluated using *Cutibacterium acnes.* Devil's Claw was the most active, as reflected by the MIC of 31.25 μg/mL obtained. Two of the tested extracts (*H. procumbens* and *Ipomoea oblongata*) were strongly cytotoxic towards the non-cancerous human keratinocyte (HaCat) cell line when tested using the 2,3-*bis*-(2-methoxy-4-nitro-5-sulphophenyl)-2H-tetrazolium-5-carboxyanilide salt (XTT) assay.

8.1.3 Central nervous system activity

The anticholinesterase (ACE) activity of an aqueous secondary tuber extract of Devil's Claw tested at concentrations ranging from 10 to 1000 mg/mL was investigated by Mahomed et al. (2005). They found that the extract displayed ACE activity, and also induced significant concentration-dependent atropine-sensitive contractions of oesophagus muscle isolated from chicks and of ileum isolated from guinea pigs. The contractile effects observed in the smooth muscle of the ileum treated with the extract were partly attributed to the ACE activity observed. An ethyl acetate extract tested *in vitro* at 100 μg/mL, indicated that the plant has ACE and butyrylcholinesterase activity (Bae et al., 2014). A water extract of Devil's Claw roots (1.5% harpagoside), evaluated in an experimental Alzheimer's Disease model, was found to reduce oxidative stress and prevented the reduction in dopamine, norepinephrine and serotonin (5-HT) concentrations induced by amyloid β-peptide in the synaptosomes of the cortex of rats (Ferrante et al., 2017). Evidence of the beneficial effects of Devil's Claw in mitigating neurodegenerative conditions through its anti-oxidant effect has been reported, although the compounds responsible have not been identified. Harpagoside may be involved since the compound has demonstrated protective effects in both *in vitro* and in *vivo* assays.

8.1.4 Other activities

The *in vitro* antiviral activity of some metabolites of *H. procumbens*, including harpagide and harpagoside, was determined against herpes simplex virus type 1, the vesicular stomatitis virus and the poliovirus (Bermejo et al., 2002). Harpagoside displayed activity against the vesicular stomatitis virus with 43.3% cellular viability when treated with the non-toxic concentration of 450 mg/mL. Two diterpenes, (+)-8,11,13-totaratriene-12,13-diol and (+)-8,11,13-abietatrien-12-ol, isolated from *H. procumbens*, were found to exhibit significant ($IC_{50} < 1$ µg/mL) *in vitro* antiplasmodial activity towards chloroquine-sensitive and chloroquine-resistant strains of *P. falciparum* in the dehydrogenase (pLDH) assay (Clarkson et al., 2003). At concentrations ranging from 10 to 1000 µg/mL, an aqueous *H. procumbens* root extract induced strong atropine-sensitive contractions in esophageal and ileum muscle isolated from chicks and guinea pigs, respectively (Mohamed and Ojewole, 2005). The effects were found to be concentration-dependent. Further studies (Mahomed and Ojewole, 2006a) indicated that at 200–1000 µg/mL, the extract induced the same effect in longitudinal, tubular uterine horn muscle isolated from non-pregnant and pregnant female rats. Together these findings prove the spasmogenic, uterotonic action of the extract on mammalian uterine muscles (Mahomed and Ojewole, 2006a), and justify the traditional obstetric uses of the secondary root infusion to induce the onset of and/or accelerate labour, and expel retained placentas after delivery (Van Wyk, 2008). Mahomed and Ojewole (2009) went further to study the effect of the aqueous root extract on uterine horn muscle excised from stilboesterol-pretreated non-pregnant and pregnant adult female rats. Longitudinal, tubular strips, isolated from the non-pregnant rats, and treated with 10–800 µg/mL of the extract, underwent significant increases in the baseline tone and strong oestrogen-related rhythmic, myogenic contractions. The same test concentrations induced the same concentration-dependent effects in excised strips from the pregnant rats in the early, middle and late stages of pregnancy. Moderate to high concentrations (200–1000 µg/mL) of the aqueous root extract were able to consistently bring about strong contractions in the smooth horn muscles isolated from both pregnant and non-pregnant rats. A strong ferrous ion-chelating capacity was displayed by methanol extracts prepared from the cell and hairy root cultures of *H. procumbens*. The capacity was 1.5–2 times higher than that of butylated hydroxyanisole, which was used as the positive control (Georgiev et al., 2012). The ability of harpagoside to mitigate osteoporosis was tested in cell cultures. The compound enhanced bone formation by inducing osteoblast proliferation, alkaline phosphatase activity, and mineralisation in osteoblastic MC3T3-E1 cells. Through regulation of the BMP2 and Wnt signaling pathway in MC3T3-E1 cells, harpagoside demonstrated the ability to increase the mRNA and protein expression of bone formation biomarkers. It also suppressed the RANKL-induced osteoclastogenesis of cultured mouse bone marrow cells (Chung et al., 2017).

8.2 *In vivo* studies and clinical trials

8.2.1 Anti-inflammatory, analgesic and anti-arthritis activity

The effect of taking 2.0g *H. procumbens* powder (500mg/capsule) containing 3% total gluco-iridoids on arachidonic acid metabolism was tested in healthy volunteers ($n=25$) (Moussard et al., 1992). After daily intake for 21 days, the effect of *H. procumbens* was not found to be as pronounced as that of the non-steroidal anti-inflammatory drugs (NSAIDs) used in the trial, since no statistically significant changes in the biochemical parameters monitored were recorded. The following results (ng/mL serum), before and after treatment, were obtained: $PGE_2=2.1$ *vs* 3.2; thromboxane (TX) $B_2=147$ *vs* 143; leukotriene (LT)$B_4=3.4$ *vs* 3.8 and 6-keto-prostaglandin (PG)F_1 alpha=4.4 *vs* 4.2. To validate the anti-inflammatory and analgesic effects of *H. procumbens* and to establish the role of harpagoside, the dried aqueous root extract (100mg/kg) and pure compound were administered to mice and rats. Significant concentration-dependent anti-inflammatory and analgesic effects were reported using the carrageenan-induced oedema assay in rats (acute inflammatory activity) and the writhing test in mice (chemical pain stimulus). At 5 and 10mg/kg, harpagoside had no protective effect in the carrageenan assay, suggesting that it is not involved in the anti-inflammatory effects of the roots. However, the main iridoid glycoside of *H. procumbens* appeared to be key in the peripheral analgesic activity observed. It was deduced from the results that other compounds must also contribute to the significant protective effect. Loss of activity of *H. procumbens* following acid treatment (0.1M HCl), indicates that formulations containing the plant should be designed to protect the active principles from being exposed to the acidic conditions in the stomach (Lanhers et al., 1992).

A randomised double-blind study to evaluate the therapeutic effect of Devil's Claw on lower back pain was carried out over 4weeks (Chrubasik et al., 1999). A characterised *Harpagophytum* extract (WS1351) was administered bidaily as a 600mg (Group 1) or 1200mg dose (Group 2) containing 50 and 100mg of harpagoside, respectively, to 197 subjects with chronic back pain and current exacerbations with intense pain. Six of Group 1 and 10 of Group 2 were pain-free by the end of the trial. However, analysis of the data of the 183 subjects that completed the trial, indicated that patients in the lower dose group (Group 1) with less severe pain and without radiation or neurological deficit benefitted more. Those with more severe pain used Tramadol® (an opioid rescue pain remedy) more frequently, but at a lower dose than the maximum permitted dose. In a clinical trial involving 25 patients suffering from rheumatoid arthritis, 20 diagnosed with osteoarthritis were treated with a daily dose of 2.46g root extract of *H. procumbens* formulated as Pagosid® (Szczepanski et al., 2000). Initially, the extract was added to NSAIDs, as combined therapy, but after 2weeks, the drug was taken on its own for a period of 4weeks. A small reduction in the C-reactive protein (CRP) concentration was observed in the rheumatoid arthritis patients and a significant reduction in creatinine concentration in the osteoarthritis patients, after the period of treatment by Pagosid® alone. However, no significant difference between the intensity of pain and early morning stiffness was recorded for the treatment group using Pagosid® without NSAIDs, compared to those on NSAIDs. Both patients and physicians rated the therapeutic effect of the drug as acceptable. In two cases, treatment was terminated due to some adverse effects. In most cases, Pagosid® acted as a suitable replacement for NSAIDs, mainly because it was tolerated well, had no deleterious effects on kidney function, and relieved pain.

Patients with hip and/or knee osteoarthritis ($n = 122$) took part in a double-blind, multicentre, randomised, parallel-group study to evaluate the therapeutic effects of *H. procumbens* over a 4-month period (Leblan et al., 2000). The most important evaluation criterion was the pain score according to a visual analogue scale. The treatment group received a daily dose of *Harpagophytum* (2610 mg) compared to the drug control, diacerein at 100 mg daily. At the end of the study, considerable improvements in symptoms associated with osteoarthritis were evident in both groups, with no significant differences in pain, functional disability, or the Lequesne score. The need for an analgesic drug (acetaminophen-caffeine) and NSAIDs (diclofenac) was significantly reduced in the *Harpagophytum* group, which was also associated with fewer side effects. It was concluded that *Harpagophytum* was equally effective as diacerein in the treatment of osteoarthritis affecting the knee or hip, and lowered the use of analgesics and NSAIDs. A randomised, double-blind, placebo-controlled study to investigate the effects of *H. procumbens* on the sensory, motor and vascular mechanisms of muscle pain was conducted over a 4-week period, using experimental algesimetric methods (Göbel et al., 2001). By the end of the study, the clear clinical efficacy was reflected by the treatment (verum) group on the clinical global score and by the patient and physician scores. The visual analogue scale indicated highly significant effects, together with the pressure algometer test, the muscle stiffness test and the muscular ischaemia test. However, the antinociceptive muscular reflexes and electromyography (EMG) surface activity did not differ from the placebo. The drug was well tolerated and no serious side effects were recorded. Treatment with *Harpagophytum* dry extract LI 174 for 4 weeks at a bidaily dose of 480 mg achieved significant clinical efficacy in cases where patients experienced slight to moderate muscular pain. It was concluded from the mode-of-action investigations that *Harpagophytum* extract LI 174 probably has a significant effect on sensory and vascular muscular responses and alleviates muscle stiffness. No effects on the central nervous system were reported.

A 2400 mg dose of an aqueous extract of Devil's Claw (Doloteffin™), equivalent to 50 mg harpagoside, was tested for 12 weeks in 75 patients presenting with arthrosis of the hip or knee (Wegener and Lüpke, 2003). The Western Ontario and McMaster Universities (WOMAC) osteoarthritis index (10 point scale), as well as the 10 cm visual analogue scale (VAS) for pain, were used to standardise the evaluation of the effects of the treatment. The results indicated that the drug alleviated pain and some of the symptoms of osteoarthritis. Each WOMAC subscale showed improvement, namely 23.8% for the pain subscale, 22.2% for the stiffness subscale, and 23.1% for the physical function subscale. The total WOMAC index was reduced by 22.9%. In addition, VAS pain scores were reduced by 25.8% for actual pain, 25.2% for average pain, 22.6% for the worst pain, and 24.5% for the total pain score. A continuous improvement in symptoms such as pain on palpation (45.5% lower), limitation of mobility (reduced by 35%), and joint crepitus (25.4% lower) were reported by physicians. Possible adverse effects were reported in only two cases.

The inhibitory effects of *H. procumbens* on tumour promoter-induced COX-2 expression was investigated by Na et al. (2004) in mouse skin. They found that the methanolic extract inhibited DNA-binding of nuclear factor kappa B cells (NF-κB) activated by 12-*O*-tetradecanoylphorbol-13-acetate (TPA). Their results were consistent with those of Kundu et al. (2005), who reported that ethanol extracts inhibited TPA-induced COX-2 expression when applied topically at doses of 200–400 mg in a mouse-skin model. The inhibition of COX-2 expression appears to be the result of inhibition of the catalytic activity of ERK and prevention of the activation of AP-1 and cAMP response element binding (CREB). An aqueous extract of *H. procumbens* (800 mg/kg) was administered intraperitoneally to study the effect of a single dose on acute and chronic inflammation in rats (Ahmed et al., 2005). The NSAID, indomethacin, was administered at 10 mg/kg, and served as the reference drug. Arthritis was first induced in the rats using Freund's adjuvant, and caused significant increases in the thickness of the paws and of C-reactive protein, together with significant decreases in serum cortisol and serum albumin. Subsequent administration of *H. procumbens* and indomethacin resulted in a significant decrease in paw thickness. The intraperitoneal (i.p.) administration of *H. procumbens* and indomethacin in rats reduced inflammation, which was indicated by a significant reduction in the weight of the pellet in the cotton pellet-induced granuloma test (Catelan et al., 2006). An extract of Devil's Claw, administered intraperitoneally 30 min before a carrageenan injection, caused a reduction in the intensity of the inflammatory response by approximately 88%, 80%, 70% and 60%, at doses of 100, 200, 400 or 800 mg/kg bw), respectively, 4 h after inflammation was induced. The number of circulating mononuclear leucocytes was also reduced in normal rats (Catelan et al., 2006). Oral administration did not have the same effect as when the extract was injected intraperitoneally or intraduodenally. It was proposed that acid-hydrolysis or denaturation of active constituents in the stomach may be responsible for the differences observed.

The pain-relieving effect of an aqueous extract of *H. procumbens* was investigated using a writhing test in mice (Ahmed et al., 2005). Results obtained using the cotton pellet-induced granuloma test indicated that administration of *H. procumbens* at 400 mg/kg (i.p.), significantly lowered the number of writhing reactions. A 50–800 mg/kg dose of a water extract of the secondary tuber extract had significant analgesic effects in mice against nociceptive pain stimuli, which were thermally or chemically induced by hotplate or acetic acid, respectively (Mahomed and Ojewole, 2005). Uchida et al. (2008) reported that significant antinociceptive effects in mice resulted from the administration of Devil's Claw extract in the formalin test at a dose of 30–300 mg/kg. It was reported that the extract reduced the length of licking/biting following formalin injection, in both the first and second phases, in a dose-dependent manner. Formalin injection caused a significant increase in the concentration of nitrites/nitrates (NOx) in the spinal cords of the mice, but this was significantly reduced by the herbal extract. The possibility that the opioidergic system is involved in the antinociceptive effect of *H. procumbens* was postulated.

A large number of patients ($n=259$) suffering from arthritis and other rheumatic-related disorders took part in a clinical trial in the UK (Warnock et al., 2007). Patients were selected based on the criterion that pain (rated 2–7 out of 10) had been experienced in the affected area for at least 2 days per week over the previous 8 weeks. The herbal preparation A. Vogel Rheuma Tabletten®, containing 480 mg of *H. procumbens* dried extract each, was taken bidaily with meals. The effectiveness, assessed in 207 patients, reflected a significant reduction in the global mean scores for pain, stiffness and function from the start of the trial to weeks 4 and 8. Mean scores for pain in the back, hip, knee, hand, wrist and elbow reduced significantly from baseline to week 8. A large percentage (54.1%) of the patients rated the treatment as good or excellent. Although 11 patients (4.2%) terminated the treatment due to adverse side effects, which were related mainly to gastro-intestinal conditions, the dosage form was well tolerated. The concomitant use of painkillers was also investigated with 26.0% of 154 patients not requiring any additional drugs, 44.8% reducing their dosage, 16.9% indicating the same intake, and the remainder (9.1%) increasing their use of pain-killers (Warnock et al., 2007). A 12-week multicentre clinical trial was conducted to test the efficacy of Doloteffin™, a Devil's Claw aqueous extract, in 75 patients diagnosed with arthritis of the hip or knee. Improvements in pain on palpation, limitation of mobility and joint crepitus in 45.5%, 35.0% and 25.4% of the patients, respectively, indicated the therapeutic benefits of the herbal drug (Warnock et al., 2007). These results prompted a further single group open study in 259 patients. Devil's Claw dry extract taken for 8 weeks at a dosage of 960 mg/day, was found to significantly reduce global pain and stiffness, with improved mobility and lower average pain scores for hand, wrist, elbow, shoulder, hip, knee and back pain. The efficacy of Devil's Claw was also evaluated in a rat model of arthritis and found to be effective (Andersen et al., 2004). Evidence was produced in rat knee joint challenged with formalin that the combination of Devil's Claw extract, containing 3% harpagoside, together with bromelain extract, glucosamine hydrochloride, chondroitin sulphate, or methylsulphonylmethane, protects the cartilage against damage (Ucuncu et al., 2015). The combined formula also reduced oxidative stress and inflammation, as reflected by lower concentrations of malondialdehyde, nitric oxide and 8-hydroxyguanine (8-OH/Gua), and pro-inflammatory cytokine gene expression in the knee joint tissue. There is sufficient scientific evidence from these preclinical and clinical studies to conclude that Devil's Claw is a promising option for the treatment of osteoarthritis.

A meta-analysis was conducted by Brien et al. (2006), encompassing 14 studies carried out over the period 1966–2006, on *H. procumbens* as a treatment for osteoarthritis. The literature included eight observational studies; two comparator trials and four double-blinded, placebo-controlled, randomised controlled trials. Although several of the published studies did not adhere to important quality criteria in the methodology, data emanating from the better quality studies indicate that the herbal drug is effective in reducing pain associated with osteoarthritis. Overall, the numbers of patients included in the clinical trials were too few to permit credible safety assessments, but the authors concluded that *H. procumbens* poses a smaller risk than NSAIDs, and recommended further longer-term studies to assess safety. A Cochrane Review of herbal medicine used for pain in the lower back reported on two clinical trials, rated as high quality, utilising *H. procumbens* (Gagnier et al., 2007). The first provided strong evidence that doses of *H. procumbens*, standardised to 50 or 100 mg harpagoside, and taken daily, resulted in the short-term management of pain. The second trial demonstrated that a *H. procumbens* product had the same efficacy as a daily dose containing 12.5 mg of the anti-inflammatory drug, rofecoxib (Gagnier et al., 2007). A later Cochrane review, with the same aim as the first, retrieved three randomised clinical trials (Oltean et al., 2014). Two of these compared the effect of a *H. procumbens* product to a placebo (a total of 315 volunteers), while a third study compared the effect to that elicited by rofecoxib. The Arhus (or modified Arhus) pain index was used to monitor pain. The studies, using placebo as a comparison, made use of a 50 mg dose for the first, and a 50 and 100 mg dose for the second study. A significant reduction in pain score was reported over placebo. However, a low score was attained for the quality of evidence when the Grading of Recommendations Assessment, Development and Evaluation (GRADE) was applied (Oltean et al., 2014). Similar pain reduction scores were obtained for Devil's Claw and rofecoxib in the third study involving 88 participants. Although systematic reviews indicate that there is proof that preparations containing Devil's Claw benefit inflammatory/painful conditions, more rigorous studies are required to fully substantiate its efficacy. The Herbal Medicinal Products Committee (HMPC) of the European Medicines Agency (EMA), approved the use of Devil's Claw for the relief of pain in joints on the basis of its longstanding use.[c]

The potential role of the heme oxygenase (HO)/carbon monoxide (CO) pathway in the pain-relief elicited by *H. procumbens* in carrageenan-induced hyperalgesia in rats, was investigated by Parenti et al. (2015). Von Frey filaments and the plantar test were applied to study mechanical allodynia and thermal hyperalgesia, respectively. Pretreatment of the carrageenan-induced rats with the HO inhibitor ZnPP IX, caused a significant reduction of the antihyperalgesic effect induced after administration of 800 mg/kg (i.p.) *H. procumbens*. Pretreatment with hemin, a HO-1 substrate, before a low dose of *H. procumbens* (300 mg/kg, i.p.), induced a clear anti-allodynic response in carrageenan-injected rats. The same result was obtained after pretreatment with CORM-3, a CO releasing molecule. These results reveal the involvement of the HO-1/CO system in the anti-allodynic and antihyperalgesic effects of *H. procumbens* in carrageenan-induced inflammatory pain. A study in male Sprague–Dawley (SD)

[c] http://www.ema.europa.eu; EMA/571858/2016.

rats was conducted to determine the pain-relieving effects of *H. procumbens* extracts in the plantar incision and spared nerve injury (SNI) (Lim et al., 2014). A significant increase in the mechanical withdrawal threshold (MWT) values of the group treated with *H. procumbens* extract (300 mg/kg) was reported. However, fewer 22–27 kHz ultrasonic vocalisations (USVs) were recorded at 6 and 24 h after the plantar incision operation. Continuous treatment with 300 mg/kg of *H. procumbens* extract over a period of 21 days, caused a reduction in SNI-induced hypersensitivity responses as measured by the MWT in the treated group, compared with the control group. The benefit of simultaneously administering a low dose of *H. procumbens*, followed by a subanalgesic dose of morphine, was investigated in a neuropathic pain model (Parenti et al., 2016). A synergistic relationship between the two drugs was evident from the well-defined anti-allodynic and antihyperanalgesic effects observed, despite the dosage of *H. procumbens* being unable to induce an antinociceptive effect, followed by a subanalgesic dose of morphine. Two common symptoms of neuropathic pain, namely hyperalgesia and allodynia, were successfully resolved due to the dual-drug system.

The ingredients of the commercial formulation MA212 (Rosaxan) are *Rosa canina* L. (rosehip) puree/juice concentrate, *Urtica dioica* L. (nettle) leaf extract, and *H. procumbens* (Devil's Claw) or *H. zeyheri* root extract (Moré et al., 2017). The product is marketed as a medicinal food ([EU] No 609/2013) designed to manage pain in people afflicted with gonarthritis. Patients suffering from the condition were involved in a 12-week randomised, placebo-controlled double-blind parallel-design study to evaluate the safety and efficacy of MA212. The WOMAC and quality-of-life scores were recorded at the start and at 6 and 12 weeks, and the use of painkillers by the patients was documented. Initially, the WOMAC subscores/scores did not differ significantly between the treatment and placebo groups. However, the average scores improved significantly for both groups as the study progressed. The average pre-post change of the WOMAC pain score (primary endpoint) was 29.87 for the treatment group and 10.23 for the placebo group. The difference in the values reflects that MA212 is superior. All of the WOMAC subscores/scores at 6 and 12 weeks for the comparison of the two groups had the same level of significance. Not only was there an improvement in the physical quality of life within the MA212 group, but they also benefitted mentally, compared to the placebo group. The treatment group also consumed fewer analgesics. Physicians and patients alike rated the efficacy of MA212 superior to placebo in treating gonarthritis and found it to be well tolerated.

8.2.2 Anti-osteoporotic activity

The remodelling of bone is a physiological process that is controlled by the fine balance between osteoclasts and osteoblasts, and involves the receptor activator of NF-kB (RANK)/receptor activator of NF-kB ligand (RANKL)/osteoprotegerin pathway. Osteoporosis is initiated when this process is disrupted. The protective effect of harpagide against the loss of bone was demonstrated by Chung et al. (2016) in ovariectomised (OVX) mice. This animal model is used to simulate postmenopausal osteoporosis caused by oestrogen insufficiency. The compound was found to effectively stimulate osteoblast and suppress osteoclast differentiation induced by RANKL. Oral intake of harpagide was found to stimulate bone mineral density, trabecular bone volume, and trabecular number in the femur, while simultaneously lowering alkaline phosphatase, osteocalcin, C-terminal telopeptide and tartrate-resistant acid phosphatase concentrations in the serum. These markers are directly associated with bone loss. Harpagoside was also reported to contribute to the protection of bone. The compound suppressed bone loss attributed to both RANKL-induced osteoclastogenesis and inflammation (Kim et al., 2015). However, harpagoside was ineffective in preventing bone erosion in OVX-mice. In contrast, Chung et al. (2016) demonstrated that harpagoside was able to reverse the destruction of trabecular bone in OVX mice, while also stimulating osteoblast proliferation. The difference in the design of this study compared to that of Kim et al. (2015) could, to some degree, explain the contrasting results obtained by the two research groups. Although both studies administered the same doses of harpagoside (2–10 mg/kg), the study of Chung et al. (2016) continued for 12 weeks, compared to the trial of Kim et al. (2015), of which the duration was only 4 weeks. The duration of treatment may impact the pharmacological response, *in vivo*. In this regard, several studies recommend a treatment duration not shorter than 12 weeks in OVX mice for identifying significant protective effects induced by herbal drugs (Lai et al., 2015). Further research by Chung et al. (2017) revealed that oral intake of harpagoside could reverse trabecular bone depletion in OVX mice. A significant increase in the bone mineral density of the femur was also reported. The elevated concentrations of osteocalcin, C-terminal telopeptide and tartrate-resistant acid phosphatase in the serum of OVX mice were reduced following harpagoside treatment. The protection against bone loss offered by harpagoside in OVX-mice was attributed to the stimulation of osteoblast differentiation and the inhibition of osteoclast resorption. It can thus be concluded that both harpagide and harpagoside contribute to the treatment of postmenopausal osteoporosis and bone disorders related to inflammation.

As part of a study to determine cartilage turnover in 6-month-old rabbits after treatment with *H. procumbens*, a 7.1T MRI scanner was used to derive measurements of the tibial condylar cartilage (Wachsmuth et al., 2011). The thickness and surface area was measured and the volume of the cartilage obtained was compared with values determined through water displacement of the dissected cartilage to enable calculation of precision. Quantitative measurements were made in 16 rabbits after unilateral medial meniscectomy and transection of the back cruciate ligament. Half of the group was treated with a *H. procumbens* extract. Good precision reflected by a relative standard deviation of $\leq$6.4% was determined for the MRI-based measurement of the cartilages, and the values were similar to those obtained after dissection. The thickness and volume of the medial tibial cartilage were approximately 35% less in the operated knees than in the intact knees. The difference between operated and non-operated knees for both thickness and volume of the tibial cartilage was smaller, but not significantly so, in animals treated with the herbal drug, compared to the untreated group. An analysis of systematic reviews indicated that at least two studies on Devil's Claw preparations containing more than 50mg harpagoside, yielded strong evidence of a clinically relevant effect (Chrubasik et al., 2007). Three studies were mentioned in a systematic review, which included randomised controlled trials involving patients with osteoarthritis that compared different dosage forms containing Devil's Claw with either placebo or reference drugs (Cameron et al., 2009). The herbal drug was administered as an aqueous extract, an alcoholic extract or a cryo-ground powder. The water-based extracts were effective in suppressing pain caused by osteoarthritis, but the alcoholic extract was ineffective. Compared to the control drug diacerein, a drug used to treat joint diseases, the powdered sample of Devil's Claw was equally effective. A more recent systematic review set out to evaluate the effectiveness and safety of oral preparations used in Brazil for the treatment of osteoarthritis involved participants ($n=122$) diagnosed with osteoarthritis of the knees or hips. The efficacy of diacerein and Devil's Claw extract was rated as similar according to the global assessment of efficacy (Del Grossi et al., 2017).

8.2.3 Antimicrobial and anti-oxidant properties

A significant anti-oxidant effect of an extract prepared from *H. procumbens* was reported after testing, in the brain frontal cortex and striatum of rats (Bhattacharya and Bhattacharya, 1998). The extract was administered at a dose of 100 or 200mg/kg i.p. for 14days. Dose-dependent increases in superoxide dismutase, catalase and glutathione peroxidase activities were found in both regions of the brain, together with a reduction in lipid peroxidation activity. The authors suggested that the anti-inflammatory effect of *H. procumbens* may be associated partly with its anti-oxidant properties. Results from a study involving a cell-free oxidant-generating system and biopsy tissue from inflamed human colorectum indicated that exposure of the tissue to *H. procumbens* results in the scavenging of superoxide peroxyl radicals in a dose-dependent manner (Langmead et al., 2002). A further study to determine the anti-oxidant properties of *H. procumbens* extract offered various explanations for the activity observed towards stannous ions, tested as $SnCl_2$, namely that some of the extract constituents (i) chelate Sn^{2+}, thereby restricting the generation of free radicals, (ii) act as free radical scavengers, preventing cells from being oxidised and/or (iii) act as a reducing agent(s) upon Sn^{2+}, thereby mitigating the cytotoxicity of $SnCl_2$ (Almeida et al., 2007). Since flavonoids are well-known free radical scavengers, they could be involved in the anti-oxidant activity of *H. procumbens*.

8.2.4 Antidiabetic and anti-obesity activity

A dose-dependent reduction in blood glucose concentrations, in both control and streptozotocin (STZ)-induced diabetic rats, was reported by Mahomed and Ojewole (2004), following i.p. injection of a water extract of the secondary roots of *H. procumbens*. Analgesic, anti-inflammatory, as well as hypoglycaemic activities, were displayed by the extract, confirming the traditional uses. Harpagoside, in contrast, had no effect on blood glucose levels in diabetic rats, although it was effective in combating carrageenan-induced inflammation. The Chinese Traditional Medicine,

Fufang Xueshuantong Capsule, which contains harpagoside, successfully reduced retinal lesions in STZ-induced diabetic rats (Jian et al., 2016), thereby indicating that Devil's Claw may benefit diabetic patients by controlling inflammatory components associated with diabetes. Further study by Mahomed and Ojewole (2005) revealed that the aqueous extract (50–800 mg/kg) resulted in a significant dose-dependent hypoglycaemic effect in both normal and diabetic rats. The hypoglycaemic agent, chlorpropamide (250 mg/kg), was used as the positive control. A reduction in blood glucose following intake of *H. procumbens* root justified its traditional use as a treatment for adult-onset, type-2 diabetes mellitus in some communities of South Africa. The ability of a *H. procumbens* dry tuber extract to activate the ghrelin (GHS-R1a) receptor was evaluated using calcium mobilisation and receptor internalisation assays in human embryonic kidney cells (Hek) (Torres-Fuentes et al., 2014). These cells express the GHS-R1a receptor consistently. The food intake of male C57BL/6 mice was also recorded following i.p. injection of the root extract of *H. procumbens*, both with and without food restriction. A substantial increase in cellular calcium influx occurred following the injection, but full receptor activation did not take place, since GHS-R1a receptor internalisation did not occur. The mice displayed a significant anorexigenic effect following peripheral administration of the extract, indicating that *H. procumbens* root extract is a potential natural source of anti-obesity compounds (Torres-Fuentes et al., 2014). Cholecystokinin (CCK) has been identified as an important hormone associated with weight loss. The effect of Devil's Claw extract on the CCK concentration in serum and on the body weight of male rats was investigated after oral administration for 28 consecutive days (Saleh et al., 2018). The rats were weighed 1 day after the final injection, and blood taken. The CCK concentrations were determined in the serum and found to increase significantly in rats treated with 300 and 600 mg/kg Devil's Claw extract. In addition, the treatment group had a lower body weight than the control group. It can be concluded that Devil's Claw extracts reduce body weight through stimulation of CCK hormone production.

8.2.5 Central nervous system activity

Dose-dependent increases in superoxide dismutase, catalase and glutathione peroxidase activities, with a simultaneous reduction of tissue lipid peroxidation, was recorded in the cortex of rats, following 14 days of treatment with *H. procumbens* at 100 or 200 mg/kg (Bhattacharya and Bhattacharya, 1998). Cell damage was prevented by an ethyl acetate fraction of the extract after it was induced in isolated rat cortex specimens using Fe^{2+} or sodium nitroprusside (Schaffer et al., 2013). Harpagoside, harpagide, procumbide and 8-*p*-coumaroyl-harpagide were linked to the high anti-oxidant capacity in the brain (Baghdikian et al., 1997). Furthermore, harpagoside was demonstrated by Kim et al. (2002) to exert protective effects on rat cortical neurons, exposed to glutamate. The compound also exhibited cognitive-stimulating and anti-oxidant activities in mice with amnesia, induced by treatment with scopolamine (Jeong et al., 2008). It was reported that harpagoside was able to attenuate dopaminergic degeneration caused by 1-methyl-4-phenylpyridinium (MPP^+), in cultured rat mesencephalic neurons (Sun et al., 2012). It also improved the locomotor ability as evaluated in a 1-methyl-4-phenyl-1,2,3,6-tetrahydropyridine mouse model. The protective effect of harpagoside was attributed to higher concentrations of glial cell line-derived neurotrophic factor. Treatment of rats in an amyloid β-peptide (1–40)-injected Alzheimer's disease model with harpagoside, resulted in neuroprotective effects on learning and memory deficit (Li et al., 2015). These effects were attributed in part to increased expression of brain-derived neurotrophic factor, in conjunction with the activation of MAPK/ERC and PI3K/Akt pathways, which play important roles associated with learning and memory.

In contrast to Alzheimer's disease, effective drugs to treat vascular dementia (VaD) have yet to be identified. The neuroprotective effects of harpagoside have been investigated with regard to Aβ- and MPTP-induced neurotoxicity. Results from a well-known VaD model, namely chronic cerebral hypoperfusion (CCH) rats, indicated that chronic intake of harpagoside over a 2-month period restored the spatial learning/memory, as well as the fear memory impairments. The protective effects of the compound did not arise from physiological or metabolic changes, or from changes to the locomotor abilities of the rats. Instead, the compound suppressed the overstimulation of phosphatase and tensin homolog deleted on chromosome 10 (PTEN) induced by CCH, by increasing PTEN phosphorylation. In addition, harpagoside enhanced the activity of Akt and reduced the activity of GSK-3β, which are downstream effectors of PTEN (Chen et al., 2018). The anticonvulsant activity of an aqueous extract of Devil's Claw tuber was evaluated after inducing seizures in mice with pentylenetetrazole (PTZ), picrotoxin (PCT) and bicuculline (BCL) (Mahomed and Ojewole, 2006b). Phenobarbitone and diazepam were used as reference drugs. The herbal extract delayed the onset of, and antagonised, PTZ-induced seizures significantly at doses of 100–800 mg/kg. It also notably antagonised PCT-induced seizures, but was only partially and weakly antagonising towards BCL-induced seizures. A delay in the onset of convulsions was recorded and seizure duration was shorter on average. The anticonvulsant activity and its ability to suppress the CNS may be linked. The beneficial effects of *H. procumbens* were investigated on specific aspects of spinal cord injury (SCI), a condition with loss of locomotor function and sensory abnormalities that lead to incapacitation. The influence of herbal drug treatment on locomotor function was studied in a modified rodent contusion model of SCI, as well as responses to mechanical stimuli after treatment. Neurochemical changes associated with SCI-induced allodynia were also explored. The experimental protocol was as follows: spinal cord contusion at T10 level, dosage herbal drug administered p.o. at 300 mg/kg daily or vehicle (water), drug given 24 h after surgery, measurements to assess behavior every 48 h, and sacrifice (Day 21). The herbal drug caused an increase in sensitivity towards physical stimuli and mitigated the decrease in locomotor function caused by the surgery. The infiltration of microglia into spinal cord tissue was monitored by Iba1 expression and found to start 3 days after injury. Higher concentrations of 4-hydroxynonenal (a product of oxidative stress) and pro-algesic resulting from SCI, reduced after 7 days of treatment with *H. procumbens*. The spinal injury also upregulated the anti-oxidant heme oxygenase-1 (HO-1) expression. In a simultaneous study, the herbal drug was found to inhibit oxidative/nitrosative stress, as reflected by a decrease in the production of NO and ROS, in cultured murine BV-2 microglial cells. In addition, suppression of inflammatory responses, including phosphorylation of cytosolic phospholipases A2, and upregulation of the anti-oxidative stress pathway involving the nuclear factor erythroid 2-related factor 2 and HO-1, was also reported. It can be concluded that the results provide evidence that Devil's Claw is beneficial in the management of allodynia by reducing neuro-inflammation and pain associated with neuropathological conditions, including SCI (Ungerer et al. 2020).

8.2.6 Cardiovascular properties

The protective effects of crude methanolic *H. procumbens* root extracts were reported by Circosta et al. (1984) towards arrhythmia induced by aconitine, calcium chloride or chloroform-epinephrine in rats and rabbits. High doses caused a significant and dose-dependent reduction in arterial blood pressure and heart rate in conscious rats with normal blood pressure. A significant, protective effect, which was dose-dependent, was caused by methanol extracts and harpagoside in an HVA-induced reperfusion model of hyperkinetic ventricular arrhythmias (HVA) using Langendorff preparations of rat heart (Costa De Pasquale et al., 1985). An aqueous extract administered (10–400 mg/kg) to rats, while anaesthetised with pentobarbitone, caused dose-dependent hypotensive and cardiodepressant changes in the systemic arterial blood pressure and heart rate, respectively (Mahomed and Ojewole, 2004). Initial slight, transient and strong contractions of isolated rat portal veins were followed by significant relaxation of longer duration in the cardiac muscles, depending on the dose, after exposure to 10–1000 mg/mL of the extract. It also displayed a negative inotropic effect on isolated rabbit hearts. In rats, the extract was reported to reduce the heart rate and blood pressure; effects that may be related to QT prolongation and abnormal heart rhythms, as well as disruption of calcium currents (verapamil-like effect).

8.2.7 Other effects

Longitudinal, tubular strips of uterine horn muscle were excised from pregnant and non-pregnant adult rats (Mahomed and Ojewole, 2006a). It was demonstrated that exposure of these strips to moderate to high concentrations (200–1000 mg/mL) of *H. procumbens* induced pronounced contractions, consistent with the traditional use. In addition, uterine horn muscle strips taken from stilboesterol-pretreated non-pregnant female rats underwent concentration-dependent oestrogen-dominated contractions, when exposed to 10–800 mg/mL extracts. Significant increases in baseline tone, and strong and rhythmic myogenic contractions were observed. Similar effects were reported for muscle strips excised during the early, middle and late stages of pregnancy. These results confirmed the spasmogenic and uterotonic effects of *H. procumbens* on mammalian uterine muscles.

8.3 Safety

An evaluation report was prepared by the European Medicines Agency (EMEA, 2009) on the safety of the tubers of *H. procumbens* and *H. zeyheri* for human use.

They reported lethal dose to kill 50% (LD_{50}) values determined at 4.6 and 1.0 g/kg, for oral and intravenous administration, respectively, of aqueous, methanolic and butanolic extracts, reflecting low toxicity. For the pure compounds, harpagoside and harpagide, i.p. administration to mice yielded LD_{50} values of 1.0 and 3.2 g/kg, respectively. Sub-acute toxicity studies involving repeated dosing did not reveal haematological or pathological findings of note, or any indications of hepatotoxicity. However, they concluded that the lack of study details brings the validity of the study into question (EMEA, 2009). The cytotoxicity of *H. procumbens* extracts and their pure constituents were determined by Gyurkovska et al. (2011) using murine peritoneal macrophages and the 3-(4,5-dimethyl-thaizol-2-yl)-2,5-diphenyl tetrazolium bromide (MTT) assay. They reported that β-OH-verbascoside, martynoside and harpagide at 1.0 mg/mL resulted in fewer viable cells. Harpagide was found to be the most toxic. Preparations containing Devil's Claw to treat osteoarthritis and back pain were assessed for their safety by Vlachojannis et al. (2008). They evaluated studies from 1985 onward reported that a total of 6892 patients used such products for up to 1 year, in double-blind ($n = 615$) or observational ($n = 6277$) trials. Only 20 of the 28 clinical trials included in the study reported minor adverse events, which translated to 3% of the participants, and included mainly gastro-intestinal complaints, such as diarrhoea. The use of *H. procumbens* is contraindicated in patients with a history of stomach or duodenal ulcers (Chantre et al., 2000; Vlachojannis et al., 2008). It is known that patients with sensitive digestive systems may be affected by the increased production of gastric juice caused by the bitter principles of *H. procumbens*. A negative inotropic effect on isolated rabbit heart and a reduction in arterial blood pressure and heart rate in rats was documented in trials involving *H. procumbens* (Chantre et al., 2000; Vlachojannis et al., 2008). The possibility of the herbal drug causing QT prolongation (delayed ventricular repolarisation), abnormal heart rhythms, and interfering with calcium currents has been suggested. Based on current evidence of *H. procumbens* use, cardiovascular effects have a low probability of occurring, yet it may be prudent to include a warning for patients treated for cardiovascular conditions on product labels (EMEA, 2009). Both the assessment report and systematic review mentioned, pointed out that toxicology data for extracts of *H. procumbens* are lacking and do not confirm safety for human use. Both advocated for additional studies, including repeated-dose and chronic toxicity trials and reproductive, genotoxicity, mutagenicity and carcinogenicity studies (Vlachojannis et al., 2008).

Harpagophytum procumbens was found to be cytotoxic towards a hepatic cell line (HepG2/C3A) (Biazi et al., 2017). The pure compound, harpagoside, was lethal towards cells in the S phase, but caused an increase in the number of cells in the G2/M phase, and induced apoptosis. Harpagoside also inhibited the expression of CDK6 and CTP3A4. Neither of the test substances was genotoxic, but both inhibited CYP1A2 and CYP3A4 expression significantly. It is possible that the cytotoxicity caused by both test substances is related to the inhibition of metabolism, rather than through transcriptional regulation of the cyclins and CDKs tested. This deduction was made after reviewing the results of an MTT assay and the changes in the expression of genes related to drug metabolism, leading to cell death. Exposure to the plant extract and harpagoside slowed the rate of cell proliferation. The findings that both the whole extract and the pure compound can be cytotoxic should be taken into account when considering the treatment of rheumatic diseases with *H. procumbens*. Further toxicity studies of capsules containing Devil's Claw were conducted in mice by Ibrahim et al. (2010). They investigated potential biochemical, haematological and histopathological changes brought about in acute, subacute and chronic toxicity studies. Mice were treated with a single dose of 81 mg/kg body weight (bw) (acute toxicity), with 27 mg/kg bw, administered orally every second day for 7 days (subacute toxicity), or with 5.4 mg/kg bw daily for 90 days (chronic toxicity). No signs of toxicity were apparent in any of the animals and none died during the observation period. There were also no significant haematological or biochemical changes when comparing the treated animals and those in the control group.

9. Phytochemistry

9.1 Non-volatile constituents

A large number of phytoconstituents has been isolated and identified from *H. procumbens* by a host of researchers. Several iridoid glycosides are produced by the plant and include harpagoside, procumbide and harpagide. Phenylpropanoid glycosides, such as acteoside (verbascoside) and isoacteoside (isoverbascoside), as well as other compound classes, including harpagoquinones, amino acids, flavonoids, phytosterols and carbohydrates, have been reported (Gruenwald, 2002). The iridoid glycosides are regarded as the main biologically active constituents of Devil's Claw. Two acetyl phenolic glycosides, namely 6-acetylacteoside and 2,6-diacetylacteoside, were isolated from the dichloromethane:methanol (1:1 v/v) extract of commercial secondary tubers (Munkombwe, 2003). These compounds comprise two aromatic moieties linked to two sugars (glucose and rhamnose) and are similar in structure to acteoside. 6-Acetylacteoside has been proven to be a reliable marker for distinguishing *H. procumbens* and *H. zeyheri* since it is absent in the latter species. Boje et al. (2003) isolated several compounds from the aqueous extract of secondary tubers of *H. procumbens,* including 8-feruloylharpagide, 8-cinnamoylmyoporoside, pagoside, cinnamic acid and caffeic acid. Clarkson et al. (2003) reported the isolation of two diterpenes from a petroleum ether secondary tuber extract of the plant. These were identified as (+)-8,11,13-totaratriene-12,13-diol and (+)-8,11,13-abietatrien-12-ol (ferruginol).

With the aid of a sophisticated liquid chromatography-diode array detection-mass spectrometry/solid phase extraction-nuclear magnetic resonance (LC-DAD-MS/SPE-NMR) technique, Seger et al. (2005) were able to identify isobaric iridoid glycoside regio-isomers as the (*E/Z*) pairs of 6′-*O*-*p*-coumaroylharpagide (6′-PCHG) and 8-*p*-coumaroylharpagide (8-PCHG), from a methanol secondary tuber extract. While 6′-PCHG (*E/Z*) and 8-PCHG (*E*) had been previously identified in very few natural products, 8-PCHG (*Z*) was reported as a new metabolite. It was also the first report of 6′-PCHG (*E/Z*) from *H. procumbens*. Clarkson et al. (2006) used high-performance liquid chromatography (HPLC)-SPE-NMR to isolate new, but unstable chinane-type tricyclic diterpenes from a petroleum ether extract of secondary tubers. 12,13-Dihydroxychina-8,11,13-trien-7-one and 6,12,13-trihydroxychina-5,8,11,13-tetraen-7-one are characterised by an isopropyl group at C-11, whereas the isopropyl group is positioned at C-13 and C-14 in the skeletons of the common diterpenes, abietane and totarane. The instability of these structures is probably due to degradation as a result of oxidation. Two more novel iridoid glycosides, harprocumbide A (6″-*O*-α-D-galactopyranosyl harpagoside) and harprocumbide B (6″-*cis*-*p*-coumaroylprocumbide), were identified from the tubers (Qi et al., 2006b). In addition, the presence of 6-*O*-α-D-galactopyranosyl harpagoside was reported for the first time from *H. procumbens* (Qi et al., 2006b) and nigaichigoside F1, nigaichigoside F2, chebuloside II, 7α-hydroxysitosterol, 7β-hydroxysitosterol, martynoside, 7α,23-dihydroxytormentic acid ester glucoside, ethyl ferulate and pentacosanoic acid in subsequent studies (Qi et al., 2006a, 2007). The same group (Qi et al., 2010) later isolated a new triterpenoid glycoside, named harproside, as well as a new iridoid glycoside, referred to as pagide. Six known compounds and a new iridoid diglucoside were isolated from a water extract of the secondary roots. Spectroscopic techniques were used to elucidate the structure of the novel compound, reported as 6′-*O*-glucopyranosyl-8-*O*-*trans*-coumaroylharpagide (Tomassini et al., 2016).

The natural intra- and interpopulation phytochemical variation within and between *H. procumbens* ($n=241$) and *H. zeyheri* ($n=107$) was investigated using both UHPLC–MS and proton NMR (^{1}H NMR) spectroscopy, in combination with multivariate data analysis (Mncwangi et al., 2014). Quantitative determination of harpagoside using UHPLC–MS revealed significant variation in the content, with the concentrations in *H. procumbens* ranging from 0.17% to 4.37% and from not detected to 3.07% in *H. zeyheri*. The specification of >1.2% harpagoside as set out in the European Pharmacopeia was met by only 41% and 17% of the *H. procumbens* and *H. zeyheri* samples, respectively. It was subsequently deduced from the results that the chemistry of the two species is different and that there is no basis for their interchangeable use.

An iridoid glucoside-rich organic extract of the dried and ground secondary tubers of *H. procumbens* was obtained using methanol:acetonitrile (1:1, v/v) (Steenkamp and Steenkamp, 2019). A UPLC–MS profiling method was developed to enable the identification of the extract constituents using high-resolution mass spectral detection. Six extract constituents were confirmed in the extract, namely harpagide, acteoside, isoacteoside, harpagoside and 6-acetylacteoside, after analysing reference standards. Another three compounds were identified tentatively from the accurate masses determined using the time-of-flight (ToF) mass spectrometer. Based on the accurate masses obtained and the fragmentation patterns, the three compounds were reported as dihydrichinatrienone, totaratrienediol, and a possible isomer of 6-acetylacteoside.

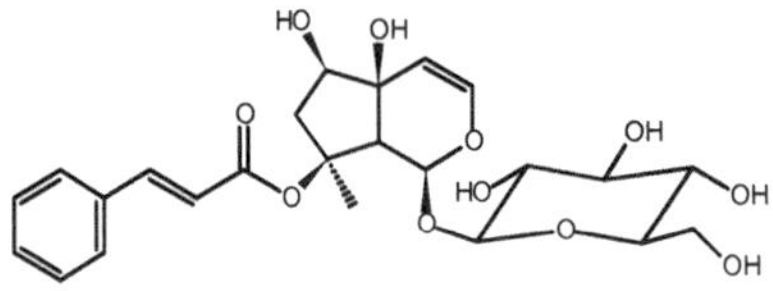

Harpagoside

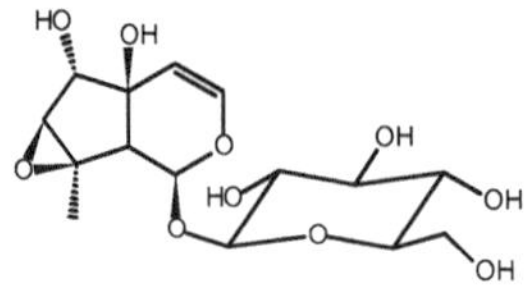

Harpagide

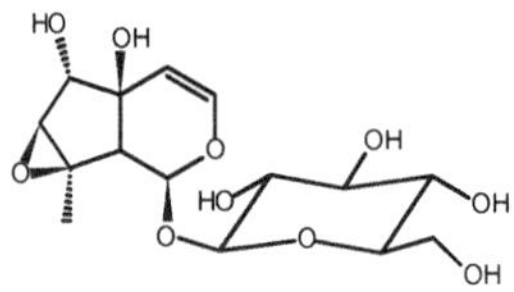

Procumbide

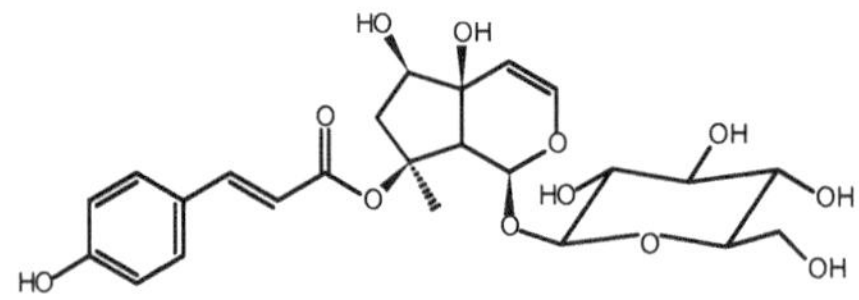

8-*O*-*p*-Coumaroylharpagide

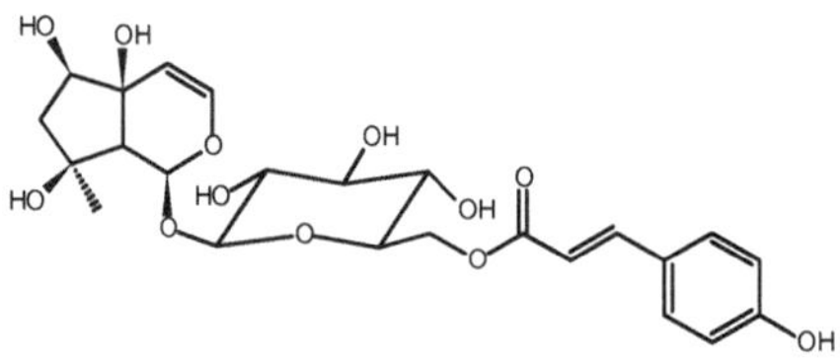

6'-*O*-*p*-Coumaroylharpagide

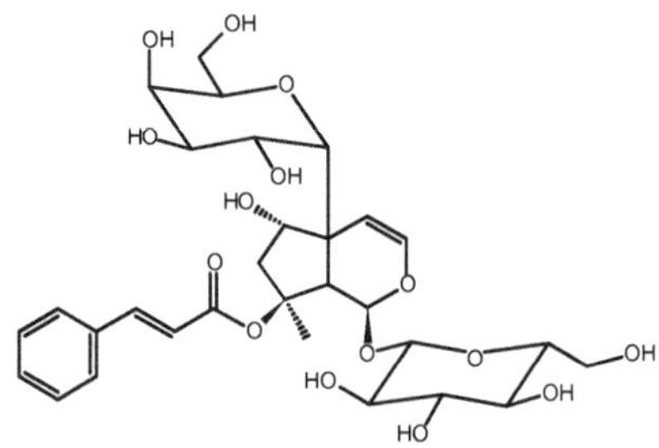

Harprocumbide A

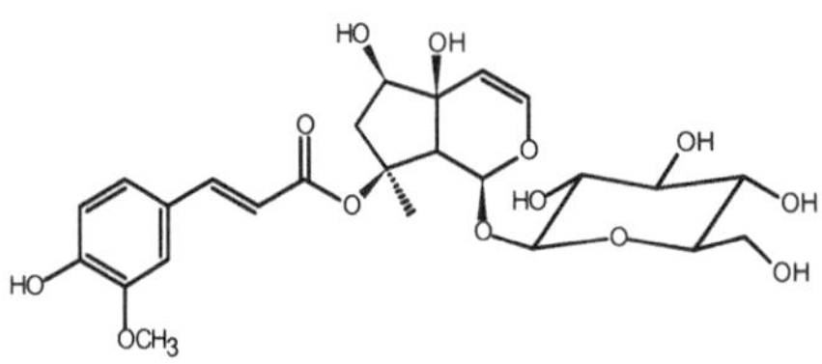

8-Feruloylharpagide

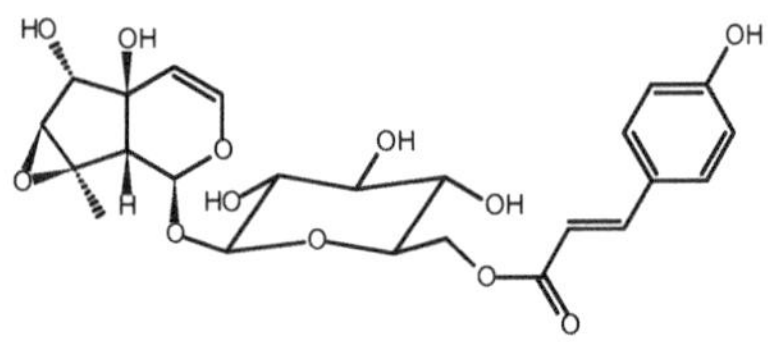

6'-*O*-*p*-Coumaroylprocumbide

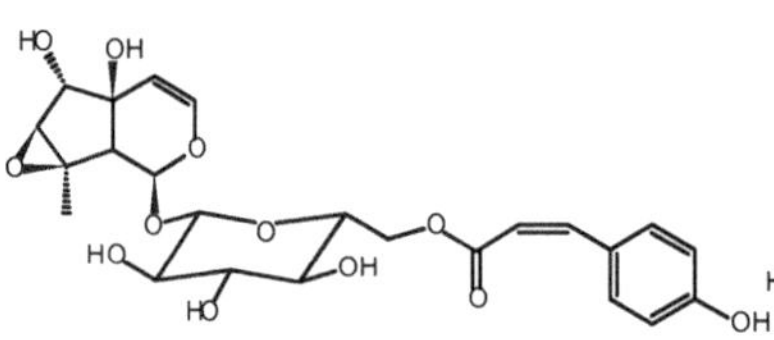

Harprocumbide B

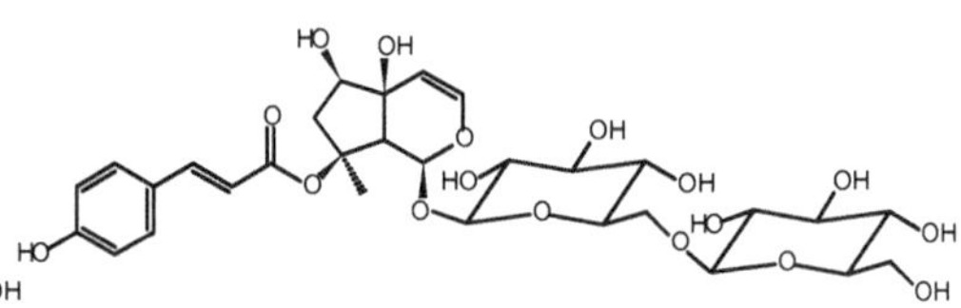

6′-*O*-Glucopyranosyl-8-*O*-trans-coumaroylharpagide

Part B: Chemical profiling and quality control

10. Chromatography analysis

10.1 High-performance thin-layer chromatography (HPTLC) fingerprint analysis

General instrumentation: CAMAG HPTLC instrument consists of an automatic TLC sampler (ATS 4), automatic developing chamber (ADC 2), CAMAG TLC visualiser 2, CAMAG derivatiser, and TLC plate heater. *HPTLC plates:* Silica gel glass plates 60 F_{254} (Merck). *Plant part:* Secondary tubers, methanol extract. *Sample application:* Application volume of 2 μL methanol extract (100 mg/mL) and standards (1 mg/mL) spotted as 10 mm bands. Plates were developed in a 20 × 10 × 4 cm glass twin-trough chamber to a migration distance of 70 mm. *Tank saturation:* 20 min at 15 °C and 33% RH, with 25 mL of the mobile phase. *Mobile phase:* Ethyl acetate: water: formic acid: acetic acid (8:1:1:1, v/v/v/v). *Derivatisation:* Vanillin-sulphuric acid reagent. The plate is sprayed with 3 mL of vanillin reagent followed by heating the plate for 3 min at 100 °C, and then visualised. *Visualisation:* The plate was viewed under 366 nm fluorescent light.

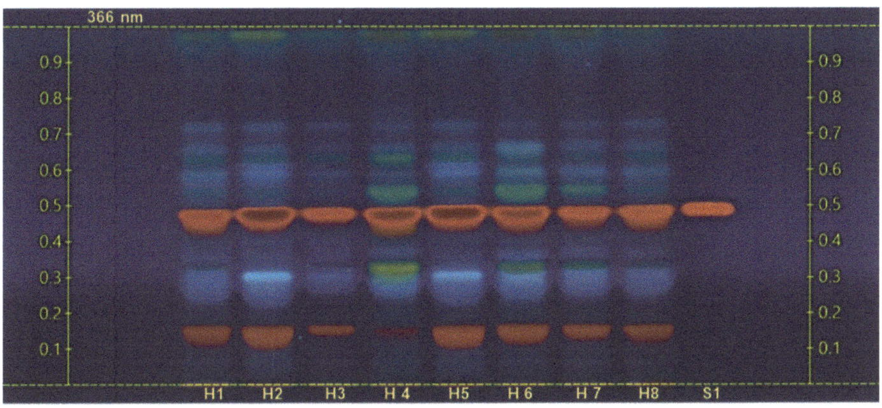

HPTLC plate of *Harpagophytum procumbens* methanol extracts (n = 8) (H1–H8) and the standard (S1). The samples are characterised by a brown band for harpagoside (S1) (R_f = 0.50), under 366 nm radiation.

10.2 Ultra-performance liquid chromatography (UPLC) analysis

General instrumentation: Waters Acquity Ultra-Performance Liquid Chromatography system with photodiode array (PDA) detector combined with Xevo G2QToF mass spectrometer (Waters, USA). *Plant part:* Secondary root tubers, methanol extract. *Sample application:* Injection volume of 2 μL (full-loop injection) at 1 mg/mL. *Column:* Acquity UPLC BEH C_{18} column (150 mm × 2.1 mm, i.d., 1.7 μm particle size, Waters). *Mobile phase:* 0.1% formic acid in water (solvent A) and acetonitrile (solvent B). *Analysis conditions:* Gradient elution at a flow rate of 0.3 mL/min, changing as follows: 85% A: 15% B, changed to 65% A: 35% B in 4 min, to 50% A: 50% B in 2 min, to 20% A: 80% B in 1 min, held for 1 min, back to initial ratio in 0.5 min, equilibrating the system for 1.5 min, total run time 10 min. *Mass spectrometry:* ESI^- (negative ionisation mode), N_2 used as the desolvation gas, desolvation temperature 350 °C at a flow rate of 500 L/h, source temperature 100 °C. Capillary and cone voltages 2800 and 30 V, respectively. Data was collected between *m/z* 100 and 1500.

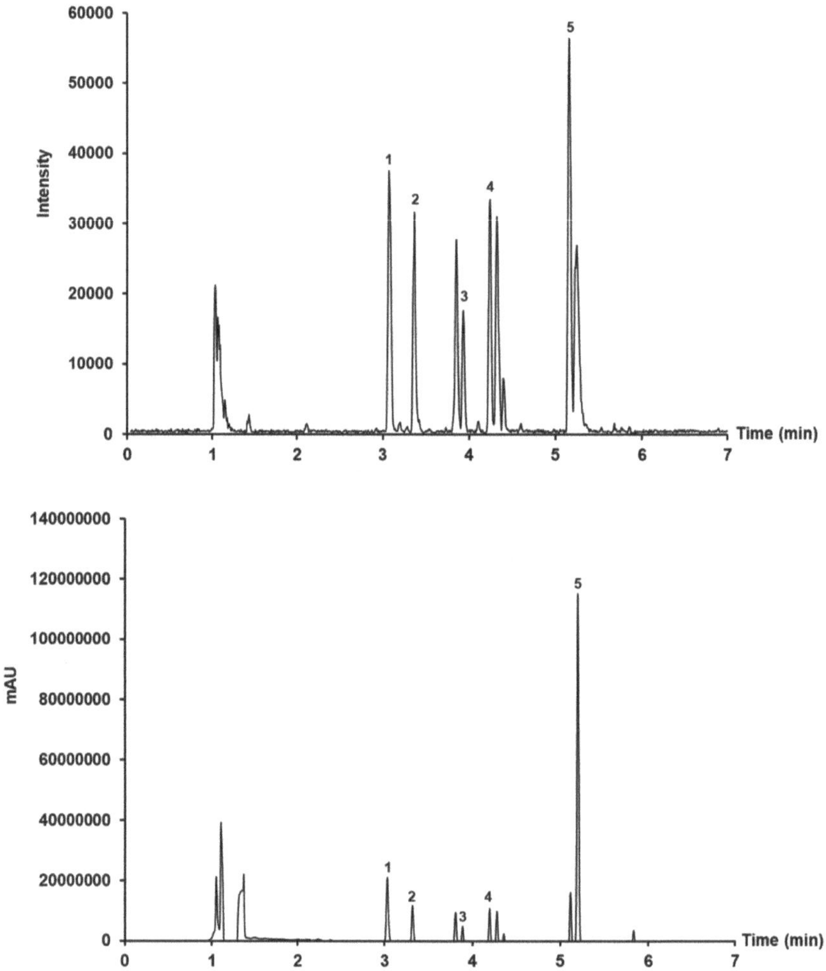

UPLC-ToF-MS ESI^- (upper) and PDA (lower) chromatograms of *Harpagophytum procumbens* methanol extract: [1] = acteoside (verbascoside) *m/z* 623.1990; [2] = isoacteoside (isoverbascoside) *m/z* 623.1970; [3] = 8-*O*-*p*-coumaroyl-harpagide *m/z* 509.1665; [4] = acetylacteoside *m/z* 665.2095; [5] = harpagoside *m/z* 493.1712.

11. Mid-infrared (MIR) spectroscopy analysis

General instrumentation: Alpha-P Bruker spectrometer, mounted with an attenuated total reflectance (ATR) diamond crystal. *Spectral acquisition:* Spectrum obtained in absorbance mode, with a spectral resolution of 4 cm^{-1} over the range 4000–550 cm^{-1} and captured using OPUS 6.5 software. *Plant part:* Secondary root tubers. *Sample preparation:* Secondary tubers are powdered, sieved (<500 μm) and placed directly onto the surface of the diamond crystal.

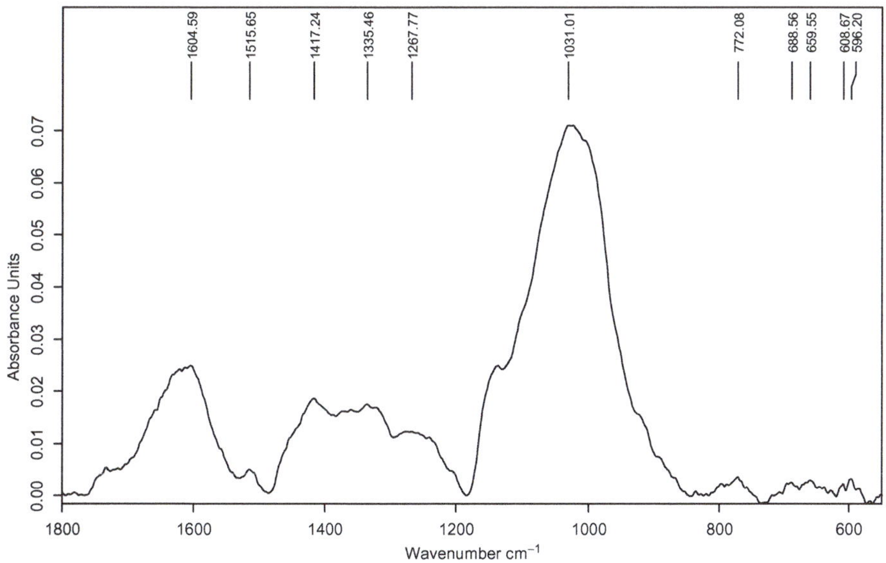

Mid-infrared spectrum of *Harpagophytum procumbens* powder displaying the fingerprint region (1800–550 cm^{-1}).

References

Abdelouahab, N., Heard, C.M., 2008. J. Nat. Prod., 71:746–749.

Aberham, A., Schwaiger, S., Stuppner, H., Ganzera, M., 2007. J. Pharm. Biomed. Anal., 45:437–442.

Ahmed, M.I., Afifi, M.I., Younos, I.H., 2005. Iran. J. Pharmacol. Ther., 4:54–63.

Almeida, M.C., Soares, S.F., Abreu, P.R., Jesus, L.M., Brito, L.C., Bernardo-Filho, M., 2007. Cell. Mol. Biol. (Noisy-le-Grand), 923–927. (53 Supply, OL).

Anauate, M.C., Torres, L.M., Veríssimo de Mello, S.B., 2010. Phytother. Res., 24 (9):1365–1369.

Andersen, M.L., Santos, E.H., de Seabra, M.L., Da Silva, A.A., Tufik, S., 2004. J. Ethnopharmacol., 91:325–330.

Bae, Y.H., Cuong, T.D., Hung, T.M., Kim, J.A., Woo, M.H., Byeon, J.S., Min, B.S., 2014. Arch. Pharm. Res., 37:1124–1129.

Baghdikian, B., Lanhers, M.C., Fleurentin, J., Ollivier, E., Maillard, C., Balansard, G., Mortier, F., 1997. Planta Med., 63:171–176.

Bermejo, P., Abad, M.J., Diaz, A.M., Fernandez, L., Santos, J.D., Sanchez, S., Villaescusa, L., Carrasco, L., Irurzun, A., 2002. Planta Med., 68:106–110.

Berthod, A., Maryutin, T., Spivakov, B., Shipgun, O., Sutherland, A.A., 2009. Pure Appl. Chem., 81:355–387.

Betancor-Fernandez, A., Perez-Galvea, A., Sies, H., Stahl, W., 2003. J. Pharm. Pharmacol., 55:981–986.

Bhattacharya, A., Bhattacharya, S., 1998. Br. J. Phytother., 5:68–71.

Biazi, B.I., D'Epiro, G.F.R., Zanetti, T.A., De Oliveira, M.T., Ribeiro, L.R., Mantovani, M.S., 2017. Phytother. Res., 31:387–394.

Boje, K., Lechtenberg, M., Nahrstedt, A., 2003. Planta Med., 69:820–825.

Brien, S., Lewith, G.T., McGregor, G., 2006. J. Altern. Complement. Med., 12:981–993.

Cameron, M., Gagnier, J.J., Little, C.V., Parsons, T.J., Blümle, A., Chrubasik, S., 2009. Phytother. Res., 23:1497–1515.

Catelan, S.C., Belentani, R.M., Marques, L.C., Silva, E.R., Silva, M.A., Caparroz-Assef, S.M., Cuman, R.K.N., Bersani-Amado, C.A., 2006. Phytomedicine, 13:446–451.

Chantre, P., Cappelaere, A., Leblan, D., Guedon, D., Vandermander, J., Fournie, B., 2000. Phytomedicine, 7:177–183.

Chen, C., Zhang, H., Xu, H., Xue, R., Zheng, Y., Wu, T., Lian, Y., 2018. J. Alzheimers Dis., 63:445–455.

Chrubasik, S., Junck, H., Breitschwerdt, H., Conradt, C., Zappe, H., 1999. Eur. J. Anaesthesiol., 16:118–129.

Chrubasik, J.E., Roufogalis, B.D., Chrubasik, S., 2007. Phytother. Res., 21:675–683.

Chung, H.J., Kyung Kim, W., Joo Park, H., Cho, L., Kim, M.R., Kim, M.J., Kook Lee, S., 2016. J. Ethnopharmacol., 179:66–75.

Chung, H.-J., Kim, W.K., Oh, J., Kim, M.-R., Shin, J.-S., Lee, J., Ha, I.-H., Lee, S.K., 2017. J. Nat. Prod., 80:434–442.

Chung, H.-J., Koh, W., Kim, W.K., Shin, J.-S., Lee, J., Lee, S.K., Ha, I.-H., 2018. Mediat. Inflamm., 2018, Art. No. 4514329.

Circosta, C., Occiuto, F., Ragusa, S., Trovato, A., Tumino, G., Briguglio, F., 1984. J. Ethnopharmacol., 11:259–274.

Clarkson, C., Campbell, W.E., Smith, P., 2003. Planta Med., 8:720–724.

Clarkson, C., Staerk, D., Hansen, S.H., Smith, P.J., Jaroszewski, J.W., 2006. J. Nat. Prod., 69:527–530.

Cole, D., 2003. The Impact of Certification on the Sustainable use of Devil's Claw (*Harpagophytum procumbens*) in Namibia. Non-Wood Forest Products Programme. Available at: http://foris.fao.org/static/pdf/NWFP/Namibia_devils_claw.pdf.

Costa De Pasquale, R., Busa, G., Circosta, C., Iauk, L., Ragusa, S., Ficarra, P., Occhiuto, F., 1985. J. Ethnopharmacol., 13:193–199.

Del Grossi, M.M., Lopes, L.C., Biavatti, M.W., Kennedy, S.A., De Oliveira, E., Silva, M.C., De Cássia Bergamaschi, C., 2017. Phytother. Res., 31:1676–1685.

Ebrahim, N., Uebel, R.A., 2011. Afr. J. Pharm. Pharmacol., 5:2209–2212.

EMEA (European Medicines Agency), 2009. Assessment Report on *Harpagophytum procumbens* DC. and/or *Harpagophytum zeyheri* Decne, Radix. Available at: http://www.ema.

europa.eu/docs/en_GB/document_library/Herbal_HMPC_assessment_report/2010/01/WC500059019.pdf.
Ernst, W.H.O., Tietema, T., Veenedaal, E.M., Nasene, R., 1988. J. Trop. Ecol., 4:185–198.
ESCOP (European Scientific Cooperative on Phytotherapy), 2003. Monography Harpagophyti radix. In: ESCOP (Ed.), Monographs on the Medicinal Uses of Plant Drugs. Centre of Complemetary Health Studies, University of Exeter, Exeter, UK, pp. 233–240.
Ferrante, C., Recinella, L., Locatelli, M., Guglielmi, P., Secci, D., Leporini, L., Orlando, G., 2017. Phytother. Res., 31:1257–1264.
Fiebich, B.L., Heinrich, M., Hiller, K.O., Kammerer, N., 2001. Phytomedicine, 8:28–30.
Fiebich, B.L., Muñoz, E., Rose, T., Weiss, G., McGregor, G.P., 2012. Phytother. Res., 26:806–811.
Frum, Y., Viljoen, A.M., 2006. Pharmacol. Physiol., 19:329–335.
Gagnier, J.J., Van Tulder, M.W., Bergman, B., Bombardier, C., 2007. Cochrane Collab., 32:82–92.
Georgiev, M., Alipieva, K., Pashova, S., Denev, P., Angelova, M., Kerns, G., Bley, T., 2010. Food Chem., 121:967–972.
Georgiev, M.I., Alipieva, K., Orhan, I.E., 2012. Phytother. Res., 26:313–316.
Göbel, H., Heinze, A., Ingwersen, M., Niederberger, U., Gerber, D., 2001. Schmerz, 15:10–18.
Grant, L., McBean, D.E., Fyfe, L., Warnock, A.M., 2009. Phytother. Res., 23:104–110.
Grote, K., 2003. The Increased Harvest and Trade of Devil's Claw (*Harpagophytum procumbens*) and Its Impacts on the Peoples and Environment of Namibia, Botswana and South Africa. Global Facilitation Unit for Underutilized Species, Italy. Available at: http://www.underutilized-species.org/documents/publications/devils_claw.pdfS.
Gruenwald, J., 2002. Expanding the market for Devil's Claw in Europe. In: Namibian National Devil's Claw Conference. Available at: http://www.criaasadc.org/pdf/DEVCLW_conf2002.PDF.
Gyurkovska, V., Alipieva, K., Maciuk, A., Dimitrova, P., Ivanovska, N., Haas, C., Bley, T., Georgiev, M., 2011. Food Chem., 125:171–178.
Hachfeld, F., Schippmann, U., 2002. Occurrence and density of *Harpagophytum procumbens* in Namibia and South Africa. In: Paper Presented at the Regional Devil's Claw Conference, Windhoek, Namibia, pp.157–163.
Haseeb, A., Ansari, M.Y., Haqqi, T.M., 2017. J. Orthop. Res., 35:311–320.
Hostanska, K., Melzer, J., Rostock, M., Suter, A., Saller, R., 2014. J. Pharm. Pharmacol., 66:1606–1614.
Huang, T.H.-W., Tran, V.H., Duke, R.K., Tan, S., Chrubasik, S., Roufogalis, B.D., Duke, C.C., 2006. J. Ethnopharmacol., 104:149–155.
Ibrahim, K.E., Al-Ashban, R.M., El-Sammani, S.A., 2010. Res. J. Pharmacol., 4:69–73.
Ihlenfeldt, H.D., Hartmann, H., 1970. Dié gattung *Harpagophytum* (Burch.) Devil's Claw ex Meissn (Monographie der afrikanischen Pedaliaceae II). Mitteilungen aus dem Institut für Allgemeine Botanik Hamburg, vol. 13, pp. 15–69.
Inaba, K., Murata, K., Naruto, S., Matsuda, H., 2010. J. Nat. Med., 64:219–222.
Jang, M.H., Lim, S., Han, S.M., Park, H.J., Shin, I., Kim, J.W., Kim, N.J., Lee, J.S., Kim, K.A., Kim, C.J., 2003. J. Pharmacol. Sci., 93:367–371.
Jeong, E.J., Lee, K.Y., Kim, S.H., Sung, S.H., Kim, Y.C., 2008. Europ. J. Pharmacol., 588:78–84.
Jian, W., Yu, S., Tang, M., Duan, H., Huang, J., 2016. J. Ethnopharmacol., 182:50–55.
Kaszkin, M., Becka, K.F., Kochb, E., Erdelmeierb, C., Kuscha, S., Pfeilschiftera, J., Loew, D., 2004. Phytomedicine, 11:585–595.

Kathe, W., Barch, F., Honnef, S., 2003. Trade in Devil's Claw (*Harpagophytum* spp.) in Germany—status, trends and certification. Prepared for the Food and Agriculture Organisation of the United Nations, Non-Wood Forest Products Programme, pp. 1–40. Available at: http://foris.fao.org/static/pdf/NWFP/Germany_devils_claw.pdf.

Kim, S.R., Lee, K.Y., Koo, K.A., Sung, S.H., Lee, N.G., Kim, J., Kim, Y.C., 2002. J. Nat. Prod., 65:1696–1699.

Kim, J.Y., Park, S.H., Baek, J.M., Erkhembaatar, M., Kim, M.S., Yoon, K.H., Lee, M.S., 2015. J. Nat. Prod., 78:2167–2174.

Kundu, J.K., Mossanda, K.S., Na, H.-K., Surh, Y.-J., 2005. Cancer Lett., 218:21–31.

Lai, N., Zhang, Z., Wang, B., Miao, X., Guo, Y., Yao, C., Jiang, G., 2015. J. Ethnopharmacol., 166:228–239.

Lall, N., Blom van Staden, A., Rademan, S., Lambrechts, I., De Canha, M.N., Mahore, J., Winterboer, S., Twilley, D., 2019. S. Afr. J. Bot., 126:241–249.

Langmead, L., Dawson, C., Hawkins, C., Banna, N., Loo, S., Rampton, D.S., 2002. Aliment. Pharmacol. Ther., 16:2.

Lanhers, M.-C., Fleurentin, J., Mortier, F., Vinche, A., Younos, C., 1992. Planta Med., 58:117–123.

Leblan, D., Chantre, P., Fournie, B., 2000. Joint Bone Spine, 67:462–467.

Li, J., Ding, X., Zhang, R., Jiang, W., Sun, X., Xia, Z., Hu, Y., 2015. Neuroscience, 303:103–114.

Lim, D.W., Kim, J.G., Han, D., Kim, Y.T., 2014. Molecules, 19:1060–1068.

Locatelli, M., Ferrante, C., Carradori, S., Secci, D., Leporini, L., Chiavaroli, A., Menghini, L., 2017. Phytother. Res., 31:937–944.

Loew, D., Möllerfeld, J., Schrödter, A., Puttkammer, S., Kaszkin, M., 2001. Clin. Pharmacol. Ther., 69:356–364.

Mahomed, I.M., Ojewole, J.A., 2004. Phytother. Res., 18:982–989.

Mahomed, I.M., Ojewole, J.A.O., 2005. Phytother. Res., 18:982–989.

Mahomed, I.M., Ojewole, J.A.O., 2006a. Afr. J. Tradit. Complement. Altern. Med., 3:82–89.

Mahomed, I.M., Ojewole, J.A.O., 2006b. Brain Res. Bull., 69:57–62.

Mahomed, I.M., Ojewole, J.A.O., 2009. J. Smooth Muscle Res., 45:231–239.

Mahomed, I.M., Nsabimana, A.M., Ojewole, J.A.O., 2005. Afr. J. Tradit. Complement. Altern. Med., 2:31–45.

Menghini, L., Leporini, L., Vecchiotti, G., Locatelli, M., Carradori, S., Ferrante, C., Orlando, G., 2018. Food Res. Int., 109:91–98.

Mncwangi, N., Chen, W., Vermaak, I., Viljoen, A.M., Gericke, N., 2012. J. Ethnopharmacol., 143:755–771.

Mncwangi, N.P., Viljoen, A.M., Zhao, J., Vermaak, I., Chen, W., Khan, I., 2014. Phytochemistry, 106:104–115.

Moatti, R., Fauron, R., Donadieu, Y., 1983. La phytothérapie. Librairie Maloine, Paris, France.

Moré, M., Gruenwald, J., Pohl, U., Uebelhack, R., 2017. Planta Med., 83:1384–1391.

Moussard, C., Alber, D., Toubin, M.M., Thevenon, N., Henry, J.C., 1992. Prostaglandins Leukot. Essent. Fat. Acids, 46:283–286.

Munkombwe, N.M., 2003. Phytochemistry, 62:1231–1234.

Muzila, M., Rumpunen, K., Wright, H., Roberts, H., Grant, M., Nybom, H., Sehic, J., Ekholm, A., Widén, C., 2016. Oxid. Med. Cell. Longev., 2016, Art. No. 3841803.

Na, H.K., Mossanda, K.S., Lee, J.Y., Surh, Y.J., 2004. Biofactors, 21:149–153.

Oltean, H., Robbins, C., Van Tulder, M.W., Berman, B.M., Bombardier, C., Gagnier, J.J., 2014. Cochrane Database Syst. Rev., 12, CD004504.

Ouitas, N.A., Heard, C.M., 2009. Int. J. Pharm., 376:63–68.
Parenti, C., Aricò, G., Chiechio, S., Di Benedetto, G., Parenti, R., Scoto, G.M., 2015. Molecules, 20:16758–16769.
Parenti, C., Aricò, G., Pennisi, M., Venditti, A., Scoto, G.M., 2016. Nat. Prod. Res., 30:1248–1255.
Qi, J., Zhou, J.-H., Chen, L., Chen, J.-J., Yu, B.-Y., Qiu, S.-X., 2006a. Chin. Pharm. J., 41:1613–1615.
Qi, J., Chen, J.-J., Cheng, Z.-H., Zhou, J.-H., Yu, B.-Y., Qiu, S., 2006b. Phytochemistry, 67:1372–1377.
Qi, J., Chen, J.-J., Tu, Y., Chen, L., Yu, B.-Y., 2007. Chin. J. Nat. Med., 5:105–107.
Qi, J., Li, N., Zhou, J.-H., Yu, B.-Y., Qiu, S.X., 2010. Planta Med., 76:1892–1896.
Rabovsky, A.B., Ivie, J., Nielson, S., 2011. Dietary Supplements and Methods for Treating Pain and Inflammation. US Patent 20110038962 A1.
Rahimi, A., Razmkhah, K., Mehrnia, M., Mohamadnia, A., Sahebjamee, H., Salehi, S., Asl, E.A., Tahmasebi, H., Shandiz, S.A.S., Davouodbeglou, F., Ghasemi, S., Ardalan, N., Kordkandi, Z.G., 2016. Asian Pac. J. Trop. Dis., 6:227–231.
Raimondo, D., Fell, C., Donaldson, J., Newton, D., Dickson, B., 2003. Devil's Claw in South Africa: Conservation and Livelihood Issues. Whitley Laing Foundation for International Nature Conservation. Available at: https://cites.org/sites/default/files/ eng/com/pc/14/E-PC14-06-02.pdf.
Ridgway, R., Krugmann, H., 2011. Indigenous Natural Products Producer and Processor Organisations Sub-Activity EIA for Devil's Claw Report Reference Number 5a. Available at: https://www.nbri.org.na/sites/default/files/Devil%27s%20Claw%20-%20Environmental%20Impact%20Assessment.pdf.
Saleh, S., Jahromi, H.K., Jahromi, Z.K., Kamfiruzi, S., Zahediniya, F., 2018. Asian J. Pharm., 12:S170–S172.
Schaffer, L.F., Peroza, L.R., Boligon, A.A., Athayde, M.L., Alves, S.H., Fachinetto, R., Wagner, C., 2013. Neurochem. Res., 38:2256–2267.
Schopohl, P., Grüneberg, P., Melzig, M.F., 2016. Fitoterapia, 110:157–165.
Schulze-Tanzil, G., Hansen, C., Shakibaei, M., 2004. Arzneimittelforschung, 54:213–220.
Seger, C., Godejohann, M., Tseng, L.-H., Spraul, M., Girtler, A., Sturm, S., Stuppner, H., 2005. Anal. Chem., 77:878–885.
Shikhman, A.R., 2010. Compositions Containing Harpagoside and Peaoniflorin and Methods for Treatment of Conditions Associated With Pain, Inflammation, Arthritis and Symptoms Thereof. US Patent 2010/0261663 A1.
Steenkamp, P.A., Steenkamp, L.H., 2019. S. Afr. J. Bot., 124:138–143.
Stewart, K.M., Cole, D., 2005. J. Ethnopharmacol., 100:225–236.
Strobach, M., Cole, D., 2007. Population Dynamics and Sustainable Harvesting of the Medicinal Plant Harpagophytum procumbens in Namibia. BfN—Skripten 203 Budesamt fur Naturschutz (BfN), Germany. Available at: http://www.bfn.de/fileadmin/MDB/documents/service/skript203.pdfS.
Sun, X., Xiong, Z., Zhang, Y., Meng, Y., Xu, G., Xia, Z., Hu, Y., 2012. J. Neurochem., 120: 1072–1083.
Szczepanski, L., Chudzik, D., Mazurek, M., Soroka, P., 2000. Reumatologia, 38:67–73.
Tomassini, L., Serafini, M., Foddai, S., Ventrone, A., Nicoletti, M., 2016. Nat. Prod. Res., 30:157–161.
Torres-Fuentes, C., Theeuwes, W.F., McMullen, M.K., McMullen, A.K., Dinan, T.G., Cryan, J.F., Schellekens, H., 2014. PLoS ONE, 9 (7), Art. No. e103118.

Uchida, S., HiraiI, K., Hatanaka, J., Hanato, J., Umegaki, K., Yamada, S., 2008. Biol. Pharm. Bull., 31:240–245.
Ucuncu, Y., Celik, N., Ozturk, C., Turkoglu, M., Cetin, N., Kockara, N., Suleyman, H., 2015. Life Sci., 130:31–37.
Ungerer, G., Cui, J., Ndam, T., Bekemeier, M., Song, H., Li, R., Siedhoff H.R., Yang, B., Appenteng, M.K., Greenlief, C.M., Miller, D.K., Sun, G.Y., Folk, W.R., Gu, Z., 2020. Neuromolecular Med., 22:278–292.
Van den Eynden, V., Vernemmen, P., Van Damme, P., 1992. The Ethnobotany of the Topnaar. Universiteit Gent, Commission of the European Community. Available at: http://the-eis.com/elibrary/sites/default/files/downloads/literature/The%20ethnobotany%20of%20the%20topnaar.pdf.
Van Wyk, B.-E., 2008. J. Ethnopharmacol., 119:342–355.
Van Wyk, B.-E., Gericke, N., 2000. People's Plants: A Guide to Useful Plants of Southern Africa. Briza Publications, Pretoria, South Africa.
Van Wyk, B.-E., Van Oudtshoorn, B., Gericke, N., 1997. Medicinal Plants of South Africa. Briza Publications, Pretoria, South Africa.
Vlachojannis, J., Roufogalis, B.D., Chrubasik, S., 2008. Phytother. Res., 22:149–152.
Von Koenen, E., 1996. Edition Namibia 2 Heil-, Gift- und esβare Pflanzen in Namibia. Klaus Hess Verlag, Gottingen, Germany.
Von Willert, D.J., Sanders, J., 2004. Devil's claw: conservation through cultivation – results of worldwide ecological studies. In: Breckle, S.W., Schweizer, B., Fangmeier, A. (Eds.), Proceedings of the Second Symposium of the A.S.W. Schimper Foundation, pp. 27–44.
Wachsmuth, L., Lindhorst, E., Wrubel, S., Hadzhiyski, H., Hudelmaier, M., Eckstein, F., Chrubasik, S., 2011. Phytother. Res., 25:1133–1140.
Warnock, M., McBean, D., Suter, A., Tan, J., Whittaker, P., 2007. Phytother. Res., 21:1228–1233.
Watt, J.M., Breyer-Brandwijk, M.G., 1962. The Medicinal and Poisonous Plants of Southern and Eastern Africa, second ed. E. & S. Livingstone Ltd, Edinburgh and London, UK.
Weckesser, S.E., Simon-Haarhaus, K.B., Wittmer, A., Pelz, K., Schempp, C.M., 2007. Phytomedicine, 14:508–516.
Wegener, T., Lüpke, N.-P., 2003. Phytother. Res., 17:1165–1172.
Wynberg, R., 2004. Achieving a fair and sustainable trade in Devil's Claw (*Harpagophytum* spp.) In: Sunderland, T., Ndoye, O. (Eds.), Forest Products, Livelihoods and Conservation: Case Studies of Non-Timber Forest Product Systems. Volume 2 – Africa. Centre for International Forestry Research, Indonesia.

CHAPTER

Helichrysum odoratissimum 10

Khotso Serabele, Weiyang Chen and Sandra Combrinck
Department of Pharmaceutical Sciences, Tshwane University of Technology, Pretoria, South Africa

Abstract

Helichrysum odoratissimum (L.) Sweet (Asteraceae), also known as 'African incense', 'kooigoed' and 'imphepho' is a perennial herb that reaches 1.75 m in height. The plant has a silver appearance and bears pale golden-yellow flowers. It is abundant throughout southern Africa, where it is one of the most popular traditional remedies. It occurs in six provinces of South Africa, from sea level to altitudes of over 3000 m above sea level. Helichrysum odoratissimum is of great cultural significance in South Africa. The aerial parts are burnt to rebuke evil spirits, or inhaled as a steam to attract good luck. Medicinal uses include the treatment of heart diseases, relief of chest pains, and for calming. Furthermore, H. odoratissimum is used to treat coughs, fever and urinary tract infections, suggesting that it possesses antimicrobial properties. Helichrysum odoratissimum is one of the most frequently harvested and traded plants in South Africa, with potential for commercialisation. The chemical profiles of individual plants harvested from different locations were obtained using semi-automated high-performance thin-layer chromatography (HPTLC) and ultra-performance liquid chromatography coupled to mass spectrometry (UPLC–MS). Mid-infrared (MIR) spectroscopy analysis was performed to obtain a characteristic spectrum. 4,5-Dicaffeoylquinic acid was isolated as a marker compound, and its presence confirmed in samples through HPTLC and UPLC–MS analysis.

Keywords: *Helichrysum odoratissimum*, Imphepho, Everlasting, Aerial parts, Smoke inhalants, HPTLC, UPLC–MS, MIR spectroscopy, 4,5-Dicaffeoylquinic acid

The South African Herbal Pharmacopoeia. https://doi.org/10.1016/B978-0-323-99794-2.00013-1

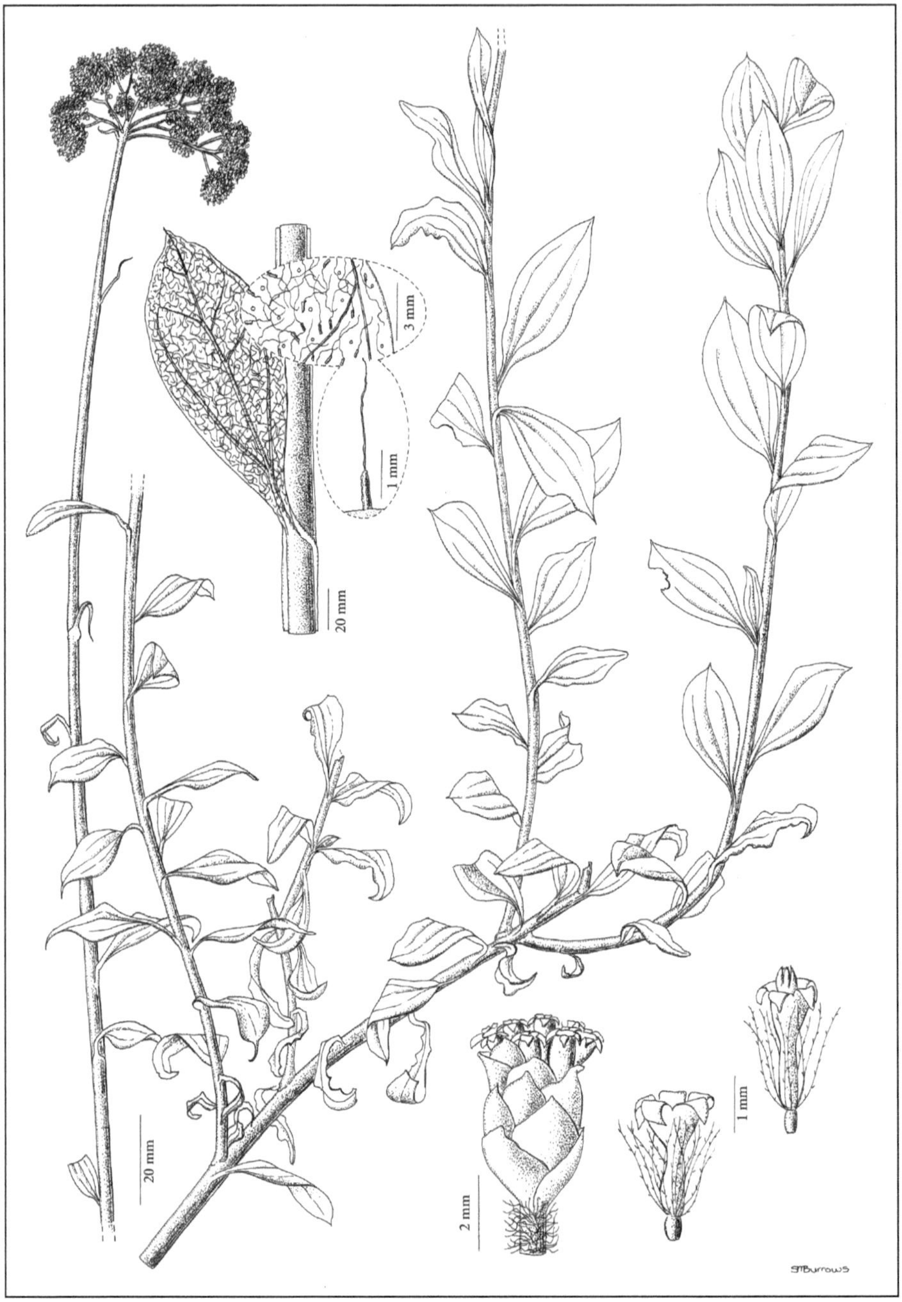
3 mm
1 mm
20 mm
20 mm
2 mm
1 mm

Part A: General overview

1. Synonyms

Gnaphalium odoratissimum L., *Helichrysum odoratissimum* var. *odoratissimum, Helichrysum odoratissimum* (L.) Sweet var. *lanatum* Sond.[a,b]

2. Common name(s)

African incense, our incense, everlasting (English) (Van Wyk et al., 2000); *'Imphepho'* (isiXhosa/isiZulu), *'phefo-ea-setlolo'*, *'tooane'* (Sesotho), *'kooigoed'*, *'hottentotskruie'*, *'hotnotskooigoed'*, *'hottentotskooigoed'* (Afrikaans).[a]

3. Conservation status

Least concern.[a]

4. Botany

Helichrysum odoratissimum is a strongly aromatic perennial herb. The name refers to the intense fragrance of the crushed leaves. Plants reach heights of 0.2–1.75 m. The species is characterised by white-woolly, erect or straggling, winged branches and leaves that have a silver appearance and are generally woolly on both surfaces (A). The leaves are described as linear oblong, with an obtuse apex (Van Wyk and Gericke, 2000). A multitude of pale golden-yellow, small flower heads (B) are borne between August and December in winter rainfall areas, and from January to June in summer rainfall regions. The seeds have a dull brown colour. The four species (*H. odoratissimum*, *Helichrysum petiolare, Helichrysum cymosum* and *Helichrysum nudifolium*) are collectively referred to as *'Imphepho'* (Van Wyk et al., 2000).

[a] The Red List of South African Plants (http://redlist.sanbi.org).
[b] World Flora Online (http://www.worldfloraonline.org).

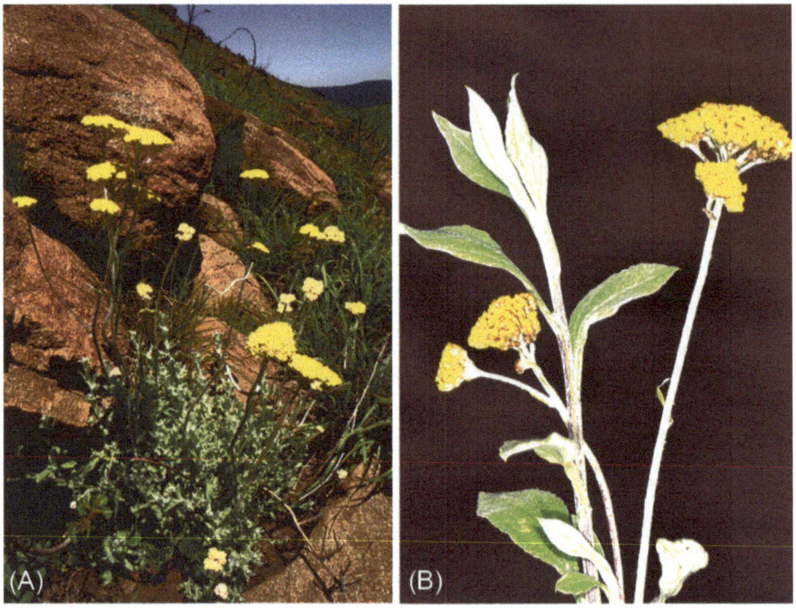

Helichrysum odoratissimum shrub in natural habitat (A) with white-woolly and erect branches that bear silvery leaves (B) and small golden-yellow flowers at the tips.

5. Geographical distribution

Helichrysum odoratissimum is not endemic to South Africa. It is widely distributed throughout southern Africa from sea level to altitudes of over 3000 m above sea level. The species occurs abundantly in Swaziland, Lesotho and in the

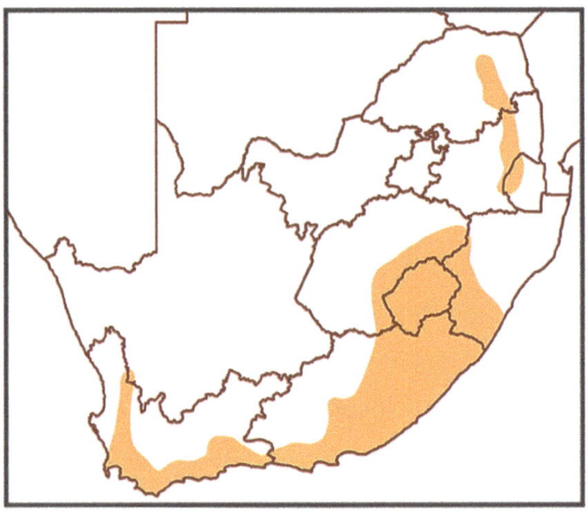

Geographical distribution of *Helichrysum odoratissimum* in South Africa.

Limpopo, Mpumalanga, the Free State, KwaZulu-Natal, and Western Cape and Eastern Cape provinces of South Africa (Germishuizen et al., 2006). It also grows in the mountainous regions of Mozambique, Zambia and Zimbabwe (Van Wyk et al., 2000).

6. Ethnopharmacology

The leaves of *H. odoratissimum* are burnt to rebuke evil spirits, or inhaled as a steam to promote good fortune (Cocks and Møller, 2002). Sometimes the stems and leaves are chewed, or are placed under the pillow to relieve bad dreams (Hutchings, 2007). Medicinal uses of *H. odoratissimum* include the treatment of heart diseases, relief of chest pains, stress reduction, and for alleviating hypertension, anxiety and overexcitement (Olorunnisola et al., 2011). *Helichrysum odoratissimum* possibly contains antimicrobial compounds, as it is used to treat coughs and colds, catarrh, headaches, fever and urinary tract infections (Lall and Meyer, 1999; Lourens et al., 2008; Heyman et al., 2015). It is also used to treat menstrual disorders. Wounds are normally dressed by applying a poultice prepared from the leaves to enhance healing and prevent infections (Kuiate et al., 1999; Lourens et al., 2008). The whole plant is crushed and boiled, and the resulting decoction is taken orally to treat diabetes (Erasto et al., 2005). *Helichrysum odoratissimum* is used interchangeably with *H. petiolare* and the species used is determined primarily by availability, rather than by preference (Van Vuuren et al., 2014).

7. Commercialisation

Although *H. odoratissimum* has not been formally commercialised, it is one of the most frequently harvested and traded plants in South African herbal shops (Dold and Cocks, 2002). The high demand for the plant indicates that it is a suitable candidate for commercialisation. Van Wyk (2011) described *H. odoratissimum* as a plant of high prominence with regard to its historic and current use, and the potential to be developed as a commercial medicinal plant in South Africa.

8. Pharmacological evaluation

8.1 *In vitro* studies

Antimicrobial studies involving *H. odoratissimum* have been carried out using the micro-dilution assay (Eloff, 1998). The acetone extract of *H. odoratissimum* was found to have noteworthy antimicrobial activity against Gram-positive bacteria with a minimum inhibitory concentration (MIC) of 0.01 mg/mL (Mathekga and Meyer, 1998). Hexane extracts exhibited better activity, with MICs ranging from 0.125 to 0.5 mg/mL, as compared to the methanol extract (MICs 0.5–1 mg/mL) against three Gram-positive bacteria and one Gram-negative bacterium (Ocheng et al., 2014). An acetone extract of *H. odoratissimum* also displayed moderate activity (MIC 0.5 mg/mL) towards *Mycobacterium tuberculosis* (Lall and Meyer, 1999). A flavonoid isolated from *H. odoratissimum* proved to be active against a wide range of micro-organisms, including Gram-negative bacteria (MIC 0.050 mg/mL), Gram-positive bacteria (MIC 0.00625 mg/mL) and fungi (MIC 0.0125 mg/mL) (Lourens et al., 2008). Serabele et al. (2021) investigated the antimicrobial activity of *H. odoratissimum* against pathogens causing respiratory and gastro-intestinal ailments. *Escherichia coli* was found to be the most susceptible pathogen (MIC 0.063 mg/mL), whilst moderate activity (average MIC of 0.786 mg/mL) was obtained against the respiratory tract pathogens, *Moraxella catarrhalis* and *Streptococcus agalactiae*.

8.2 *In vivo* studies and clinical trials

A volatile monoterpene component of *H. odoratissimum*, 1,8-cineole, was reported to reduce inflammation by up to 62% in trinitrobenzene sulphonic acid-induced colitis rats (De Cássia da Silveira e Sá et al., 2013). An aqueous leaf extract of *H. odoratissimum* induced hypoglycaemic activity of up to 75% (similar to that of insulin) in the management of diabetes mellitus in alloxan-induced diabetic mice (Njagi et al., 2015).

8.3 Safety

No toxicity studies have been reported for *H. odoratissimum*.

9. Phytochemistry

9.1 Volatile constituents

Essential oil constituents of *H. odoratissimum* from Zimbabwe were identified using gas chromatography–mass spectrometry (GC–MS) by Gundidza and Zwaving (1993). The oils comprised 66% sesquiterpenes and 31% monoterpenes. The major compounds were identified as α-pinene (15.0%), α-humulene (13.0%), β-caryophyllene (9.6%), elemol (8.7%), β-himachalene (8.2%), 1,8-cineole (7.7%), limonene (3.6%), δ-cadinene (2.0%), valencene (1.9%), β-caryophyllene epoxide (1.5%), ledene (1.2%), α-curcumene (1.2%), β-pinene (1.2%) and β-cedrene (1.1%). Kuiate et al. (1999) reported the major constituents of essential oils from *H. odoratissimum* growing in Cameroon as α-pinene (47.0%), α-curcumene (20.3%), β-caryophyllene (14%), δ-cadinene (5.8%), α-humulene (4.9%), (*Z*)-β-ocimene (2.7%), germacrene-D (2.6%), valencene (2.3%), (*E*)-β-farnesene (2.1%), β-bisabolene (2.0%) and T-cadinol (1.8%), indicating intraspecies variation. α-Pinene (43.4%), (*E,E*)-farnesol (16.8%) and α-humulene (14.6%) were identified as major constituents of essential oils isolated from flowers of *H. odoratissimum* growing in Kenya (Lwande et al., 1993). The essential oil extracted from fresh plants of *H. odoratissimum* grown in South Africa (Asekun et al., 2007) was characterised by oxygenated monoterpenes such as *p*-menthone (35.4%), pulegone (34.2%) and 1,8-cineole (13.0%). The essential oil of flowers studied in this work confirmed the presence of 1,8-cineole. High concentrations of α-pinene (18.4%) were determined herein, together with those of germacrene A (10.7%), β-caryophyllene (9.7%), δ-cadinene (9.7%), bifloratriene (7.4%) and α-himachalene (5.3%).

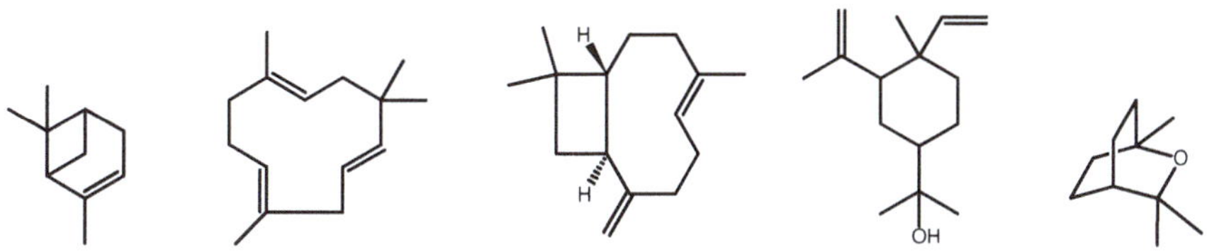

α-Pinene α-Humulene β-Caryophyllene Elemol 1,8-Cineole

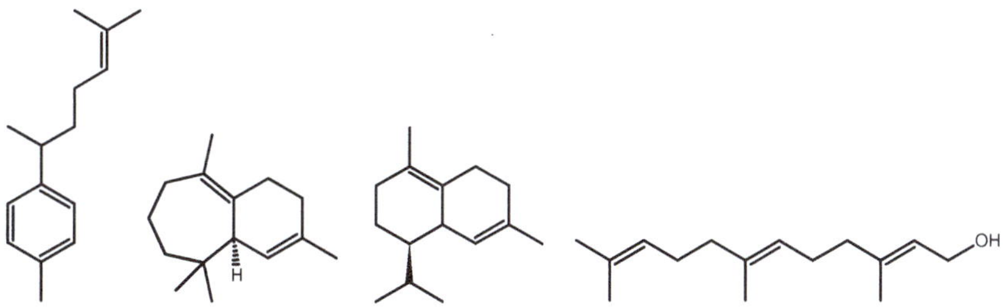

α-Curcumene β-Himachalene δ-Cadinene (*E,E*)-Farnesol

9.2 Non-volatile constituents

Van Puyvelde et al. (1989) isolated two flavonoids, namely 3,5-dihydroxy-6,7,8-trimethoxyflavone and 3-*O*-methylquercetin, and one chalcone, helichrysetin ((*E*)-1-(2,4-dihydroxy-6-methoxyphenyl)-3-(4-hydroxyphenyl)-2-Oropen-1-one). The flavonoid, 3,5-dihydroxy-6,7,8-trimethoxyflavone, was isolated from a petroleum ether extract in 0.38% yield as yellow-brown crystals, whilst helichrysetin was isolated from the methanol extract as yellow-orange crystals (0.48% yield).

Following optimisation of the extracting solvent, aqueous methanol extracts of the aerial parts of 12 *H. odoratissimum* and 15 *H. petiolare* samples, representing several wild populations, were analysed using ultra-performance liquid chromatography coupled to mass spectrometry (UPLC–MS). Chemometric modelling of the aligned UPLC–MS data indicated that the two species could be distinguished by their chemical profiles. Within the *H. odoratissimum* samples, a large degree of interpopulation variation in the chemistry was evident, with the samples loosely clustered into two main groups. Discriminant analysis revealed four distinguishing marker compounds for each species. 4,5-Dicaffeoylquinic acid was isolated from *H. odoratissimum* and identified using nuclear magnetic resonance (NMR) spectroscopy. It represented one of the three isomeric compounds common to both species. The concentration of the compound was highly variable and ranged from 3.89 to 31.1 μg/g in *H. odoratissimum* and from 2.3 to 13.4 μg/g in *H. petiolare*. The chemical variation within *H. odoratissimum* was also reflected by high-performance thin-layer chromatography (HPTLC) fingerprints of the individual sample extracts.

Helichrysum odoratissimum and *H. petiolare* are both used as smoke inhalants during traditional rites (Lourens et al., 2008). Five major compounds in the UPLC profiles of smoke condensates of the two species, obtained under controlled conditions, were common to both species (Serabele et al., 2021). Four compounds were present in the photodiode array (PDA) profile, whilst the fifth compound was only visible in the MS profile. The five corresponding compounds in the smoke condensates of the two species offer an explanation for their interchangeable use as smoke inhalants. This finding should be investigated further, since most of the compounds present in the solvent extracts of the two species were different, yet the smoke condensates were similar.

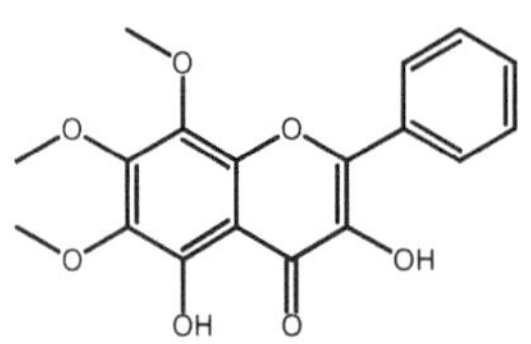

3,5-Dihydroxy-6,7,8-trimethoxyflavone

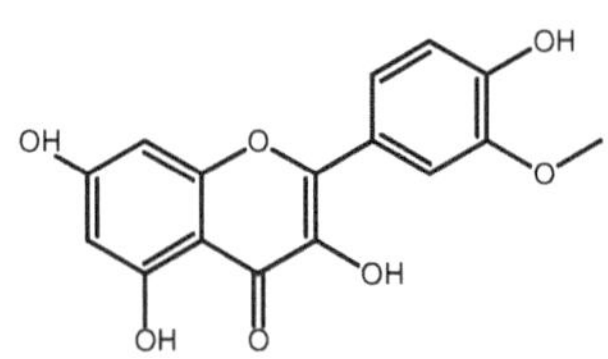

3-*O*-Methylquercetin

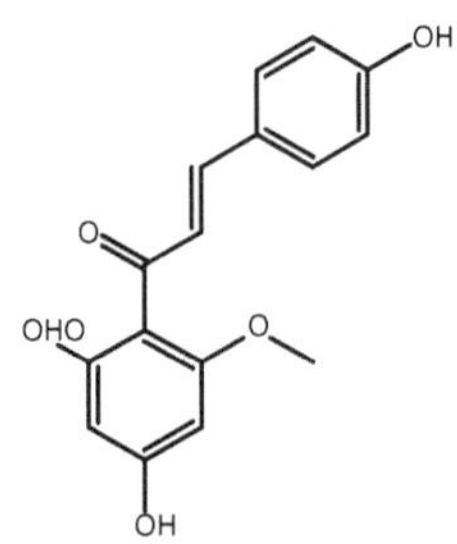

Helichrysetin

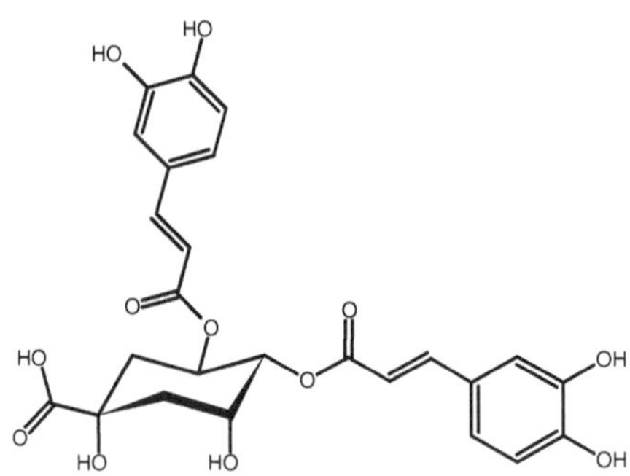

4,5-Dicaffeoylquinic acid

Part B: Chemical profiling and quality control

10. Chromatography analysis

10.1 High-performance thin-layer chromatography (HPTLC) fingerprint analysis

General instrumentation: CAMAG HPTLC instrument consisting of an automatic TLC sampler (ATS 4), automatic developing chamber (ADC 2), CAMAG TLC visualiser 2, CAMAG derivatiser, and TLC plate heater. *HPTLC plates*: Silica gel glass plates 60 F_{254} (Merck). *Plant part*: Aerial parts, methanol:water extract (80:20, v/v). *Sample application*: Application volume of 10 µL methanol extract (10 mg/mL) and standard (1 mg/mL) spotted as 10 mm bands. Plates developed in a 20 × 10 × 4 cm glass twin-trough chamber to a migration distance of 85 mm. *Tank saturation*: 20 min at 15 °C and 33% RH, with 25 mL of mobile phase. *Mobile phase*: Ethyl acetate:formic acid:acetic acid:water (100:11:11:27, v/v/v/v). *Derivatisation*: Natural Product reagent followed by polyethylene glycol reagent. The plate was heated for 3 min at 100 °C on a TLC plate heater sprayed with 3 mL of the reagent mixture and then visualised. *Visualisation*: The plate was viewed under 366 nm radiation.

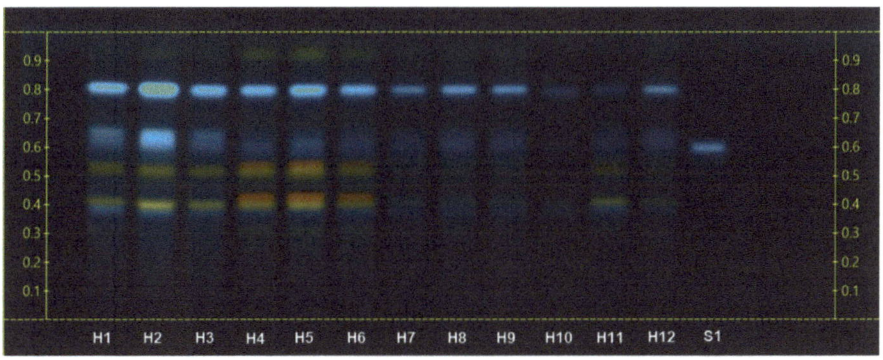

HPTLC plate of *Helichrysum odoratissimum* methanol:water extracts (n = 12) (H1–H12) and the standard (S1). The samples are characterised by a blue fluorescent band of 4,5-dicaffeoylquinic acid (S1) (R_f = 0.60).

10.2 Ultra-performance liquid-chromatography (UPLC) analysis

General instrumentation: Waters Acquity Ultra-Performance Liquid Chromatography system with photodiode array (PDA) detector combined with Xevo G2QToF mass spectrometer (Waters, United States). *Plant part*: Aerial parts, methanol:water (80:20, v/v) extract. *Sample application*: Injection volume: 1.0 µL (full-loop injection) at 1 mg/mL. *Column:* Acquity UPLC HSS T3 column (150 mm × 2.1 mm, i.d., 1.8 µm particle size, Waters). *Mobile phase*: 0.1% formic acid in water (solvent A) and acetonitrile (solvent B). *Analysis conditions*: Gradient elution at a flow rate of 0.3 mL/min, changing as follows: 90% A: 10% B changed to 65% A: 35% B in 6 min, to 35% A: 65% B in 4 min, to 5% A: 95% B in 4.5 min, held for 1 min, back to initial ratio in 0.5 min, equilibrating the system for 2 min, total run time 18 min. *Mass spectrometry*: ESI$^-$ (negative ionisation mode), N_2 used as the desolvation gas, desolvation temperature 350 °C at a flow rate of 500 L/h, and source temperature 100 °C. Capillary and cone voltages 2500 and 45 V, respectively. Data collected between *m/z* 100 and 1500.

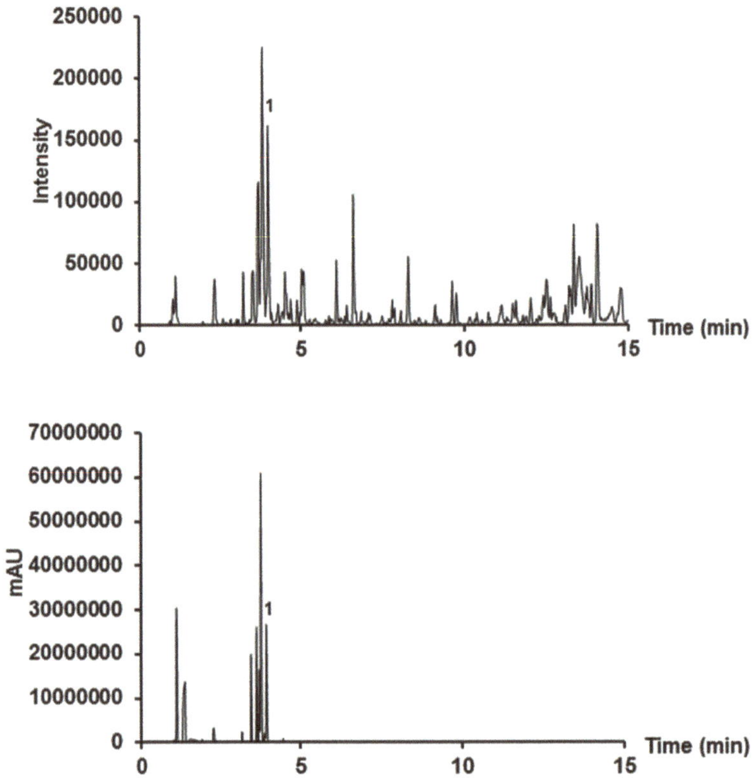

UPLC–ToF–MS ESI$^-$ (upper) and PDA (lower) chromatograms of *Helichrysum odoratissimum* methanol:water extracts. [1] = 4,5-dicaffeoylquinic acid (*m/z* 515.1312).

11. Mid-infrared (MIR) spectroscopy analysis

General instrumentation: Alpha-P Bruker spectrometer, mounted with an attenuated total reflectance (ATR) diamond crystal. *Spectral acquisition*: Spectrum obtained in absorbance mode, with a spectral resolution of 4 cm^{-1} over the range 4000–550 cm^{-1} and captured using OPUS 6.5 software. *Plant part*: Aerial parts.

Sample preparation: Aerial parts powdered, sieved (<500 μm) and placed directly onto the surface of the diamond crystal.

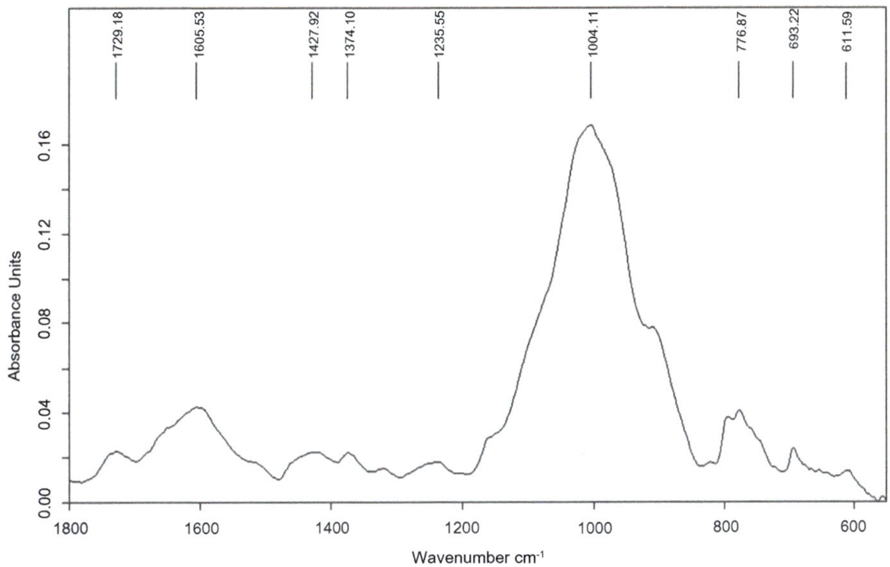

Mid-infrared spectrum of *Helichrysum odoratissimum* powder displaying the fingerprint region (1800–550 cm^{-1}).

References

Asekun, O.T., Grierson, D.S., Afolayan, A.J., 2007. J. Appl. Sci., 7:1005–1008.

Cocks, M., Møller, V., 2002. Soc. Sci. Med., 54:387–397.

De Cássia da Silveira e Sá, R., Andrade, L.N., De Sousa, D.P., 2013. Molecules, 18:1227–1254.

Dold, A.P., Cocks, M.L., 2002. S. Afr. J. Sci., 98:589.

Eloff, J.N., 1998. Planta Med., 64:711–713.

Erasto, P., Adebola, P.O., Grierson, D.S., Afolayan, A.J., 2005. Afr. J. Biotechnol., 4:1458–1460.

Germishuizen, G., Meyer, N.L., Steenkamp, Y., Keith, M. (Eds.), 2006. A Checklist of South African Plants. Southern African Botanical Diversity Network, No. 41, Pretoria, South Africa.

Gundidza, M.G., Zwaving, J.H., 1993. J. Essent. Oil Res., 5:341–343.

Heyman, H.M., Senejoux, F., Seibert, I., Klimkait, T., Maharaj, V.J., Meyer, J.J.M., 2015. Fitoterapia, 103:155–164.

Hutchings, A., 2007. Alternation, 14:189–218.

Kuiate, J.R., Amvam Zollo, P.H., Nguefa, E.H., Bessière, J.M., Lamaty, G., Menut, C., 1999. Flavour Fragr. J., 14:82–84.

Lall, N., Meyer, J.J.M., 1999. J. Ethnopharmacol., 66:347–354.

Lourens, A.C.U., Viljoen, A.M., Van Heerden, F.R., 2008. J. Ethnopharmacol., 119:630–652.

Lwande, W., Hassanali, A., Wanyama, O.B., Ngola, S., Mwangi, J.W., 1993. J. Essent. Oil Res., 5:93–95.

Mathekga, A.D.M., Meyer, J.J.M., 1998. S. Afr. J. Bot., 64:293–295.
Njagi, J.M., Ngugi, M.P., Kibiti, C.M., Ngeranwa, J., Njue, W.N., Gathumbi, P., Njagi, E.N., 2015. J. Pharmacol., 4:30–33.
Ocheng, F., Bwanga, F., Joloba, M., Borg-Karlson, A.K., Gustafsson, A., Obua, C., 2014. J. Ethnopharmacol., 155:852–855.
Olorunnisola, O.S., Bradley, G., Afolayan, A.J., 2011. J. Med. Plant Res., 5:4256–4260.
Serabele, K., Chen, W., Tankeu, S., Combrinck, S., Veale C.G.L., Van Vuuren, S., Chaudhary, S.K., Viljoen A., 2021. S. Afr. J. Bot., 137:117–132.
Van Puyvelde, L., De Kimpe, N., Costa, J., Munyjabo, V., Nyirankuliza, S., Hakizamungu, E., Schamp, N., 1989. J. Nat. Prod., 52:629–633.
Van Vuuren, S., Williams, V.L., Sooka, A., Burger, A., Van der Haar, L., 2014. S. Afr. J. Bot., 94:95–100.
Van Wyk, B.E., 2011. S. Afr. J. Bot., 77:812–829.
Van Wyk, B.-E., Gericke, N., 2000. People's Plants. A Guide to Useful Plants of Southern Africa. Briza Publications, Pretoria, South Africa.
Van Wyk, B.E., Van Oudtshoorn, B., Gericke, N., 2000. Medicinal Plants of South Africa. Briza Publications, Pretoria, South Africa.

CHAPTER

Helichrysum petiolare

11

Khotso Serabele, Sandra Combrinck and Weiyang Chen

Department of Pharmaceutical Sciences, Tshwane University of Technology, Pretoria, South Africa

Abstract

Helichrysum petiolare Hilliard & B.L.Burtt (Asteraceae), also known as 'African incense', 'kooigoed', and 'imphepho', is a perennial plant of 0.3–1 m in height, with round aromatic leaves that are tightly matted with hairs. The shrub occurs in the Western and Eastern Cape provinces of South Africa. The plant is burnt as incense to invoke the ancestors during cultural rites. Medicinal uses include the treatment of coughs, colds, catarrh, headache, fever, menstrual disorders and urinary tract infections. The species is used interchangeably with Helichrysum odoratissimum. Although H. petiolare is widely traded and used traditionally, there are no commercial products available. The phytochemistry of the plant remains largely unexplored. This monograph is a summary of the available literature on the plant. Semi-automated high-performance thin-layer chromatography (HPTLC) and ultra-performance liquid chromatography coupled to mass spectrometry (UPLC–MS) were used to obtain the chemical profiles of H. petiolare. Mid-infrared (MIR) spectroscopy analysis was used to establish a characteristic spectrum for the powdered material. A marker compound, which was present in all the H. petiolare samples, was identified as 4,5-dicaffeoylquinic acid and is visible on the HPTLC plates and on the UPLC–MS chromatograms.

Keywords: *Helichrysum petiolare*, Imphepho, Kooigoed, African incense, Leaves, Smoke inhalants, HPTLC, UPLC–MS, MIR spectroscopy, 4,5-Dicaffeoylquinic acid

The South African Herbal Pharmacopoeia. https://doi.org/10.1016/B978-0-323-99794-2.00021-0

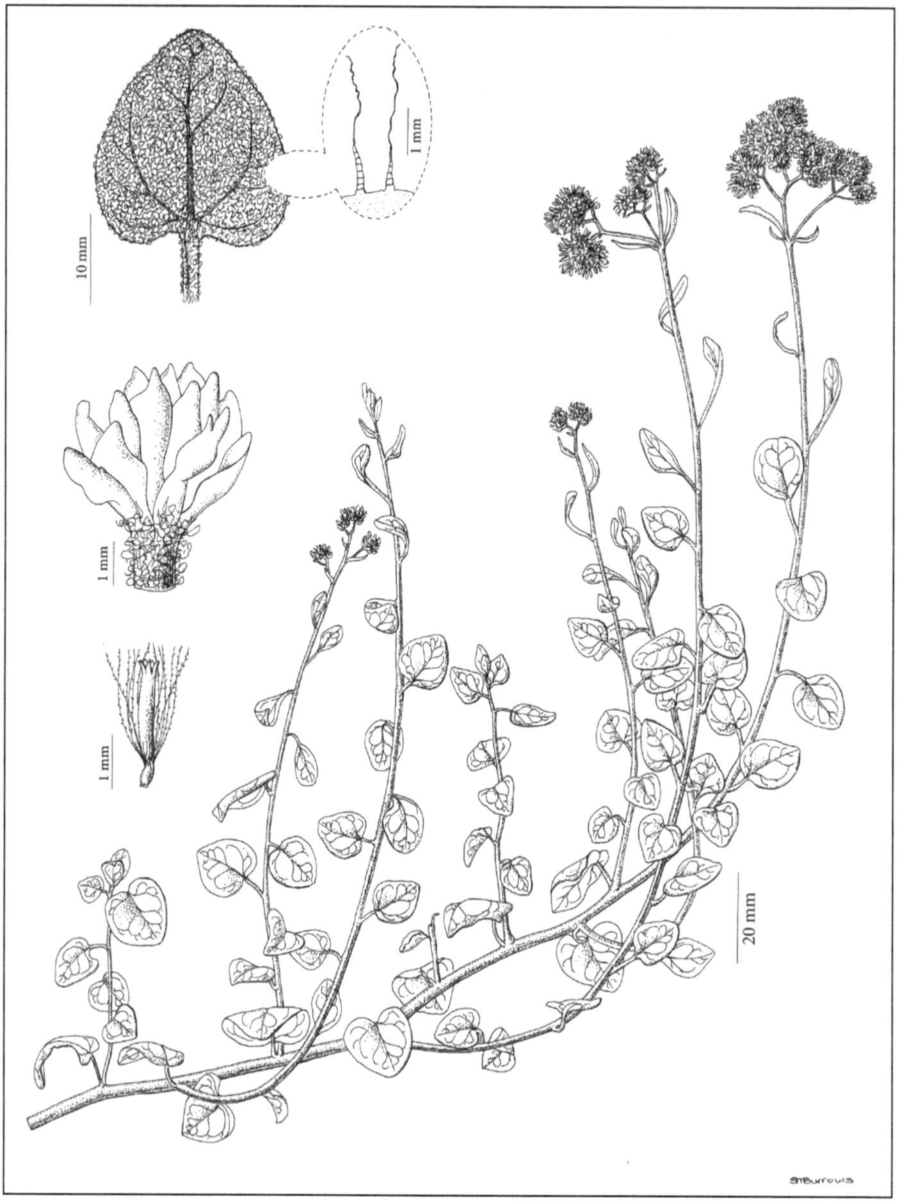
10 mm
1 mm
1 mm
1 mm
20 mm
STBurrows

Part A: General overview

1. Synonyms

Helichrysum petiolatum (L.) DC.[a]

2. Common name(s)

African incense, our incense, everlasting (Van Wyk and Gericke, 2000), silver bush everlasting (English); '*hottentotskooigoed*', '*hottentotskruie*', '*kooigoed*' (Afrikaans)[b]; '*imphepho*' (isiXhosa/ isiZulu) (Van Wyk and Gericke, 2000).

3. Conservation status

Least concern.[b]

4. Botany

The genus *Helichrysum*, belonging to the Asteraceae family, consists of about 600 species worldwide. The name of the genus is derived from the Greek words '*helios*' and '*chryos*', which mean '*sun*' and '*gold*', respectively. This nomenclature refers to the typical bright yellow inflorescences of the flowers of most *Helichrysum* species. '*Imphepho*' is a collective name for four *Helichrysum* species (*H. odoratissimum, H. petiolare, H. cymosum* and *H. nudifolium*) (Van Wyk and Gericke, 2000) that are used interchangeably. *Helichrysum petiolare* is a perennial shrub of 0.3–1 m in height. The plant is characterised by round aromatic leaves that are densely matted with hairs, giving the plant a whitish appearance (A & C). Small, clustered yellow flower heads of about 5 mm in diameter appear in summer (B) (Randall, 1997).

[a] World Flora Online (http://www.worldfloraonline.org).
[b] The Red List of South African Plants (http://redlist.sanbi.org).

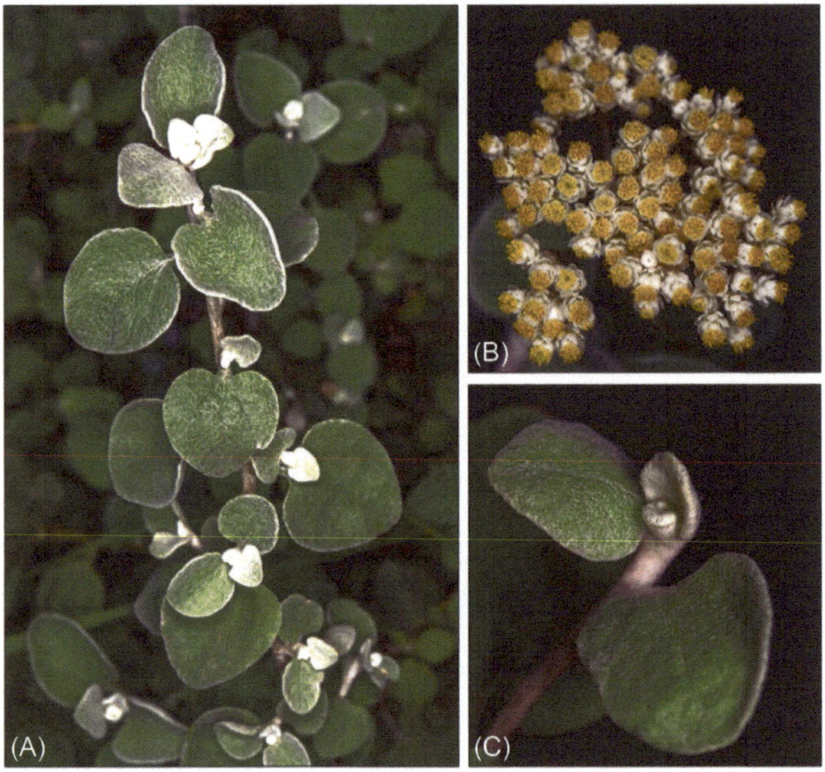

Helichrysum petiolare shrub characterised by round hairy leaves (A and C) and small clustered yellow flowers (B).

5. Geographical distribution

Helichrysum petiolare grows mainly in the Western and Eastern Cape provinces of South Africa, occurring at sea level to altitudes of 2000 m above sea level (Germishuizen et al., 2006).

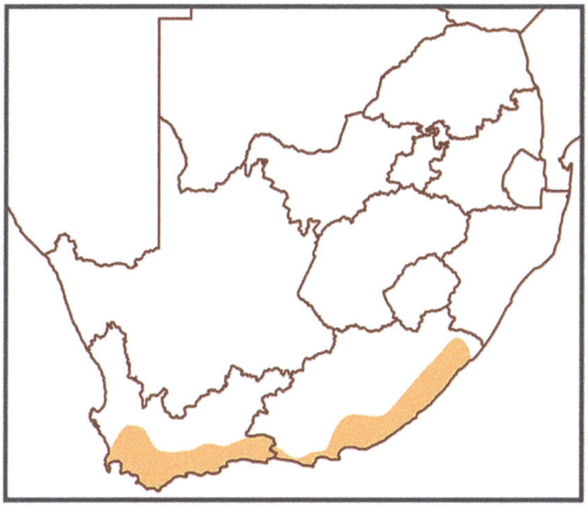

Geographical distribution of *Helichrysum petiolare* in South Africa.

6. Ethnopharmacology

Helichrysum petiolare has spiritual significance in many cultures. It is burnt as incense to invoke the ancestors, protect the home from evil spirits, and for body cleansing. The plant is used as an antifungal agent and as an insect repellent (Hutchings, 2007). Its traditional medicinal uses include the treatment of coughs, colds, catarrh, headache, fever, menstrual disorders and urinary tract infections. The plant is used as an antiseptic wound dressing and to treat burns. A decoction prepared from the aerial parts is taken to alleviate heart conditions, stress, hypertension, anxiety, overexcitement and diabetes (Erasto et al., 2005; Lourens et al., 2008). Of the four '*imphepho*' species, *H. petiolare* and *H. odoratissimum* are often used interchangeably and they are the most commonly harvested and traded plant species in South Africa (Dold and Cocks, 2002; Van Vuuren et al., 2014).

7. Commercialisation

Helichrysum petiolare is sold in '*muthi*' markets, and very little scientific research has been done to facilitate formal commercialisation.

8. Pharmacological evaluation

8.1 *In vitro* studies

The antibacterial activities of the essential oil, acetone and methanol extracts of *H. petiolare* were evaluated using the disc diffusion assay and the microplate dilution serial assays (Lourens et al., 2004). For the disc diffusion assay, neomycin

(30 µg/disc) and nystatin (100 IU/disc) were used as positive controls for antibacterial and antifungal activities, respectively. Some growth inhibition was reported as zones of inhibition for the acetone (4 and 2.5 mm) and methanol extracts (9 and 7 mm) towards *Bacillus cereus* and *Staphylococcus aureus*, respectively. For the positive controls, 6 mm zones were recorded for both bacteria. The minimum inhibitory concentrations (MICs) for the acetone extract were 500 and 312.5 µg/mL towards *B. cereus* and *S. aureus*, respectively. The acetone and methanol extracts exhibited good anti-oxidant activity with half maximal inhibitory concentration (IC_{50}) values of 44.28 and 28.70 µg/mL, respectively, as assessed using the 2,2-diphenyl-1-picrylhydrazyl (DPPH) assay. No activity was noted for the essential oil. More recently, Serabele et al. (2021) determined the antibacterial activity of methanol and dichloromethane:methanol (1:1) extracts of 15 samples of *H. petiolare* towards six pathogens associated with urinary tract, gastrointestinal and respiratory infections to confirm the traditional use for infectious conditions. Both Gram-negative and Gram-positive pathogens were selected. The MIC serial dilution assay was used, and the values obtained were compared to those obtained for *H. odoratissimum*. The average MICs for the methanol extracts of *H. petiolare* ranged from 1.4 to 6.7 mg/mL, and from 1.4 to 4.4 mg/mL for the chloroform:methanol extracts, indicating poor antibacterial activity. The best MIC value (0.50 mg/mL) was obtained for the methanol extracts against *Moraxella catarrhalis* and *Streptococcus agalactiae*. The antibacterial activity of *H. odoratissimum* was substantially higher than that of *H. petiolare*. Only 5.6% of the methanol extracts, and none of the chloroform:methanol extracts of *H. petiolare*, yielded moderate to noteworthy activity (≤ 160 µg/mL) against the pathogens, whilst 40% of the methanol and 43% of the dichloromethane:methanol extracts of *H. odoratissimum* yielded moderate to noteworthy activity. There was no correlation between the MICs and the concentrations of the marker compound, 4,5-dicaffeoylquinic acid, identified in the extracts, indicating that the compound does not contribute to the antibacterial activity. The authors concluded that the antibacterial activities of *H. petiolare* and *H. odoratissimum* do not justify their interchangeable use for the treatment of infectious diseases. The acetone and methanol extracts of the aerial parts had no anti-inflammatory activity when tested using the 5-lipoxygenase assay. However, the essential oil proved to have significant anti-inflammatory activity with an IC_{50} value of 25.03 µg/mL) (Lourens et al., 2004).

8.2 *In vivo* studies and clinical trials

A dichloromethane:methanol extract of *H. petiolare* administered to mice lowered their mean blood pressure by 21% and resulted in a 6% reduction in heart rate, compared to the control group (Lourens et al., 2008). To date, there are no documented clinical trials on *H. petiolare*.

8.3 Safety

No toxicity studies have been reported for *H. petiolare*.

9. Phytochemistry

9.1 Volatile constituents

A study by Giovanelli et al. (2018) involving the essential oils of *Helichrysum* species revealed that monoterpenes are the dominant class of compounds present, with 95.1% in *Helichrysum tenax*, 77.9% in *H. cymosum,* 68.7% in *H. petiolare,* 68.3% in *H. odoratissimum* and 59.2% in *H. saxatile* essential oils. The major compounds identified in *H. petiolare* by Lourens et al. (2004) were 1,8-cineole (22.4%), α-caryophyllene (14.0%), *p*-cymene (9.8%), α-pinene (6.8%), α-terpineol (5.1%), borneol (3.3%), limonene (3.1%), caryophyllene oxide (2.5%), γ-muurolene (2.2%), α-muurolene (2.2%), α-humulene (2.0%), α-caryophyllene alcohol (1.9%), fenchyl alcohol (1.5%), kaur-16-ene (1.3%) and α-copaene (1.3%). Caser et al. (2016) reported the presence of non-terpenic derivatives (2.3%–8.2%), monoterpene hydrocarbons (55.7%–66.4%), oxygenated monoterpenes (4.8%–9.8%), sesquiterpene hydrocarbons (11.8%–12.0%) and oxygenated sesquiterpenes (12.5%–13.3%) in drought-induced *H. petiolare*. The major constituents reported were sabinene (40.4%–51.1%), dihydro-agarofuran (18.3%–19.5%), α-pinene (8.1%–10.4%), longipinanol (7.1%–8.4%), lavandulyl acetate (1.5%–5.1%), β-dihydro-agarofuran (4.6%–4.9%), α-humulene (4.1%–4.5%), limonene (3.6%–4.0%), δ-cadinene (2.9%–3.1%), γ-cadinene (2.3%–3.0%), selin-11-en-4-α-ol (1.9%–2.4%), lavandulyl isovalerate (1.2%–1.7%), prenopsan-8-ol (1.3%–1.5%) and α-calacorene (1.2%–1.3%).

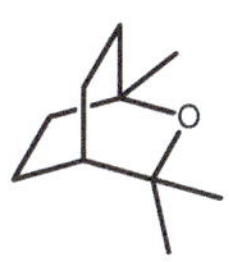

1,8-Cineole

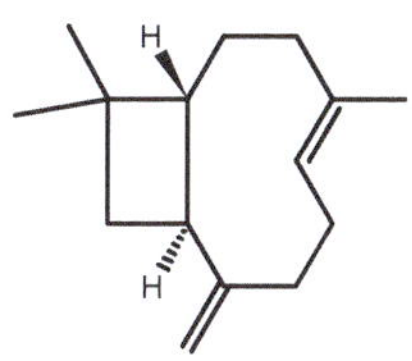

β-Caryophyllene

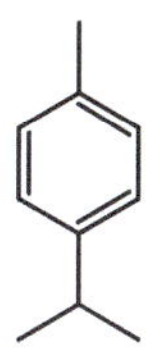

p-Cymene

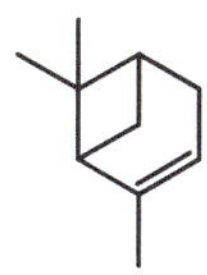

α-Pinene

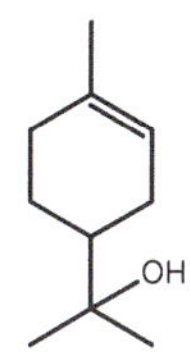

α-Terpineol

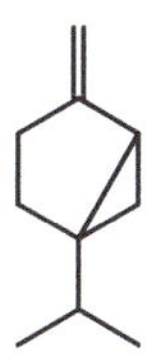

Sabinene

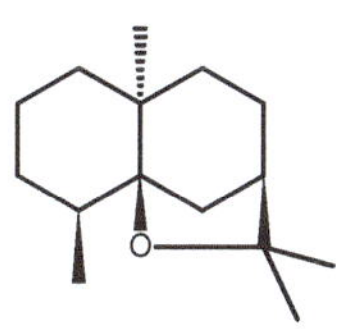

Dihydro-agarofuran

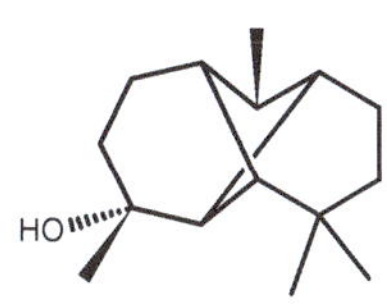

Longipinanol

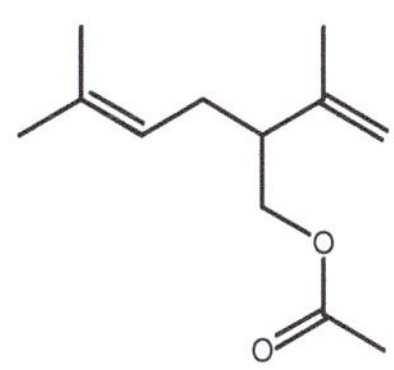

Lavandulyl acetate

9.2 Non-volatile constituents

Not much attention has been paid to the non-volatile constituents of this species. The chemical profiles of aqueous methanol extracts of the aerial parts of 15 *H. petiolare* samples and 12 samples of *H. odoratissimum*, harvested from different sites, were obtained using ultra-performance liquid chromatography coupled with mass spectrometry (UPLC–MS) (Serabele et al., 2021). The construction of chemometric models from the data indicated that the chemistry of *H. petiolare* was consistent, and that the chemical profiles of the extracts could be used to distinguish the species from *H. odoratissimum*. Four discriminating markers were revealed for each species. The compound 4,5-dicaffeoylquinic acid was isolated from the aqueous methanol extract of the aerial parts. The concentrations of the compound in the individual samples ranged from 2.3 to 13.4 µg/g (Serabele et al., 2021). Dicaffeoylquinic acids have been reported to have antiviral, anti-oxidant and anti-inflammatory activities and may protect against cardiovascular disease, Alzheimer's disease and diabetes.

'*Sangomas*' inhale the smoke of burning *H. petiolare* or *H. odoratissimum* during traditional rites (Lourens et al., 2008). Serabele et al. (2021) burned plant material from both species under controlled conditions and obtained the resulting smoke condensates. Analysis using ultra-performance liquid chromatography revealed the presence of five major compounds, common to both species. One compound was visible in the UPLC–MS chromatogram, whilst the other four could be seen in the UPLC–PDA chromatogram. Although the solvent extracts of the two species were very different, the smoke condensates were found to be similar. Three dicaffeoylquinic acid isomers (including the isolated 4,5-dicaffeoylquinic acid) were found to be present in both species. The authors speculated that the compounds common to the smoke condensate of both species are possibly derived from these dicaffeoylquinic acid isomers. These findings provide a plausible explanation for the use of both species as smoke inhalants. The pyrolysis products should be further investigated to determine if they have hallucinogenic effects.

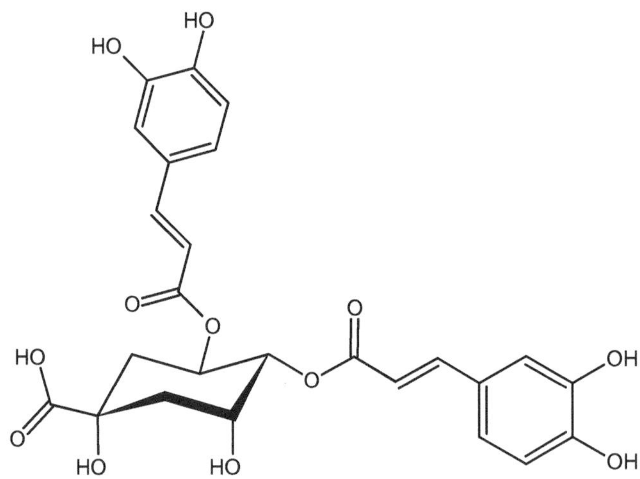

4,5-Dicaffeoylquinic acid

Part B: Chemical profiling and quality control

10. Chromatography analysis

10.1 High-performance thin-layer chromatography (HPTLC) fingerprint analysis

General instrumentation: CAMAG HPTLC instrument consisting of an automatic TLC sampler (ATS 4), automatic developing chamber (ADC 2), CAMAG TLC visualiser 2, CAMAG derivatiser and TLC plate heater. *HPTLC plates:* Silica gel glass plates 60 F_{254} (Merck). *Plant part:* Aerial parts, methanol:water (80:20, v/v). *Sample application:* Application volume of 10 μL extract (10 mg/mL) and standards (1 mg/mL) spotted as 10 mm bands. Plates developed in a 20×10×4 cm glass twin-trough chamber to a migration distance of 85 mm. *Tank saturation:* 20 min at 15 °C and 33% RH, with 25 mL of mobile phase. *Mobile phase:* Ethyl acetate:formic acid:acetic acid:water (100:11:11:27, v/v/v/v). *Derivatisation:* Natural Product reagent followed by polyethylene glycol reagent. The plate was heated for 3 min at 100 °C on a TLC plate heater, sprayed with 3 mL of the reagent mixture and then visualised. *Visualisation:* The plate was viewed under 366 nm radiation.

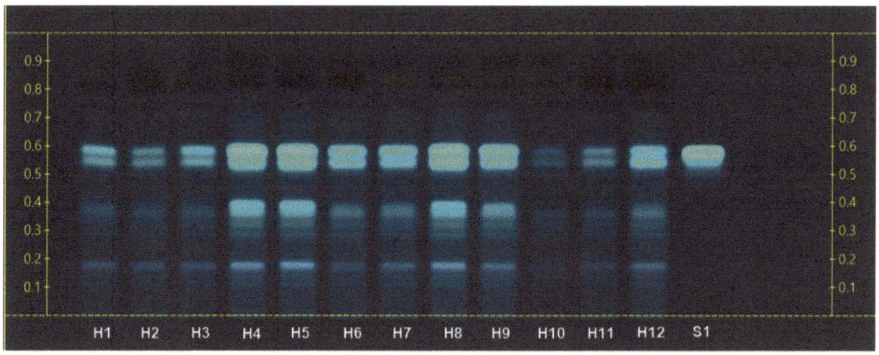

HPTLC plate of *Helichrysum petiolare* methanol:water extracts (n=12) tracks (H1–H12) and the standard (S1). The samples are characterised by a light blue band for 4,5-dicaffeoylquinic acid (S1) (R_f=0.60).

10.2 Ultra-performance liquid chromatography (UPLC) analysis

General instrumentation: Waters Acquity Ultra-Performance Liquid Chromatography system with photodiode array (PDA) detector combined with Xevo G2QToF mass spectrometer (Waters, United States). *Plant part:* Aerial parts, methanol:water extract (80:20, v/v). *Sample application:* Injection volume: 1.0 μL (full-loop injection) at 1 mg/mL. *Column:* Acquity UPLC HSS T_3 column (150 mm×2.1 mm, i.d., 1.8 μm particle size, Waters). *Mobile phase:* 0.1% formic acid in water (solvent A) and acetonitrile (solvent B). *Analysis conditions:* Gradient elution at a flow rate of 0.3 mL/min, changing as follows: 90% A: 10% B changed to 65% A: 35% B in 6 min, to 35% A: 65% B in 4 min, to 5% A: 95% B in 4.5 min, held for 1 min, back to the initial ratio in 0.5 min, equilibrating the system for 2 min, total run time 18 min. *Mass spectrometry:* ESI$^-$ (negative ionisation mode), N_2 used as the desolvation gas, desolvation temperature 350 °C at a flow rate of 500 L/h and source temperature 100 °C. Capillary and cone voltages 2500 and 45 V, respectively. Data collected between *m/z* 100 and 1500.

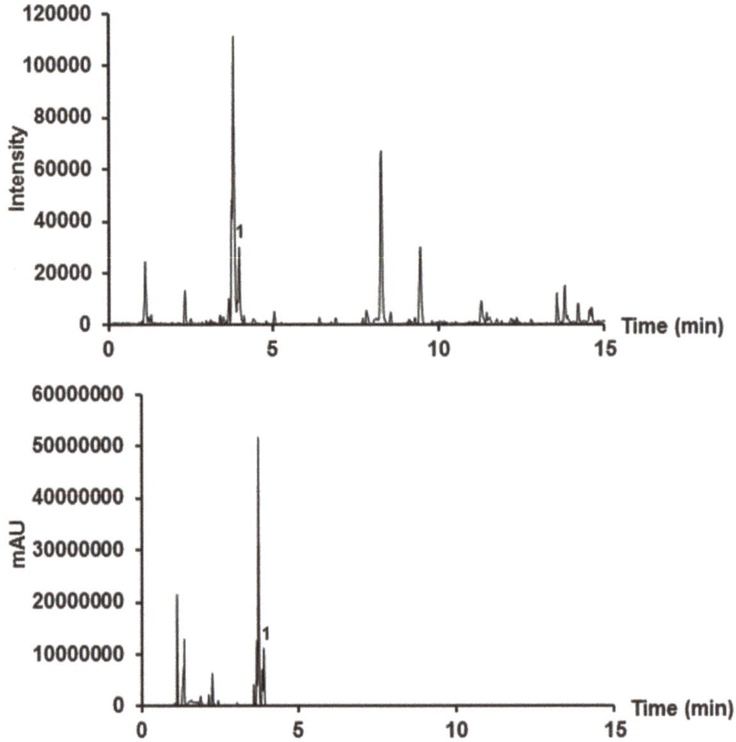

UPLC–ToF–MS ESI$^-$ (upper) and PDA (lower) chromatograms of *Helichrysum petiolare* methanol:water extract. [1] = 4,5-Dicaffeoylquinic acid (*m/z* 515.1312).

11. Mid-infrared (MIR) spectroscopy analysis

General instrumentation: Alpha-P Bruker spectrometer, mounted with an attenuated total reflectance (ATR) diamond crystal. *Spectral acquisition:* Spectrum obtained in absorbance mode, with a spectral resolution of 4 cm^{-1} over the range 4000–550 cm^{-1} and captured using OPUS 6.5 software. *Plant part:* Aerial parts. *Sample preparation:* Aerial parts powdered, sieved (< 500 µm) and placed directly onto the surface of the diamond crystal.

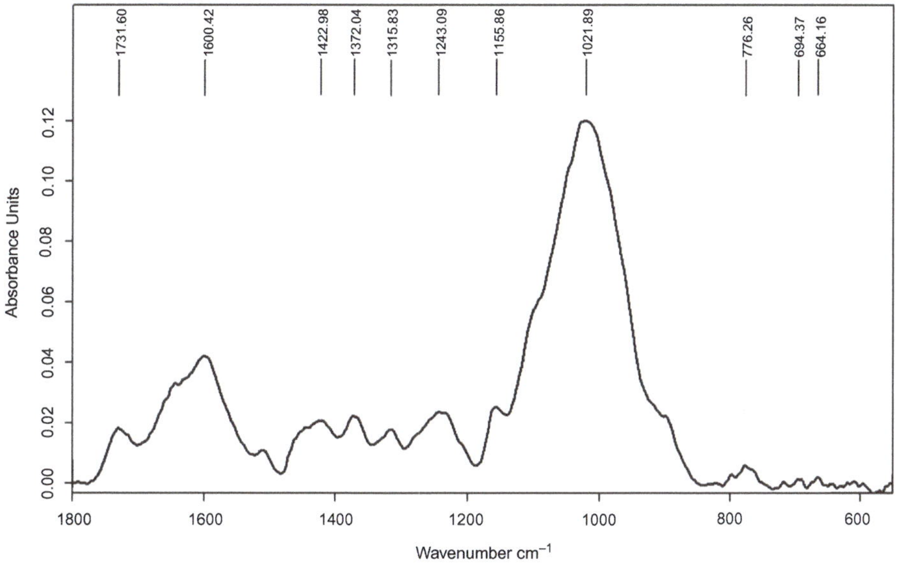

Mid-infrared spectrum of *Helichrysum petiolare* powder displaying the fingerprint region (1800–550 cm^{-1}).

References

Caser, M., D'Angiolillo, F., Chitarra, W., Lovisolo, C., Ruffoni, B., Pistelli, L., Pistelli, L., Scariot, V., 2016. Ind. Crops Prod., 83:680–692.

Dold, A.P., Cocks, M.L., 2002. S. Afr. J. Sci., 98:589.

Erasto, P., Adebola, P.O., Grierson, D.S., Afolayan, A.J., 2005. Afr. J. Biotechnol., 4:1458–1460.

Giovanelli, S., De Leo, M., Cervelli, C., Ruffoni, B., Ciccarelli, D., Pistelli, L., 2018. Chem. Biodivers., 15 (5), Art. No. e1700545, https://doi.org/10.1002/cbdv.20170054.

Germishuizen, G., Meyer, N.L., Steenkamp, Y., Keith, M. (Eds.), 2006. A Checklist of South African Plants. Southern African Botanical Diversity Network, No. 41, Pretoria, South Africa.

Hutchings, A., 2007. Alternation, 14:189–218.

Lourens, A.C.U., Reddy, D., Başer, K.H.C., Viljoen, A.M., Van Vuuren, S.F., 2004. J. Ethnopharmacol., 95:253–258.

Lourens, A.C.U., Viljoen, A.M., Van Heerden, F.R., 2008. J. Ethnopharmacol., 119:630–652.

Randall, J.M., 1997. In Symposium Proceedings of the California Exotic Pest Plan Council. California Exotic Pest Plan Council, Sacramento, CA, pp. 1–6.

Serabele, K., Chen, W., Tankeu, S., Combrinck, S., Veale C.G.L., Van Vuuren, S., Chaudhary, S.K., Viljoen A., 2021. S. Afr. J. Bot., 137:117–132.

Van Vuuren, S., Williams, V.L., Sooka, A., Burger, A., Van der Haar, L., 2014. S. Afr. J. Bot., 94:95–100.

Van Wyk, B.-E., Gericke, N., 2000. People's Plants. A Guide to Useful Plants of Southern Africa. Briza Publications, Pretoria, South Africa.

CHAPTER

Hoodia gordonii 12

Ilze Vermaak[a,b], Nduvho Mulaudzi[a] and Gerda Fouche[c]

[a]*Department of Pharmaceutical Sciences, Tshwane University of Technology, Pretoria, South Africa*

[b]*SAMRC Herbal Drugs Research Unit, Faculty of Science, Tshwane University of Technology, Pretoria, South Africa*

[c]*Chemistry Department, University of Pretoria, Pretoria, South Africa*

Abstract

Hoodia gordonii (Masson) Sweet ex Decne. (Apocynaceae), commonly known as bitterghaap, is a spiny succulent plant with rows of small thorns visible along the fairly hard and fleshy, glabrous, grey-brown to grey-green stems. The plant has a narrow geographical distribution, but is widely distributed throughout the dry, desert areas of South Africa and Namibia. Traditionally, the Khoisan people in southern Africa sucked on Hoodia stems while on long hunting trips to quench hunger and thirst. It is also said that the stems were used traditionally in the treatment of tuberculosis, and honey from the flowers was used to treat cancer. The commercialisation of this plant as an anti-obesity agent has been highly controversial due to benefit-sharing issues and intellectual property rights. Although no commercial product has been developed due to efficacy and safety concerns, some Hoodia herbal products are available on the market. The Council for Scientific and Industrial Research (CSIR) isolated and patented the pregnane glycoside P57 in 1995. Since then the phytochemistry has been extensively researched. In vitro and in vivo biological activities investigated include appetite-suppressant, antidiabetic, anti-inflammatory and antidepressant activities, as well as the pharmacokinetics and biopharmaceutics of various compounds. Using semi-automated high-performance thin-layer chromatography (HPTLC), ultra-performance liquid chromatography coupled with mass spectrometry (UPLC–MS), and mid-infrared (MIR) spectroscopy, the chemical profiles of H. gordonii methanol extracts were obtained. The marker compound P57 of H. gordonii was identified in the chemical fingerprints of all the samples on HPTLC plates viewed under 366 nm radiation, and UPLC–MS chromatograms confirmed the presence of the compound.

Keywords: *Hoodia gordonii*, Bitterghaap, P57, Pregnane glycosides, Appetite suppressant, HPTLC, UPLC–MS, MIR spectroscopy

The South African Herbal Pharmacopoeia. https://doi.org/10.1016/B978-0-323-99794-2.00018-0

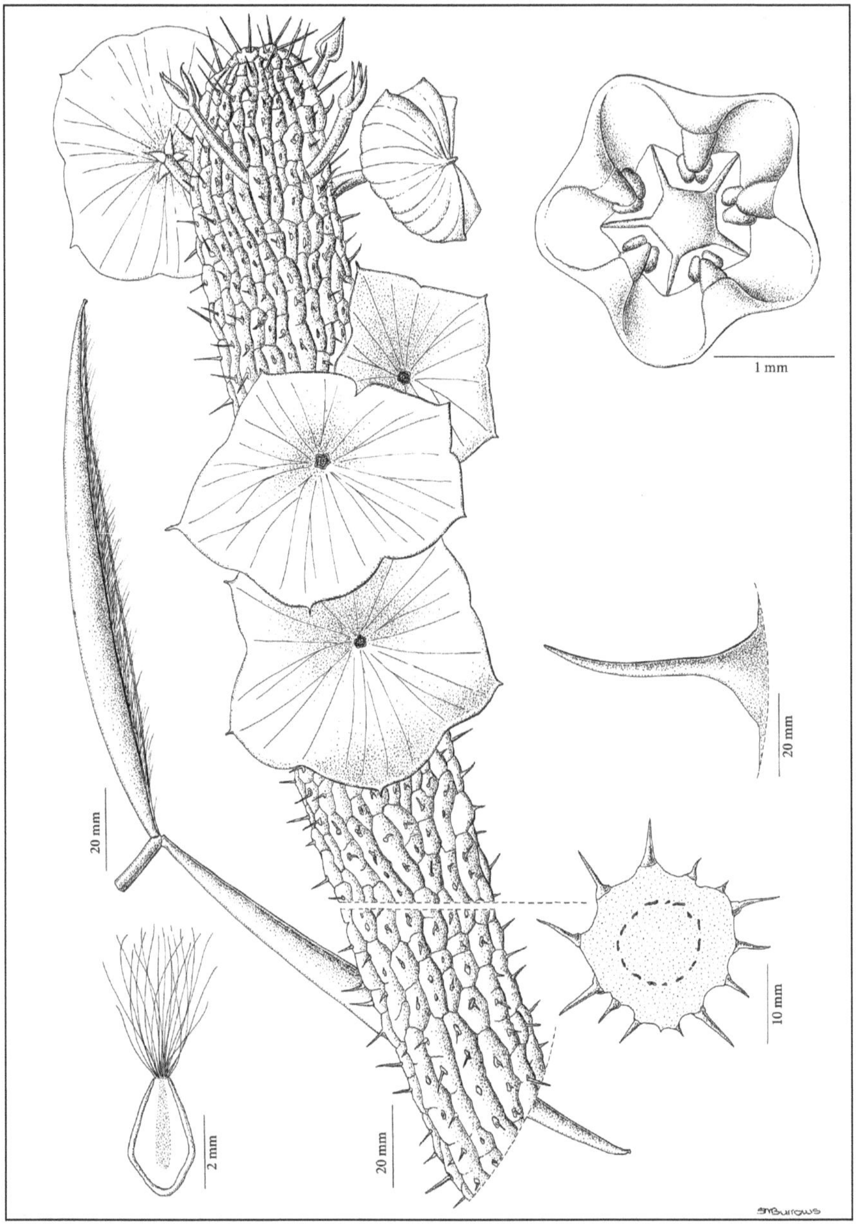
1 mm
20 mm
20 mm
10 mm
2 mm
20 mm
SMBurrows

Part A: General overview

1. Synonyms

Hoodia longispina Plowes, *Hoodia bainii* Dyer, *Hoodia burkei* N.E.Br., *Hoodia albispina* N.E.Br., *Hoodia whitesloaneana* Dinter ex A.C.White and B.Sloane, *Hoodia rosea* Oberm. & Letty, *Hoodia barklyi* Dyer, *Hoodia pillansii* N.E.Br., *Hoodia langii* Oberm. & Letty, *Hoodia husabensis* Nel.[a,b]

2. Common name(s)

Bitterghaap or Bushman's hat (English); *'bitterghaap', 'bobbejaanghaap', 'bokhorings', 'jakkalsghaap', 'muishondghaap', 'wildeghaap, 'bergghaap', 'wolweghaap'* (Afrikaans); *'khobab'*, *'guaap'* (Khoi).[a]

3. Conservation status

Protected and listed as a CITES Appendix II species. Permits are required for cultivation, collection, export and transport of the plant.[c]

4. Botany

The genus *Hoodia* is listed as one of the stapeliads, belonging to the family Apocynaceae, a group of stem succulents that was previously part of the family Asclepiadaceae. *Hoodia* is currently classified within the tribe Ceropegieae, of the sub-family Asclepiadoideae (Apocynaceae). The genus name '*Hoodia*' was designated after Van Hood, a keen succulent grower. The plant species *H. gordonii* was first published in 1844 by Joseph Decaisne after the former generic names were announced invalid (Bruyns, 2005). *Hoodia gordonii* (Masson) Sweet ex Decne. is a succulent, spiny plant with rows of small thorns visible along the fairly hard and fleshy, glabrous, grey-brown to grey-green stems (B). Only one stem is formed in the early stages of development, but as the plant grows, as many as 50 individual branches are produced from the one base (A). The tubercles are fused in the lower halves into 11–17 obtuse angles along the stem, prominent, each tipped with a sharp spine, 6–12 mm long. The flowers are large, borne close or on the terminal apex and are usually flesh-coloured (A). The flower size varies between 50 and 100 mm and the flowers reduce in size as the flowering stage advances. The plant usually flowers from August to September, and a multitude of flowers almost entirely covers the stems. An unpleasant smell that resembles decaying flesh attracts blowflies to the

[a] Red List of South African Plants (http://redlist.sanbi.org).
[b] World Flora Online (http://www.worldfloraonline.org).
[c] CITES (Convention of Illicit Trade of Endangered Species) (https://cites.org).

flowers for pollination. The seed capsules, formed in October to November, resemble goat or antelope horns (B) and contain many light brown, flat seeds with silky hairs attached to one end of the seed (Oliver, 2008).

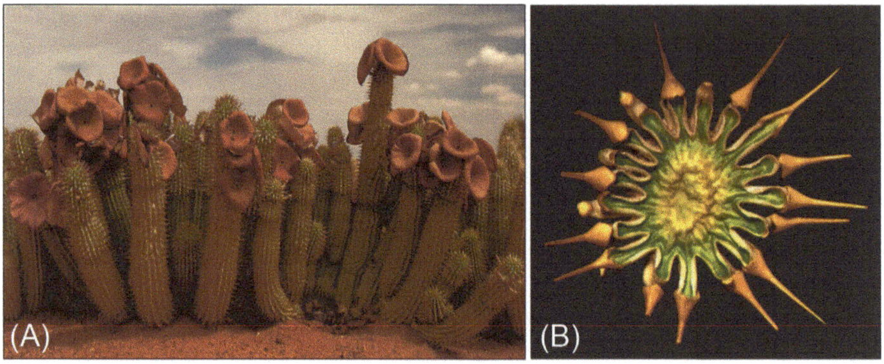

Hoodia gordonii, a succulent, spiny plant with large, flesh-coloured flowers at the tips (A) and a cross-section of the stem with rows of small thorns at the edges (B).

5. Geographical distribution

Plants belonging to the genus *Hoodia* are indigenous to the dry, desert areas of southern Africa, occurring only in Namibia, South Africa, Zimbabwe, Botswana and south-west Angola. *Hoodia gordonii* grows in south-western Namibia, and in South Africa in the southern parts of the Free State Province, the north-western and northern areas of the Northern Cape, as far as Kimberley and regions of the Western Cape. The plant has a broad growing habitat, which includes barren flats or dry stony slopes and the deep

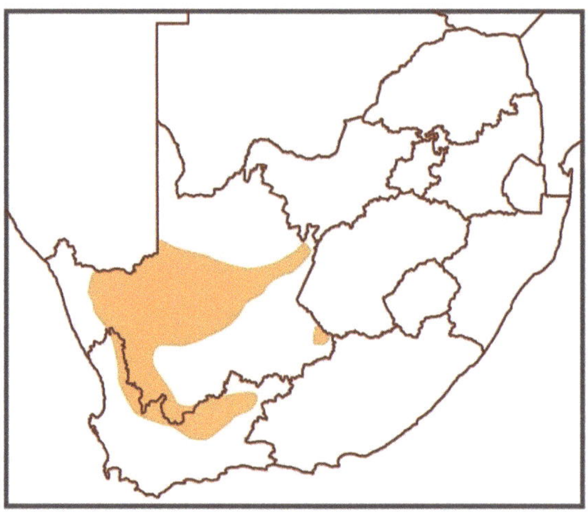

Geographical distribution of *Hoodia gordonii* in South Africa.

Kalahari dry sands, as well as under the protection of xerophytic bushes. It can survive extreme climatic conditions, such as very low temperatures (−3 °C) and temperatures above 40 °C, although it is susceptible to frost and mostly grows in summer rainfall areas. In the wild, the plant does not live longer than 15 years, although it can survive for as many as 25 years when cultivated. Cultivation is done from seeds, which is challenging, as the plant requires a great deal of attention and is slow to mature (Oliver, 2008).

6. Ethnopharmacology

The first document reporting on the application of *Hoodia* dates back to 1796, although its use as a thirst quencher was only documented centuries later. Glasl (2009) reported that *Hoodia* species were utilised by the Khoisan people of Namibia and South Africa when food supplies were low and for sustenance during long hunting trips. The term '*veldkos*' has been used to refer to *Hoodia* species, which means food from the veld. It is clear from early literature that *H. pilifera* (= *Stapelia pilifera* = *Trichocaulon piliferum*) was the superior plant species of use by the San people. Pappe (1862) reported that the plant has an insipid, yet cool and watery taste, and is eaten by the natives who call it "*guaap*", for quenching their thirst. However, Marloth (1932) documented that *T. piliferum* is the real ghaap of the natives, who use it as a substitute for food and water when both were scarce. The sweet sap reminds one of liquorice, and when consumed, it removes pangs of hunger very efficiently. It is stated that after good rains, the bitterness of the plant is less notable, and the juicy stems can then be eaten cooked or raw. Van Heerden (2008) reported that the honey from the flowers of *H. gordonii* is used to treat cancer, and that the plant is also used for the treatment of tuberculosis. Marloth (1932) examined the history of use of *Hoodia* and reported that the plant *T. piliferum* (Linn fil.) N.E.Brown was used traditionally as a source of water and food. White and Sloane (1933) documented that the plant is edible, either preserved in sugar or in its raw state. Other reports of Francis Masson (1796) and Rudolf Marloth (1932) indicate that *Hoodia* was used by the San as a thirst quencher and hunger suppressant, especially in harsh environments and on hunting trips (Wynberg and Chennels, 2009).

7. Commercialisation

In 1963, the Council for Scientific and Industrial Research (CSIR) in Pretoria, South Africa, initiated a research programme to investigate more than a thousand indigenous plant species used as food. The list included *Hoodia* species. An early experiment using mice to examine the thirst-quenching properties of the plant demonstrated the appetite-suppressant effects of the extracts (Pappe, 1862). Further studies were conducted on the appetite-suppressant activity of the extracts of *Hoodia* species and the structure of the active oxypregnane steroidal glycoside compound P57AS3, also referred to as P57, was elucidated and subsequently patented by the CSIR in 1995. In 1998, a further patent was granted by the World Intellectual Property Organisation, focusing on the appetite-suppressant activity of pharmaceutical compositions. This led to the subsequent signing of a license agreement with the company, Phytopharm®, for the commercialisation and development of *Hoodia* (P57), and the sublicensing to Pfizer for clinical development. As a result of a merger between Pharmacia and Pfizer in 2003, the nutraceutical branch managing the development of P57 was discontinued at Pfizer and further interest in *Hoodia*-related research was terminated (Wynberg et al., 2009). A campaign spearheaded by the Non-Governmental Organisations Action Aid and Biowatch notified the British media in 2001 of the commercial development of *Hoodia* without the involvement or consent of the San people. This prompted the San to contact the CSIR, and negotiations followed that led to the eventual signing of a benefit-sharing agreement in 2003 (Wynberg and Van Niekerk, 2014). The publicity emanating from the CSIR patent, as well as the agreements and marketing opportunities created by the San's use of the plant, opened up a frantic interest in *Hoodia* among plant traders. Non-patented *Hoodia* supplements emerged on the market, based on exported wild-harvested, dried *Hoodia.* The mass of harvested, wet plant material escalated in an exponential manner from 1 to 2 tons in 2002 to over 600 tons in 2005.

A *Hoodia* patent was licensed to the international company, Unilever in 2004, for the inclusion of extracts of *H. gordonii* into food products to manufacture functional foods (Wynberg et al., 2009). At that stage, *Hoodia* was successfully cultivated, and growers were in compliance with South Africa's CBD (Convention on Biological Diversity) and ABS (Access and Benefit Sharing) laws. Conservation authorities in South Africa, Namibia and Botswana reinforced permitting, border and export controls, in a bid to improve standardisation, policy cohesion, and to ensure cultivation of the plant species. The South African San Council became an integral part of the commercialisation of *Hoodia.* It was decided by the San that their tradition was mutually owned, and that any financial benefits arising from commercialisation of the plant be shared equally among countries with San populations. This laid the foundation for the establishment of a Trust in 2006 to allocate benefits to the San communities. The South African *Hoodia* Growers Association and the South African San Council compiled and signed a benefit-sharing agreement with the *Hoodia* Growers Association of Namibia, and the Nama and San communities of Namibia in 2010. Wynberg and Van Niekerk (2014) reported that a resolution was passed to allocate 75% of all Trust income (a total of US $60,000 or ZAR 600,000) equally between the San Councils of Botswana, Namibia and South Africa, and the rest to be used for the administration of the Trust. A huge cultivation programme was initiated, including over 300 ha (hectare) of *Hoodia* in Namibia and South Africa, manufacturing, clinical safety trials as well as an agreement to build a R750 million extraction facility (approximately US$75 million). However, Unilever decided in 2008 to abandon further development of *Hoodia* as a functional food, because of efficacy and safety concerns. All activities linked to *Hoodia* in South Africa were terminated from 31 March 2009. At that time, Phytopharm remained hopeful about the *Hoodia* project and continued to seek other partners for further development. However, in November 2010, Phytopharm removed the South African succulent from its research portfolio and returned all rights, commercialisation and development of P57 to the CSIR. Even though some *Hoodia* herbal products are still available on the market, mostly from cultivated material, the multi-million-dollar forecasts of profit remain evasive.

8. Pharmacological evaluation

8.1 *In vitro* studies

8.1.1 Appetite-suppressant activity

It was shown that the steroid glycoside, P57 from *H. gordonii,* activates the human bitter receptor TAS2R14 from HuTu-80 cells and induces cholecystokinin (CCK) release (Le Nevé et al., 2010). It is known that CCK exerts central actions on appetite suppression through receptors located on vagal afferent terminals in the gut wall. Results revealed that the G protein-coupled receptors (T2Rs), signalling bitter taste, are demonstrated in both human and rodent gastro-intestinal tracts. P57-activated TAS2R14 and TAS2R7 are both expressed in a heterologous manner in HEK 293 cells. The experiments displayed supplementary verification that bitter taste-sensing mechanisms are linked to hormone release in the intestine from human enteroendocrine cells. The structure–activity relationships, effects and mode of action of the pregnane glycosides from *Hoodia* on steroidogenesis in human adrenocortical H295R cells were also researched (Komarnytsky et al., 2013). Addition of pregnane glycosides over 24 h lowered the forskolin and basal-stimulated release of corticosterone, androstenedione and cortisone from H295R cells. The conversion of 17-hydroxyprogesterone to either androstenedione or 11-deoxycortisol, and progesterone to 11-deoxycorticosterone, was highly affected, with tigloyl-, 12-cinnamoyl- and benzoyl-containing pregnanes exhibiting the strongest effects. Incubation of pregnane glycosides for 24 h showed no activity on steroidogenic acute regulatory (StaR) protein and mRNA transcripts of CYP21A1, CYP11A1, CYP11B1 cytochrome enzymes, yet a twofold reduction in HSD3B1 mRNA levels was reported. Pregnane glycosides displayed weak K^+/Na^+ ATPase and glucocorticoid receptor binding, but had no effect on the CYP3, 2 or 1 drug or on steroid metabolism enzymes. The data revealed that pregnane glycosides suppressed steroidogenesis *via* potent inhibition of steroid 17-alpha-mono-oxygenase and 11β-hydroxylase, and weakly inhibited 21β-hydroxylase and cytochrome P450 side-chain division enzymes, but not 3β-hydroxysteroid isomerase/dehydrogenase.

8.1.2 Anti-HIV activity

Ethyl acetate and ethanol extracts of *H. gordonii* were screened for anti-HIV-1 reverse transcriptase (HIV-RT), integrase (HIV-I) and protease (HIV-PR) activity *in vitro* (Kapewangolo et al., 2016). The extracts exhibited strong activity against HIV-RT and HIV-PR with IC_{50} values of 69.81±9.45 and 63.76±9.01 μg/mL for the ethyl acetate extract and 73.55±0.04 and 97.29±0.01 μg/mL for the ethanol extract, respectively. Furthermore, *H. gordonii* was reported to display strong anti-oxidant activity, with IC_{50} values of 126.2±3.15 and 124.6±11.3 μg/mL reported for the ethyl acetate and ethanol extracts, respectively. Phytochemical screening of the extracts revealed the presence of terpenes, steroids, phenolic compounds, cardiac glycosides, alkaloids and tannins in the ethanol extract, while the ethyl acetate extract was composed of cardiac glycosides, phenolic compounds and steroids.

8.1.3 Other activities

Various compounds from *Hoodia*, namely P57 and hoodigosides A–K, were screened for their *in vitro* anti-oxidant and cytotoxic activities (Pawar et al., 2007). The compounds were not cytotoxic and did not inhibit the growth of cells, including BT-549, SK-MEL, KB, VERO, LLC-PK1 and SKOV-3 cells, at a concentration of 25 μg/mL. They reported that intracellular reactive oxygen species (ROS) generation was not constrained, and no anti-oxidant effect was observed in HL-60 cells. In another study, Vermaak et al. (2011) investigated the *in vitro* transport of pure P57, and P57 in an acetonitrile crude extract, across buccal and excised porcine intestinal mucosa in a Sweetana–Grass diffusion apparatus. The transport of pure P57 revealed efflux by membrane transporters, since more effective transport across intestinal tissue was seen in the secretory direction compared to the absorptive direction. Significant intestinal transport was observed for P57 in both directions when administered as a crude plant extract. This might be due to repression of efflux by other compounds in the extract as shown by decreased secretory transfer in comparison with absorptive transport. The buccal tissue experiment demonstrated high transfer of the P57 applied as crude extract, while pure P57 was not transported. The intestinal transfer of P57 was substantially decreased when prepared in simulated gastro-intestinal fluid (containing enzymes and acid) compared to a buffer solution. Significantly, the transport of P57 when prepared in artificial saliva was higher than that when buffer solution was used. This highlights the ethnopharmacological use, as it is chewed or sucked to provide its perceived biological effect. Clearly, exposure to simulated *in vivo* conditions has a significant effect on P57 transport.

8.2 *In vivo* studies and clinical trials

8.2.1 Appetite-suppressant properties

Studies on the properties of the active metabolite, P57, showed that intraventricular injection of 0.4–40 nmol of P57 significantly increased hypothalamic adenosine triphosphate (ATP) production and decreased food intake in rats (MacLean and Luo, 2004). A solution of P57 was injected intracerebroventricularly (i.c.v.) into the third ventricle of the brain. Food intake was reduced by 40%–60% with dose-dependent effects over a period of 24 h. The P57 analogues, P57NS5 and P57ASA, screened in dimethylsulphoxide (DMSO) at 40 nmol, showed no activity. The expected decrease in ATP in hypocaloric rats, kept on a normal diet, was inhibited by injection of P57, while the hypothalamic ATP content was raised after i.c.v. injection. The results indicate that P57 has a possible mode of action in the central nervous system, as reflected by the activities on the hypothalamus and hypothalamic neurons. The hypothalamus is a region in the brain responsible for the control of temperature, appetite and hunger. Van Heerden et al. (2007) reported a decrease in food intake after 3 days in rats, when *H. gordonii* glycosides were administered at 6.25–50 mg/kg body mass/day. However, no statistical analysis was conducted due to the small scale of the study (three rats per group). No indication of variability was reported (e.g. standard deviations), although normal data were reported for body mass. Daily supplementation of Ross 308 broiler chickens with 300 mg, *H. gordonii* did not result in changes in digestibility, growth or feed intake, but a decrease in fat pad weights by 40% was noted. Mohlapo et al. (2009) reported that since feed efficiency and carcass quality were decreased by a high percentage fat, the administration of *H. gordonii* can be beneficial to the industry, although the mode of action is still unknown. The effect of *H. gordonii* (organic extract) on body weight and food intake of Sprague Dawley rats (males) was investigated at three dosages of 50, 100 and 150 mg/kg body weight, administered orally over a period of 5 days. From the experiments, the dose of 100 mg/kg body weight was chosen for continued investigation on biochemical variables and regulatory hormones. A dose-dependent decrease in food intake (12%–26%) was seen at a dosage of 100 and 150 mg/kg body weight. Appetite reduction continued for 6 h and the intake of food was reinstated within 24 h after termination of treatment. An increase in the activity of mitochondrial CPT-1, liver glycogen stores, and thyroid hormones in animals administered with *H. gordonii* was observed. The circulating levels of IGF-1 and NPY were decreased with a marginal increase in CCK and leptin levels. Insulin levels were not significantly changed and blood glucose levels remained unchanged. The metabolic and hormonal changes due to the administration of the extract of *H. gordonii* were thought to be the reason for its anorectic properties (Jain and Singh, 2013).

Male Wistar rats (12 obese and 12 lean) were administered separate doses of *H. gordonii* extract (twice daily with 80 or 160 mg/kg body mass) in a placebo-controlled study over 14 days (Smith and Krygsman, 2014). All the rats given *H. gordonii* extract demonstrated noteworthy weight loss. This may be due to a reduction in both skeletal muscle fibre and adipose cell size following the administration of *H. gordonii*. GPR119, a G protein-coupled receptor, expressed mostly in intestinal L and pancreatic β cells, represents an attractive and new target for the treatment of metabolic disorders, and was proven to assist in glucose-stimulated insulin secretion (GSIS) (Zhang et al., 2014). It was demonstrated that a steroid glycoside identified in the extract of *H. gordonii*, namely gordonoside F, activated the GPR119 receptor. Gordonoside F decreased the intake of food and stimulated GSIS, both *in vivo* (mice) and *in vitro*. It was proven that the effects are linked to GPR119, because knockout of GPR119 blocked the restorative activity of gordonoside F. The appetite-suppressant activity of the extract of *Hoodia* was also partly stopped by GPR119 knockout.

The data revealed that GPR119 is one of the major mechanisms and a direct target responsible for the therapeutic activity of *H. gordonii*. Jain and Singh (2016) investigated the combined effect of L-carnitine and *H. gordonii* supplementation on appetite regulatory peptides and metabolic changes during calorie restriction. In the study, male albino rats were separated into two groups (*Hoodia*-treated and control) and an oral dosage of 100 mg/kg was administered for 5 days with <25% calorie restriction. Biochemical variables with regulatory peptides were evaluated along with physical efficiency tests. Significant changes in corticosterone, ghrelin, thyroid and leptin hormone levels were reported when compared to the control group. An increase in CPT-1 activity was observed in the treated group, while AMP-kinase and blood glucose concentrations decreased significantly when compared to the control.

Various clinical studies have been conducted on *Hoodia* species as an appetite suppressant. However, the most important one was conducted by the licensee Unilever (Blom et al., 2011). In this study, *Hoodia* extract was not tolerated as well as the placebo, with adverse effects, i.e., emesis, nausea and disturbance of skin sensation reported, although no serious adverse events (SAE) were documented. Heart rate, blood pressure, bilirubin, pulse-rate and alkaline phosphatase increased markedly in the *Hoodia*-treated group. Body weight and *ad libitum* energy intake did not differ significantly between the *Hoodia* extract treatment and placebo groups. Other clinical studies (14 in total) were conducted, but not reported in peer-reviewed journals in a work done by Pfizer, as a prior licensee. Maharaj (2011) reported on one of these and contradicting efficacy results were obtained in this study. A randomised, placebo-controlled, double-blind, repeat dose (15 days) study was conducted, with a single dose escalation stage, to investigate the safety, pharmacokinetics, effects and tolerability of the *Hoodia* extract in healthy candidates (males). In this study, the mean calorie intake in all meals was reduced for the *Hoodia-treated* group compared to the placebo. Statistically significant differences were observed for total intake of calories and for dinner calorie intake. Furthermore, a noteworthy difference was seen for the variation from baseline in the body fat content (BFC) between the different groups, with the *H. gordonii* extract having the lowest BFC on day 16. It was concluded that *H. gordonii* concentrated extract, given orally (short-term), led to a definite decrease in food intake. When the extract was administered for 15 days a considerable calorie intake reduction was seen, however, mild side effects were observed, such as headache, paraesthesia, vasodilatation, taste perversion, isolated reversible hyperbilirubinemia and somnolence. Placebo-controlled, double-blinded studies were also conducted by Phytopharm on obese, free-feeding volunteers ($n = 20$) (Holt and Taylor, 2006a). Participants were given *H. gordonii* extract and were counselled not to keep to any specific exercise or eating plan. In spite of the fact that food intake was not restricted, participants using the extract decreased their caloric intake by about 1000 cal/day. The decreased food intake revealed a favourable decrease in triglycerides and blood glucose with an additional 2 kg weight loss.

In an observational, open-label study, a capsule containing 400 mg of raw plant material of *H. gordonii* (Hoodia Supreme®) was given bidaily to eight obese candidates for a period of 4 weeks. The study included questioning participants on weight measurement as well as eating habits. Weight loss (0.91–6.8 kg), an optional decrease in calorie intake (500–1000 cal/day), reduction in appetite, a mild energising effect, and a lowering in cravings for food containing carbohydrates, were documented. Holt and Taylor (2006b) also reported that seven candidates given DEX-L10®, comprising *H. gordonii* (500 mg), for 28 days lost 4.5 kg of body weight on average, with no changes in daily activity or dietary habits. The information on clinical studies is scarce and sometimes the original sources cannot be located. Jain and Singh (2014) demonstrated that an oral dosage of 100 mg/kg of *H. gordonii* for a period of 5 days regulated the CCK activities with 25% calorie restriction. However, because there was no *Hoodia*-treated group without caloric restriction, the data cannot be used for extrapolation to advise on the mechanism/s or level of efficacy by which *H. gordonii* may have key appetite-suppressant activities when a normal diet is applied. Even so, the results contributed to the interpretation of biological targets of the plant. In another study, the glycaemic responses, glycaemic index (GI) and appetite effects of brown rice bars containing *H. gordonii* and *Kappaphycus alvarezii* were determined (Ghani et al., 2018). After overnight fasting, 12 healthy volunteers consumed HK1 (*H. gordonii*: 0 g, *K. alvarezii*: 0 g), HK2 (*H. gordonii*: 0 g, *K. alvarezii*: 2.8 g), HK3 (*H. gordonii*: 1.6 g, *K. alvarezii*: 0 g), or a reference (white bread) containing 50 g carbohydrates, in five sessions. In each session, blood glucose and appetite assessments were performed at 0, 15, 30, 45, 60, 90 and 120 min after food consumption. The energy intake (EI) assessment was performed at 120 min, and results showed that only HK3 was a medium GI food, while others were categorised as high GI foods. Consumption of HK3 provided the highest satiety and the lowest motivation to eat, and prospective food intake scores showed no significant differences when compared with other groups. Intake of HK3 also significantly reduced EI compared with HK1 and HK2, but not significantly when compared to HK4 and the reference food. It was concluded that consumption of *H. gordonii* affected GI, appetite and EI, which may have potential effects on body weight regulation.

8.2.2 Antidepressant properties

Antidepressant-like effects of extracts of *H. gordonii* were investigated using the forced swimming test (FST) in mice after repeated and acute administration (15 days) (Citó et al., 2015). The involvement of the mono-aminergic system was examined *via* neurochemical analysis of brain mono-amines to determine these effects. The administration of *H. gordonii* extracts reduced the immobility of mice in the forced swimming test without linked variations in activity in the open-field test during acute treatment, indicating antidepressant-like activity. The anti-immobility activity observed for *H. gordonii* was blocked by pretreating mice with NAN-190 (a 5-HT1A antagonist), PCPA (an inhibitor of 5-HT, serotonin synthesis), ondansetron (a 5-HT3A antagonist), ritanserin (a 5-HT2A/2C antagonist), SCH23390 (a D1 receptor antagonist), prazosin (an a1-adrenoceptor antagonist), sulpiride (a D2 receptor antagonist), and yohimbine (an alpha-2-adrenoceptor antagonist). After acute administration, significant increases in 5-HT levels were observed in the striatum, while norepinephrine, dopamine and 5-HT were remarkably raised after chronic treatment. The data demonstrated that *H. gordonii* exhibited antidepressant-like effects in the forced swimming test, by affecting the serotonergic, noradrenergic and dopaminergic systems.

8.2.3 Anti-inflammatory properties

The effects of the plant species *Hoodia parviflora* on animal models of insulin resistance and non-alcoholic steatohepatitis (the sand rat, *Psammomys obesus* and ob/ob mouse) were evaluated (Mizrahi et al., 2019). The secretion of IL-6 was determined by hepatic signal transducer and ELISA, and an activator of transcription 3 by Western blot. Oral administration of extracts raised insulin resistance displayed by enhanced glucose tolerance tests. Treatment reduced liver injury as demonstrated by a reduction in total hepatic fat, liver enzyme levels, enhanced hepatic histology and intrahepatic triglyceride content. Treatment with extracts of *H. parviflora* also decreased hepatic inflammation in mice with concanavalin A-induced hepatitis. These activities were not linked to weight and food consumption. Mizrahi et al. (2019) concluded that the data supported the plant's use as a liver protector.

8.2.4 Antidiabetic properties

A chronic (60–160 mg/kg) and acute (20–160 mg/kg) study was conducted to investigate the effect of P57 on diabetes (Rubin et al., 2006). Water and food intake, glucose, body weight, leptin and insulin content were determined in diabetic ZDF (Zucker diabetic fatty) male rats. During the chronic study, the dosages of P57 were decreased to 30–60 mg/kg on day 7, because a high reduction (50%) in food intake of the rats was observed. The data demonstrated that P57 exhibited beneficial activity on body weight, reduced water intake and sustained normal glycaemia in diabetic rats within a period of 4 days compared to the lean control rats.

8.2.5 Other properties

Hakkinen et al. (2005) described the gastroprotective properties of P57, activities on gastric motility and gastric acid secretion in a US patent application. In the study, gastric scarring caused by aspirin (orally administered) was decreased by 93.2% for cimetidine and by 91.5% for P57. When a spray-dried extract of *Hoodia* was orally administered, at 50 mg/kg dose, gastric emptying was inhibited by 26% and acid output by 50%. Further studies on P57 indicated that subcutaneous administration decreased acid output by 43%. When P57 was administered intraduodenally, acid output fell by 88% at a dosage of 10 mg/kg. Madgula et al. (2010a) reported on the gastroprotective effects of a spray-dried extract of *Hoodia*, as well as of P57. Nonetheless, in simulated gastric fluid, 100% degradation of P57 was observed, which questioned the validity of the actual active molecule. Another study investigated the pharmacokinetics, bioavailability and tissue distribution of P57 in female CD1 mice after oral administration of an enhanced methanol extract of *H. gordonii* (a single dose, similar to a dose of 25mg of P57/kg) or a single dose of 25 mg/kg of P57, intravenously. Analysis using ultra-performance liquid chromatography coupled with mass spectrometry (UPLC-MS) was employed to examine the levels of P57 in tissues (liver, brain, intestine and kidneys) and plasma. The peak plasma level of P57 was reached within 0.6h after oral administration of the extract of *Hoodia*. When intravenously administered, the plasma clearance rate of P57 was 1.09L/h/kg. It was shown that P57 was quickly eliminated and distributed from the tissues within a period of 4h. The content of tissue distribution was highly elevated in the kidneys, followed by the brain and liver. After oral intake, a low content of P57 was found in the kidneys, intestine and liver, but could not be detected in the brain. The ratio of tissue/plasma was calculated to be 0.33 for the brain, 0.75 the kidneys, and 0.57 for the liver, after intravenous (IV) administration, and 0.02 for liver, 0.11 for intestine, and 0.04 for the kidneys, following oral administration. Both routes showed a similar half-life for the elimination phase. The half-life of the absorption phase was 0.13h and the oral bioavailability was calculated as 47.5%. Pure P57 was moderately bioavailable and was shown to be rapidly eliminated (Madgula et al., 2010b).

8.3 Safety

Published data concerning the safety/toxicity of *H. gordonii* are limited. Menniti-Ippolito et al. (2008) described a 5-year study in Italy that included 233 reports on the side effects of the natural products that were investigated. An anticholinergic effect was recorded for one product containing 100mg of *H. gordonii* raw material. However, this preparation also included *Ephedra sinica* raw material (200mg), which in high likelihood was responsible for the effect. In another report linked to a case of acute hepatitis, six pharmaceutical preparations were consumed simultaneously, with one preparation containing *Hoodia*. Van Heerden et al. (2002) reported on acute toxicity studies conducted on *Hoodia*, in a patent application. The extract of the plant given to mice orally, at dosages of 100–3028.5mg/kg, displayed no toxicity. Reversible histopathological liver variations (dose-related) in the formation of hydropic degeneration of hepatocytes and cloudy, moderate swelling were documented from a dosage of 200mg/kg. A small group of animals (two animals per dosage group) were used in this study, but from all the groups, only one demonstrated liver variations upon histopathological investigation, and therefore further research is warranted. Tulp and Harbi (2002) reported that during anti-obesity studies in obese and congenic lean rats, high concentrations of *H. gordonii* (oral administration) exhibited no side effects. Dent et al. (2012a) showed that in a prenatal developmental toxicology experiment in rabbits, no adverse effects were observed on foetal development following administration of 12 mg/kg/day of *H. gordonii* extract over a period of 25days. Clinical toxicity data in the adult animals were obtained and the 6 and 12mg/kg/day doses caused a dose-dependent decrease in weight gain and food intake, while a dose of 3mg/kg/day did not affect the food intake by pregnant mothers and litters. A dosage of 12mg/kg/day was linked to a sharp decrease in water and food intake, as well as a thickening of stomach contents in animals (50%). This dosage was considered unendurable. The same group (Dent et al., 2012b) conducted a similar study in mice and demonstrated that of the dosages of 0, 5, 15 and 50 mg/kg/day of *H. gordonii* extract given over 12 days, only the 50 mg/kg/day dose decreased maternal weight gain and food intake. In addition, delayed foetal development was observed, with low foetal body mass. In another toxicity study in rodents, *H. gordonii* extracts did not cause genotoxicity in mice fed 400 mg/kg of the herbal drug (Scott et al., 2012). The high dose for administration of 400 mg/kg was selected from a tolerance study using four rats per dosage group. This study included dosages of up to 2000 mg/kg. Rodents given >350 mg/kg presented with clinical signs of toxicity, such as body mass loss, swollen abdomens and higher mortality within 48 h of administration.

In vivo studies in rodents demonstrated vast variations in results concerning the intolerable concentrations of extracts of *H. gordonii* (Smith and Krygsman 2014). These differences might be due to differences in plant material source, methods of collection of plant material, locality and timing of harvests, and the same differences probably occurred between supplement manufacturers. There were no side effects noted for the clinical study conducted on humans, but it should be stated that few were documented, probably due to the proprietary nature of the plant. A report of adverse effects will not be good for a company developing a product from *Hoodia* as this would attract negative attention. The long history of the use of *H. gordonii* (fresh plant material) by the Khoisan demonstrates its safety, but this is certainly not applicable to compounds isolated from the plant extracts, or even the extracts, as these are in concentrated forms. Roza et al. (2013) reported alarming adverse effects of products from *H. gordonii,* revealing an elevated pulse rate and increased blood pressure. Sympathomimetic effects using isolated organ experiments on rat uterine rings demonstrated smooth muscle relaxant effects of *H. gordonii*-containing products, with a considerable component mediated through β-adrenergic receptors. Chromatographic comparison of authentic plant material and the analysed product verified that the herbal product contained an extract of a *Hoodia* species, suggesting that the compounds of the plant were responsible for the observed cardiovascular activities.

9. Phytochemistry

9.1 Non-volatile constituents

Van Heerden et al. (2007) initiated phytochemical studies on *Hoodia* and isolated two steroidal glycosides from *H. gordonii* and *H. pilifera* extracts. Research conducted on the aerial parts of *H. gordonii* by Shukla et al. (2009) led to the isolation of seven pregnane glycosides, namely hoodigosides W–Z and hoodistanalosides A–B. Structure elucidation was done using spectroscopic methods, namely circular dichroism (CD) spectroscopy and one- (1D) and two-dimensional (2D) nuclear magnetic resonance (NMR) spectroscopy, as well as through chemical degradation studies. Subsequently, several novel structural derivatives were identified from *H. gordonii*, including pregnane glycosides, oxypregnane glycosides and hoodistanaloside (Vermaak et al., 2011). The core chemical structures of the compounds isolated are the aglycones calogenin, hoodigogenin A, isoramanone, dehydrohoodistanal and hoodistanal, and these were formed as a result of enzymatic and/or acid hydrolysis. Hoodigogenin A is a unique compound from *Hoodia* with a tigloyl ester group at position 12, also named 3β,12β,14β-trihydroxy-pregn-5-en-20-one. Derivatives of hoodigogenin A constitute 3β-*O*-glycosides with a chain consisting of two to five sugar components named hoodigosides W, X and A–K, as well as gordonosides A–L. A key characteristic of *Hoodia* is the rare 6–5–6-5 fused ring sterols, hoodistanaloside B and A, which are considered the first two naturally occurring glycosides comprising a 5(6 → 7)-abeosterol aglycone. P57, a complex molecule with the chemical name of 3β-[β-D-thevetopyranosyl-(1 → 4)-β-D-cymaropyranosyl-(1 → 4)-β-D-cymaropyranosyl-oxy]-12β-tigloyloxy-14β-hydroxy-pregn-5-en-20-one, is known as an active constituent of *H. gordonii* with proven appetite-suppressant activity. The chemical synthesis of P57 was attempted and required incorporation of a β-cymarosyl linkage onto the steroid aglycone (Liu et al., 2018). The stereoselective formation of this unique 2-deoxy-β-glycosidic linkage was shown to be a challenge and thus a limiting step in the synthesis of P57 and its congeners. Liu et al. (2018) investigated the glycosylation reactions with triphenylphosphine hydrobromide as promoter and glycals as donors, and a convergent synthesis of P57 through a β-selective glycosylation with a trisaccharide glycal donor. Zhang et al. (2012) also synthesised P57, *via* the synthesis of the aglycone hoodigogenin A from digoxin and the construction of the deoxytrisaccharide with glycosyl-*O*-alkynylbenzoates as donors.

Analytical methods including hyphenated chromatographic techniques were employed to investigate the chemical composition of an extract of *H. gordonii* (Russell and Swindells, 2012). The extract consisted of a mixture of plant sterols, steroid glycosides, polar organic material and fatty acids. High-performance liquid chromatography (HPLC) coupled with mass spectrometry (MS) and ultraviolet (UV) detection was employed to quantify various steroid glycosides in the extract (73.7%, w/w). Gas chromatography (GC) with flame ionisation detection (FID) and MS was utilised to determine the sterol (0.39%, w/w), fatty acid (3.12%, w/w) and alcohol (0.03%, w/w) content of a saponified sample of the extract. For indication and verification of raw materials, the concentration of P57 is usually determined. Vermaak et al. (2010) used Fourier Transform (FT)-Raman spectroscopy to quantify P57 in *H. gordonii* plant material. It was demonstrated that FT-Raman spectroscopy can be employed to quantify P57 in *H. gordonii* plant material with a high degree of accuracy as an alternative method to LC-MS analysis. Furthermore, the spatial distribution of P57 in a cross-section of a *H. gordonii* stem sample was investigated, and results showed that P57 is concentrated throughout the cortex. A study involving HPLC coupled with electrospray ionisation time-of-flight mass spectrometry (HPLC/ESI-ToF-MS) and electrospray ion-trap tandem mass spectrometry (ESI-MS/MS) resulted in the characterisation of eight C-21 steroidal glycosides present in *H. gordonii* (Avula et al., 2008). The spectra obtained for the eight C-21 steroidal glycosides were compared and a postulated fragmentation pathway suggested. The steroidal glycosides in *H. gordonii* were grouped into two major categories: calogenin and hoodigenin A. The results demonstrated the ability of ESI^+ to distinguish between calogenin and hoodigenin A glycosides, including the type of saccharide moiety and the number of sugar residues present, as well as the nature of the calogenin and hoodigenin A core.

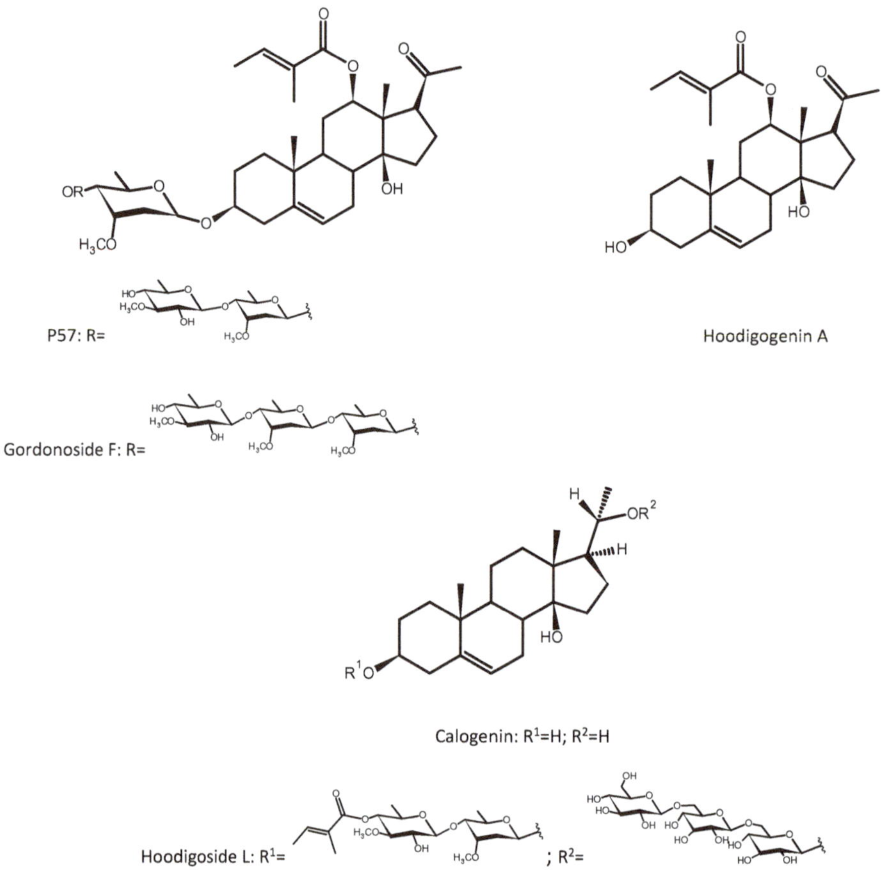

Part B: Chemical profiling and quality control

10. Chromatography analysis

10.1 High-performance thin-layer chromatography (HPTLC) fingerprint analysis

General instrumentation: CAMAG HPTLC instrument consisting of an automatic TLC sampler (ATS4), automatic developing chamber (ADC 2), CAMAG TLC visualiser 2, CAMAG derivatiser, and TLC plate heater. *HPTLC plates:* Silica gel glass plates 60 F_{254} (Merck). *Plant part:* Stems, methanol extract. *Sample application:* Application volume of 2 μL methanol extract (100 mg/mL) and standards (1 mg/mL) spotted as 10 mm bands. Plates developed in a 20×10×4 cm glass twin-trough chamber to a migration distance of 70 mm. *Tank saturation:* 20 min at 15 °C and 33% RH, with 25 mL of mobile phase. *Mobile phase:* Dichloromethane: ethyl acetate: formic acid: acetic acid: water (60:40:2:2:1, v/v/v/v/v). *Derivatisation:* Vanillin-sulphuric acid reagent. The plate was sprayed with 3 mL of the reagent and heated for 3 min at 100 °C on a TLC plate heater, then visualised. *Visualisation:* The plate was viewed under 366 nm radiation.

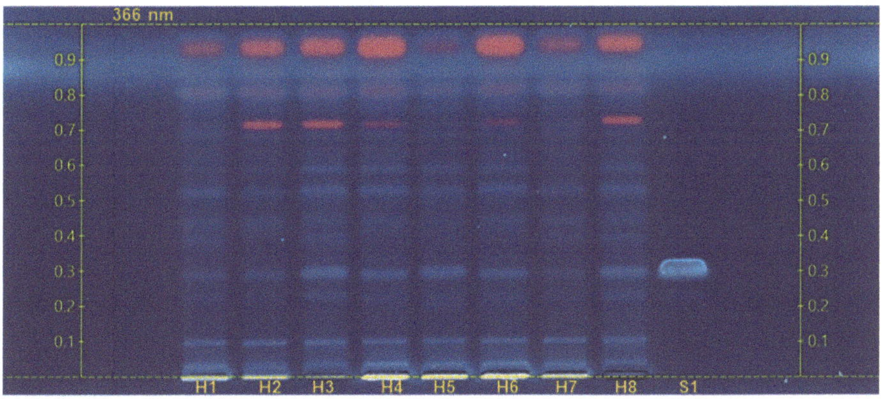

HPTLC plate of *Hoodia gordonii* methanol extracts ($n = 8$) (H1–H8) and the standard (S1). The samples are characterised by a light blue band for P57 (S1) ($R_f = 0.30$).

10.2 Ultra-performance liquid chromatography (UPLC) analysis

General instrumentation: Waters Acquity Ultra-Performance Liquid Chromatography system with photodiode array (PDA) detector combined with a Xevo G2QToF mass spectrometer (Waters, USA). *Plant part:* Stem, methanol extract. *Sample application*: Injection volume: 2.0 μL (full-loop injection) at 1 mg/mL. *Column*: Acquity UPLC BEH C_{18} column (150 mm × 2.1 mm, i.d., 1.7 μm particle size, Waters). *Mobile phase:* 0.1% formic acid in water (solvent A) and acetonitrile (solvent B). *Analysis conditions:* Gradient elution at a flow rate of 0.3 mL/min, changing as follows: 85% A: 15% B, changed to 50% A: 50% B in 2 min, to 25% A: 75% B in 8 min, to 10% A: 90% B in 3 min, held for 2 min, back to initial ratio in 0.5 min. Total running time is 16 min. *Mass spectrometry:* ESI^+ (positive ionisation mode), N_2 used as the desolvation gas. Desolvation temperature 400 °C at a flow rate of 550 L/h, source temperature 100 °C. Capillary and cone voltages, 3500 and 45 V, respectively. Data collected between *m/z* 100 and 1500.

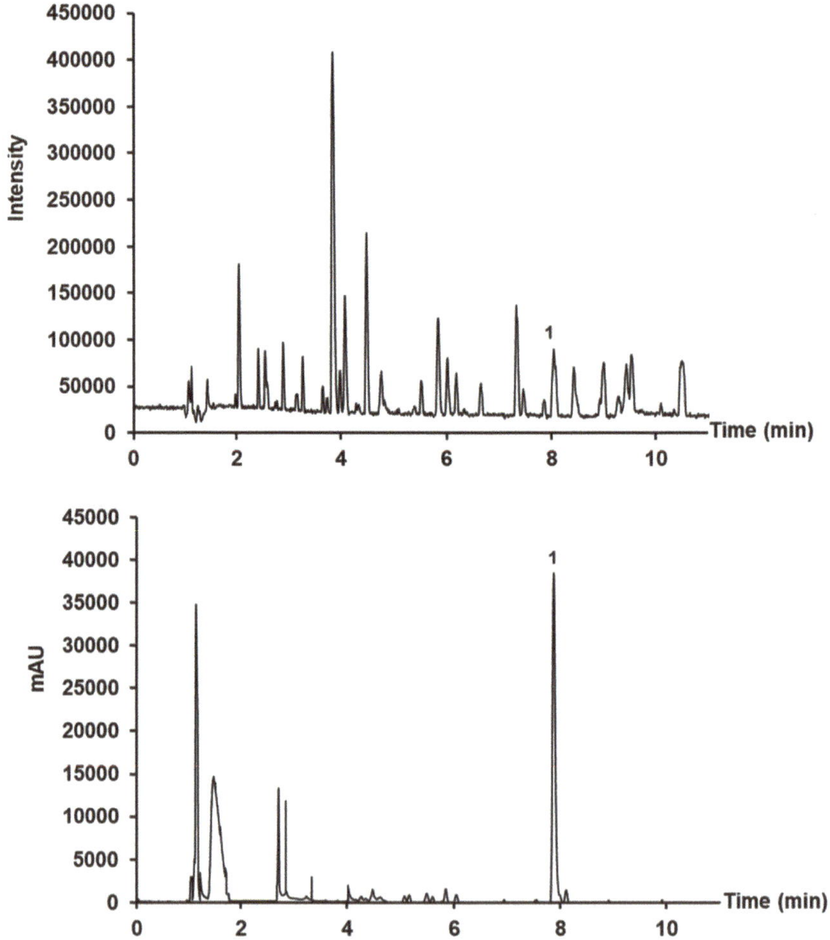

UPLC-ToF-MS ESI$^+$ (upper) and PDA (lower) chromatograms of *Hoodia gordonii* methanol extract. [1] = P57 *m/z* = 880.5504.

11. Mid-infrared (MIR) spectroscopy analysis

General instrumentation: Alpha-P Bruker spectrometer, mounted with an attenuated total reflectance (ATR) diamond crystal. *Spectral acquisition:* Spectrum obtained in absorbance mode, with a spectral resolution of 4 cm^{-1} over the range 4000–550 cm^{-1} and captured using OPUS 6.5 software. *Plant part:* Stems. *Sample preparation:* Stems powdered, sieved (< 500 μm) and placed directly onto the surface of the diamond crystal.

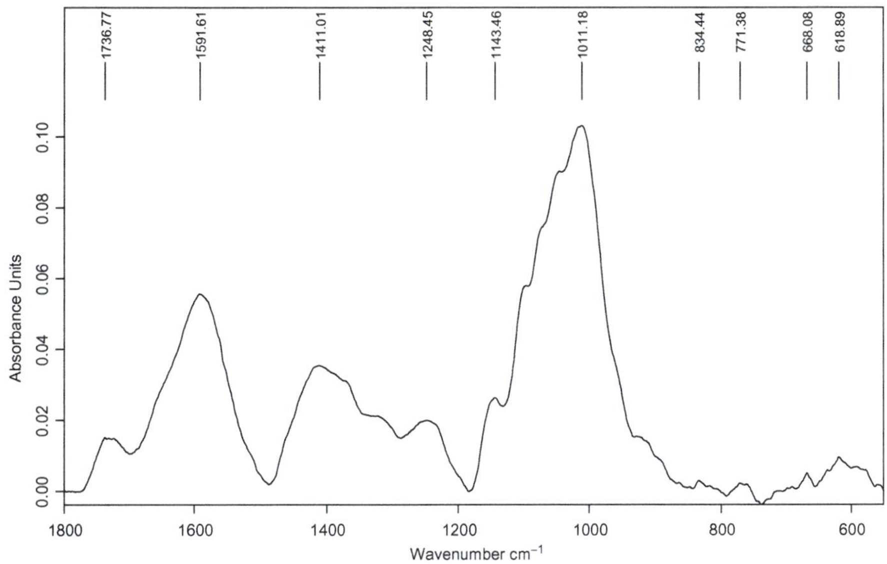

Mid-infrared spectrum of *Hoodia gordonii* powder displaying the fingerprint region (1800–550 cm^{-1}).

References

Avula, B., Wang, Y.-H., Pawar, R.S., Shukla, Y.J., Smillie, T.J., Khan, I.A., 2008. Rapid Commun. Mass Spectrom., 22:2587–2596.

Blom, W.A., Abrahamse, S.L., Bradford, R., Duchateau, G.S., Theis, W., Orsi, A., Ward, C.L., Mela, D.J., 2011. Am. J. Clin. Nutr., 94:1171–1181.

Bruyns, P.V., 2005. Stapeliads of Southern Africa and Madagascar, Vol 1. Umdani Press, Pretoria, South Africa.

Citó, M.C.O., Silva, M.I.G., Santos, L.K.X., Fernandes, M.L., Melo, F.H.C., Aguiar, J.A.C., Lopes, I.S., Sousa, P.B., Vasconcelos, S.M.M., Macêdo, D.S., Sousa, F.C.F., 2015. Braz. J. Med. Biol. Res., 48:57–64.

Dent, M.P., Wolterbeek, A.P., Russell, P.J., Bradford, R., 2012a. Food Chem. Toxicol., 50:S26–S33.

Dent, M.P., Wolterbeek, A.P., Russell, P.J., Bradford, R., 2012b. Food Chem. Toxicol., 50:S20–S25.

Ghani, M.A., Hajal, M.E., Daud, N.M., 2018. Malays. Appl. Biol., 47:55–62.

Glasl, S., 2009. Schweiz. Z. Ganzheitsmed., 21:300–306.

Hakkinen, J., Horak, R.M., Maharaj, V., 2005. Gastric Acid Secretion. US Patent 0079233 A1.

Holt, S., Taylor, T.V., 2006a. Townsend Lett., 280:104–113.

Holt, S., Taylor, T.V., 2006b. Townsend Lett., 281:99–104.

Jain, S., Singh, S.N., 2013. S. Afr. J. Bot., 86:51–55.

Jain, S., Singh, S.N., 2014. S. Afr. J. Bot., 92:73–77.

Jain, S., Singh, S.N., 2016. Def. Sci. J., 66:11–18.

Kapewangolo, P., Knott, M., Shithigona, R.E.K., Uusiku, S.L., Kandawa-Schulz, M., 2016. BMC Complement. Altern. Med., 16 (1):411.

Komarnytsky, S., Esposito, D., Poulev, A., Raskin, I., 2013. J. Cell. Physiol., 228:1120–1126.

Le Nevé, B.L., Foltz, M., Daniel, H., Gouka, R., 2010. Am. J. Physiol. Gastrointest. Liver Physiol., 299:G1368–G1375.

Liu, C., Ma, Y., Pei, C., Li, W., Yu, B., 2018. Chin. J. Chem., 36:1007–1010.

MacLean, D.B., Luo, L.G., 2004. Brain Res., 1020:1–11.

Madgula, V.L.M., Avula, B., Pawar, R.S., Shukla, Y.J., Khan, I.A., Walker, L.A., Khan, S.I., 2010a. Planta Med., 76:62–69.

Madgula, V.L.M., Ashfaq, M.K., Wang, Y.-H., Avula, B., Khan, I.A., Walker, L.A., Khan, S.I., 2010b. Planta Med., 76:1582–1586.

Maharaj, V., 2011. Summary Reports for Key *Hoodia* Clinical Studies. Retrieved from https://researchspace.csir.co.za/dspace/handle/10204/5375 (Accessed 23 May 2019).

Marloth, R., 1932. The Flora of South Africa: With a Synopsis of the South African Genera of Phanerogamous Plants. Section 2: Myoporaceae-Compositae. Darter Bros, W. Wesley & Son, London, UK.

Masson, F., 1796. *Stapelia* Novae: On a Collection of Several New Species of That Genus. W. Bulmer and Co. for George Nicol, London, UK.

Menniti-Ippolito, F., Mazzanti, G., Santuccio, C., Moro, P.A., Calapai, G., Firenzuoli, F., Valeri, A., Raschetti, R., 2008. Pharmacoepidemiol. Drug Saf., 17:626–635.

Mizrahi, M., Ben Ya'Acov, A., Adar, T., Levy Sklair, M., Gaska, S., Ilan, Y., 2019. J. Med. Food, 22:1189–1198.

Mohlapo, T.D., Ng'ambi, J.W., Norris, D., Malatje, M.M., 2009. Trop. Anim. Health Prod., 41:1591–1596.

Olivier, I., 2008. Hoodia gordonii (Masson) Sweet ex Decne. Available at http://www.plantzafrica.com/planthij/hoodgord.htm.

Pappe, K.W.L., 1862. Silva Capensis; or, a Description of South African Forest-Trees and Arborescent Shrubs Used for Technical and Economical Purposes by the Colonists of the Cape of Good Hope, second ed. Ward & Co, London, UK, pp. 54–55.

Pawar, R.S., Shukla, Y.J., Khan, S.I., Avula, B., Khan, I.A., 2007. Steroids, 72:524–534.

Roza, O., Lovász, N., Zupkó, I., Hohmann, J., Csupor, D., 2013. BioMed Res. Int., 2013, Art. No. 171059, https://doi.org/10.1155/2013/171059.

Rubin, I.D., Bindra, J.S., Cawthorne, M.A., 2006. Extracts, Compounds and Pharmaceutical Compositions Having Anti-Diabetic Activity and Their Use. US Patent 0159779 A1.

Russell, P.J., Swindells, C., 2012. Food Chem. Toxicol., 50:S6.

Scott, A.D., Orsi, A., Ward, C., Bradford, R., 2012. Food Chem. Toxicol., 50:S34–S40.

Shukla, Y.J., Pawar, R.S., Ding, Y., Li, X.-C., Ferreira, D., Khan, I.A., 2009. Phytochemistry, 70:675–683.

Smith, C., Krygsman, A., 2014. J. Ethnopharmacol., 155:1284–1290.

Tulp, O.L., Harbi, N., 2002. FASEB J., 16, Art. No. 654.

Van Heerden, F.R., 2008. J. Ethnopharmacol., 119:434–437.

Van Heerden, F.R., Vleggaar, R., Horak, R.M., Learmonth, R.A., Maharaj, V., Whittal, R.D., 2002. Pharmaceutical Compositions Having Appetite-Suppressant Activity. US Patent 6376657 B1.

Van Heerden, F.R., Horak, R.M., Maharaj, V.J., Vleggaar, R., Senabe, J.V., Gunning, P.J., 2007. Phytochemistry, 68:2545–2553.

Vermaak, I., Viljoen, A.M., Hamman, J.H., Baranska, M., 2010. Phytochem. Lett., 3:156–160.

Vermaak, I., Viljoen, A.M., Chen, W., Hamman, J.H., 2011. Phytomedicine, 18:783–787.

White, A., Sloane, B.L., 1933. The Stapelieae. Abbey San Encino Press, Pasadena, USA, pp. 152–163.
Wynberg, R., Chennells, R., 2009. Indigenous Peoples, Consent and Benefit Sharing: Lessons from the San-Hoodia Case. Springer, New York, USA.
Wynberg, R., Van Niekerk, J., 2014. For. Trees Livelihoods, 23:19–35.
Wynberg, R., Schroeder, D., Chennels, R., 2009. Indigenous Peoples, Consent and Benefit Sharing. Lessons from the San-Hoodia Case. Springer Publications, London, UK, Vols. 11–26, 89–121.
Zhang, J., Shi, H., Ma, Y., Yu, B., 2012. Chem. Comm., 48:8679–8681.
Zhang, S., Ma, Y., Li, J., Ma, J., Yu, B., Xie, X., 2014. P. Natl. Acad. Sci. USA, 111:14571–14576.

CHAPTER

13

Hypoxis hemerocallidea

Kokoette Bassey, Sandra Combrinck and Weiyang Chen

Department of Pharmaceutical Sciences, Tshwane University of Technology, Pretoria, South Africa

Abstract

Hypoxis hemerocallidea Fisch., C.A.Mey. & Avé-Lall. (Hypoxidaceae) is known as African potato. It is described as an herbaceous perennial plant, with a scythe-like appearance and bright yellow star-shaped flowers. It occurs in tropical and southern Africa, growing abundantly throughout the summer rainfall areas of South Africa. The rootstock is traditionally used for the treatment of a wide range of conditions, including urinary tract infections, common cold, influenza, nausea, heart weakness, infertility, depression and anxiety, but is best known for the treatment of benign prostate hypertrophy and HIV. A range of products including creams, capsules, tinctures and tonics prepared from H. hemerocallidea are available commercially. In vitro and in vivo investigations have proven anti-oxidant, anti-inflammatory, antidiabetic, anticonvulsant, antibacterial and CD4-count reduction potential for African potato and/or its metabolites. Semi-automated high-performance thin-layer chromatography (HPTLC) and ultra-performance liquid chromatography hyphenated with mass spectrometry (UPLC–MS) have been used to determine the chemical profiles of H. hemerocallidea. The chemical marker compound hypoxoside (R_f 0.32) was identified by HPTLC and UPLC–MS. In addition, hemerocalloside (R_t = 3.50 min; m/z 519) and geraniol glycoside (R_t = 7.60 min; m/z 447) were also identified as marker compounds in the methanol extract of H. hemerocallidea.

Keywords: *Hypoxis hemerocallidea*, African potato, Hypoxoside, Hemerocalloside, HPTLC, UPLC–MS, MIR spectroscopy

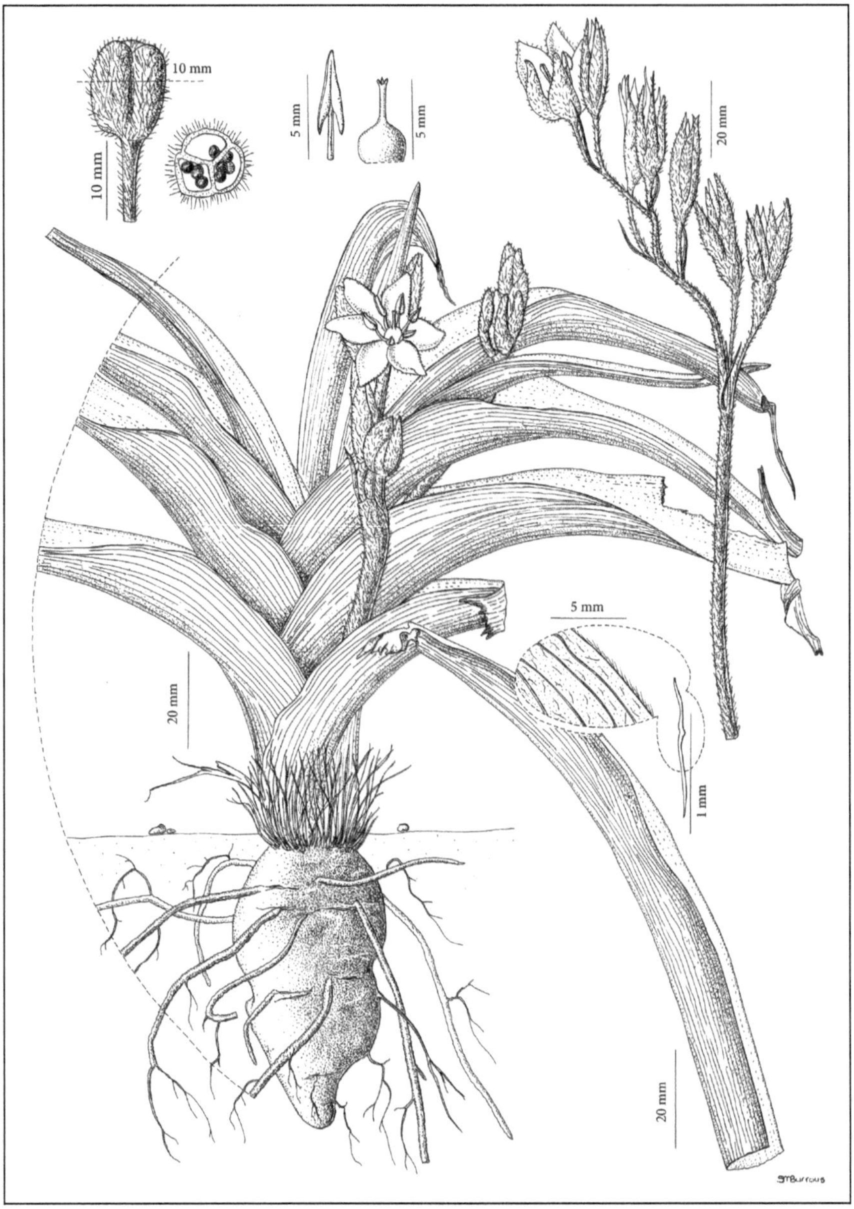
10 mm
10 mm
5 mm
5 mm
20 mm
5 mm
20 mm
1 mm
20 mm
SMBurrows

Part A: General overview

1. Synonyms

Hypoxis rooperi T.Moore, *Hypoxis obconica* Nel, *Hypoxis patula* Nel, *Hypoxis rooperi* var. *forbesii* Baker.[a]

2. Common name(s)

Star flower, yellow star, star lily, or magic muthi (English), *'inkomfe', 'ilabetheka'* (isiZulu), *'sterblom', 'sterretjie', 'Afrika patat', 'gifbol'* (Afrikaans), *'moli kharatsa', 'lotsane'* (Southern Sotho), *'inongwe', 'ilabatheka', 'ixhalanxa', 'ikhubalo lezithunzela'* (isiXhosa) and *'tshuka'* (Setswana).[a,b]

3. Conservation status

Least concern.[c]

4. Botany

The genus *Hypoxis*, representing about 90 species, is the largest in the family Hypoxidaceae R.Br. (Singh, 2009). Based on similarities with species of the Amaryllidaceae and Orchidaceae, the genus was previously classified in and alongside these families. Currently, the Hypoxidaceae represents the African branch of the Asparagales. The genus name *'hypoxis'* is derived from the Greek words *'hypo'* meaning below, and *'oxy'* meaning 'sharp', which describe the pointed base of the capsule. *Hypoxis hemerocallidea* Fisch., C.A.Mey & Avé-Lall., previously known as *H. rooperi* T.Moore, is one of the most frequently traded medicinal plants in southern Africa (Dold and Cocks, 2002). The plant grows as a stemless, perennial geophyte that reaches a height of up to 500 mm. It is characterised by 6–12 linear-lanceolate leaves, which are organised typically into three ranks and are hairy (Singh, 2009). The silhouette of the plant is scythe-shaped, whilst the leaves are usually surrounded by a dense mass of fibrous bristles resulting from the remains of dead leaves (A). Flowers, which appear between October and January, are star-shaped and bright yellow (A), and the number per inflorescence may vary from 2 to 12. The smooth, black, glossy seeds are ovoid and about 2 mm in length. The plant has large, oblong, dark fibrous corms and tuberous roots (B) that are bright yellow inside when freshly cut, but rapidly change colour.

[a] World Flora Online (www.worldfloraonline.org).
[b] PlantZAfrica (http://pza.sanbi.org).
[c] Red List of South African Plants (http://redlist.sanbi.org).

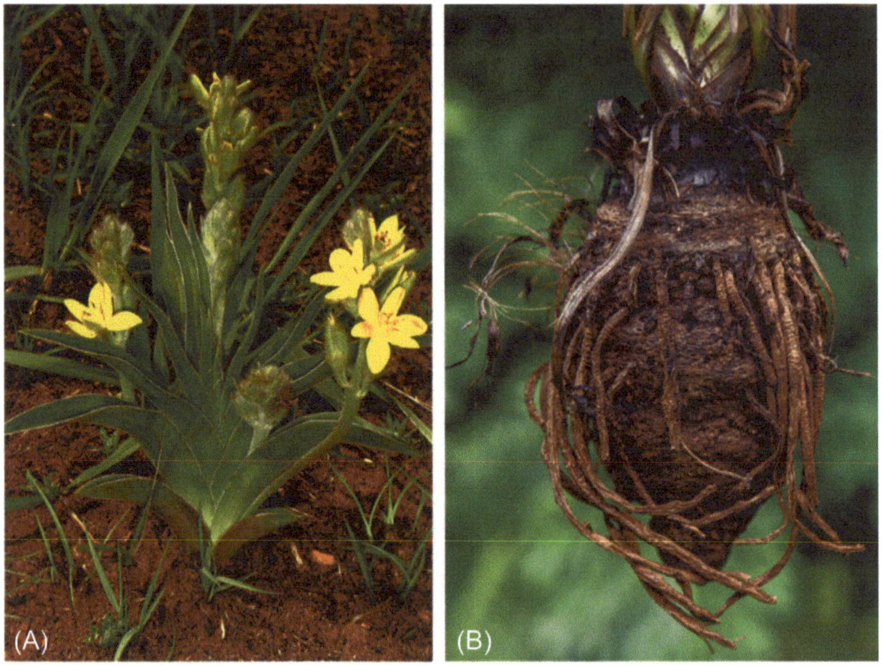

Hypoxis hemerocallidea plant displaying bright yellow, star-shaped flowers (A), and the large, oblong corm with protruding roots (B).

5. Geographical distribution

Hypoxis hemerocallidea is widespread in Africa, also occurring in tropical and southern Africa. The plant occurs abundantly along the east coast and interior of the

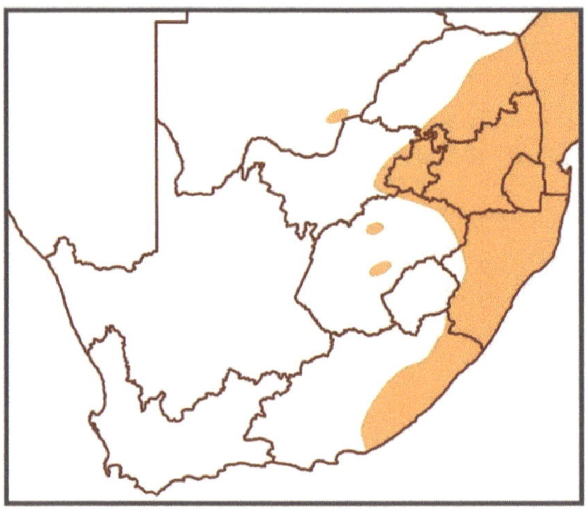

Geographical distribution of *Hypoxis hemerocallidea* in South Africa.

summer rainfall regions of South Africa at altitudes of 50–1800 m. It is also found in Botswana, Swaziland (Eswatini), Mozambique and Zimbabwe (Germishuizen et al., 2006). These frost-resistant and drought-tolerant plants grow in woodlands, rocky grasslands, and on grassy slopes that are vulnerable to fires. Corms are wild-harvested and as a result, the populations are dwindling.

6. Ethnopharmacology

Hypoxis hemerocallidea is one of the most popular medicinal plants in southern Africa. It is used for the treatment of a wide variety of symptoms and conditions. Decoctions prepared from the corms are used to treat respiratory tract infections, influenza, headaches, diabetes, benign prostate hypertrophy and prostate cancer, stomach disorders, dysentery, dermatitis, burns, hypertension, skin rashes, anxiety and acne (Watt and Breyer-Brandwijk, 1962; Hutchings, 1996; Ncube et al., 2013). Infusions of the corms are taken as a general tonic, particularly by people diagnosed with HIV or tuberculosis, to boost the immune system. Such infusions are also applied as emetics to treat dizziness and urinary tract infections (Hutchings, 1996). The plant is used interchangeably with other *Hypoxis* species, some of which have similar morphological features (Singh, 2009).

7. Commercialisation

Commercial interest in products from *H. hemerocallidea* is traceable to 1967 (Drewes and Khan, 2004). Harzol®, the first commercial product launched in 1974 and marketed in Germany, and Moducare®, which was marketed in South Africa, are probably the best known of these (Bouic et al., 2001; Boukes et al., 2008; Drewes et al., 2008). These over-the-counter drugs are marketed mainly for the treatment of prostate disorders, for which there is increasingly good evidence of efficacy. Creams containing extracts of *H. hemerocallidea* are marketed to treat eczema, whilst commercial capsules, tinctures and tonics are also available (Ncube et al., 2013). Due to the high phytosterol content, *H. hemerocallidea* products are also widely marketed for their putative antilipidemic, antidiabetic and anti-inflammatory activities. An efficient *in vitro* plant regeneration system was established *via* somatic embryogenesis of *H. hemerocallidea* by Kumar et al. (2017) for commercial production. The protocol developed will be helpful in conserving germplasm and reducing stress on natural populations, allowing regeneration of large numbers of high-value clonal plants, and enabling genetic transformational studies, as well as the further investigation of bio-active compounds.

8. Pharmacological evaluation

8.1 *In vitro* studies

Polar extracts of *H. hemerocallidea* have been evaluated in a large number of assays, and were reported to have anti-oxidant (Albrecht et al., 1995; Matotoka and Masoko, 2017), analgesic, antidiabetic (Mahomed and Ojewole, 2004), anticonvulsant (Risa et al.,

2004), uterolytic, bronchorelaxant (Nyinawumuntu et al., 2008), antiviral (Liebenberg et al., 1997), antifungal and antibacterial activities against a range of infective human pathogens (Ncube et al., 2013). The antibacterial activity may be attributed to rooperol, since exposure of *Escherichia coli* to the compound resulted in the disruption of the bacterial cell membrane (Laporta et al., 2007). Ethyl acetate corm extracts were found to inhibit the enzyme mono-amine oxidase, which is associated with several neurological conditions (Stafford et al., 2007). The anti-inflammatory activities of *H. hemerocallidea* and rooperol have been determined using various assays (Laporta et al., 2007; Drewes et al., 2008). Biogenic gold nanoparticles (GNPs) were synthesised from *H. hemerocallidea* extracts, and evaluated for their antibacterial activity against bacterial strains that are known to infect wounds (Elbagory et al., 2017). The toxicity of the biogenic GNPs to non-cancerous human fibroblast cells (KMST-6) was also investigated. The GNPs from *H. hemerocallidea* exhibited antibacterial activity against all the tested bacterial strains, but did not display any significant toxicity towards KMST-6 cells, suggesting that these nanoparticles can be safely applied to wound dressings.

8.2 *In vivo* studies and clinical trials

8.2.1 Anti-HIV activity

More clinical trials have been conducted on the active metabolites rooperol and β-sitosterol than on extracts from *H. hemerocallidea*. The effect of Moducare® (100:1 sterol/sterolin mixture) on HIV-infected individuals was evaluated (Breytenbach et al., 2001). After 6 months, the T-cell expression of interferon gamma (INF-γ) was enhanced in the treatment group, reflecting a stabilisation of the CD+ T-cell count. Furthermore, the rate of progression of the HIV-positive patients to full-blown AIDS was inhibited in the treatment group. In an animal study by Azu et al. (2016), the protective effects of *H. hemerocallidea* extracts were investigated against highly active antiretroviral therapy (HAART)-induced hepatotoxicity. Adjuvant *H. hemerocallidea* with HAART caused a reduction in low-density lipoprotein (LDL) and increased the high-density lipoprotein (HDL) and triglyceride levels. These results warrant caution on the adjuvant use of *H. hemerocallidea* together with HAART. In other studies, adjuvant treatment with the aqueous extract of *H. hemerocallidea* did not attenuate the nephrotoxicity, or show any deleterious effect on morphometric data with HAART in rat models (Jegede et al., 2017; Offor et al., 2017).

8.2.2 Antidiabetic and cardiovascular effects

In vivo data indicates that daily and consistent intake of infusions of *H. hemerocallidea* may be beneficial for the management of specific cardiac conditions, since the infusion caused bradycardia and brief hypotension in guinea pigs and rats (Ojewole et al., 2006). These findings lend pharmacological support to anecdotal uses in the management and control of certain cardiac dysfunctions and hypertension in some rural communities of southern Africa. The effects of *H. hemerocallidea* extracts were evaluated on oxidative stress biomarkers, hepatic injury, and other selected biomarkers in the liver and kidneys of healthy non-diabetic and streptozotocin-induced diabetic male Wistar rats. A significant reduction in blood glucose levels and an increase in the activities of liver enzymes were observed (Oguntibeju et al., 2016). The antidiabetic property of an aqueous extract of *H. hemerocallidea* was investigated in rats undergoing HAART. Treatment with the extracts did not change serum testosterone levels, nor did it mitigate the altered expression of collagen fibres and androgen receptors, resulting from streptozotocin-nicotinamide-induced diabetes (Ismail et al., 2017).

8.2.3 Anti-inflammatory and immune-modulating effects

An *in vivo* trial conducted in rats, to which a 50 mg/kg extract of *H. hemerocallidea* had been administered, demonstrated a significant anti-inflammatory effect compared to the controls (Ncube et al., 2013). A comparative study of the activities of β-sitosterol and a chloroform extract of *H. hemerocallidea* revealed that the pure compound appeared to be far better at modulating the immune system than the extract (De Caires et al., 2011).

8.2.4 Pharmacokinetics and drug interactions

The impact of selected *H. hemerocallidea* materials (a commercial product, an aqueous extract, and a reference plant material) on the bidirectional permeability of indinavir, an antiretroviral drug, across Caco-2 cell monolayers, as well as the bio-availability of indinavir during an acute, single administration study in Sprague–Dawley rats, were investigated (Havenga et al., 2018). An increase in the bio-availability of indinavir was observed *in vivo* when administered concomitantly with the *H. hemerocallidea* materials. All the test materials inhibited efflux of indinavir across Caco-2 cell monolayers in the following order: commercial product > aqueous extract > reference plant material. The change in bio-availability correlated directly with the *in vitro* permeability results.

8.2.5 Other effects

Phase 1 trials indicated that hypoxoside, the glycosylated form of rooperol, was effective as an oral prodrug for cancer therapy (Mills et al., 2005). An ethanolic extract of *H. hemerocallidea* used in a sexual behaviour and reproductive rat study indicated that libido and serum testosterone levels increased after 56 days treatment. An increase in epididymal sperm count was associated with the 300 mg/kg dose, and testicular oxidative status improved (Tiya et al., 2017).

8.3 Safety

Several short- and long-term studies have indicated that *H. hemerocallidea* is safe for therapeutic use (Drewes and Khan, 2004; Verschaeve et al., 2013). However, Musabayane et al. (2005) reported that an aqueous extract of *H. hemerocallidea* corms induced possible deleterious effects on kidney function. The safety of *Hypoxis* products and its purified metabolites raised concerns when a clinical trial involving HIV-positive patients was prematurely terminated by the former Medicines Control Council of South Africa, due to issues of bone marrow suppression in some of the participants (Mills et al., 2005). Apart from these findings, the use of *H. hemerocallidea* as a traditional remedy over a long time period has produced no evidence of toxicity, suggesting that the herbal drug may be safe for use (Drewes and Khan, 2004).

9. Phytochemistry

9.1 Non-volatile constituents

The norlignan glycoside, hypoxoside [(*E*)-1,5-*bis*(4′-β-D-glucopyranosyloxy-3′-hydroxyphenyl)pent-4-en-1-yne] was first isolated by Marini-Bettolo et al. (1982) from *H. obtusa*. However, this prodrug was also isolated from *H. hemerocallidea* by Drewes et al. (1984) and has since been identified in most *Hypoxis* species. Upon hydrolysis, hypoxoside is converted to the therapeutically active aglycone, known as rooperol. High concentrations of hypoxoside are mainly localised in the rootstock (Vinesi et al., 1990), but the concentrations are variable. Dehydroxyhypoxoside and *bis*-dehydroxyhypoxoside were also reported to be present in rootstock. Bassey (2015) identified a new phenolic glycoside, 1,5-*bis*(3,4-dihydroxyphenyl)-1,2-dihydroxy-4-pentyne-2-*O*-acetoxy-β-D-glucopyranoside (hemerocalloside) and geraniol glycoside from the corms of *H. hemerocallidea*. He reported that a number of plant sterols i.e. β-sitosterol, stigmasterol and their glycosides, campesterol, as well as stanols, including sitostanol (syn. stigmastanol) are also produced by *H. hemerocallidea* (Bassey, 2015). Fatty acids, including oleic and palmitic acids, and 2-hydroxyethyl linoleate were also detected using GC–MS in the chloroform extracts.

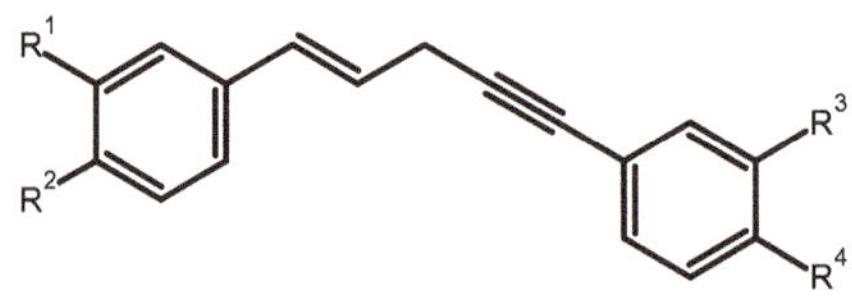

Hypoxoside: R^1=OH, R^2=*O*-β-D-glucose, R^3=OH, R^4=*O*-β-D-glucose
Dehydroxyhypoxoside: R^1=H, R^2=*O*-β-D-glucose, R^3=OH, R^4=*O*-β-D-glucose
bis-Dehydroxyhypoxoside: R^1=H, R^2=*O*-β-D-glucose, R^3=H, R^4=*O*-β-D-glucose
Rooperol: R^1=OH, R^2=OH, R^3=OH, R^4=OH

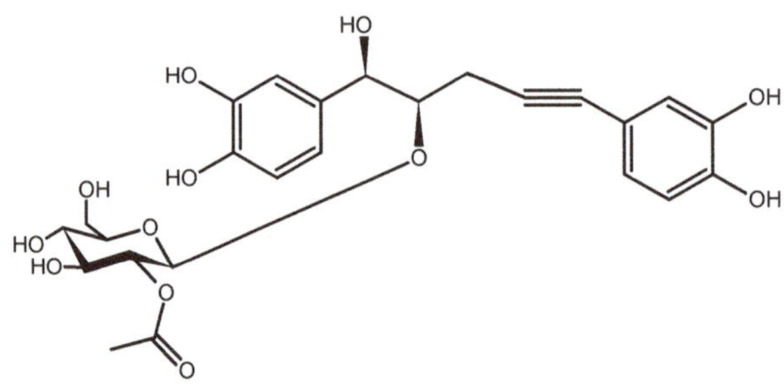

1,5-*bis*(3,4-Dihydroxyphenyl)-1,2-dihydroxy-4-pentyne-2-*O*-acetoxy-β-D-glucopyranoside
(Hemerocalloside)

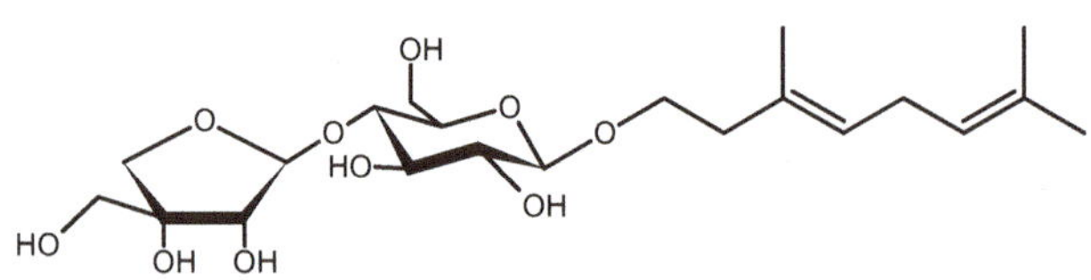

Geraniol glycoside

Part B: Chemical profiling and quality control

10. Chromatography analysis

10.1 High-performance thin-layer chromatography (HPTLC) fingerprint analysis

General instrumentation: CAMAG HPTLC instrument consisting of an automatic TLC sampler (ATS 4), automatic developing chamber (ADC 2), CAMAG TLC visualiser 2, CAMAG derivatiser, and TLC plate heater. *HPTLC plates*: Silica gel glass plates 60 F_{254} (Merck). *Plant part*: Corms, methanol extract. *Sample application*: Application volume of 2μL methanol extract (10mg/mL) and 10μL standard (1mg/mL) spotted as 10mm bands. Plates developed in a 20×10×4cm glass twin-trough chamber to a migration distance of 70mm. *Tank saturation*: 20min at 20.8°C and 30.4% RH, with 25mL of mobile phase. *Mobile phase*: Chloroform:methanol:water (70:30:4, v/v/v). *Derivatisation*: 10% sulphuric acid in methanol. The plate was dipped in the derivatising reagent and heated for 5min at 100°C on a TLC plate heater, then visualised. *Visualisation*: The plate was viewed under white reflectance light.

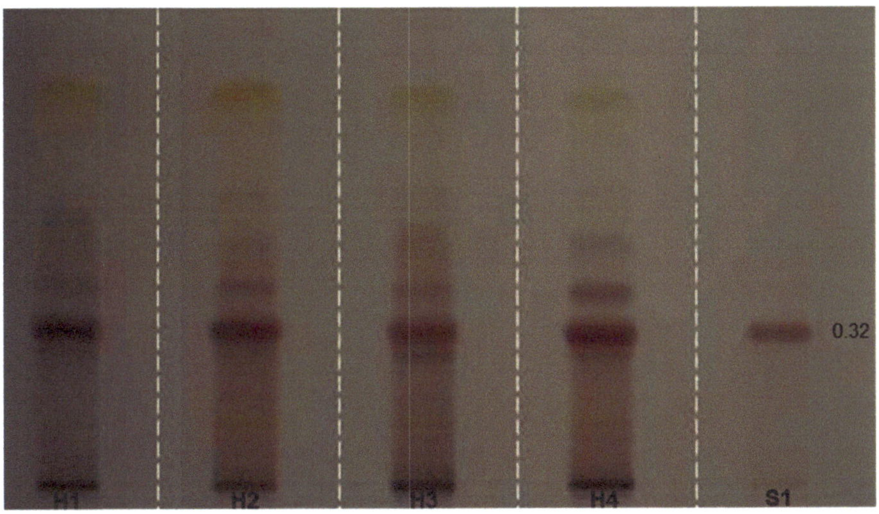

HPTLC plate of *Hypoxis hemerocallidea* methanol extracts ($n=4$) (H1–H4) and the standard (S1). The samples are characterised by a dark brown band for hypoxoside ($R_f=0.32$).

10.2 Ultra-performance liquid chromatography (UPLC) analysis

General instrumentation: Waters Acquity Ultra-Performance Liquid Chromatography system with photodiode array (PDA) detector combined with a Xevo G2QToF mass spectrometer (Waters, United States). *Plant part*: Corms, methanol extract. *Sample application*: Injection volume: 1.0μL (full-loop injection) at 1mg/mL. *Column*: Acquity UPLC BEH

C_{18} column (150 mm × 2.1 mm, i.d., 1.7 μm particle size, Waters). *Mobile phase*: 0.1% formic acid in water (solvent A) and acetonitrile (solvent B). *Analysis conditions*: Gradient elution at a flow rate of 0.3 mL/min, changing as follows: 85% A: 15% B changed to 65% A: 35% B in 7 min, to 50% A: 50% B in 1 min, held for 0.5 min, back to initial ratio in 0.5 min, equilibrating the system for 2 min, total run time 11 min. *Mass spectrometry*: ESI^- (negative ionisation mode), N_2 used as the desolvation gas. Desolvation temperature 350 °C at a flow rate of 500 L/h, source temperature 100 °C. Capillary and cone voltages 2500 and 45 V, respectively. Data collected between *m/z* 100 and 1000.

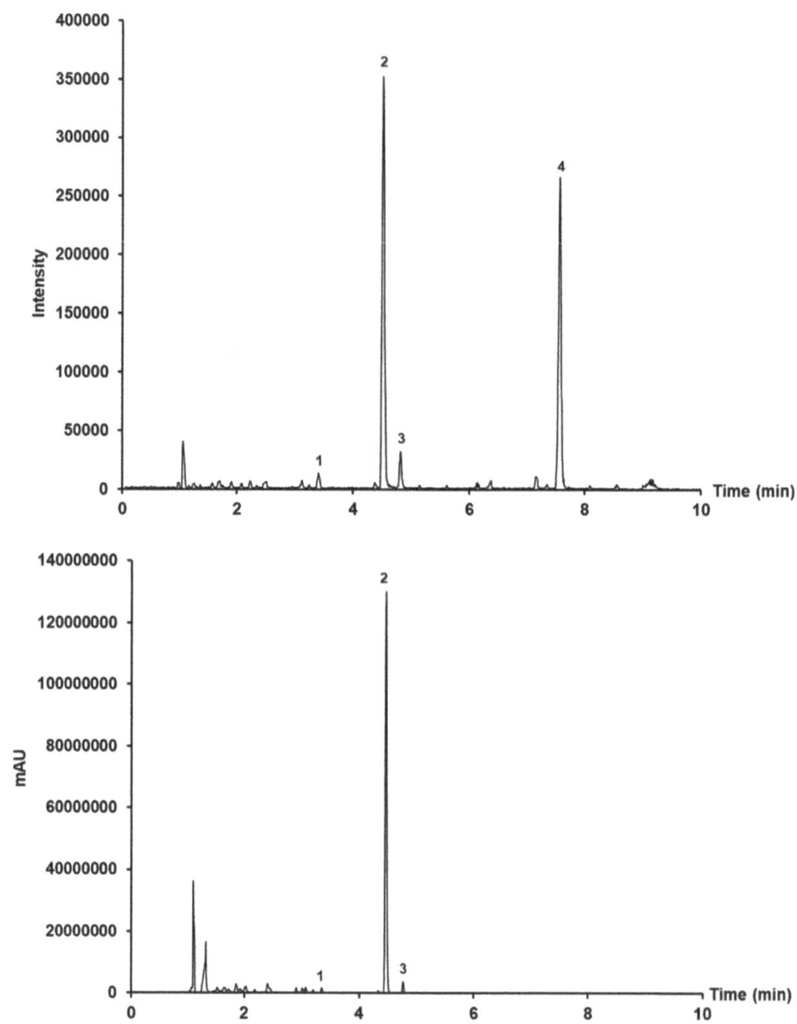

UPLC–ToF–MS ESI^- (upper) and PDA (lower) chromatograms of *Hypoxis hemerocallidea* methanol extract. [1] = hemerocalloside *m/z* 519.1550, [2] = hypoxoside *m/z* 605.1862, [3] = dehydroxyhypoxoside *m/z* 589.1920, [4] = geraniol glycoside *m/z* 447.2231.

11. Mid-infrared (MIR) spectroscopy analysis

General instrumentation: Alpha-P Bruker spectrometer, mounted with an attenuated total reflectance (ATR) diamond crystal. *Spectral acquisition*: Spectrum obtained in absorbance mode, with a spectral resolution of 4 cm^{-1} over the range 4000–550 cm^{-1} and captured using OPUS 6.5 software. *Plant part*: Corms. *Sample preparation*: Corms powdered, sieved (<500 µm) and placed directly onto surface of diamond crystal.

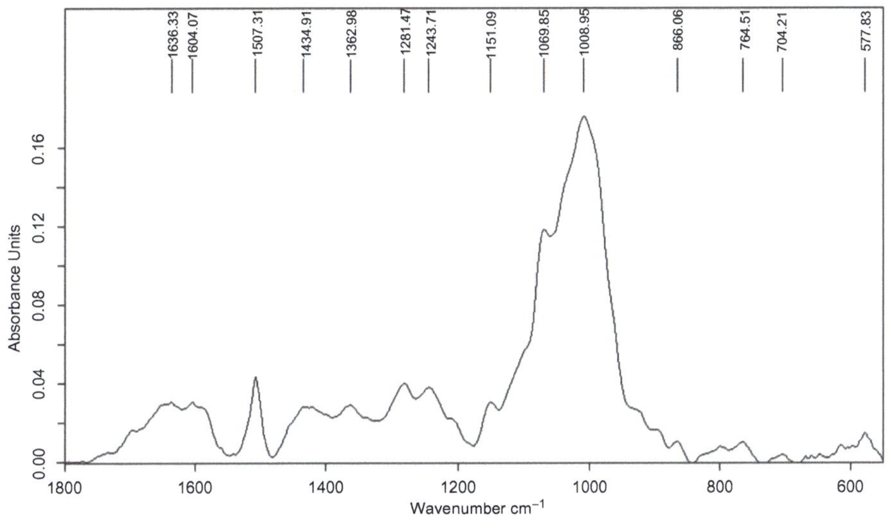

Mid-infrared spectrum of *Hypoxis hemerocallidea* corms displaying the fingerprint region (1800–550 cm^{-1}).

References

Albrecht, C.F., Kruger, P.B., Smit, B.J., Freestone, M., 1995. S. Afr. Med. J., 85:861–865.

Azu, O.O., Jegede, A.I., Ugochukwu, O., Onanuga, I.O., Kharwa, S., Naidu, E.C., 2016. Toxicol. Rep., 3:114–122.

Bassey, K.N., 2015. Phytochemical Profiling and Quality Control of *Hypoxis hemerocallidea* and Related Species. D.Tech thesis, Tshwane University of Technology, Pretoria, South Africa.

Bouic, P.J.D., Clark, A., Brittle, W., Lamprecht, J.H., 2001. S. Afr. Med. J., 91:848–850.

Boukes, J.G., Van de Venter, M., Oosthuizen, V., 2008. Afr. J. Biotechnol., 7:1624–1629.

Breytenbach, U., Clark, A., Lamprecht, J., Bouic, P., 2001. Cell Biol. Int., 25:43–49.

De Caires, S.G., Cromaty, A.D., Steenkamp, V., 2011. Lat. Am. J. Pharm., 30:1574–1581.

Dold, A.P., Cocks, M.L., 2002. S. Afr. J. Sci., 98:589–597.

Drewes, S.E., Khan, F., 2004. S. Afr. J. Sci., 100:425–430.

Drewes, S.E., Hall, H.J., Learmonth, R.A., Upfold, U.J., 1984. Phytochemistry, 23:1313–1316.

Drewes, S.E., Elliot, E., Khan, F., Dlamini, J.T.B., Gcumisa, M.S.S., 2008. J. Ethnopharmacol., 119:593–598.

Elbagory, A., Meyer, M., Cupido, C., Hussein, A.A., 2017. Nanomaterials, 7 (12), https://doi.org/10.3390/nano7120417.

Germishuizen, G., Meyer, N.L., Steenkamp, Y., Keith, M. (Eds.), 2006. A Checklist of South African Plants. Southern African Botanical Diversity Network Report 41. SABONET, Pretoria, South Africa.

Havenga, K., Abay, E., Wiesner, L., Viljoen, A., Steyn, D., Hamman, J., 2018. Planta Med., https://doi.org/10.1055/a-0607–2743.

Hutchings, A., 1996. Zulu Medicinal Plants. Natal University Press, Pietermaritzburg, South Africa.

Ismail, O.O., Isaac, J.A., Ugochukwu, O., Oluwatosin, O.O., Aniekan, P.I., Edwin, N.C.S., Onyemaechi, A.O., 2017. Folia Histochem. Cytobiol., 55:149–158.

Jegede, A.I., Offor, U., Onanuga, I.O., Naidu, E.C.S., Azu, O.O., 2017. Andrologia, 49 (2), https://doi.org/10.1111/and.12640.

Kumar, V., Moyo, M., Van Staden, J., 2017. S. Afr. J. Bot., 108:331–336.

Laporta, O., Perez-Fons, L., Mallavia, R., Caturla, N., 2007. Food Chem., 101:1425–1437.

Liebenberg, R.W., Kruger, P.B., Albrecht, C.F., Bouic, P.J.D., 1997. Method of Treating Viral Infections. Virostat (NA) NVQ (Kralendijk, Patentee LLP. US Patent 5,609,874).

Mahomed, I.N., Ojewole, J.A., 2004. Phytother. Res., 18:982–989.

Marini-Bettolo, G.B., Nicoletti, P.M., Galeffi, C., Messana, L., 1982. Tetrahedron, 38:1683–1687.

Mills, E., Cooper, C., Seely, D., Kanfer, I., 2005. Nutr. J., 4:19.

Matotoka, M.M., Masoko, P., 2017. JEBCAM, 22:805–815.

Musabayane, C.T., Xozwa, K., Ojewole, J.A.O., 2005. Ren. Fail., 2:763–770.

Ncube, B., Ndhlala, R., Okem, A., Van Staden, J., 2013. J. Ethnopharmacol., 150:818–827.

Nyinawumuntu, A., Awe, E.O., Ojewole, J.A.O., 2008. J. Smooth Muscle Res., 44:167–176.

Offor, U., Jegede, A.I., Onanuga, I.O., Naidu, E.C., Azu, O.O., 2017. Minerva Urol. Nefrol., 69:391–399.

Oguntibeju, O.O., Meyer, S., Aboua, Y.G., Goboza, M., 2016. EBCAM, 2016, https://doi.org/10.1155/2016/8934362.

Ojewole, J.A.O., Kamadyaapa, D.R., Musabayane, C.T., 2006. Cardiovasc. J. S. Afr., 17:166–171.

Risa, J., Risa, A., Adsersen, A., Gauguin, B., 2004. J. Ethnopharmacol., 93:177–182.

Singh, Y., 2009. Systematics of *Hypoxis* (Hypoxidaceae) in Southern Africa. PhD thesis, University of Pretoria, Pretoria, South Africa.

Stafford, G.I., Pedersen, P.D., Jäger, A.K., Van Staden, J., 2007. S. Afr. J. Bot., 73:384–390.

Tiya, S., Sewani-Rusike, C.R., Shauli, M., 2017. Andrologia, 49:e12742, https://doi.org/10.1111/and.12742.

Verschaeve, L., Mertens, B., Ndhlala, A.R., Anthonissen, R., Gorissen, B., Van Staden, J., 2013. Phytother. Res., 27:350–356.

Vinesi, P., Serafini, M., Nicoletti, M., Spano, L., 1990. J. Nat. Prod., 53:196–199.

Watt, J.M., Breyer-Brandwijk, M.G., 1962. The Medicinal and Poisonous Plants of Southern and Eastern Africa, second ed. E. & S. Livingstone Ltd, Edinburgh and London, UK.

CHAPTER

Leonotis leonurus

14

Baudry Nsuala, Guy Kamatou and Gill Enslin

Department of Pharmaceutical Sciences, Tshwane University of Technology, Pretoria, South Africa

Abstract

Leonotis leonurus (L.) R.Br. (Lamiaceae), commonly known as 'wild dagga', is a broad-leaf evergreen plant indigenous to southern Africa. It is naturally distributed throughout the Eastern and Western Cape, KwaZulu-Natal and Mpumalanga provinces of South Africa, as well as certain parts of Zimbabwe and Mozambique. The plant is widely known for its medicinal and psychoactive properties. The leaves or flowers are administered in various forms such as decoctions or infusions. It is smoked for its mild euphoric effects, which are believed to be similar to that of cannabis, but with less potency. A decoction is used to relieve coughs, colds, bronchitis, and as a strong purgative and emmenagogue whilst infusions are used to treat chest infections, fever, headache, influenza and delayed menstruation. Gas chromatography coupled to mass spectrometry (GC–MS) analysis of the essential oils obtained by hydro-distillation revealed eight major constituents (trans-β-ocimene, cis-β-ocimene, β-caryophyllene, caryophyllene oxide, α-humulene, γ-elemene, α-cubebene and germacrene D), which represent about 50% of the total oil composition. Ultra-performance liquid chromatography coupled to mass spectrometry (UPLC–MS) and photodiode array detection profiles from dichloromethane:methanol (50:50 v/v) extracts revealed the presence of leoleorin A, leoleorin D, luteolin, 6-methoxyluteolin-4′-methyl ether and 9,13-epoxylabda-6(19),15(14)diol dilactone in samples collected from distinct populations. Using a semi-automated high-performance thin-layer chromatography (HPTLC) system, the chemical profiles of both the volatile oils and extracts were obtained. The marker compound, marrubiin, was identified in the chemical fingerprints of all the non-volatile samples on HPTLC plates viewed under white reflectance light, whilst the standard caryophyllene oxide appeared in all the volatile oils viewed under 366nm radiation.

Keywords: *Leonotis leonurus*, Wild dagga, Aerial parts, Psychoactive, HPTLC, UPLC–MS, GC–MS, MIR spectroscopy, Marrubiin, Leoleorin A

The South African Herbal Pharmacopoeia. https://doi.org/10.1016/B978-0-323-99794-2.00004-0

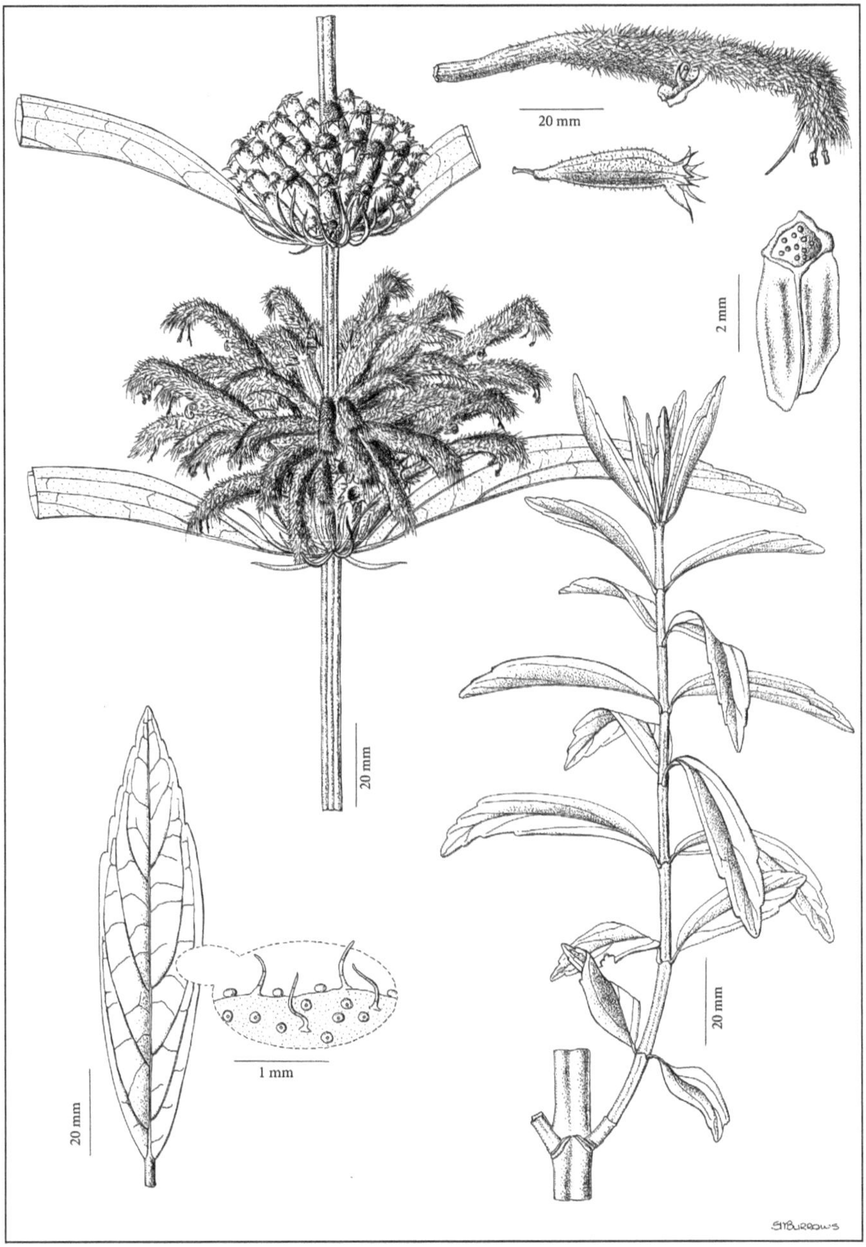
20 mm
2 mm
20 mm
20 mm
1 mm
20 mm
STBURROWS

Part A: General overview

1. Synonyms

Leonotis africanus Mill., *Leonotis grandiflorus* Moench, *Leonotis leonurus* (L.) R.Br. var. *albiflora* Benth., *Phlomis leonurus* L.[a]

2. Common name(s)

Cape hemp, leonotis, lion's ear, lion's tail, minaret flower, narrow-leafed leonotis, red dacha, red dagga, wild dagga, wild hemp (English); '*bulderdagga*', *dagga*, '*duiwelstabak*', '*duiwelstwak*', '*klipdagga*', '*koppiesdagga*', '*wildedagga*', '*rooidagga*', '*rivierdagga*' (Afrikaans); '*i-munyamunyane*', '*utshwala-bezinyoni omncane*' (isiZulu); '*imvovo*', '*utywala bengcungcu*', '*umfincane*' (isiXhosa); '*lebake*' (Sesotho).[a]

3. Conservation status

Least concern.[a]

4. Botany

Leonotis leonurus (L.) R.Br. is a woody multibranched shrub that grows to a height of 2.0–5.0 m and is about 1.5 m wide (D) (Iwarsson and Harvey, 2003; Van Wyk and Gericke, 2003). The velvety, square-shaped stem is greyish-green in colour when young, and pale brown and brittle when mature (A). The leaves are aromatic, bright yellow–green, roughly textured with toothed margins, and have sessile glands. Short hairs that appear dense on the lower surface, cover the leaves, which appear narrowly ovate to linear, with narrowly acute apex and cuneate base, and a serrated margin on opposite sides of the stem (A). The flowers are arranged in clusters of 2–11 verticils per branch and are borne along stems at 7 cm internodes, with orange tubular corollas of up to 5 cm long that are covered with orange hairs (B & C). Bracts are leaf-like and bractioles are linear and densely pubescent with sessile glands. The calyx is 12–16 mm long, 4 mm in diameter at the mouth and pale green to yellowish. The corollas bend forwards, widening at the mouth with 1–3 fringes and a hair fringe at the margin, sparsely covered with short orange hairs on the outer surface (C). The posterior lip of the corolla is significantly longer than the anterior lip, which is deflexed and withering (Iwarsson and Harvey, 2003; Hurinanthan, 2009).

[a] Red List of South African Plants (http://redlist.sanbi.org).

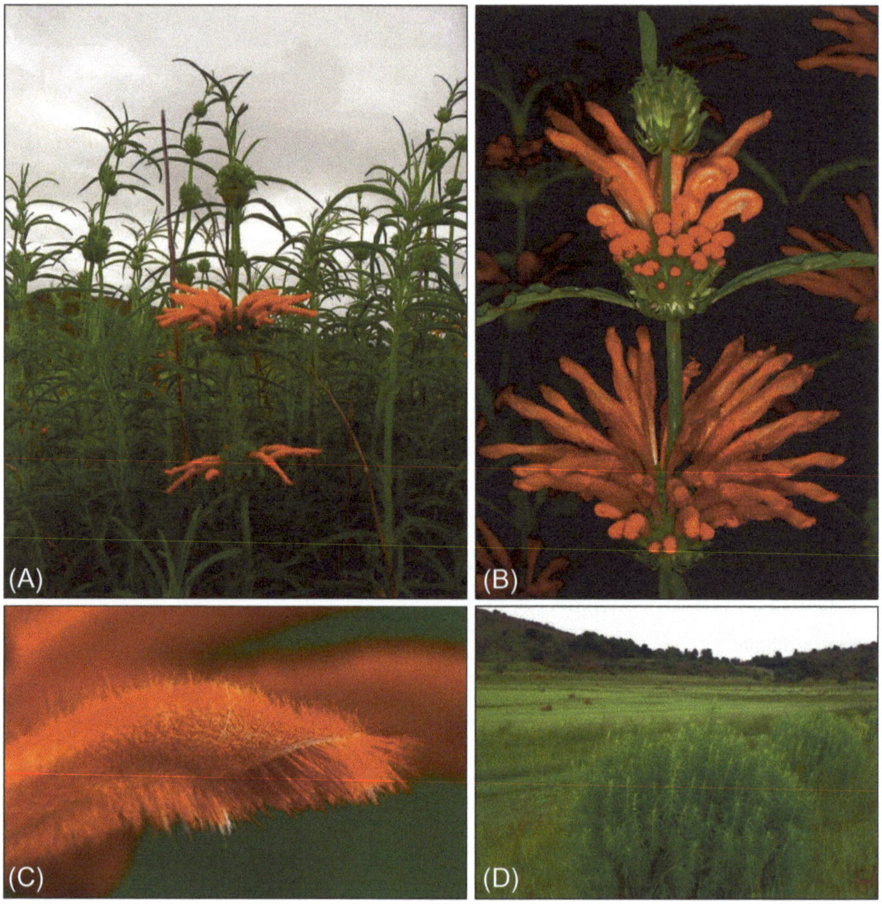

Woody *Leonotis leonurus* plants in flower (A), hairy orange corolla that resembles a lion's ear (C), the *Leonotis leonurus* bush in habitat (D), and flower clusters of orange tubular corollas (B).

5. Geographical distribution

Leonotis leonurus is naturally distributed throughout the Eastern and Western Cape, as well as the KwaZulu-Natal and Mpumalanga provinces of South Africa. It is also found in certain parts of Zimbabwe and Mozambique. The plant grows on forest margins, river banks, rocky hillsides, and in grasslands (Iwarsson and Harvey, 2003).

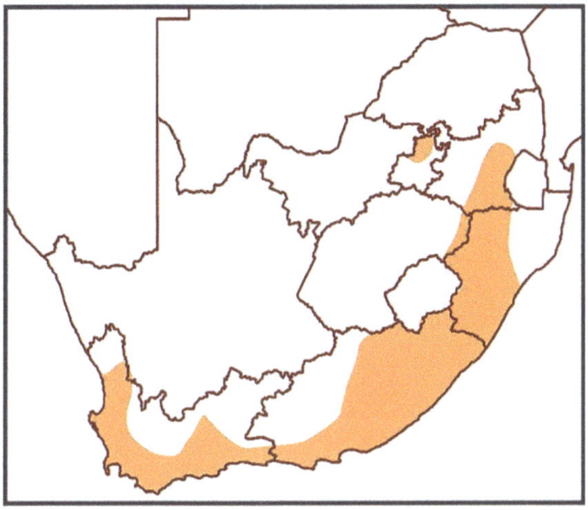

Geographical distribution of *Leonotis leonurus* in South Africa.

6. Ethnopharmacology

Traditional healers in the southern African region have used *L. leonurus* preparations for the treatment of a wide range of conditions for many years (Scott et al., 2004). A decoction, which is prepared by boiling a tablespoon of dried leaves in three cups of water for 10min, is cooled overnight, filtered, and the filtrate used topically and orally (Mugabo et al., 2012). Topical application of the decoction has assisted in the management of skin disorders such as eczema, skin rashes, boils, itching, as well as piles and muscular cramps. Orally, the decoction is taken to relieve coughs, colds and bronchitis, as a strong purgative and emmenagogue. The aerial parts of the plant, in the form of infusions, are used for chest infection, fever, dysentery, influenza, constipation, headache, epilepsy, snake bites, delayed menstruation, intestinal worms, hypertension and scorpion stings (Bryant, 1966; Jäger et al., 1996; Van Wyk et al., 2000; Stafford et al., 2008). A cold infusion of the leaves is used as a nasal douche for headaches and fever by the Zulu (Watt and Breyer-Brandwijk, 1962). Various plant parts used either as decoctions or inhalants are reported to treat the common cold, epilepsy, leprosy and cardiovascular conditions (Duke, 2001). Leaf powder is added into ointments and applied topically to relieve pain above the eye (Hutchings et al., 1996). A decoction of the powdered stem or seed is taken orally to treat haemorrhoids, and topically as a lotion for leg and head sores (Watt and Breyer-Brandwijk, 1962). A mixture of ground *L. leonurus* roots and *Strychnos spinosa* (roots and green fruits), prepared as a hot infusion, is taken to treat snakebite (Bryant, 1966). The leaves of '*mutodzvo*' are chewed and the sap is swallowed for the treatment of ulcers in Zimbabwe (Maroyi, 2013). A minty tea brewed from *L. leonurus* leaves is taken for obesity and as a diuretic (Watt and Breyer-Brandwijk, 1962; Hutchings et al., 1996; Van Wyk et al., 2000). Dried aerial parts are smoked for the relief of epileptic seizures and partial paralysis (Watt and Breyer-Brandwijk, 1962; Van Wyk et al., 2000). Indigenous ethnic groups of South Africa are reported to smoke 'wild cannabis' instead of tobacco, as it gives them intense feelings of well-being, elation and happiness, which may be linked to possible psychoactive properties. Numerous side effects have been reported where smokers have experienced changes in vision, nausea, dizziness, sedation, sweating, lightheadedness, lung and throat irritation. Smoking of the flowers has been reported to cause hallucinations (Richard et al., 2001). Ethnoveterinary uses of the plant include treatment of eye inflammation in livestock by the direct application of leaf sap; pounded roots and leaves are added to poultry drinking water to prevent sickness and to treat gallsickness in cattle (Hulme, 1954) as quoted by Hutchings et al. (1996) and McGaw and Eloff (2008), and it is used to control worm infestations in livestock (Maphosa and Masika, 2011).

7. Commercialisation

Leonotis leonurus is commercially marketed for smoking, due to its purported psychoactive properties (Hutchings et al., 1996; Van Wyk et al., 2000). A mild euphoric effect similar to that of cannabis, but with a less potent high, has been reported (Wu et al., 2013). Zuba et al. (2013) reported that *L. leonurus*, *Nymphaea caerulea*, *Turnera diffusa* and *Zornia latifolia* are marketed as legal alternatives to cannabis on the internet. Although the products were claimed to be 'pure', reports of adulteration of the herbal material with synthetic psychoactive compounds, such as cannabinoids, were made public in 2008. Cornara et al. (2013) referred to these aromatic plants as a 'green shuttle', with the chief role of disguising the synthetic cannabinoids to produce a 'legal high', whilst posing a serious threat to public health.

8. Pharmacological evaluation

8.1 *In vitro* studies

Several *in vitro* studies have been conducted to scientifically validate the traditional uses reported for *L. leonurus*. McGaw et al. (2000) reported slight anthelmintic activity of an ethanolic and aqueous extract of the plant against *Caenorhabditis elegans* at concentrations of 1 and 2 mg/mL, respectively. Aqueous and methanol extracts of the stems and leaves were moderately active towards test pathogens (*Staphylococcus aureus*, *Streptococcus pyogenes*, *Escherichia coli* and *Pseudomonas aeruginosa*) with minimum inhibitory concentrations (MICs) ≥4 mg/mL (Steenkamp et al., 2004). Oyedeji and Afolayan (2005) profiled *L. leonurus* essential oils and identified the major constituents as limonene (7.2%–15.6%), β-ocimene (7.5%–10.8%), γ-terpinene (4.0%–4.7%), β-caryophyllene (15.2%–19.6%), α-humulene (4.6%–6.5%) and germacrene D (18.9%–20.0%). The oil was active against a range of Gram-positive (*Bacillus subtilis*, *Bacillus cereus*, *Micrococcus kristinae*, *S. aureus*, *Staphylococcus epidermidis*) and Gram-negative (*E. coli*, *P. aeruginosa*, *Shigella sonnei*) bacteria, with MICs of 0.039–1.25 mg/mL recorded. Jimoh et al. (2010) reported moderate antibacterial activity of acetone and methanol leaf extracts against *B. cereus*, *Staphylococcus epidermidis*, *M. kristinae*, *S. aureus*, *Streptococcus pyogenes*, *E. coli*, *Salmonella poona*, *Serratia marcescens* and *P. aeruginosa*, whilst the water extract was inactive against *Klebsiella pneumoniae*. Naidoo et al. (2011) reported 90% growth inhibition of *Mycobacterium tuberculosis* exposed to the aqueous and methanol:dichloromethane (1:1) extracts of *L. leonurus*. Maphosa and Masika (2011) reported the potential use of *L. leonurus* aqueous leaf extract as an anthelmintic and antiprotozoal agent, after noteworthy activity was recorded against gastro-intestinal parasites in goats using the faecal egg count method. The antiviral activity of an ethanol leaf extract of *L. leonurus* was reported as producing a 33% reduction in HIV-1 p24 core protein, in a human T-lymphoblastic cell culture (CEM.NKR-CCR5) (Klos et al., 2009). The aqueous extract inhibited HIV-1 reverse transcriptase activity; however, activity was lost following the removal of common non-specific tannins and polysaccharides. A crude ethanolic extract of *L. leonurus* inhibited HIV-1 protease, with a half maximal inhibitory concentration (IC_{50}) value of 120.6 μg/mL. Agnihotri et al. (2009) reported the antimalarial activity of luteolin-7-*O*-glucoside against the *Plasmodium falciparum* D2 clone (IC_{50} = 2.2 μg/mL) and the *Plasmodium falciparum* W2 clone (IC_{50} = 1.8 μg/mL) (Kirmizibekmez et al., 2004). In another study, the aqueous extract of *L. leonurus* displayed strong *in vitro* 2,2-diphenyl-1-picrylhydrazyl radical (DPPH) scavenging activity, demonstrating anti-oxidant potential of the plant (Oyedemi et al., 2011).

8.2 *In vivo* studies and clinical trials

Results from a study conducted to investigate the anticonvulsant activity of an aqueous leaf extract of *L. leonurus* in mice, indicated seizure prevention in 37.5% and 50% of the animals at 200 and 400 mg/kg doses, respectively (Bienvenu et al., 2002). A significant delay of pentylenetetrazole (PTZ)-induced tonic seizure onset was recorded at a 90 mg/kg dose of the extract. Two compounds were isolated from *L. leonurus* extracts and tested for their anticonvulsant activity. At 400 mg/kg, the diterpene lactone, 20-acetoxy-9α,13α-epoxylabda-14-en-6β(19)-lactone, delayed onset of seizures in 50% of the mice, whilst a quinone, isolated from the methanol extract, protected 75% and 87.5% of the mice at 200 and 400 mg/kg, respectively. An aqueous leaf extract of *L. leonurus* was evaluated for its antidiabetic activity at doses of 125, 250 and 500 mg/kg for 15 days in streptozotocin (STZ)-induced (45 mg/kg intraperitoneal) diabetic rats (Oyedemi et al., 2011). A reduction in elevated glucose, cholesterol, high density lipoprotein (HDL) and triglycerides levels, accompanied by weight loss, was recorded following treatment. Maphosa and Masika (2011) reported on the antiparasitic activity of aqueous *L. leonurus* extracts towards gastro-intestinal worms and *Coccidia* species in goats.

8.3 Safety

In a study of the safety profile of *L. leonurus*, female rats fed with aqueous shoot extracts of the plant displayed decreased respiratory rate and motor activity, respiratory failure, skeletal muscle paralysis, ataxia and convulsions (Maphosa et al., 2008). In another study, 70% aqueous methanol and chloroform extracts exhibited hepatoprotective activity in a paracetamol-induced liver damage rat model (El-Ansari et al., 2009).

9. Phytochemistry

9.1 Volatile constituents

The composition of the volatile fractions isolated from both leaves and flowers of *L. leonurus* have been studied and reported, due to their widespread use in traditional medicine for the treatment of epilepsy and partial paralysis (Watt and Breyer-Brandwijk, 1962; Inouye et al., 1974; Van Wyk et al., 2000). The oil is light yellow in colour, with a strong minty odour. Nsuala et al. (2017) investigated the essential oil of the aerial parts of *L. leonurus*, obtained from three provinces of South Africa. Twenty-six compounds were identified with eight major constituents in the oil, representing about 50% of the total oil composition, using both gas chromatography coupled to mass-spectrometry and flame ionisation detection (GC-MS-FID) and comprehensive two-dimensional gas chromatography-time-of-flight-mass spectrometry (GCxGC-ToF-MS). These major compounds were *trans*-β-ocimene (0.1%–5.0%), *cis*-β-ocimene (0.1%–31.5%), β-caryophyllene (0.3%–15.0%), caryophyllene oxide (0.1%–5.0%), α-humulene (0.4%–18.2%), γ-elemene (0.4%–10.6%), α-cubebene (0.2%–12.0%) and germacrene D (0.1%–22.1%). Compositional similarities between populations were observed with some quantitative differences.

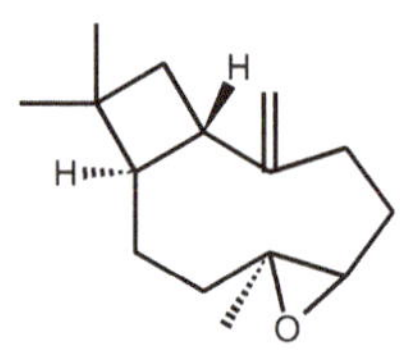

Caryophyllene oxide

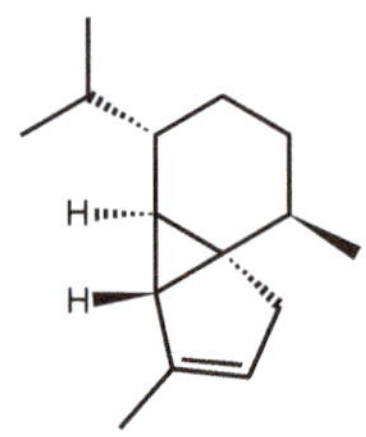

α-Cubebene

9.2 Non-volatile constituents

The phytochemistry of the non-volatile constituents of *L. leonurus* has been investigated and a number of compounds have been isolated and characterised. *Leonotis leonurus* contains mainly terpenoids, particularly labdane diterpenes, with the major diterpene reported as marrubiin (Nsuala et al., 2015). Various other compounds have been reported by some authors to have been isolated from the plant, including the mildly psychoactive alkaloid, leonurine. Leonurine has, however, never been reported by any scientific analysis of the extracts of *L. leonurus* (Nsuala et al., 2015). Organic extracts of the flowering parts of the plant provided flavonoids and acyclic diterpene esters, whilst the leaves contained mostly labdane diterpenoids. Wu et al. (2013) reported the major constituents of the non-volatile fraction to be labdane diterpenoids, leoleorins A–J and 16-epi-leoleorin F. Two new labdane-type diterpenoids were also isolated by Naidoo et al. (2011), namely 9,13-epoxy-6-hydroxy-labdan-16,15-olide and 9,13:15,16-diepoxy-6,16-labdanediol from the methanol:dichloromethane (1:1) leaf extract. The structures of the compounds were identified by one- and two-dimensional nuclear magnetic resonance (1D and 2D NMR) spectroscopy. Phenolic compounds were detected by Kuchta et al. (2016) from the aqueous extract of the aerial parts of *L. leonurus*. Chlorogenic, caffeic, cichoric acids, rutoside, lavandulifolioside and isoquercitrin were identified and quantified using a reversed phase high-performance liquid chromatography (RP-HPLC) method.

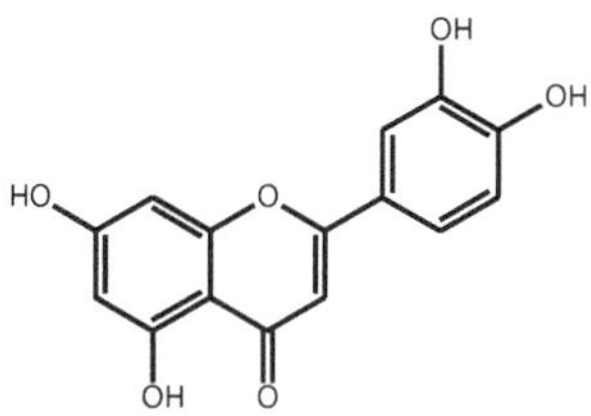

Luteolin

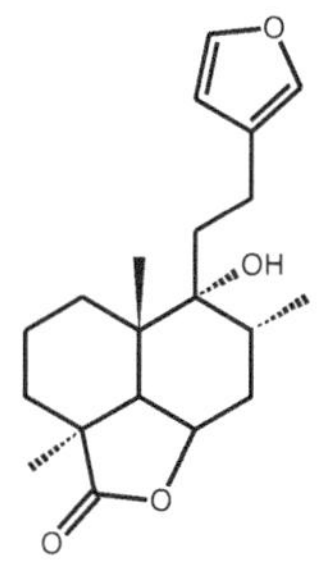

Marrubiin

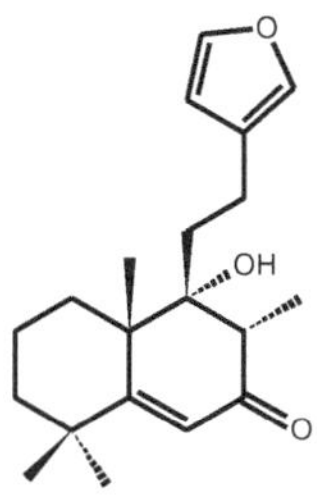

Leoleorin A

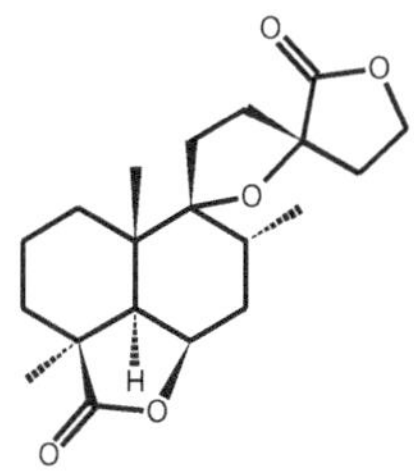

9,13-epoxylabda-6(19),15(14)-dioldilactone (EDD)

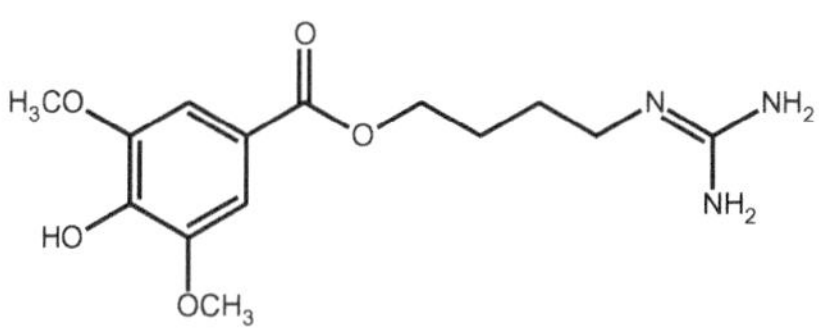

Leonurine

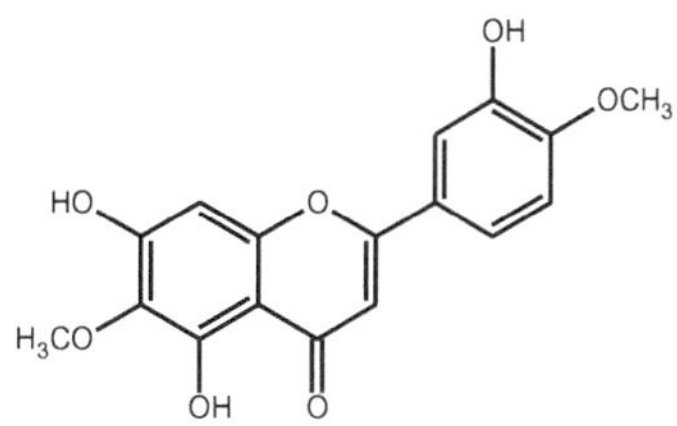

6-Methoxyluteolin-4′-methyl ether

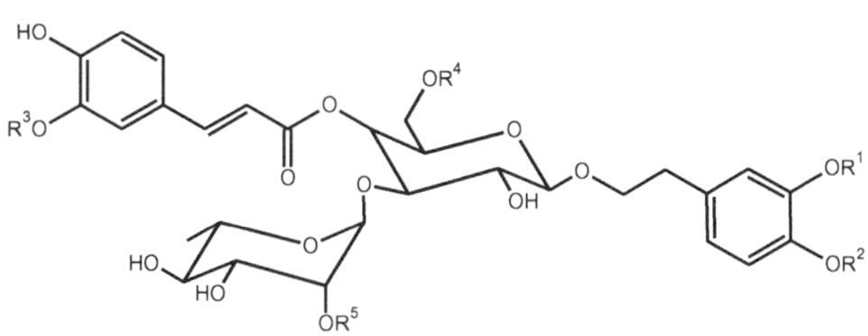

Lavandulifolioside: R^1,R^2,R^3,R^4=H; R^5=arabinose

Part B: Chemical profiling and quality control

10. Chromatography analysis

10.1 High-performance thin-layer chromatography (HPTLC) fingerprint analysis

General instrumentation: CAMAG HPTLC instrument consisting of an automatic TLC sampler (ATS 4), automatic developing chamber (ADC 2), CAMAG TLC visualiser 2, CAMAG derivatiser and TLC plate heater. *HPTLC plates*: Silica gel glass plates 60 F_{254} (Merck).

10.1.1 Non-volatile fraction analysis

Plant part: Aerial parts, dichloromethane:methanol (80:20 v/v) extract. *Sample application*: Application volume of 2 µL methanol extract (10 mg/mL) and standards (1 mg/mL) spotted as 10 mm bands. Plates developed in a 20 × 10 × 4 cm glass twin-trough chamber to a migration distance of 80 mm. *Tank saturation*: 20 min at 15 °C and 45% RH, with 10 mL of mobile phase. *Mobile phase*: Hexane:ethyl acetate (80:20 v/v). *Derivatisation*: *p*-Anisaldehyde/sulphuric acid reagent. The plate was sprayed with 3 mL of the reagent, heated for 2 min at 100 °C on a TLC plate heater and visualised. *Visualisation*: The plate was viewed under white reflectance light.

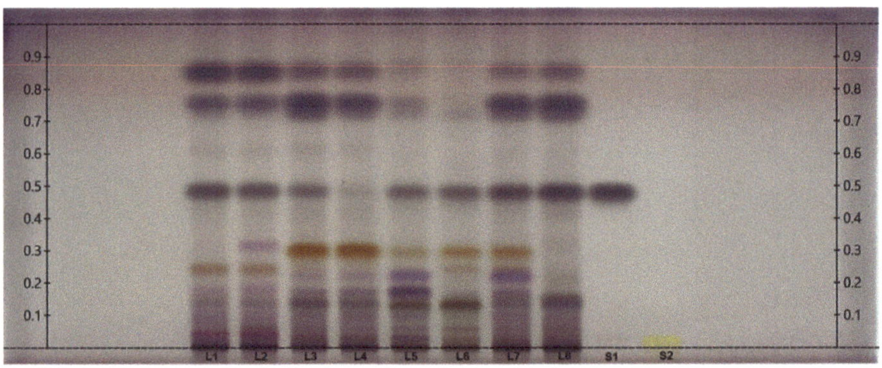

HPTLC plate of *Leonotis leonurus* dichloromethane:methanol (80:20) extracts ($n = 8$) (L1–L8) and the standards (S1–S2). The samples are characterised by a dark blue band for marrubiin (S1) ($R_f = 0.49$) and a yellow band for luteolin (S2) ($R_f = 0.02$), under white reflectance light.

10.1.2 Essential oil analysis

Plant part: Aerial parts, essential oil. *Sample application*: Application volume of 2 µL essential oil (25 µL/mL in toluene) and standards (1 mg/mL in methanol) spotted as 10 mm bands. Plates developed in a 20×10×4 cm glass twin-trough chamber to a migration distance of 70 mm. *Tank saturation*: 20 min at 15 °C and 45% RH, with 10 mL of mobile phase. *Mobile phase*: Toluene:ethyl acetate (95:5 v/v). *Derivatisation*: *p*-Anisaldehyde/sulphuric acid reagent. The plate was sprayed with 3 mL of the reagent and heated for 2 min at 100 °C on a TLC plate heater and visualised. *Visualisation*: The plate was viewed under 366 nm fluorescent light.

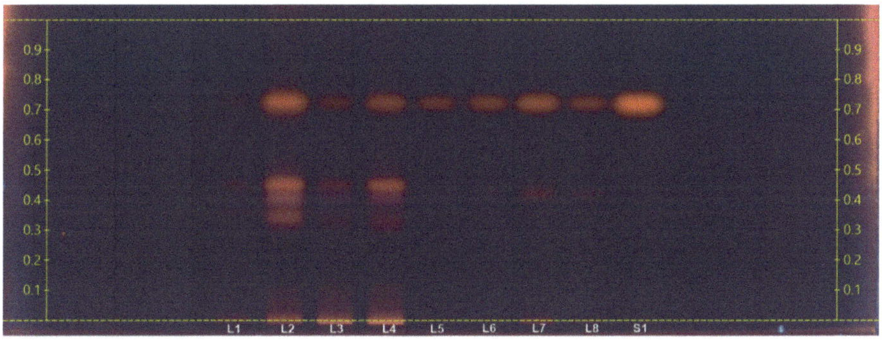

HPTLC plate of *Leonotis leonurus* essential oil ($n=8$) (L1–L8) and the standard caryophyllene oxide (S1) characterised by an orange band at $R_f=0.72$ under 366 nm fluorescent light.

10.2 Ultra-performance liquid chromatography (UPLC) analysis

General instrumentation: Waters Acquity Ultra-performance Liquid Chromatography system with photodiode array (PDA) detector combined with a Xevo G2QToF mass spectrometer (Waters, United States). *Plant part*: Aerial parts, dichloromethane:methanol (80:20) extract. *Sample application*: Injection volume: 1.0 µL (full-loop injection) at 1 mg/mL. *Column*: Acquity UPLC BEH C_{18} column (150 mm × 2.1 mm, i.d., 1.7 µm particle size, Waters). *Mobile phase*: 0.1% formic acid in water (solvent A) and acetonitrile (solvent B). *Analysis conditions*: Gradient elution at a flow rate of 0.4 mL/min, changing as follows: 90% A:10% B changed to 60% A: 40% B in 2 min, to 30% A: 70% B in 10 min, to 5% A: 95% B in 2 min, held for 0.5 min, back to initial ratio in 0.5 min, equilibrating the system for 1.5 min, total run time 16.5 min. *Mass spectrometry*: ESI^+ (positive ionisation mode), N_2 used as the desolvation gas, desolvation temperature 350 °C at a flow rate of 500 L/h, source temperature 100 °C. Capillary and cone voltages 3300 and 40 V, respectively. Data collected between *m/z* 100 and 1200.

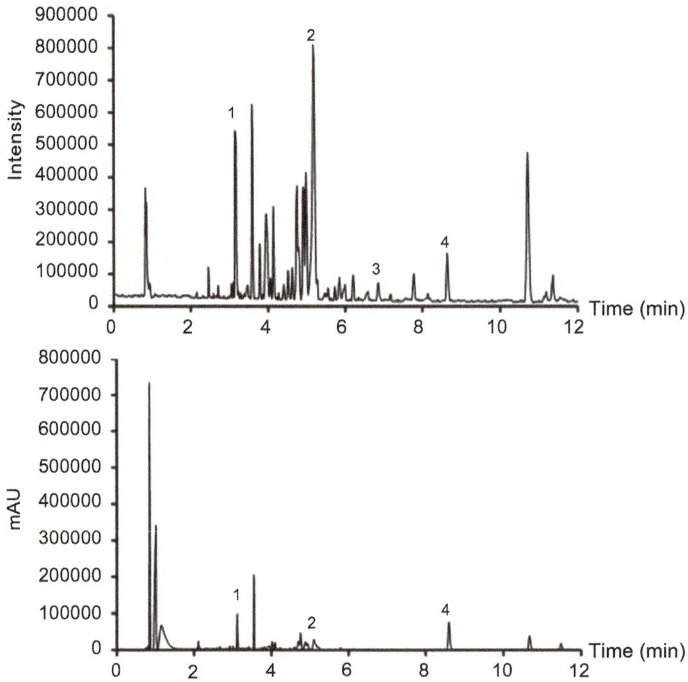

UPLC–ToF–MS ESI$^+$ (upper) and PDA (lower) chromatograms of *Leonotis leonurus* dichloromethane: methanol extract: [1] = 6-methoxyluteolin-4′-methyl ether *m/z* 331.0823, [2] = 9,13-epoxylabda-6(19),15(14)-dioldilactone (EDD) *m/z* 349.2027, [3] = marrubiin *m/z* 333.2059, [4] = leoleorin A *m/z* 317.2118.

10.3 Gas chromatography (GC) analysis

General instrumentation: An Agilent 6860N chromatograph (Agilent Technologies, Hanova, United States) fitted with a flame ionisation detector and a mass spectrometer. *Column*: HP-Innowax, 60 m × 250 µm × 0.25 µm (polyethylene glycol column, Agilent Technologies, Hanova, United States). *Plant part*: Aerial parts, essential oil. *Sample application*: Injection volume of 1 µL (split) at 20% (v/v) in hexane. *Analysis conditions*: Inlet temperature 250 °C, split ratio: 1:200, helium carrier gas, flow rate: 1.2 mL/min, pressure: 24.79 psi. Starting oven temperature at 60 °C and then rise to 220 °C at 4 °C/min, holding for 10 min and increased to 240 °C at 1 °C/min. *Mass spectrometry conditions*: Chromatograms obtained on electron impact at 70 eV using an Agilent 5973 mass selective detector, scanning range: *m/z* 35–550 (Agilent Technologies, Hanova, United States). *Identification*: Authentic standards, NIST®, Mass Finder®.

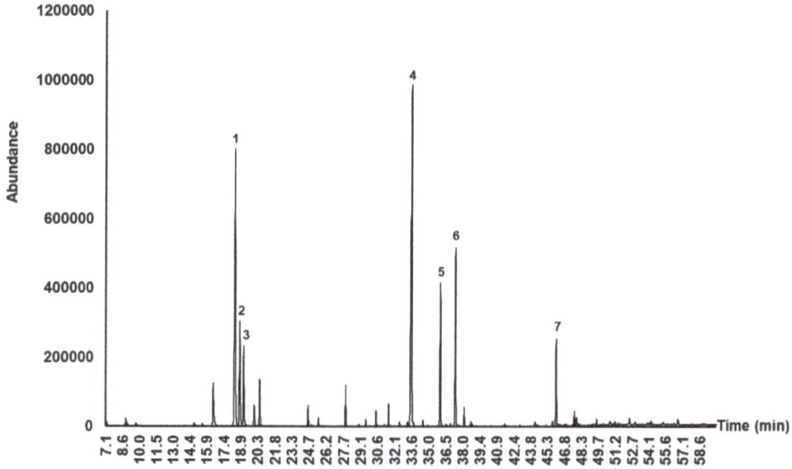

Total ion chromatogram (TIC) of *Leonotis leonurus* essential oil indicating major compounds. [1] = *Z*-β-ocimene (R_t 18.30, *m/z* 136.1252), [2] = γ-terpene (R_t 18.79, *m/z* 136.1252), [3] = *E*-β-ocimene (R_t 19.10, *m/z* 136.1252), [4] = β-caryophyllene (R_t 33.51, *m/z* 204.1878), [5] = α-humulene (R_t 36.05, *m/z* 204.1878), [6] = germacrene D (R_t 37.32, *m/z* 204.1878), [7] = caryophyllene oxide (R_t 46.10, *m/z* 220.1827).

11. Mid-infrared (MIR) spectroscopy analysis

General instrumentation: Alpha-P Bruker spectrometer, mounted with an attenuated total reflectance (ATR) diamond crystal. *Spectral acquisition*: Spectrum obtained in absorbance mode, with a spectral resolution of 4 cm^{-1} over the range 4000–550 cm^{-1} and captured using OPUS 6.5 software.

11.1 Powder analysis

Plant part: Aerial parts. *Sample preparation*: Aerial parts powdered, sieved (<500 μm), and placed directly onto the surface of the diamond crystal.

11.2 Essential oil analysis

Plant part: Aerial parts, essential oil. *Sample preparation*: Aerial parts, hydro-distillation to obtain essential oil, placed directly onto the surface of the diamond crystal.

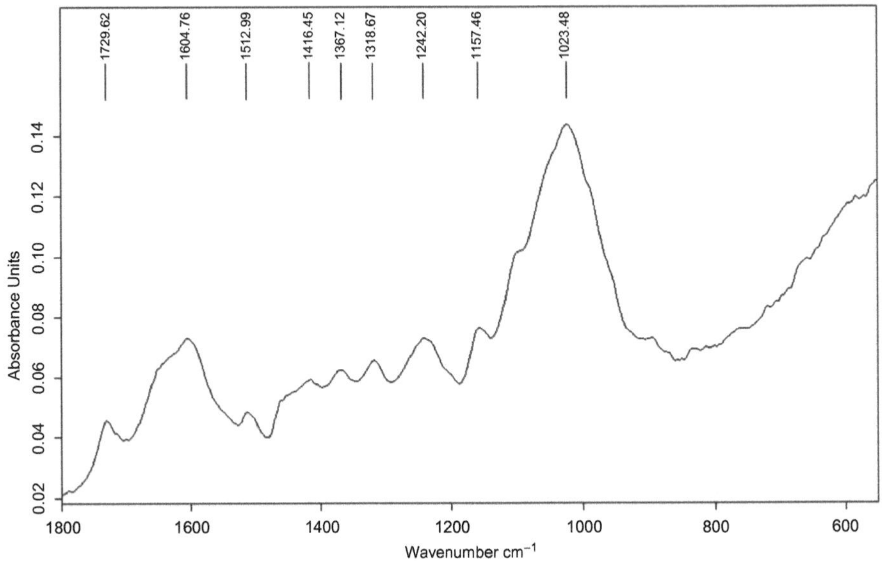

Mid-infrared spectrum of *Leonotis leonurus* powder displaying the fingerprint region (1800–550 cm^{-1}).

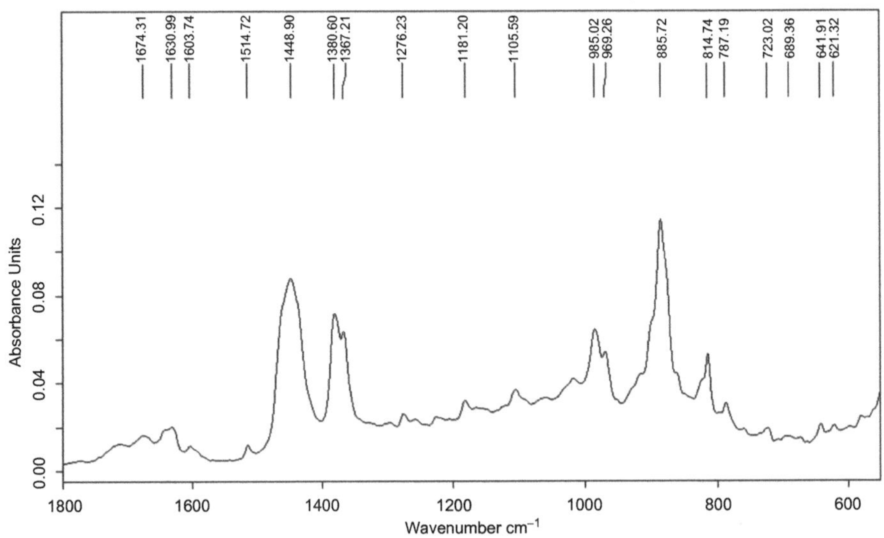

Mid-infrared spectrum of *Leonotis leonurus* essential oil displaying the fingerprint region (1800–550 cm^{-1}).

References

Agnihotri, V.K., Elsohly, H.N., Smillie, T.J., Khan, I.A., Walker, L.A., 2009. Phytochem. Lett., 2:103–105.

Bienvenu, E., Amabeoku, G.J., Eagles, P.K., Scott, G., Springfield, E.P., 2002. Phytomedicine, 9:217–223.

Bryant, A.T., 1966. Zulu Medicine and Medicine Men. Struik, Cape Town, South Africa.

Cornara, L., Borghesi, B., Canali, C., Andrenacci, M., Basso, M., Frederici, S., Labra, M., 2013. Int. J. Legal Med., 127:1109–1123.

Duke, J.A., 2001. Handbook of Medicinal Herbs, second ed. CRC Press, Boca Raton, Florida, USA.

El-Ansari, M.A., Aboutabl, E.A., Farrag, A.R.H., Sharaf, M., Hawas, U.W., Soliman, G.M., El-Seed, G.S., 2009. Pharm. Biol., 47:894–902.

Hulme, M.M., 1954. Wild Flowers of Natal. Shuter & Shooter, Pietermaritzburg, South Africa.

Hurinanthan, V., 2009. Immune Modulatory Effect of *Dichrostachys cinerea*, *Carpobrotus dimidiatus*, *Capparis tomentosa* and *Leonotis leonurus*. M.Sc. dissertation, Durban University of Technology, Durban, South Africa.

Hutchings, A., Scott, A.H., Lewis, G., Cunningham, A.B., 1996. Zulu Medicinal Plants: An Inventory. University of Natal Press, Pietermaritzburg, South Africa.

Inouye, H., Takeda, Y., Uobe, K., Yamauchi, K., Yabuuchi, N., Kuwano, S., 1974. Planta Med., 25:285–288.

Iwarsson, M., Harvey, Y., 2003. Monograph of the genus *Leonotis*. Kew Bull., 58:597–645.

Jäger, A.K., Hutchings, A., Van Staden, J., 1996. J. Ethnopharmacol., 52:95–100.

Jimoh, F.O., Adedapo, A.A., Afolayan, A.J., 2010. Food Chem. Toxicol., 48:964–971.

Kirmizibekmez, H., Calis, I., Perozzo, R., Brun, R., Doenmez, A.A., Linden, A., Rueedi, P., Tasdemir, D., 2004. Planta Med., 70:711–717.

Klos, M., Van De Venter, M., Milne, P.J., Traore, H.N., Meyrer, D., Oosthuizen, V., 2009. J. Ethnopharmacol., 124:182–188.

Kuchta, K., Ortwein, J., Çali, A., Volk, R.B., Rauwald, H.W., 2016. Nat. Prod. Commun., 11:1129–1133.

Maphosa, V., Masika, P.J., 2011. Parasitol. Res., 110:103–108.

Maphosa, V., Masika, P.J., Adepapo, A.A., 2008. Hum. Exp. Toxicol., 27:837.

Maroyi, A., 2013. J. Ethnobiol. Ethnomed., 9:31.

McGaw, L.J., Eloff, J.N., 2008. J. Ethnopharmacol., 119:559–574.

McGaw, L.J., Jäger, A.K., Van Staden, J., 2000. J. Ethnopharmacol., 72:247–263.

Mugabo, P., Khan, F., Burger, A., 2012. J. Med. Aromat. Plants, 2:281–292.

Naidoo, D., Maharaj, V., Crouch, N.R., Ngwane, A., 2011. Biochem. Syst. Ecol., 39:216–219.

Nsuala, B.N., Enslin, G., Viljoen, A., 2015. J. Ethnopharmacol., 174:520–539.

Nsuala, B.N., Kamatou, G.P., Sandasi, M., Enslin, G., Viljoen, A., 2017. Biochem. Syst. Ecol., 70:155 –161.

Oyedeji, O.A., Afolayan, A.J., 2005. S. Afr. J. Bot., 71:114–116.

Oyedemi, S.O., Yakubu, M.T., Afolayan, A.J., 2011. J. Med. Plant Res., 51:119–125.

Richard, E.S., Albert, H., Christian, R., 2001. Plants of the Gods. Healing Arts Press, Rochester, Vermont, USA.

Scott, G., Springfield, E.P., Coldrey, N., 2004. Pharm. Biol., 42:186–213.

Stafford, G.I., Pedersen, M.E., Van Staden, J., Jäger, A.K., 2008. J. Ethnopharmacol., 119:513–537.

Steenkamp, V., Mathivha, E., Gouws, M.C., Van Rensburg, C.E.J., 2004. J. Ethnopharmacol., 95:353–357.
Van Wyk, B.E., Gericke, N., 2003. People's Plants—A Guide to Useful Plants of South Africa. Briza Publications, Pretoria, South Africa.
Van Wyk, B.E., Van Oudshoorn, B., Gericke, N., 2000. Medicinal Plants of South Africa, second ed. Briza Publications, Pretoria, South Africa.
Watt, J.M., Breyer-Brandwijk, M.G., 1962. The Medicinal and Poisonous Plants of Southern and Eastern Africa, second ed. E. & S. Livingstone Ltd, Edinburgh and London, UK.
Wu, H., Li, J., Fronczek, F.R., Ferreira, D., Burandt, C.L. Jr., Setola, V., Roth, B.L.K., Zjawiony, J.K., 2013. Phytochemistry, 91:229–235.
Zuba, D., Geppert, B., Sekula, K., Zaba, C., 2013. Forensic Toxicol., 31:281–291.

CHAPTER

Lessertia frutescens 15

Nontobeko Mncwangi[a], Alvaro Viljoen[a,b], Nduvho Mulaudzi[a] and Gerda Fouche[c]

[a]*Department of Pharmaceutical Sciences, Tshwane University of Technology, Pretoria, South Africa*

[b]*SAMRC Herbal Drugs Research Unit, Faculty of Science, Tshwane University of Technology, Pretoria, South Africa*

[c]*Chemistry Department, University of Pretoria, Pretoria, South Africa*

Abstract

Lessertia frutescens (L.) Goldblatt & J.C.Manning (Fabaceae) previously known as Sutherlandia frutescens (L.) R.Br. is a small, soft-wooded shrublet, with spectacular red flowers. This species, widely known as cancer bush, is indigenous to South Africa, Lesotho, southern Namibia and south-eastern Botswana. Although extremely bitter, it has been used traditionally as a medicinal tea against internal cancers and also as a cancer prophylactic. Cancer bush is well known as an adaptogenic tonic, and commercial tablets are popular to counteract the muscle-wasting effects associated with HIV-AIDS in patients and to stimulate appetite. In vitro biological activities of the plant include anticancer, antidiabetic, analgesic, anti-inflammatory and immunomodulatory effects. Results of animal studies, as well as a phase I clinical study, have shown no indications of toxicity. Phytochemical studies of L. frutescens reported the presence of amino acids, pinitol, flavonoids and cycloartanol glycosides. The plant is unusual in having high levels of the non-protein amino acid L-canavanine in the leaves. Chemical profiles of L. frutescens aerial parts were obtained, using a semi-automated high-performance thin-layer chromatography (HPTLC) system and ultra-performance liquid chromatography coupled to mass spectrometry (UPLC–MS). The cycloartanol glycosides, sutherlandioside A and sutherlandioside B (SU1), were identified in the methanol extracts of the aerial parts.

Keywords: *Lessertia frutescens*, Cancer bush, SU1, Sutherlandioside A, Sutherlandioside B, Pinitol, Cycloartanol glycosides, HPTLC, UPLC–MS, MIR spectroscopy

The South African Herbal Pharmacopoeia. https://doi.org/10.1016/B978-0-323-99794-2.00008-8

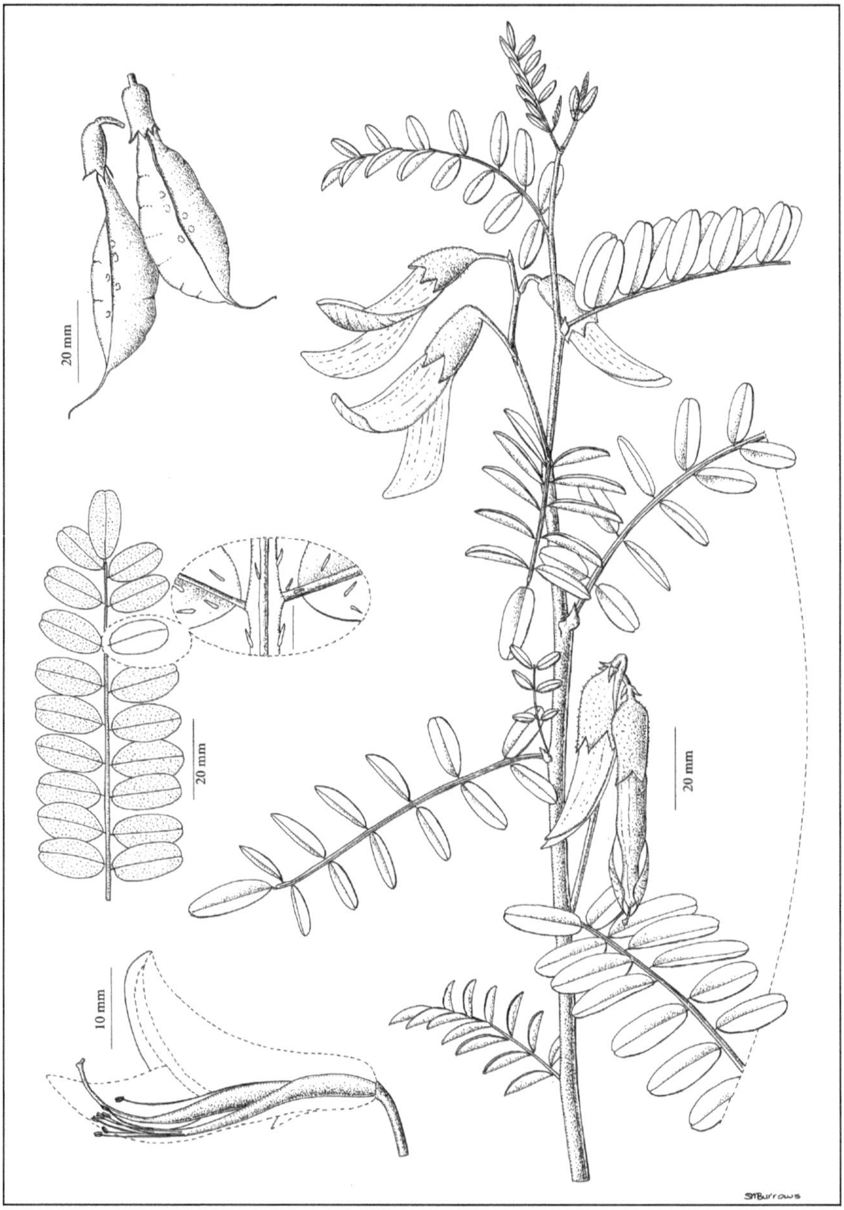
20 mm
20 mm
20 mm
10 mm
SMBurrows

Part A: General overview

1. Synonyms

Sutherlandia frutescens (L.) R.Br., *Colutea frutescens* L., *Sutherlandia montana* E. Phillips & R.A.Dyer, *Sutherlandia humilis* E. Phillips & R.A. Dyer.[a]

2. Common name(s)

Cancer bush, balloon pea, belletjie heath, camphor bush, Turkey flower (English); *'blaasbossie'*, *'blaas-ertjie'*, *'belbos'*, *'belletjie'*, *'belletjieheide'*, *'bergkankerbos'*, *'bergkankerbossie'*, *'blaasbossie'*, *'eendjies'*, *'eendjiesblom'*, *'gansbossie'*, *'gansies'*, *'gansiesblom'*, *'gansiesbos'*, *'gansieskeur'*, *'gansiekeurtjie'*, *'hoenderbelletjie'*, *'hoenderkloek'*, *'jantjie-bêrend'*, *'jantjiebarend'*, *'kalkoenbelletjieblom'*, *'kalkoenbelletjie'*, *'kalkoenbos'*, *'kalkoenbelletjiebos'*, *'kalkoentjiebos'*, *'kankerbossie'*, *'kankerbos'*, *'kipkippers'*, *'kiepiebos'*, *'klappers'*, *'kleingansiesbossie'*, *'kleingansies'*, *'rooi-ertjie'*, *'kleinkankerbossie'*, *'rooi-ertjiebos'*, *'wildekeur'* (Afrikaans); *'umnwele'*, *'insiswa'* (isiZulu); *'umnwele'*, *'insiswa'* (isiXhosa); *'phetola'* (Tswana); *'lerumo-lamadi'* (Northern Sotho); *'motlepelo'* (Sotho); *'pethora'* (Khoi-San).[a]

3. Conservation status

Least concern.[a]

4. Botany

The genus *Lessertia* (formerly *Sutherlandia*) belongs to the Fabaceae family (pea, pod-bearing or bean family), which is the second largest flowering plant family (SANBI[b]). The family is found throughout the world and encompasses more than 600 genera and 12,000 species. According to the South African National Biodiversity Institute (SANBI[b]), this family represents 134 genera and more than 1300 species in southern Africa. The genus *Lessertia* is widely distributed in Africa, and consists of about 60 species, with about 50 occurring in southern Africa. *Lessertia frutescens* currently includes *Sutherlandia humilis* and the previously known *S. montana* or mountain cancer bush. The genus *Sutherlandia* was named after James Sutherland, who was the first superintendent of the Royal Botanic Garden Edinburgh, whilst the genus *Lessertia* is named after Jules Paul Benjamin de Lessert, a French industrialist (SANBI[b]), banker, and owner of a private herbarium used by De Candolle. The Latin name for the species *'frutescens'* means bushy. *Lessertia frutescens* is a small, attractive, soft-wooded shrublet, 0.5–1 m in height. The leaves are pinnately compound, the leaflets are grey–green in colour, 4–10 mm long, giving the bush a silvery appearance (A). Spectacular red flowers (A) are borne in few-flowered axillary racemes. Each flower is tubular, markedly compressed laterally, with boat-shaped, oblong

[a] Red List of South African Plants (http://redlist.sanbi.org).
[b] SANBI, South African National Biodiversity Institute (http://pza.sanbi.org).

keel petals, two minute wing petals and an apically, large, recurved standard petal, typically marked with white lines (Van Wyk and Albrecht, 2008). The plant species does not have typical pea flowers, but the wing petals are concealed in the calyx and are very small, with the petal much shorter than the keel. The fruit is a large bladder-like inflated papery pod, and is almost transparent (B). Each pod bears numerous pale brown seeds (pale to dark brown). The seeds are laterally compressed, kidney shaped, and smooth to markedly rugose. The dry flowers are used in flower arrangements as they dry well and maintain their form and colour.

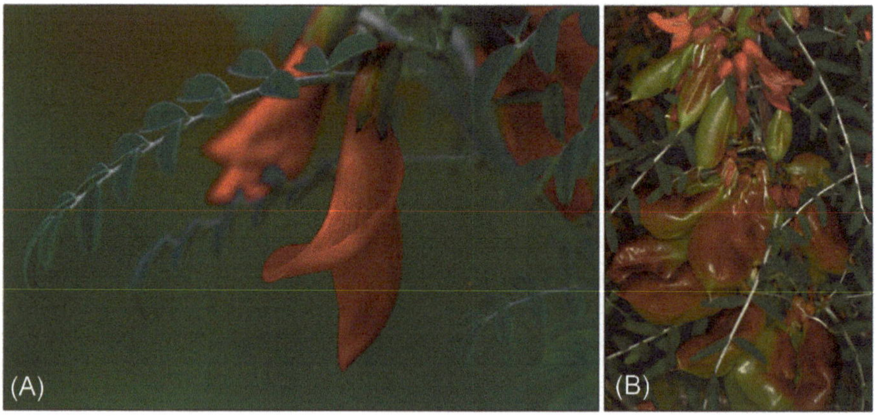

Lessertia frutescens with strikingly red flowers and pinnately compound leaves (A), inflated papery pods (B).

5. Geographical distribution

Lessertia frutescens occurs naturally throughout the dry parts of southern Africa, up the west coast as far north as Namibia and into Botswana, in the Western Cape region, and in the

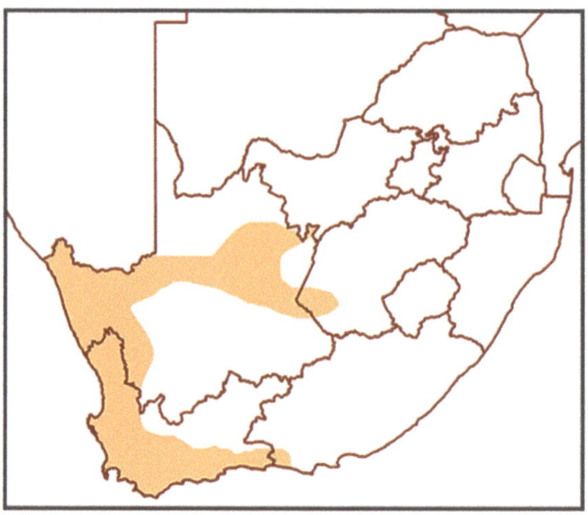

Geographical distribution of *Lessertia frutescens* in South Africa.

Western Karoo as far as the Eastern Cape Province. It is also found in the Mpumalanga and KwaZulu-Natal provinces, and it shows remarkable variation within its distribution (SANBI[b]).

6. Ethnopharmacology

The plant has long been known, respected, and used as a medicinal plant in southern Africa. The Nama and Khoi-San people, as the original inhabitants of the Cape, used the plant mainly in the form of a decoction for washing of wounds and consumed it to reduce fever. The early colonists regarded it as giving successful results in the treatment of stomach problems, chicken pox, and in the treatment of internal cancers (Van Wyk and Albrecht, 2008). It is also known to have been used as a treatment of eye troubles, the eyes being bathed with a decoction of the plant. Farm workers in the Cape still use it to treat eye conditions (Xaba, 2007), as well as to wash wounds, treat chicken pox, bring down fevers, and for internal cancers. Other traditional applications of the plant include the treatment of upper respiratory tract infections (URTIs), bronchitis, asthma, rheumatoid arthritis, rheumatism, osteoarthritis, haemorrhoids, piles, liver problems, uterus and women's complaints, bladder conditions, dysentery, diarrhoea, stomach ailments, peptic ulcers, heartburn, diabetes, backache, inflammation and varicose veins (Colling, 2009). It is also used in the treatment of emotional stress and mental problems, including anxiety, irritability and depression, and is considered a mild tranquilliser. It is a useful bitter tonic, and a little taken before meals improves appetite and aids digestion. Overall, it is considered a good general medicine. Cancer patients, as well as AIDS patients, tend to lose weight (Van Wyk and Albrecht, 2008). This plant dramatically stimulates the appetite, with patients starting to gain weight. It is also known to induce an enhanced sense of well-being and improve energy levels.

7. Commercialisation

In the late 1990s, commercial plantations of *L. frutescens* were established, such as at Sannieshof in the North West Province (Van Wyk, 2011). Commercialisation and small-scale cultivation started when air-dried leaves were supplied to a health shop in Port Elizabeth (now Gqeberha) in the Eastern Cape Province. Large-scale cultivation and contract manufacturing started in 2000 by the company Phyto Nova (Pty) Ltd. with the production of tablets from dry, powdered leaves and stems (thin) of *Lessertia*. Tablets produced by Phyto Nova, South Africa, contain 300 mg *L. frutescens* subspecies *microphylla* and have been tested in studies (Van der Walt et al., 2016). The tablets became popular as an adaptogenic tonic, reported to counteract the muscle-wasting effects associated with HIV-AIDS, and are claimed to stimulate appetite in patients. In recent years, there has been a marked increase in the commercial interest and scientific investigation of *Lessertia*. Commercial products are mostly sold in the form of tinctures and tablets.

8. Pharmacological evaluation

8.1 *In vitro* studies

8.1.1 Anticancer activity

The plant has become widely known as cancer bush, because of the reported use against internal cancers by the Cape Dutch people, as well as the Khoi-San. *Lessertia* showed potential as an anticarcinogen or chemopreventative agent in studies conducted using the Ames test, with dichloromethane extracts of the plant exhibiting antimutagenic activity (Reid et al., 2006). An *in vitro* study provided evidence of anticancer effects by exhibiting a concentration-dependent effect of *L. frutescens* on several tumour cell lines, with 50% inhibition of proliferation of MDA-MB-468, MCF7, HL60 and Jurkat cells. *Lessertia* treatment did not induce granulocyte lineage or HL60 differentiation along the monocyte/macrophage. It exhibited anti-oxidant activity by reducing free radical cations, with an estimated activity of 0.5 μL of the extract equivalent to that of 10 μM of Trolox. However, the treatment did not significantly inhibit TNF-α and IL-1β mRNA expression in RAW 264.7 cells, nor did it suppress lipopolysaccharide (LPS)-stimulated nitric oxide (NO) production by murine monocyte/macrophage RAW 264.7 cells (Tai et al., 2004). It was also shown that the methanol extracts of *L. frutescens* inhibited the DNA binding of NF-κB, activated by 12-*O*-tetradecanoylphorbol-13-acetate (TPA) in MCF10A human breast epithelial cells in a dose-dependent manner (Na et al., 2004). Cytotoxicity was observed in Chinese Hamster Ovary (CHO) cell lines and neoplastic cells (cervical carcinoma) by the aqueous extract of *L. frutescens* (Chinkwo, 2005). Apoptotic responses were shown through monitoring and morphological observation with other biological assays involving phosphatidylserine externalisation and chromatin condensation. Biochemical assays indicated similar DNA fragmentation patterns induced by the extracts compared to other inducers of apoptosis, such as ceramide and staurosporine. Growth inhibition effects against LNCaP and PC-3 human prostate tumour cell lines were exhibited in a dose-dependent manner for non-polar and polar extracts of *Lessertia* (Chen, 2007). The extracts of *L. frutescens* decreased cell growth, observed in a statistically significant manner, of human non-tumourigenic epithelial mammary gland (MCF-12A) and human breast adenocarcinoma (MCF-7) cells by 49% and 26%, respectively, following exposure for 72 h. Hyper-condensed chromatin, membrane blebbing, cytoplasmic shrinking and apoptotic bodies were more pronounced in the MCF-7 cell line, and cell density was significantly compromised. Late stages of apoptosis were more prominent in MCF-7 *L. frutescens*-treated cells, when compared to the MCF-12A cells at a concentration of 10 mg/mL. Transmission electron microscopy revealed hallmarks of increased hypercondensed and vascularisation chromatin, suggesting apoptotic and autophagic processes. Fluorescence microscopy indicated evidence of the induction of autophagy, whilst flow cytometry revealed an increase in phosphatidylserine translocation in the MCF-7 cell line, indicative of apoptosis induction and a decrease in actively cycling cells in both cell lines (Stander et al., 2007, 2009; Vorster et al., 2012; Mqoco et al., 2014). An SNO oesophageal cancer cell line was used to investigate the apoptosis-inducing effects of two *L. frutescens* extracts. The extract-treated SNO cells presented with morphological features characteristic of apoptosis, as revealed by microscopy studies. Caspase inhibition revealed that the extracts were able to induce independent cell death, as well as caspase-dependent cell death (Skerman et al., 2011).

Colon cancer cells (Caco-2) exposed to the ethanolic extracts of *L. frutescens* were found to have a significantly decreased cell viability, reflected by increased pyknosis and reduced 3-(4,5-dimethylthiazol-2-yl)-2,5-diphenyl tetrazolium bromide (MTT) reductive capacity, as well as loss in cellular membrane integrity. The *in vitro* study demonstrated that the extract attenuated proliferation of colon cancer cells by the disruption of key molecules in the PI-3K pathway, thereby inducing apoptosis (Leisching et al., 2015). When the ethanol extract of *L. frutescens* was evaluated for the ability to inhibit Hedgehog (Hh)-signalling-driven genes in prostate cancer cells, it was found that 50% of Hh-responsive genes were repressed, including the newly distinguished Hh-responsive genes, Penk and Hsd11b1, in addition to the canonical Hh-responsive genes, Ptch1 and Gli1 (Lu et al., 2015). *Lessertia frutescens* extracts induced apoptosis in A375 melanoma cells, as evidenced by morphological features of apoptosis, nuclear condensation, phosphatidylserine exposure, caspase activation, and the release of cytochrome *c* from the mitochondria. Studies by Van der Walt et al. (2016), conducted in the presence of a pan-caspase inhibitor, alluded to caspase-independent cell death, and this appeared to be mediated by the apoptosis-inducing factor. Antimutagenesis studies were conducted with hot aqueous extracts of *L. frutescens* against the N-oxide, 4-(methylnitrosamino)-1-(3-pyridyl)-1-butanol (NNAL) and the tobacco-specific mutagens 4-(methylnitrosamino)-1-(3-pyridyl)-1-butanone (NNK). Cancer bush exhibited protection similar to that exhibited by unfermented and fermented honeybush against NNK mutagenesis, when considering the number of total polyphenols (TPP) incorporated in the assay (Gelderblom et al., 2017). Specific polyphenol-cytochrome P450 (CYP450) interactions are likely to be involved in the protection against tobacco-related mutagenesis.

8.1.2 Anti-HIV/AIDS activity

Bessong et al. (2006) and Harnett et al. (2005) reported that compounds in the aqueous extracts of *Lessertia* are responsible for the inhibitory effects observed in *in vitro* experiments of the aqueous and organic extracts on HIV reverse transcriptase and other HIV target enzymes. They recommended that further studies be undertaken to establish the mode of action. In a review by Mills et al. (2005), the likelihood of *Lessertia* interacting with antiretroviral drugs in treating HIV was deduced from the available evidence. Significant effects were shown of *Lessertia* extracts on cytochrome P450 3A4 metabolism with an approximately two-fold activation of the pregnane X receptor. Inhibition of *p*-glycoprotein expression was reported, with *Lessertia* displaying 19%–31% of activity compared to verapamil (Mills et al., 2005). The immune-enhancing potential of the extract has been recognised in South Africa, to the extent that *L. frutescens* has been recommended as an adjuvant in HIV/AIDS treatment by the South African Ministry of Health. The apoptotic effects of *L. frutescens* extracts were investigated *in vitro* on normal human lymphocytes (Korb et al., 2010). The extract caused a significant increase in apoptosis of CD4+ cells and in the total lymphocyte population at 12 h, as evidenced by increased caspase-3/7 activity, phosphatidylserine translocation, and decreased ATP content. Lymphocyte activation was also initiated by the extract in both total CD4+ and lymphocyte subpopulations, as indicated by a doubling of the number of cells expressing the CD69 activation marker. The immunomodulatory effects of *L. frutescens* extracts were determined *in vitro* on normal human peripheral blood mononuclear cells (PBMCs) (Ngcobo et al., 2012a). Changes in cytokine secretion, relative to the dose of the extract, were induced by the ethanol extracts. A significant reduction in the levels of some cytokines, including IL-1β and TNF-α, was observed for the extract at a dose of 2.5 mg/mL. The concentrations of IFNγ and IL-1β were increased by the aqueous extract, whilst that of TNF-α decreased. *In vitro* results clearly showed that *L. frutescens* extracts modulated cytokine secretion in normal unstimulated PBMCs. The effects of extracts of *L. frutescens* (aqueous and 70% ethanol) were examined on normal isolated human T cells at a concentration of 2.5 mg/mL, and the ethanolic extract induced significant depletion of ATP (76%), necrosis (95%) and inhibition of caspase-3/7 activity, following a 24-h incubation period (Ngcobo et al., 2012b). The aqueous extract (at 2.5 mg/mL) showed the same trend, but was less effective. The researchers showed in this *in vitro* study that, although high concentrations of the extracts can be toxic to normal T cells, fractions from the water extract were relatively safe for use. The potential of *L. frutescens* to inhibit the human organic anion transporting polypeptide (OATP1B3 and OATP1B1) and the human ATP-binding cassette transporter (BCRP and P-gp) activities were assessed using cell lines that overexpress the transporter proteins. Data showed that the *L. frutescens* extract shows inhibitory potency with time-dependent inhibition (irreversible). In addition, delayed production of midazolam metabolites in the hepatocytes was observed, decreasing its clearance by 40%. Furthermore, the extract of *L. frutescens* inhibited OATP1B1, P-gp and OATP1B3 (Fasinu et al., 2013). HL60 cell lines were employed to determine the immune modulating effects of extracts of *L. frutescens* on cytokines, including interleukins 4, 8, 6, 12p70, 10 and TNF (Faleschini et al., 2013). The data showed that the extracts possess both anti-inflammatory and immune-modulating effects. The study indicated that an ethanolic extract appeared to recruit the various inflammatory cytokines to the site of infection, upon stimulation with phorbol 12-myristate-13-acetate, and further showed that the non-polar compounds present in the ethanol extract contributed mostly to the activity of this extract.

8.1.3 Antidiabetic activity

The effects of extracts of *L. frutescens*, on the metabolism and absorption of the protease inhibitor, atazanavir (ATV), were investigated *in vitro* (Müller et al., 2012). Flavonol glycoside and triterpenoid glycoside fractions were isolated by solvent extraction and column chromatography, and fractions obtained showed the presence of the sutherlandins and sutherlandiosides, known to be present in *L. frutescens*. D-Pinitol, as well as the aqueous extract of *L. frutescens*, significantly reduced ATV accumulation by Caco-2 cells, implying a decrease in ATV absorption, whilst the opposite effect was seen for the triterpenoid glycoside fraction. Enhanced atazanavir metabolism was observed for the triterpenoid glycoside fraction, whilst the methanolic and aqueous extracts inhibited ATV metabolism in human liver microsomes. Müller et al. (2012) demonstrated that the compounds and extracts of *L. frutescens* affected ATV metabolism in human liver microsomes and also influenced the accumulation of ATV by Caco-2 cells. The aqueous extract of *L. frutescens* was also investigated for its capacity to prevent insulin resistance in a human liver cell culture. The insulin-resistant Chang liver cells took up significantly less 2-[^{3}H]-deoxyglucose than the controls, accumulated more intracellular lipid, and released more glucose into the culture medium. Simultaneous treatment with *L. frutescens* prevented development of these insulin resistance parameters. Significant down- and up-regulation of 27 gene targets were observed in the extract-treated insulin-resistant cells using *L. frutescens*. The gene VAMP3, which plays a role in vesicle transport, was up-regulated by *L. frutescens* and down-regulated by insulin resistance. Data confirmed that *L. frutescens* can prevent insulin resistance in hepatocytes, through regulation of 26 genes encoding receptors, vesicle transporters, transcription factors, signalling molecules and metabolic enzymes (Williams et al., 2013). Alimi and Ashafa (2017) investigated the antidiabetic and anti-oxidant activities of leaf extracts. The antidiabetic potential was evaluated through the inhibition of key carbohydrate hydrolysing enzymes (α-glucosidase and α-amylase), whilst enzyme kinetic analysis was conducted to assess the mode of the enzyme inhibition. The ethanol extract showed the best reducing power efficiency and also exhibited the best scavenging activity, when compared to silymarin (standard), whilst the decoction displayed the strongest metal chelating potential. The decoction and ethanol extracts exhibited strong and mild inhibitory effects on the specific activities of α-glucosidase and α-amylase, respectively, through non-competitive and uncompetitive modes of action.

8.1.4 Anti-inflammatory and analgesic activities

Fernandes et al. (2004) observed the link between anti-inflammatory and anti-oxidant activities, and reported that hot water *Lessertia* extracts have hydrogen peroxide- and superoxide-scavenging activities at concentrations as low as 10 μg/mL. Acetone extracts exhibited anti-oxidant activity in the 2,2-diphenyl-1-picrylhydrazyl (DPPH) free-radical scavenging assay (Katerere and Eloff, 2005).

The use of *L. frutescens*, when formulated in an oily base, appeared to have a rational basis for topical staphylococcal infections (Katerere and Eloff, 2005). The extracts of *L. frutescens* were assessed for total phenolic and flavonoid contents, total reducing power, iron chelating capacity, and free radical scavenging power, including, scavenging of hydroxyl radicals, superoxide anions, nitric oxide and hydrogen peroxide. The extracts showed significant anti-oxidant capacity, depending on the nature of the extraction solvent, against *t*BHP-induced oxidative stress in cells, by preserving intracellular oxidised glutathione/reduced glutathione ratio (GSSG/GSH) and scavenging radical oxygen species (ROS) (Tobwala et al., 2014). The efficacy of *L. frutescens* as an anti-inflammatory agent was investigated in a co-culture model of the blood–brain barrier (BBB), *in vitro*. Stimulation was conducted in single cultures of human astrocytes (HA), primary human monocytes, human umbilical cord endothelial cells (HUVECs), as well as BBB co-cultures, with HL2/3 cell secretory proteins and/or HIV-1 subtype B & C Tat protein. Significant increases were seen for CD14+ monocyte infiltration across the BBB, as well as the monocyte chemo-attractant protein-1, a major role player in HIV-associated neuro-inflammation, whilst IL-1β secretion decreased (Africa and Smith, 2015). Jiang et al. (2014) reported that the ethanol extract of *L. frutescens* suppressed NO and IFNγ- and LPS-induced ROS production in microglial cells, as well as *N*-methyl-D-aspartate receptor (NMDA)-induced ROS production in neurons. The mechanism of the extract on microglial cells appeared to be mediated through inhibition of the IFNγ-induced p-ERK1/2 signalling pathway, which is central to regulating a number of intracellular metabolic processes. These include enhancing filopodia and STAT1α phosphorylation formation. The involvement of these pathways indicates the potential of novel therapeutics for the treatment of HIV/AIDS and/or stress and prevention of stress, as well as inflammatory diseases in the brain. Lei et al. (2015a) reported that the extracts of *L. frutescens* displayed potent immune-stimulatory activities, using primary murine macrophages and a murine macrophage cell line. Short-term treatment with a polysaccharide-enriched fraction or a crude aqueous extract of *L. frutescens* increased macrophage production of NO and ROS. Evaluation of the anti-inflammatory activity of an ethanolic extract of *L. frutescens* was conducted on primary mouse macrophages and a murine macrophage cell line (RAW 264.7 cells). Further experiments were conducted on the activity of the cycloartanol glycosides and a flavonol found in large quantities within the extract. The effect did not appear to be mediated by sutherlandins or sutherlandiosides, in contrast to the extract that exhibited anti-inflammatory activities upon murine macrophages, similar to that reported for the microglia cell line (Lei et al., 2015b). The molecular action of *L. frutescens* with regard to potential functions involving inflammation and wound healing, and macrophage differentiation, was investigated *in vitro* by Camille and Dealtry (2018). The responses of cells of the RAW 264.7 murine macrophage cell line to ethanol and hot aqueous extracts of *L. frutescens* were investigated to determine the action and relative efficacy of each extract, prepared from a single plant source, previously shown to target T2D. The ethanolic extract upregulated CD206, whilst both extracts downregulated CD86 expression, indicating stimulation of the M2 phenotype over the M1 phenotype. M1 macrophage pro-inflammatory responses, including ROS and NO production, as well as cyclo-oxygenase-2 (COX-2) expression were inhibited *in vitro* by both extracts. Cytokine production patterns determined by enzyme-linked immunosorbent assays (ELISA) indicated that the M2 cytokine profile remained unchanged, but the M1 pro-inflammatory cytokine profile was downregulated. Reduced production of inflammatory mediators was associated with decreased activity of the nuclear factor kappa-light-chain-enhancer of activated B-cells (NF-κB) signalling pathways and the mitogen-activated protein kinases (MAPKs).

8.1.5 Antistress activity

The effects of aqueous and methanol extracts of *L. frutescens* on adrenal steroidogenic cytochrome P450 enzymes were investigated, since stress-related ailments are known to be linked to the endocrine system (Prevoo et al., 2008). The methanol and aqueous extracts resulted in an inhibition of the type I progesterone-induced difference spectrum, whilst inhibition of pregnenolone binding was negligible, and stronger inhibition was associated with the aqueous extract. The triterpenoid fraction resulted in the inhibition of both the type I progesterone- and pregnenolone-induced difference spectra, and elicited a type II difference spectrum in the absence of substrate. Prevoo et al. (2008) reported that both progesterone and pregnenolone metabolism were inhibited by the aqueous extract, with the inhibition of CYP17 more than that of CYP21, influencing the flux through glucocorticoid precursor pathways. An immortalised rat astrocyte (DI TNC1) cell line, expressing a luciferase reporter driven by the Nrf2/anti-oxidant response element (ARE) promoter or NF-κB, was used to assess regulation of these two pathways by *L. frutescens*. It was shown that the extract effectively inhibited LPS-induced NF-κB reporter activity. The extract also enhanced ARE activity in the presence of LPS. Ajit et al. (2016) reported that *L. frutescens* induced Nrf2 and HO-1 protein expression. Sutherlandioside B, also known as SU1, and extracts of *L. frutescens* were evaluated for their effects on key steroidogenic enzymes in COS-1 cells. Significant inhibitory effects of the extract towards progesterone conversion by CYP21A2 and CYP17A1 were recorded. The compound SU1 inhibited 3β-HSD2 and CYP17A1, but did not affect CYP21A2. It also decreased androgen and cortisol precursors significantly in H295R cells. The extract decreased mineralocorticoid metabolites significantly, as well as total steroid production (stimulated and basal) with cortisol and its precursor, deoxycortisol, under forskolin-stimulated conditions. The compound SU1 and the extracts of *L. frutescens* repressed NF-κB-driven gene expression without activating GRE-driven gene expression. Both antagonised the effects of aldosterone *via* the MR, whilst neither activated mineral corticoid receptor-mediated gene transcription. Data obtained presented evidence linking the anti-inflammatory, antistress and antihypertensive properties of *L. frutescens* to modulation of adrenal hormone biosynthesis and inhibition of steroidogenic enzymes (Sergeant et al., 2017).

8.1.6 Other activities

The leaf extract of *L. frutescens* exhibited antithrombotic activity (IC_{50} = 2.17 mg/mL) (Kee et al., 2008). A study was conducted to evaluate the mitochondrial membrane potential, anti-oxidant potential, apoptotic induction and lipid peroxidation of *L. frutescens* extracts on distal and proximal tubule epithelial cells. The extracts increased lipid peroxidation in treated MDBK and LLC-PK1 cells and significantly decreased intracellular GSH in MDBK and LLC-PK1 cells. The activity of caspase 3/7 increased in both MDBK and LLC-PK1 cells. Phulukdaree et al. (2010) showed that the aqueous extracts at high concentrations appeared to alter mitochondrial membrane integrity, increase oxidative stress and promote apoptosis in renal tubule epithelia. *Lessertia frutescens* extracts were tested against shikimate kinase enzyme (MtbSK) and the methanol:dichloromethane (1:1 v/v) extract showed good inhibition of MtbSK (IC_{50} = 0.1 μg/mL) and the purified α-linolenic acid compound exhibited antimycobacterial activity with an IC_{50} = 3.7 μg/mL (Masoko et al., 2016).

8.2 *In vivo* studies and clinical trials

8.2.1 Anticancer activity

Clinical evidence, obtained through a study of 16 cancer patients, proved that ingestion of the plant was able to reduce fatigue (Grandi et al., 2005). A diet supplemented with *L. frutescens* was fed to TRAMP mice and found to suppress the formation of poorly differentiated carcinoma in their prostate glands. The *in vivo* effect observed for the extract was linked to its inhibition of Gli/Hh signalling in prostate cancer. The data showed that sutherlandioside D was the most potent compound in the methanol extract that suppressed Gli-reporter in Shh Light II cells (Lin et al., 2016).

8.2.2 Anti-HIV/AIDS activity

The effects of chronic and short-term exposure of *Lessertia* on oral pharmacokinetics and bio-availability of nevirapine (NVP), a non-nucleoside reverse transcriptase inhibitor, were investigated (Minocha et al., 2011). Short-term co-administration of the extract resulted in non-significant differences in the pharmacokinetic parameters of NVP. A 50% decrease in the area under curve (AUC) and Cmax values of NVP were observed after 5 days of chronic exposure to *Lessertia* extracts. Minocha et al. (2011) suggested potential drug-herb interactions of NVP with *L. frutescens*. Twelve healthy male subjects were administered extracts of *L. frutescens* in a study to determine the bio-availability of ATV. Participants ingested a single dose of ATV during a phase I study, and blood samples were drawn, before and after dosing. A significant reduction in the bio-availability of ATV was observed for the extract, as indicated by the confidence interval (CI) that fell below the limits of the 'no-effect' boundary for both pharmacokinetic parameters. This may potentially result in subtherapeutic plasma concentrations, resulting in reduced anti-HIV efficacy of ATV (Müller et al., 2013). A clinical pilot study was conducted to evaluate the effects of *L. frutescens* extracts on cachexia, the muscle-wasting effects seen in patients with tuberculosis, cancer or AIDS. The primary endpoint (frequency of adverse events) and secondary endpoint (changes in vital, physical, biomarker indices and blood) were determined in the study. No adverse events or significant differences were seen in vital, physical, biomarker indices and blood between the placebo and treatment groups. However, improved appetite was reported of participants consuming *Lessertia* compared to the placebo group. The biomarker, canavanine, was undetectable in plasma of the participants (Johnson et al., 2007; Morris, 2017).

8.2.3 Antidiabetic activity

A study was undertaken in animal models to investigate the anti-inflammatory, analgesic and antidiabetic properties of the aqueous extract of the plant shoots (Ojewole, 2004). The hypoglycaemic and anti-inflammatory effects of the aqueous extract were investigated in rats, using streptozotocin (STZ)-induced diabetes mellitus and fresh egg albumin-induced pedal (paw) oedema. In addition, the analgesic effect was evaluated using the acetic acid test and hot-plate models of pain in mice. Significant analgesic effects were seen in mice for the aqueous extract against chemically and thermally induced nociceptive pain stimuli. The plant extract caused significant hypoglycaemia in rats and further significantly inhibited fresh egg albumin-induced acute inflammation. The effects of *L. frutescens* extracts in promoting glucose uptake and inducing hypoglycaemia in prediabetic rats were examined by Chadwick et al. (2007). Rats were fed a high-fat diet and crushed leaves of *L. frutescens* in drinking water were administered. Rats receiving *L. frutescens* displayed normal insulinemic levels after 8 weeks of treatment compared to the fatty controls. There was a significant decrease in intestinal glucose uptake, as well as uptake into adipose and muscle tissue in rats receiving the plant extract. The researchers demonstrated that the plant extract was a promising candidate for a type 2 antidiabetic medication, as it suppressed intestinal glucose uptake and normalised insulin levels and glucose uptake in peripheral tissues, with no weight gain observed. *Lessertia frutescens* reduced plasma free fatty acid levels in an *in vivo* study, thereby preventing the development of insulin resistance (IR) in rats fed a high-fat diet (MacKenzie et al., 2009). In comparison to rats fed high-fat diet only (positive control for IR), levels of plasma free fatty acids (FFA) were significantly reduced after 1 week. The extract reduced the level of plasma FFA in a 12-week treatment study below that of rats fed a normal diet (negative control). HOMA-IR and QUICKI indices confirmed that *L. frutescens*-treated rats over a period of 12 weeks did not develop IR when fed a high-fat diet. Chronic medication over 12 weeks decreased the low-density/high-density lipopolysaccharide (LDL/HDL) ratio and total cholesterol levels, and in addition, reduced plasma FFA and prevented IR. Results showed that *L. frutescens* is an effective medicinal remedy to prevent IR and elevated plasma free fatty acids, and therefore type 2 diabetes (MacKenzie et al., 2009). Insulin resistance is induced by a high-fat diet linked to ectopic fat deposits and dyslipidaemia in liver and skeletal muscles. An IR rat model was employed to evaluate the effects of *L. frutescens* on lipid metabolism in 3T3-pre-adipocytes (MacKenzie et al., 2012). A significant effect was seen after 4 weeks, as the extract-treated group had significantly lower body weight than the high-fat control group. Blood plasma analysis showed a decrease in free fatty acids, insulin and triglycerides, and related changes in lipid parameters were observed in the skeletal muscles, liver and adipose tissue. Lactate production and glucose consumption were increased with treatment using *L. frutescens*, whilst a simultaneous decrease in triglyceride accumulation was observed. The study indicated that *L. frutescens* directly affected lipid biosynthesis and mitochondrial activity in adipose tissue, and provided a mechanism by which the extract restored insulin sensitivity through modulating fatty acid biosynthesis (MacKenzie et al., 2012).

8.2.4 Anti-inflammatory and analgesic activities

Inhibited TPA-induced COX-2 expression was seen with topical application of a methanolic extract of *L. frutescens* (Kundu et al., 2005). The extract diminished TPA-stimulated catalytic activity of extracellular signal-regulated protein kinase (ERK), as an underlying mechanism of COX-2 inhibition, which is known to regulate the activation of eukaryotic transcription factors mediating COX-2 induction. The extract attenuated the expression of the key component c-Fos and inhibited TPA-induced activation of activator protein-1 (AP-1), whilst TPA-induced activation of NF-kB remained unchanged. In another *in vivo* study, pretreatment with the extract prevented the induction of DNA binding of cyclic AMP response element binding (CREB) protein in mouse skin compared to the control (control: topical application of TPA-induced CREB protein). Statistically significant anti-inflammatory effects were recorded for *L. frutescens* in reducing fresh egg albumin-induced pedal oedema in mice (Ojewole, 2004). *Lessertia frutescens* was included in a diet given to mice, and results indicated no changes to systemic infection by either a Gram-negative or a Gram-positive bacterium (i.e. *E. coli* and *L. monocytogenes*). No evidence was found that *L. frutescens* consumption stimulated *in vivo* inflammatory responses, as the extract rather tended to diminish *in vivo* inflammatory responses. These observations are in contrast to *in vitro* results published later (Lei et al., 2016).

8.2.5 Antistress activity

A warm water extract of *Lessertia* leaves was investigated in a model of chronic intermittent immobilisation stress in adult male Wistar rats (Smith and Myburgh, 2004). Immobilisation stress resulted in significantly increased concentrations of corticosterone in immobilisation + placebo (IP) *versus* control + placebo (CP) groups, whereas concentrations of corticosterone were significantly decreased in immobilisation + treatment (IS) group compared to IP. Neither IL-6 nor testosterone and TNF-α concentrations were significantly different amongst the groups. Smith and Myburgh (2004) reported that *L. frutescens* treatment effectively decreased the corticosterone response to chronic stress, thereby confirming the indigenous use. In another study in adult rats, the claimed stress-relieving properties of the extracts of the shrub were investigated using an *in vivo* model of chronic intermittent immobilisation stress. Immobilisation stress resulted in significantly decreased corticosterone levels of the *Lessertia* extract-treated group, whilst the control group exhibited increased corticosterone levels. Since the biosynthesis of glucocorticoids in the adrenals is catalysed by the cytochrome P450-dependent enzymes, the effect of the extracts on adrenal steroidogenesis was determined in ovine mitochondria and adrenocortical microsomes, using enzyme conversion and spectral binding assays (Prevoo et al., 2004). The aqueous extracts showed inhibition of substrate binding to cytochrome P450 11β-hydroxylase (CYP11B1) by 60% and cytochrome P450 21-hydroxylase (CYP21) by 38%. The conversion of pregnenolone and progesterone was inhibited by 30% and 34%, respectively. Negligible inhibition was observed for the methanol extract, but the chloroform extract caused 62% inhibition of the pregnenolone to CYP17. The chloroform extract also exerted a higher inhibitory effect compared to the methanol extract on pregnenolone and progesterone metabolism (20%–50%).

8.2.6 Other activities

The anticonvulsant property of the plant shoot aqueous extract was examined against picrotoxin (PCT)-, pentylenetetrazole (PTZ)-, and bicuculline (BCL)-induced seizures in mice (Ojewole, 2008). *Lessertia frutescens* aqueous extract significantly delayed the antagonised onset of PTZ-induced seizures. It also significantly antagonised PCT-induced seizures, but a weak effect was seen for antagonised BCL-induced seizures. The results suggested that the plant can be used as a natural supplementary remedy in the control, management and/or treatment of childhood epilepsy and convulsions. An *in vivo* study was conducted to investigate signalling mechanisms, atrophy and apoptosis of restraint stress in 40 adult male Wistar rats (Engelbrecht et al., 2010). Results indicated that restraint significantly increased myostatin, the levels of which were significantly reduced with treatment of an extract of *L. frutescens*. The extract also significantly counteracted the expression of MyoD attenuated in RP. Restraint also resulted in a significant increase of apoptosis attenuation and the PI3-Kinase/Akt signalling pathway, which was reversed by *L. frutescens* treatment. Engelbrecht et al. (2010) demonstrated in this study that psychological stress elevated markers of apoptosis and muscle atrophy were affected by *L. frutescens* through the inhibition of signalling pathways and apoptosis associated with muscle atrophy. A rodent model was used to evaluate *L. frutescens* extract for acute psychological stress (Smith and Van Vuuren, 2014). The extract was administered at a low dose (4 mg/kg body mass), 30 min prior to stress exposure (1 h restraint) and further investigated for its peripheral and central mechanisms of action in acute stress. After 1 h of exposure to stress, acute restraint resulted in a significant increase in anterior pituitary adrenocorticotropic hormone (ACTH) levels, as well as plasma corticosterone levels, with decreasing gamma-aminobutyric acid (GABA) (A)α1 receptor and hippocampal glucocorticoid receptor (GR) levels. Smith and Van Vuuren (2014) showed that the low dose abolished the stress-induced downregulation of GR, with a mode independent of GABA

(A)α1 receptor. It was reported (Chuang et al., 2015) that *L. frutescens* exhibited significant protective effects against neuropathological changes and global cerebral ischemia-induced functional motor deficits, including microglial activation and neuronal cell death, in mice. Results further indicated beneficial effects against ischemic damage through suppression of pro-inflammatory and oxidative pathways in microglial cells and neurons. Ethanolic extracts of *Lessertia* suppressed both IFNγ- and LPS-induced NO and ROS production by microglial cells, and production of ROS in rat primary cortical neurons stimulated by NMDA (Folk et al., 2016). Consumption of the extracts mitigated microglial activation in the striatum and hippocampus of ischemic brains of mice. RNAseq analysis indicated suppressed gene expression of inflammatory signalling, oxidative stress and toll-like receptor pathways that can reduce the host's immune response to infection and reactivation of latent *Mycobacterium tuberculosis*.

8.3 Safety

Initially, vervet monkeys were used to investigate the safety of *Lessertia* extracts at doses of up to 80 mg/kg dried powder over a period of 3 months, and no side effects were observed (Seier et al., 2002). Ojewole (2004) studied acute toxicity of aqueous extracts of *L. frutescens* (20–25 g) by intraperitoneal administration to fasted mice. It was concluded that the crude extracts are relatively safe in mammals, as the calculated median lethal dose (LD_{50}) was 1280 ± 71 mg of extract per kg. In 2004, a randomised, controlled trial was conducted in Cape Town in order to evaluate the safety of the plant in healthy humans taking 400 mg dried powder twice daily over a period of 24 weeks, and no toxicity was recorded (Johnson et al., 2007). The possibility of drug–herb interactions was investigated, since products containing *L. frutescens* may interact with insulin or other diabetes medication (Sia, 2004), or with antiretroviral drugs (Mills et al., 2005). In an adaptive, randomised, two-stage, double-blind placebo controlled study, interaction with medication was observed (Wilson et al., 2015). The safety of consuming dried *L. frutescens* by HIV seropositive adults with CD4 T-lymphocyte counts of >350 cells/µL was investigated. It was found that *L. frutescens* did not change CD4 T-lymphocyte count and HIV viral load. Similar results were seen in the two arms of the study at 24 weeks. However, total burden and mean of infection was higher in the *L. frutescens* group, attributed to two tuberculosis cases in participants taking isoniazid preventive therapy (IPT). A possible interaction between IPT and *L. frutescens* requires further investigation, although no other safety issues were observed. Possible long-term adverse effects were further investigated for methanol and ethyl acetate extracts of *L. frutescens* (Ntuli et al., 2018). The extracts were screened for antimutagenic and mutagenic activities using the Ames assay, utilising TA98, TA97a, TA102 and TA100 in the absence and presence of metabolic activation. Both extracts exhibited protective effects, with the ethyl acetate extract exhibiting higher potency.

9. Phytochemistry

9.1 Non-volatile constituents

Many members of the Fabaceae, including *Lessertia* (mainly the leaves), contain high levels of free, non-protein and protein-bound amino acids. The chemotypic variation and phytochemical content of *L. frutescens* were investigated by Mncwangi and Viljoen (2012). L-Asparagine, proline and alanine were the most abundant amino acids identified and together represented approximately 60% of the total amino acid content; however, not all samples contained all of the amino acids. Quantitative determination of the various compounds in *Lessertia* reflected tremendous variation, both between and within populations. An example of this is the compound L-canavanine (a non-protein amino acid), for which concentrations ranged from 0.14 to 13.58 mg/g. Early studies by Viljoen (1969) revealed the presence of pinitol and cyclitol in *Lessertia*. Proline, an amino acid, was detected in *L. frutescens* at levels from 0.7 to 7.5 mg/g (Van Wyk and Albrecht, 2008). Further analyses conducted by Avula et al. (2010), using liquid chromatography–mass spectrometry (LC–MS), showed the presence of flavonoids and cycloartane-type triterpenoids. Four cycloartanol glycosides (sutherlandiosides A–D) and four flavonoids (sutherlandins A–D) were separated from the aerial parts of *L. frutescens* using a reversed phase (RP-18) column, and photodiode array (PDA) and evaporative light-scattering (ELSD) detection. The method was validated for repeatability, linearity, limits of quantification and detection. Subsequent determination of the major compound, sutherlandioside B (SU1), in the products indicated considerable variation in content, ranging from 1.099 to 5.224 mg/average weight. Isolation and structure elucidation were done using chemical and spectroscopic methods (Fu et al., 2010). Flavonoid (retention time: 15.0–19.0 min) and terpenoid (retention time: 7.5–9.0 min) regions of the chromatograms were useful for distinguishing between samples, and five distinct clusters were revealed after principal component analysis (Albrecht et al., 2012). Spiral countercurrent chromatography was employed, using an optimised solvent system (ethyl acetate:*n*-butanol:acetic acid:water), to isolate the flavonol glycosides (sutherlandins A–D) from *L. frutescens* (Chen et al., 2017). The absence or the presence of sutherlandioside B and its derivatives contributed significantly to the distinction of plants collected from Gansbaai and those from the Karoo. *In vitro* generated plants, as part of a commercialisation–conservation strategy, displayed a metabolite profile similar to non-propagated plants (Mavimbela et al., 2018). The similarity of wild plants to micro-propagated plants proved that tissue culture does not have deleterious effects on the chemistry of the plants as reflected by SU1 as a chemical marker for quality control. A rapid quality control method was also developed for *L. frutescens* by Mavimbela et al. (2018) using vibrational spectroscopy, in combination with chemometric data analysis. The concentrations of SU1, determined using ultra-high-performance liquid chromatography–mass spectrometry (UHPLC–MS), were highly variable, ranging from 0.04 to 10.10 µg/mg of dried leaf material.

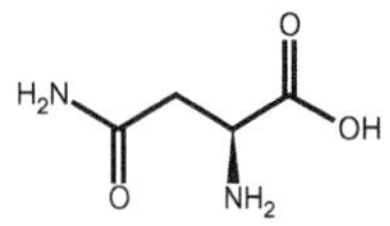
L-Asparagine

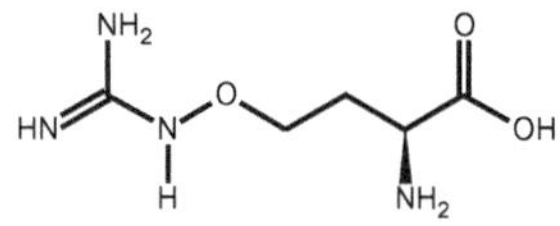
L-Canavanine

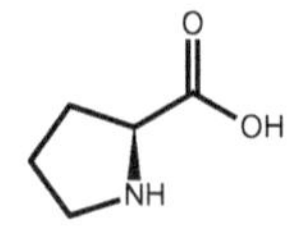
Proline

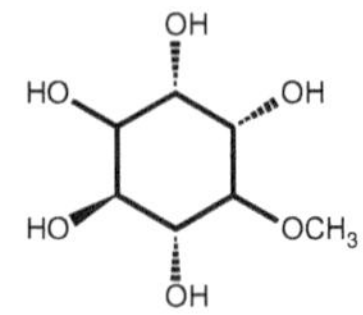
D-Pinitol

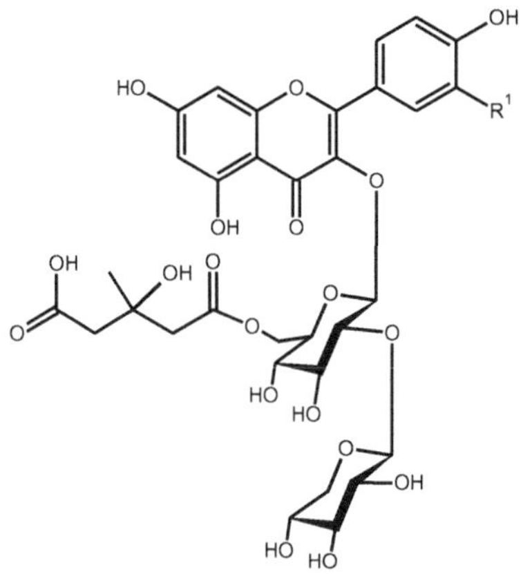
Sutherlandin A: R^1=OH
Sutherlandin C: R^1=H

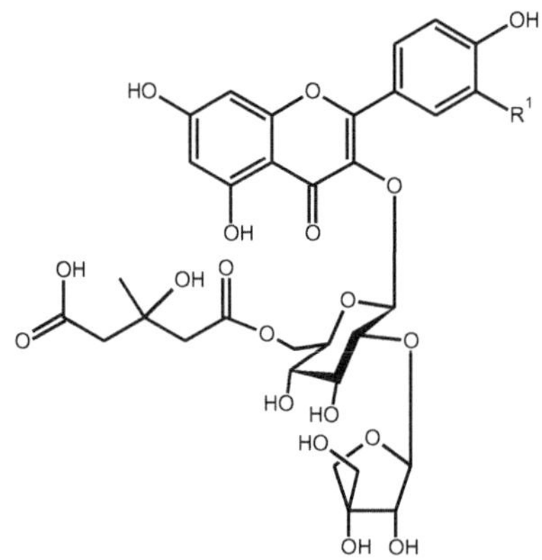
Sutherlandin B: R^1=OH
Sutherlandin D: R^1=H

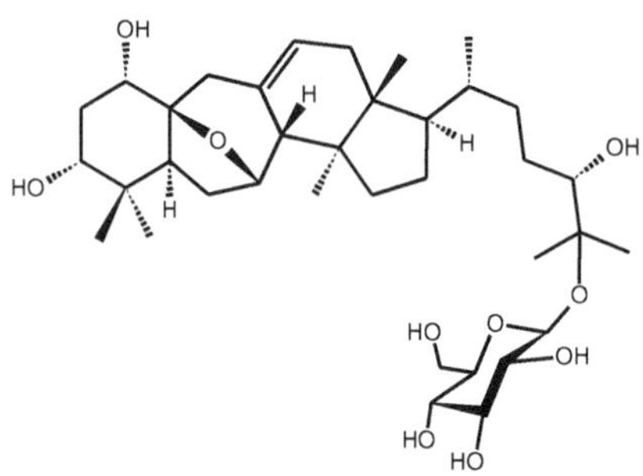
Sutherlandioside A

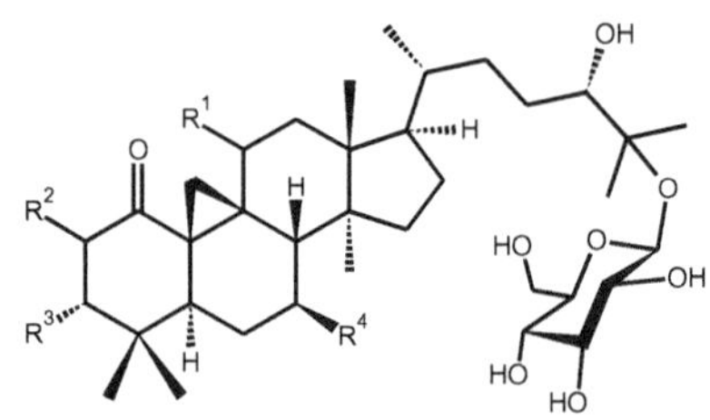
Sutherlandioside B: R^1=H, R^2=2H, R^3=OH, R^4=OH
Sutherlandioside C: R^1=O, R^2=2H, R^3=OH, R^4=H
Sutherlandioside D: R^1=H, R^2=H, R^3=H, R^4=OH

Part B: Chemical profiling and quality control

10. Chromatography analysis

10.1 High-performance thin-layer chromatography (HPTLC) fingerprint analysis

General instrumentation: CAMAG HPTLC instrument consisting of an automatic TLC sampler (ATS 4), automatic developing chamber (ADC 2), CAMAG TLC visualiser 2, CAMAG immersion device, and TLC plate heater. *HPTLC plates:* Silica gel glass plates 60 F_{254} (Merck). *Plant part:* Aerial parts, methanol extract. *Sample application:* Application volume of 10 μL methanol extract (10 mg/mL) and standard (1 mg/mL) spotted as 10 mm bands. Plates developed in a 20 × 10 × 4 cm glass twin-trough chamber to a migration distance of 80 mm. *Tank saturation:* 20 min at 20.8 °C and 30.4% RH, with 25 mL of mobile phase. *Mobile phase:* Chloroform: methanol:water (70:30:10 v/v/v). *Derivatisation:* *p*-Anisaldehyde reagent prepared by adding 5 mL of concentrated sulphuric acid to a solution of 85 mL methanol and 10 mL acetic acid and then, finally, 0.5 mL of *p*-anisaldehyde. The plate was dipped and heated for 3 min at 100 °C on a TLC plate heater and visualised. *Visualisation:* The plate was viewed under white reflectance.

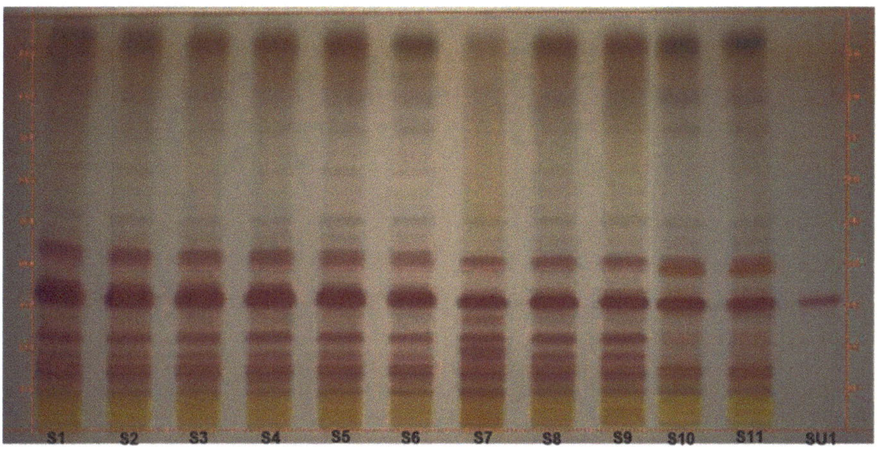

HPTLC plate of *Lessertia frutescens* methanol extracts (n = 11) (S1–S11) and the standard SU1 (sutherlandioside B) (R_f=0.30).

10.2 Ultra-performance liquid chromatography (UPLC) analysis

General instrumentation: Waters Acquity Ultra-Performance Liquid Chromatography system with photodiode array (PDA) detector combined with a Xevo G2QToF mass spectrometer (Waters, United States). *Plant part:* Aerial parts, methanol extract. *Sample application:* Injection volume: 2.0 μL (full-loop injection) at 1 mg/mL. *Column:* Acquity UPLC BEH C_{18} column (150 mm × 2.1 mm, i.d., 1.7 μm particle size, Waters). *Mobile phase:* 0.1% formic acid in water (solvent A) and acetonitrile (solvent B). *Analysis conditions:* Gradient elution at a flow rate of 0.35 mL/min, changing as follows: 80% A: 20% B, held for 0.5 min, changed to 40% A: 60% B in 13 min, to 0% A: 100% B in 2.5 min, held for 1 min, back to the initial ratio in 1 min, total run time 20 min. *Mass spectrometry*: ESI^- (negative ionisation mode), N_2 used as desolvation gas, desolvation temperature 350 °C at a flow rate of 500 L/h, and source temperature at 100 °C. Capillary and cone voltages 2500 and 45 V, respectively. Data collected between *m/z* 100 and 1500.

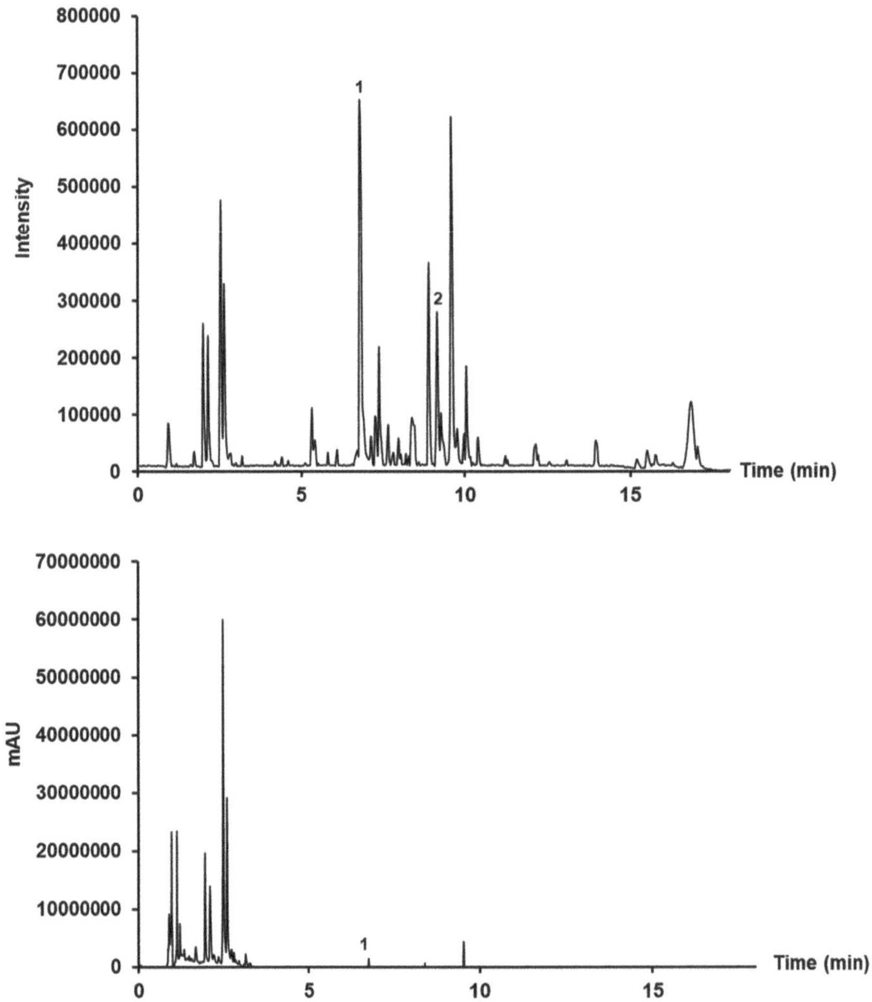

UPLC–ToF–MS ESI^- (upper) and PDA (lower) chromatograms of *Lessertia frutescens* methanol extract: [1] = sutherlandioside B *m/z* 652.4108 and [2] = sutherlandioside A *m/z* 652.4106.

11. Mid-infrared (MIR) spectroscopy analysis

General instrumentation: Alpha-P Bruker spectrometer, mounted with an attenuated total reflectance (ATR) diamond crystal. *Spectral acquisition:* Spectrum obtained in absorbance mode, with a spectral resolution of 4 cm^{-1} over the range 4000–550 cm^{-1} and captured using OPUS 6.5 software. *Plant part:* Aerial parts. *Sample preparation:* Aerial parts powdered, sieved (<500 μm), and placed directly onto the surface of the diamond crystal.

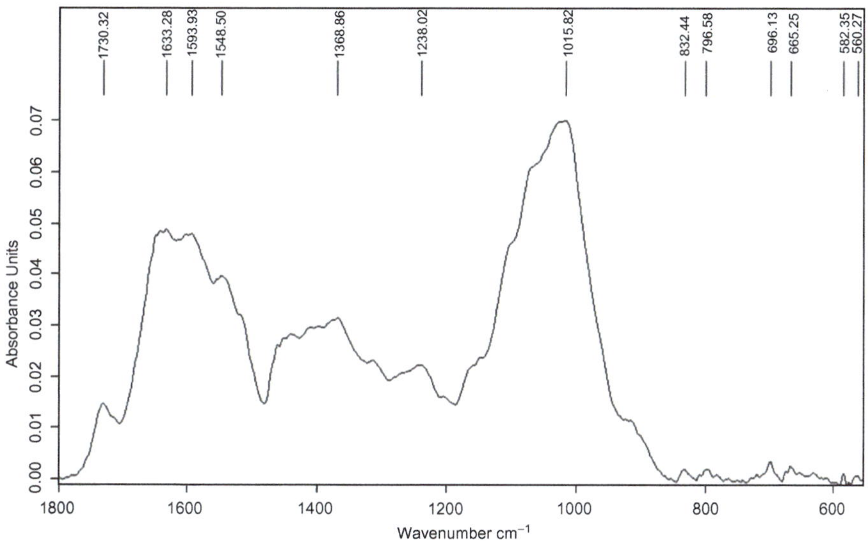

Mid-infrared spectrum of *Lessertia frutescens* leaf powder indicating the fingerprint region (1800–550 cm^{-1}).

References

Africa, L.D., Smith, C., 2015. J. Negat. Results BioMed., 14:14.

Ajit, D., Simonyi, A., Li, R., Chen, Z., Hannink, M., Fritsche, K.L., Mossine, V.V., Smith, R.E., Dobbs, T.K., Luo, R., Folk, W.R., Gu, Z., Lubahn, D.B., Weisman, G.A., Sun, G.Y., 2016. Neurochem. Int., 97:49–56.

Albrecht, C.F., Stander, M.A., Grobbelaar, M.C., Colling, J., Kossmann, J., Hills, P.N., Makunga, N.P., 2012. S. Afr. J. Bot., 82:33–45.

Alimi, A.A., Ashafa, A.O.T., 2017. Asian Pac. J. Trop. Biomed., 7:765–772.

Avula, B., Wang, Y.-H., Smillie, T.J., Fu, X., Li, X.C., Mabusela, W., Syce, J., Johnson, Q., Folk, W., Khan, I.A., 2010. J. Pharm. Biomed. Anal., 52:173–180.

Bessong, P.O., Rojas, L.B., Obi, L.C., Tshisikawe, P.M., Igunbor, E.O., 2006. Afr. J. Biotechnol., 5:526–528.

Camille, N., Dealtry, G., 2018. S. Afr. J. Bot., 116: 42–51.

Chadwick, W.A., Roux, S., van de Venter, M., Louw, J., Oelofsen, W., 2007. J. Ethnopharmacol., 109:121–127.

Chen, Y.-C., 2007. Bioactivities of Selected *Sutherlandia frutescens* (L.) R.Br. Leaf Extracts. M.Sc. dissertation, University of Missouri, Columbia, Missouri, USA.

Chen, C., Folk, W.R., Lazo-Portugal, R., Finn, T.M., Knight, M., 2017. J. Chromatogr. A, 1508:7–15.

Chinkwo, K.A., 2005. J. Ethnopharmacol., 98:163–170.

Chuang, D.Y., Cui, J., Simonyi, A., Engel, V.A., Chen, S., Fritsche, K.L., Thomas, A.L., Applequist, W.L., Folk, W.R., Lubahn, D.B., Sun, A.Y., Sun, G.Y., Gu, Z., 2015. ASN Neuro, 6:6, https://doi.org/10.1177/1759091414554946.

Colling, J., 2009. Towards Understanding *In Vitro Sutherlandia frutescens* Cultures. MSc dissertation, Stellenbosch University, Stellenbosch, South Africa.

Engelbrecht, A.-M., Smith, C., Neethling, I., Thomas, M., Ellis, B., Mattheyse, M., Myburgh, K.H., 2010. Stress, 13:132–141.

Faleschini, M.T., Myer, M.S., Harding, N., Fouchè, G., 2013. S. Afr. J. Bot., 85:48–55.

Fasinu, P.S., Gutmann, H., Schiller, H., James, A.-D., Bouic, P.J., Rosenkranz, B., 2013. Drug Metab. Dispos., 41:488–497.

Fernandes, A.C., Cromarty, A.D., Albrecht, C., Jansen Van Rensburg, C.E., 2004. J. Ethnopharmacol., 95:1–5.

Folk, W.R., Smith, A., Song, H., Chuang, D., Cheng, J., Gu, Z., Sun, G., 2016. NeuroMolecular Med., 18:483–486.

Fu, X., Li, X.-C., Wang, Y.-H., Avula, B., Smillie, T.J., Mabusela, W., Syce, J., Johnson, Q., Folk, W., Khan, I.A., 2010. Planta Med., 76:178–181.

Gelderblom, W.C.A., Joubert, E., Gamieldien, K., Sissing, L., Malherbe, C.J., Maritz, G., 2017. S. Afr. J. Bot., 110:194–200.

Grandi, M., Roselli, L., Vernay, M., 2005. Phytothérapie, 3:110–113.

Harnett, S.M., Oosthuizen, V., Van De Venter, M., 2005. J. Ethnopharmacol., 96:113–119.

Jiang, J., Chuang, D.Y., Zong, Y., Patel, J., Brownstein, K., Lei, W., Lu, C.-H., Simonyi, A., Gu, Z., Cui, J., Rottinghaus, G.E., Fritsche, K.L., Lubahn, D.B., Folk, W.R., Sun, G.Y., 2014. PLoS One, 9:2.

Johnson, Q., Syce, J., Nell, H., Rudeen, K., Folk, W., 2007. PLoS Clin. Trials, 2:16.

Katerere, D.R., Eloff, J.N., 2005. Phytother. Res., 19:779–781.

Kee, N.L.A., Mnonopi, N., Davids, H., Naudé, R.J., Frost, C.L., 2008. Afr. J. Biotechnol., 7:217–223.

Korb, V.C., Moodley, D., Chuturgoon, A.A., 2010. S. Afr. J. Sci., 106:64–69.

Kundu, J.K., Mossanda, K.S., Na, H.-K., Surh, Y.-J., 2005. Cancer Lett., 218:21–31.

Lei, W., Browning, J.D. Jr., Eichen, P.A., Lu C.H., Mossine, V.V., Rottinghaus, G.E., 2015a. J. Ethnopharmacol., 172:247–253.

Lei, W., Browning, J.D., Jr., Eichen, P.A., Brownstein, K.J., Folk, W.R., Sun, G.Y., Lubahn, D.B., Rottinghaus, G.E., Fritsche, K.L., 2015b. Int. Immunopharmacol., 29:254–262.

Lei, W., Browning, J.D., Jr., Eichen, P.A., Folk, W.R., Sun, G.Y., Lubahn, D.B., Fritsche, K.L., 2016. PLoS One, 11:8, https://doi.org/10.1371/journal.pone.0160994.

Leisching, G., Loos, B., Nell, T., Engelbrecht, A.-M., 2015. S. Afr. J. Bot., 100:20–26.

Lin, H., Jackson, G.A., Lu, Y., Drenkhahn, S.K., Brownstein, K.J., Starkey, N.J., Lamberson, W.R., Fritsche, K.L., Mossine, V.V., Besch-Williford, C.L., Folk, W.R., Zhang, Y., Lubahn, D.B., 2016. Cell Biol. Int., 40:131–142.

Lu, Y., Starkey, N., Lei, W., Li, J., Cheng, J., Folk, W.R., Lubahn, D.B., 2015. PLoS One, 10:12.

MacKenzie, J., Koekemoer, T., Van De Venter, M., Dealtry, G., Roux, S., 2009. Phytother. Res., 23:1609–1614.

MacKenzie, J., Koekemoer, T.C., Roux, S., Van De Venter, M., Dealtry, G.B., 2012. Phytother. Res., 26:1830–1837.
Masoko, P., Mabusa, I.H., Howard, R.L., 2016. BMC Complement. Altern. Med., 16:366, https://doi.org/10.1186/s12906-016-1344-1.
Mavimbela, T., Vermaak, I., Chen, W., Viljoen, A., 2018. Phytochem. Lett., 25:184–190.
Mills, E., Foster, B.C., Van Heeswijk, R., Phillips, E., Wilson, K., Leonard, B., Kosuge, K., Kanfer, I., 2005. AIDS, 19:95–97.
Minocha, M., Mandava, N.K., Kwatra, D., Pal, D., Folk, W.R., Earla, R., Mitra, A.K., 2011. Int. J. Pharm., 413:44–50.
Mncwangi, N.P., Viljoen, A.M., 2012. S. Afr. J. Bot., 82:46–52.
Morris, C., 2017. Med. Anthropol.: Cross Cult. Stud. Health Illn., 36:685–698.
Mqoco, T.V., Visagie, M.H., Albrecht, C., Joubert, A.M., 2014. S. Afr. J. Bot., 90:59–67.
Müller, A.C., Patnala, S., Kis, O., Bendayan, R., Kanfer, I., 2012. J. Pharm. Pharm. Sci., 15:221–233.
Müller, A.C., Skinner, M.F., Kanfer, I., 2013. Evid. Based Complement. Alternat. Med., https://doi.org/10.1155/2013/324618.
Na, H.-K., Mossanda, K.S., Lee, J.-Y., Surh, Y.-J., 2004. Biofactors, 21:149–153.
Ngcobo, M., Gqaleni, N., Chelule, P.K., Serumula, M., Assounga, A., 2012a. Afr. J. Tradit. Complement. Altern. Med., 9:3, https://doi.org/10.4314/ajtcam.v9i3S.6.
Ngcobo, M., Gqaleni, N., Chelule, P.K., Serumula, M., Assounga, A., 2012b. Afr. J. Tradit. Complement. Altern. Med., 9:1, https://doi.org/10.4314/ajtcam.v9i1.11.
Ntuli, S.S.B.N., Gelderblom, W.C.A., Katerere, D.R., 2018. BMC Complement. Altern. Med., 18:93.
Ojewole, J.A.O., 2004. Methods Find. Exp. Clin. Pharmacol., 26:409–416.
Ojewole, J.A.O., 2008. Brain Res. Bull., 75:126–132.
Phulukdaree, A., Moodley, D., Chuturgoon, A.A., 2010. S. Afr. J. Sci., 106:54–58.
Prevoo, D., Smith, C., Swart, P., Swart, A.C., 2004. Endocr. Res., 30:745–751.
Prevoo, D., Swart, P., Swart, A.C., 2008. J. Ethnopharmacol., 118:118–126.
Reid, K.A., Maes, J., Maes, A., Van Staden, J., De Kimpe, N., Mulholland, D.A., Verschaeve, L., 2006. J. Ethnopharmacol., 106:44–50.
Seier, J., Mdhluli, M., Dhansay, M., Loza, J., Laubscher, R., 2002. Final Report. Medical Research Council of South Africa and National Research Foundation. Available from: www.sahealthinfo.org/traditionalmeds/firststudy.htm.
Sergeant, C.A., Africander, D., Swart, P., Swart, A.C., 2017. J. Ethnopharmacol., 202:290–301.
Sia, C., 2004. Rev. Diabet. Stud., 1:145–149.
Skerman, N.B., Joubert, A.M., Cronjé, M.J., 2011. J. Ethnopharmacol., 137:1250–1260.
Smith, C., Myburgh, K.H., 2004. S. Afr. J. Sci., 100:229–232.
Smith, C., van Vuuren, M.J., 2014. Exp. Biol. Med., 239:123–128.
Stander, B.A., Marais, S., Steynberg, T.J., Theron, D., Joubert, F., Albrecht, C., Joubert, A.M., 2007. J. Ethnopharmacol., 112:312–318.
Stander, A., Marais, S., Stivaktas, V., Vorster, C., Albrecht, C., Lottering, M.-L., Joubert, A.M., 2009. J. Ethnopharmacol., 124:45–60.
Tai, J., Cheung, S., Chan, E., Hasman, D., 2004. J. Ethnopharmacol., 93:9–19.
Tobwala, S., Fan, W., Hines, C.J., Folk, W.R., Ercal, N., 2014. BMC Complement. Altern. Med., 14, https://doi.org/10.1186/1472-6882-14-271.
Van Der Walt, N.B., Zakeri, Z., Cronjé, M.J., 2016. Evid. Based. Complement. Alternat. Med., Art. No. 4921067, https://doi.org/10.1155/2016/4921067.
Van Wyk, B.-E., 2011. S. Afr. J. Bot., 77:812–829.

Van Wyk, B.-E., Albrecht, C., 2008. J. Ethnopharmacol., 119:620–629.
Viljoen, P.T., 1969. The Oxidation of Pinitol and Partial Identification of a Triterpene Glycoside From *Sutherlandia microphylla*. M.Sc. dissertation, University of the Free State, Bloemfontein, South Africa.
Vorster, C., Stander, A., Joubert, A., 2012. J. Ethnopharmacol., 140:123–130.
Williams, S., Roux, S., Koekemoer, T., Van De Venter, M., Dealtry, G., 2013. J. Ethnopharmacol., 146:482–489.
Wilson, D., Goggin, K., Williams, K., Gerkovich, M.M., Gqaleni, N., Syce, J., Bartman, P., Johnson, Q., Folk, W.R., 2015. PLoS One, 10:7.
Xaba, P., 2007. J. Bot. Soc. S. Afr., 93:234–236.

CHAPTER

Lippia javanica

16

Maxleene Sandasi[a,b], Faith Malope[a], Guy Kamatou[a] and Sandra Combrinck[a]

[a]*Department of Pharmaceutical Sciences, Tshwane University of Technology, Pretoria, South Africa*

[b]*SAMRC Herbal Drugs Research Unit, Faculty of Science, Tshwane University of Technology, Pretoria, South Africa*

Abstract

Lippia javanica (Burm.f.) Spreng (Verbenaceae), commonly known as 'fever tea', is an erect, highly aromatic, woody shrub that grows up to 2 m in height, with hairy leaves that are thinly veined. The plant is native to central, eastern and southern Africa, and occurs in Botswana, Malawi, Swaziland (Eswatini), Mozambique, Tanzania, Zambia and Kenya. It is traditionally used as a decoction or infusion to treat respiratory and gastro-intestinal conditions, as well as skin infections, and has spiritual significance. Commercially, essential oil of the plant is used as a mosquito repellent and in household fragrances, and dried aerial parts are sold as herbal tea. The in vitro and in vivo pharmacological activities (anti-oxidant, antimalarial and antimicrobial) of the plant extracts and essential oils have been studied extensively, and some of the results confirm the traditional use. The essential oil composition is highly variable and several chemotypes, characterised by carvone, piperitenone, ipsenone and myrcenone, have been identified. Phytochemicals present in the non-volatile fraction of the plant include iridoid glycosides, triterpenoids, flavones and various phenolic compounds. Chromatographic techniques, namely semi-automated high-performance thin-layer chromatography (HPTLC), ultra-performance liquid chromatography, coupled to mass spectrometry (UPLC–MS), and gas chromatography, coupled to mass spectrometry (GC–MS), were used to establish chemical profiles of the solvent extracts and essential oils of L. javanica. The analysis of the oils, using HPTLC and GC–MS/FID, confirmed different chemotypes, whilst HPTLC enabled the identification of theveside and verbascoside. Isoverbascoside, diosmetin and apigenin were further detected using UPLC analysis.

Keywords: *Lippia javanica*, Fever tea, Mosquito repellent, Essential oil, Theveside, Verbascoside, HPTLC, UPLC–MS, GC–MS, MIR spectroscopy

The South African Herbal Pharmacopoeia. https://doi.org/10.1016/B978-0-323-99794-2.00024-6

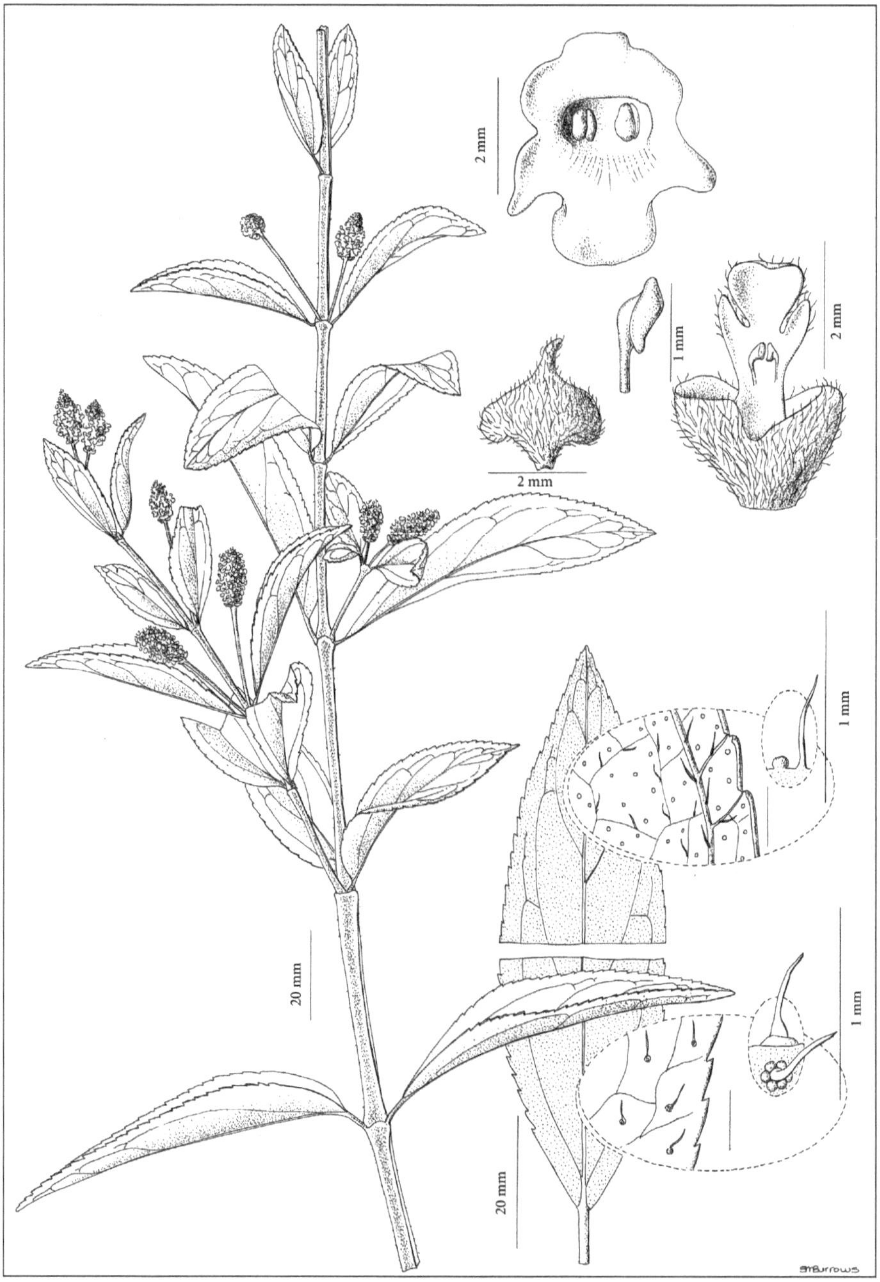
2 mm
2 mm
1 mm
2 mm
1 mm
1 mm
20 mm
20 mm
BMBurrows

Part A: General overview

1. Synonyms

Lantana galpiniana H.Pearson, *Lippia asperifolia* Rich., *Verbena javanica* Burm.f.[a]

2. Common name(s)

Fever tea, lemon bush, wild sage, wild tea (English); '*koorsbossie*', '*koorsteebossie*', '*lemoenbossie*', '*maagbossie*', '*beukesbos*' (Afrikaans); '*mumara*' (Shona); '*musukudu*', '*bokhukhwane*' (Setswana); '*inzinziniba*' (isiXhosa); '*umsuzwane*', '*umswazi*' (isiZulu); '*umsuzwana*', '*usuzwane*' (isiNdebele); '*musutswane*', '*umsutane*' (siSwati).[a]

3. Conservation status

Least concern.[a]

4. Botany

Lippia javanica (Burm.f.) Spreng belongs to the family Verbenaceae, comprising approximately eight genera and 40 species in southern Africa (Germishuizen et al., 2006). *Lippia javanica* is a woody, multistemmed shrub that grows up to 2 m in height (A). The leaves are 3–4 cm long, hairy on both sides and have dentate, lightly toothed margins. They are rough to the feel and appear on opposite sides of the stem, often in whorls of up to four. The leaves have conspicuous veins and are highly aromatic, with a range of medicinal applications in both fresh and dried forms (C). The shrub bears dense, rounded flower heads. Small flowers that vary in colour from white, cream, yellowish-white to yellow (B) adorn the shrub, which continues to flower from February to May. The nut-like seeds are small and brown in colour (Van Wyk and Gericke, 2000).

[a] Red List of South African Plants (http://redlist.sanbi.org).

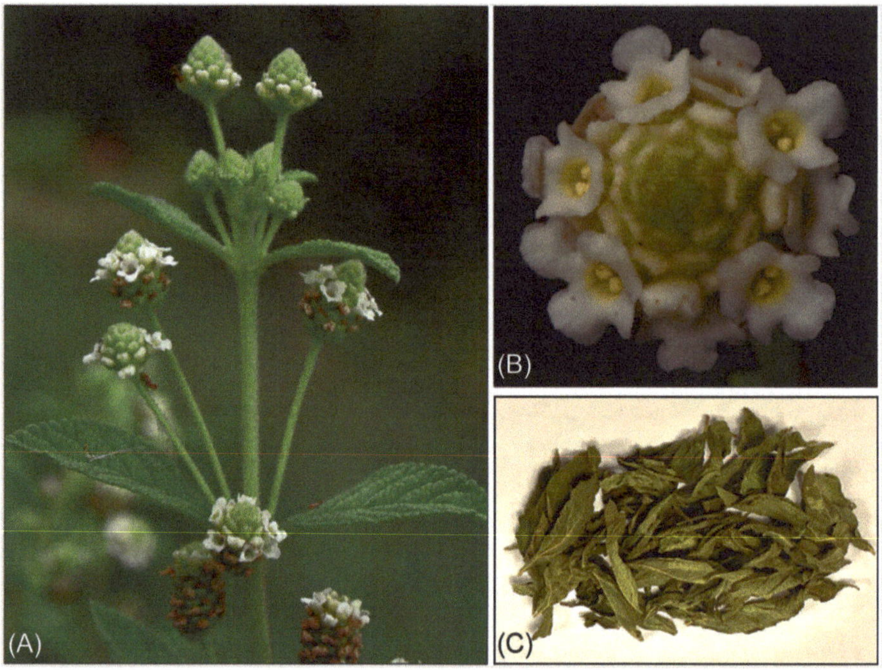

Lippia javanica plant (A), bears small white flowers on an oval flower head (B) and rough, strong-scented green leaves that are dried before use (C).

5. Geographical distribution

Lippia javanica is drought-resistant and adapts well to different soil types. The shrub is abundant on hillsides, roadsides, forest edges, stream banks, and in grasslands

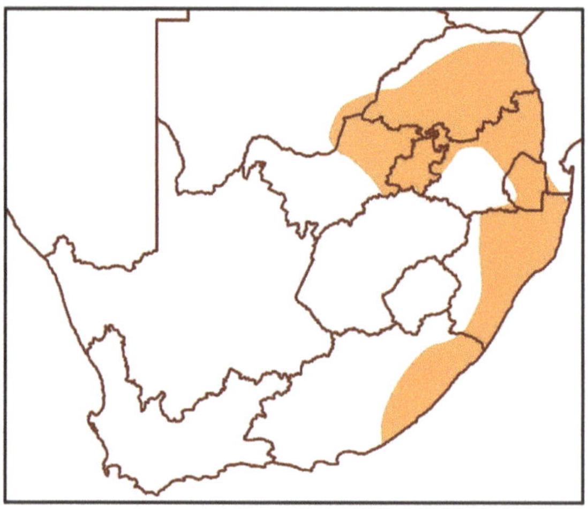

Geographical distribution of *Lippia javanica* in South Africa.

and bushveld. Its natural distribution in South Africa spans the Eastern Cape, Free State, Gauteng, KwaZulu-Natal, Limpopo, Mpumalanga and North West provinces. Its distribution extends to central, eastern and southern Africa, including Botswana, Malawi, Swaziland (Eswatini), Mozambique, Tanzania, Zambia and Kenya (Retief and Herman, 1997; Van Wyk and Gericke, 2000; Germishuizen et al., 2006).

6. Ethnopharmacology

Lippia javanica has a long history of traditional use in Africa with medicinal applications in treating a wide range of conditions, including pain, fever, infections, inflammation, coughs, colds, bronchitis, influenza, stomach problems, measles, malaria and headaches (Watt and Breyer-Brandwijk, 1962; Hutchings and Van Staden, 1994; Hutchings et al., 1996; Pascual et al., 2001; Hutchings, 2003; Manenzhe et al., 2004). The aerial parts, prepared in the form of decoctions, are usually used for medicinal purposes, but the roots are also indicated for some conditions. Leaves are crushed and mixed with cold or hot water, and the infusion is administered to combat diarrhoea in northern Maputaland, KwaZulu-Natal Province (De Wet et al., 2010). The Vhavenda people use leaf infusions as anthelmintics, for respiratory and febrile ailments and as prophylactics against dysentery, diarrhoea and malaria (Mabogo, 1990). The plant species was reported by Mavundza et al. (2011) as the most frequently used species (91.7%) to traditionally repel mosquitoes in the uMkhanyakude district of KwaZulu-Natal. It is also commonly used as a herb and spice in the Nkonkobe Municipality, Eastern Cape Province of South Africa (Asowata-Ayodele et al., 2016). Overall, traditional applications of *L. javanica* are wide-ranging and fall into the following eight categories as reviewed by Maroyi (2017): (i) respiratory complaints (leaves, stems, twigs and roots)—asthma, blocked nose, bronchitis, chest pains, cold, cough, influenza, lung infections, pneumonia, runny nose, dyspnoea and tuberculosis; (ii) gastro-intestinal diseases (leaves, twigs, roots)—amoebiasis, anthelmintics, diarrhoea, gangrenous rectitis, prophylactic against diarrhoea and vomiting, ulcers and abdominal pains; (iii) malaria (leaves, stems, twigs, roots and whole plant)—fever, prophylactic against malaria, and mosquito repellent; (iv) skin conditions (leaves, roots, twigs)—acne, boils, chicken pox, febrile rashes, inflammation, pubic sores, scabies, shingles, heat rash, scratches, stings, bites, sores, measles and wounds; (v) pain (leaves)—earache, backache, headache and migraines, sore eyes, sprained joints, sore throat and tonsillitis; (vi) ethnoveterinary uses (whole plant, leaves, twigs, stems)—disinfecting suspected anthrax-infested meat, getting rid of ticks and other ectoparasites, and insect repellent; (vii) other conditions (leaves, stems, twigs, roots)—antidote, anaemia in pregnancy, cancer, diabetes, convulsions, fatigue, HIV symptoms, kidney problems, night blindness, pre-, intra- and postpartum complications, venereal diseases, weak joints, air freshener, psychotropic behaviour, dispelling bad luck and bad spirits, combating sleeplessness, protection against dogs and lightning; and (viii) Culinary uses (leaves, stems, twigs)—herbal caffeine-free tea and general health tonic (Maroyi, 2017).

7. Commercialisation

Due to its aromatic nature, *L. javanica* is a popular garden plant that can be used to repel insects and as a household fragrance. Commercial cultivation is mainly for essential oil production (Maharaj et al., 1995). The essential oil is an important ingredient in the fragrance industry. The repellent properties of the essential oil have contributed to the successful commercialisation of the plant in South Africa. A mosquito/insect repellent formulated into candles, with a higher potency compared to other insect repellents, is branded and marketed locally by Ulwazi Botanicals. Wild-harvested leaves of *L. javanica* have been used since the mid-1990s in branded infusions (herbal teas) to treat bronchitis, colds, coughs and fever (Van Wyk, 2011). An infusion of the aerial parts is popularly marketed and consumed as herbal tea for its health benefits. 'Mosukudu' and 'Zimbani', as the tea is branded and sold in Botswana, South Africa and Zimbabwe, are popular products in Africa that are expected to expand to international markets. There is an increase in demand for *L. javanica* herbal tea in light of growing health consciousness worldwide, with the potential demand for the species and its products estimated at 100 tons per year on the local Zimbabwean market, and up to 1000 tons per year on the export market.[b]

8. Pharmacological evaluation

8.1 *In vitro* studies

8.1.1 Insect repellent and antiparasitic activity

Studies on *L. javanica* indicate a wide range of *in vitro* pharmacological activities that include anticancer, antimalarial, antimicrobial, anti-oxidant, antiplasmodial, mosquito repellence, pesticidal and various other effects. Govere et al. (2000) demonstrated the insect repellence activity of *L. javanica* where the topical application of the alcohol extract exhibited 76.7% protection against *Anopheles arabiensis* mosquitoes for a period of 4h. Lukwa et al. (2009) also reported that topical application of 5 mg/cm^2 *L. javanica* resulted in 100% protection against *Anopheles aegypti* for 8h. Ethanol extracts of the leaves of *L. javanica* exhibited larvicidal activity (21%) against *A. arabiensis* mosquitoes (Mavundza et al., 2013). Mavundza et al. (2014) reported that the dichloromethane and ethanol leaf extracts of *L. javanica* displayed adulticidal activity against *A. arabiensis*, causing 45% and 55% mortality, respectively. Extracts of *L. javanica* were also effective in killing larvae of the *A. gambiae* mosquitoes with a half maximal lethal concentration (LC_{50}) = 125.34 mg/mL (Lukwa, 1994). In line with the use of *L. javanica* for malaria, the oil demonstrated activity against *Plasmodium falciparum* with an IC_{50} value of 8 μg/mL (Manenzhe et al., 2004). It was demonstrated by Oketch-Rabah et al. (1999) that lipophilic compounds in the non-polar extract (CH_2CH_2:EtOAc, 1:1) exhibited antiplasmodial activity. A methanol extract of *L. javanica* was reported to exhibit antiplasmodial activity using the parasite lactase dehydrogenase (pLDH) assay (Clarkson et al., 2004; Ayuko

[b] http://bio-innovation.org/work/fever-tea-tree.

et al., 2009). Prozesky et al. (2001) reported an IC_{50} value of 4.26 µg/mL for the acetone leaf extract against a chloroquine-resistant strain of *Plasmodium falciparum*.

Extracts of *L. javanica* exhibited a significant dose-dependent repellence response in adults of *Hyalomma marginatum rufipes*, with 107 mg/mL of extract causing 100% repellence at 30 min and 1 h (Magano et al., 2011). In another study, *L. javanica* aqueous leaf extract at 10% and 20% (w/v) was effective at controlling cattle ticks (Madzimure et al., 2011). Peripheral blood samples collected during the study, indicated the absence of haemoparasites in treated cattle, implying that animals did not suffer from tick-borne diseases. McGaw et al. (2000) screened *L. javanica* for anthelmintic activity using the free-living nematode, *Caenorhabditis elegans*. The crude ethanol and hexane extracts were active at 2 mg/mL when tested using the 7-day incubation assay. The two extracts also exhibited good anthelmintic activity against *Paramphistomum* species at 50 mg/mL concentration, and the time taken for paralysis and death to occur was recorded as 0.56 ± 0.09 h and 1.35 ± 0.07 h, respectively (Swargiary et al., 2016). Interactions of *Cucumis myriocarpus, L. javanica* and *Ricinus communis* on suppression of the nematode, *Meloidogyne incognita*, and improving tomato (*Lycopersicon esculentum)* productivity were reported. The extracts successfully reduced nematode infection and improved fruit yield, dry shoot weight and plant height (Mashela et al., 2007).

8.1.2 Antimicrobial activity

The antimicrobial activity of *L. javanica* essential oil was reported against three strains of *Staphylococcus aureus* (including methicillin-resistant strains), two strains of *Candida albicans*, and one strain of *Cryptococcus neoformans*. All isolates were inhibited by $\leq 1\%$ of the oil (Huffman et al., 2002; Osée Muyima et al., 2004). *In vitro* antimicrobial activity of the essential oil was reported against the respiratory pathogens *Klebsiella pneumoniae, C. neoformans* and *Bacillus cereus* (Viljoen et al., 2005). Various solvent extracts, including methanol, acetone, hexane and dichloromethane, were tested and proven to exhibit good antimicrobial activity against *S. aureus*, *Enterococcus faecalis*, *Escherichia coli* and *Pseudomonas aeruginosa* (Samie et al., 2005; Shikanga et al., 2010; Lekganyane et al., 2012). When tested against *S. aureus* and *E. coli*, the oil displayed moderate activity at a concentration of 10 mg/mL (Manenzhe et al., 2004). Samie et al. (2009) demonstrated that the compound, piperitenone, isolated from *L. javanica*, displayed antibacterial activity towards *Acinetobacter calcoaceticus*, *Micrococcus kristinae*, *Salmonella typhi* and *S. aureus*, with MICs ranging from 12 to 50 µg/mL. The antimicrobial activity of crude extracts of *L. javanica* was investigated against 31 *Helicobacter pylori* strains. The strains were inhibited by all the extracts, with marked susceptibility of strains (100%) for the acetone extract, followed by the methanol extract (60%). The MICs ranged from 0.00195 to 1.25 mg/mL for the acetone and methanol extracts, respectively (Nkomo et al., 2011).

Methanol and water extracts of *L. javanica* were investigated for the ability to control a microbial trigger for ankylosing spondylitis (*K. pneumoniae*), and were found to be effective inhibitors (Cock and Van Vuuren, 2014a). The extracts were also effective against

Proteus mirabilis and *Phaseolus vulgaris* (Cock and Van Vuuren, 2014b). The essential oil and fractions were assessed for antimicrobial activity towards two bacterial strains (*B. cereus* and *K. pneumoniae*) and one fungal pathogen (*C. neoformans*). *Klebsiella pneumoniae* was found to be the most susceptible bacterium (MIC <25 μg/mL) (Endris et al., 2016). Extracts of *L. javanica* were inhibitory towards fungal growth in clinical isolates of *Candida albicans*, *Candida krusei* and *C. neoformans* (Samie et al., 2010). *Fusarium* species and other fungal pathogens have also demonstrated susceptibility to *L. javanica* extracts (Shikanga et al., 2010; Thembo et al., 2010). Organic extracts and the essential oil of *L. javanica* were also tested against resistant bacterial strains (*E. faecalis*, *S. aureus*, *B. cereus*, *K. pneumoniae*, *Acinetobacter baumannii*, *P. aeruginosa*, *E. coli* and *Serratia marcescens*). The organic extracts, followed by the essential oils, were more effective against the resistant strains than the antibiotic (ciprofloxacin) (Van Vuuren and Muhlarhi, 2017). (*E*)-2(3)-Tagetenone epoxide and piperitenone have been reported to exhibit antiviral activity against HIV-1 reverse transcriptase strain, by 91% and 53%, respectively, at 100 μg/mL (Mujovo et al., 2008). The antimycobacterial activity of organic extracts of *L. javanica* was evaluated. The acetone extract displayed activity against *Mycobacterium smegmatis* with an MIC of 0.47 mg/mL (Masoko and Nxumalo, 2013). Several researchers (York et al., 2011; Masoko and Nxumalo, 2013) have also documented the antimycobacterial activity of *L. javanica* extracts against *M. smegmatis*.

8.1.3 Anti-oxidant activity

Shikanga et al. (2010) evaluated the relationship between phenolic compounds and the anti-oxidant activities of tea infusions prepared from *L. javanica* using the 2,2-diphenyl-1-picryl-hydrazyl-hydrate (DPPH) assay. The activity of *L. javanica* compared well to popular black, green and herbal tea brands, with an EC_{50} of 358 μg/mL, and contained a high phenolic content of 14.8 mg/mL of dry weight gallic acid equivalent (Shikanga et al., 2010; Katerere et al., 2012). In other studies, *L. javanica* exhibited anti-oxidant activity in the DPPH assay (Narzary et al., 2016) with an IC_{50} value of 135.0 ± 1.49 μg/mL, whilst Swargiary et al. (2016) reported an anti-oxidant activity of 48.57 ± 3.07 μg ascorbic acid equivalent (AAE)/mg for the extract. *Lippia javanica* has a high radical scavenging activity ($83.77\% \pm 0.8\%$), which is probably due to a high total phenolic content (Maroyi, 2017). Endris et al. (2016) assessed the anti-oxidant property of the essential oil using the free radical scavenging assay and reported an IC_{50} value of 16.6 μL/mL.

8.1.4 Other activities

Fouche et al. (2008) reported the anticancer effects of a dichloromethane root extract of *L. javanica* against three human cancer cell lines, recording tumour growth inhibition (TGI) values of 1.82, 1.86 and 2.09 μg/mL for MDA-MB-435 (breast), MDA-N (breast) and MALME-3M (melanoma), respectively. A few isolated compounds, including linalool, limonene and α-pinene were also reported to exhibit antitumor activities (Yang et al., 2001; Fouche et al., 2008). Extracts of *L. javanica* demonstrated promising *in vitro* inhibition of 15-lipoxygenase (97.4% at 25 μg/mL) and nitric oxide production (97% at 25 μg/mL), but moderate anti-oxidant and poor anti-acetylcholinesterase activities (Dzoyem and Eloff, 2015).

8.2 *In vivo* studies and clinical trials

Lippia javanica was reported to exhibit antidiabetic effects in white albino diabetic mice. Following oral and intraperitoneal administration of the aqueous extract, the blood glucose levels in the mice were significantly lowered (Arika et al., 2015). Field trials conducted on 'Valencia' oranges showed that polar extracts of *L. javanica* and *Lippia rehmannii* caused significant inhibition of mycelial growth (*Penicillium digitatum*) at concentrations above 0.6 mg/mL (Shikanga et al., 2009). The observed activity was largely ascribed to the presence of verbascoside (also known as acteoside) in the plant extracts. The extract of *L. javanica* was investigated for pesticidal activity and found to effectively control key pest species on common bean plants (*Phaseolus vulgaris*), under field conditions (Mkenda et al., 2015). In another study, the inclusion of *L. javanica* in quail diets at 25 g/kg feed, promoted similar growth performance, health status and meat quality traits as the commercial grower diet containing antibiotics (Mnisi et al., 2017). *Lippia javanica* leaf meal (5 g/kg feed) was evaluated for growth performance, carcass characteristics and fatty acid profiles over a 42-day feeding period in broiler chicks' diets (Mpofu et al., 2016). The broilers fed with *L. javanica* had significantly lower feed intake compared to the negative and positive control groups, but higher average daily weight gain, lower feed conversion ratio and higher slaughter weights. Overall, the findings from the study showed that the inclusion of *L. javanica* in broiler diets at 5 g/kg feed had a positive influence on growth performance, carcass characteristics and fatty acid profiles of broiler meat. To date, there are no documented clinical trials on *L. javanica* extracts or products.

8.3 Safety

Lippia javanica is consumed as a herbal tea with no adverse reactions reported to date. Whilst anecdotal evidence suggests that *L. javanica* has low mammalian toxicity, scientific studies have not documented evidence of toxicity. Arika et al. (2015) reported alterations in biochemical and haematological parameters, following chronic and subchronic administration of *L. javanica* extracts to mice. Substantial changes in body and organ weight were observed after a dose of 450 to 1000 mg/kg was given to mice. These reports suggested potential toxicity when consumed in high doses, thus caution should be taken when using the herb. In another study, Madzimure et al. (2011) reported that all mice, within 48 h after being fed with *L. javanica* leaf aqueous extract at 12.5%–37.5% v/v, were lethargic, and the overall mortality was 37.5%. Photosensitisation effects and liver damage in livestock due to the presence of icterogenic compounds in *L. javanica* have been documented (Van Wyk et al., 2009). In contrast, the essential oil of *L. javanica* was reported to exhibit moderate toxicity towards *Artemia salina* (LC_{50} value of 129.11 μg/mL) (Adeogun et al., 2018). The oil also displayed fumigant toxicity against adult *Sitophilus zeamais*, with an increased dose. The half maximal lethal dose (LD_{50}) fumigant toxicity values at 72 and 120 h were 254 and 216 μg/cm^3 air, respectively (Kamanula et al., 2017). The oil was also toxic upon contact, with an LC_{50} value of 6.22 mg/mL, towards adult *Sitophilus zeamais*.

9. Phytochemistry

9.1 Volatile constituents

The volatile fraction of *L. javanica* contains various classes of compounds, and the profiles vary within and between populations. Generally, the following compounds have been identified in high concentrations in volatile fractions of *L. javanica*: myrcene, myrcenone, β-caryophyllene, carvone, ipsenone, limonene, linalool, ocimenone, *p*-cymene, piperitenone, sabinene, ipsenone, ipsdienone and (*E*)- and (*Z*)-tagetenone (Fujita, 1965; Neidlein and Staehle, 1974; Mwangi et al., 1991, 1992; Velasco-Negeureula et al., 1993; Terblanché and Kornelius, 1996; Van Wyk, 2008). The oil composition varies considerably within and between populations. Five chemotypes were described by Viljoen et al. (2005), with myrcenone (36%–62%), carvone (61%–73%), piperitenone (32%–48%), ipsenone (42%–61%) and linalool (>65%), identified as the major compounds corresponding to each chemotype, respectively. Philemon et al. (2015) reported a monoterpenoid chemotype, with high levels of artemisia ketone and other compounds, including *m-tert*-butylphenol, linalool, β-myrcene, tagetone and isopiperitenone. Chagonda et al. (2000) reported three chemotypes from Zimbabwe with high levels of myrcene, linalool and limonene. In a further study, Chagonda and Chalchat (2015) identified a myrcene-rich variety in the western part of Zimbabwe. Research on *L. javanica* from Tanzania revealed the presence of germacrene D, neral, geranial, camphor, as well as *cis*- and *trans*-ocimene (Mwangi et al., 1992; Ngassapa et al., 2003).

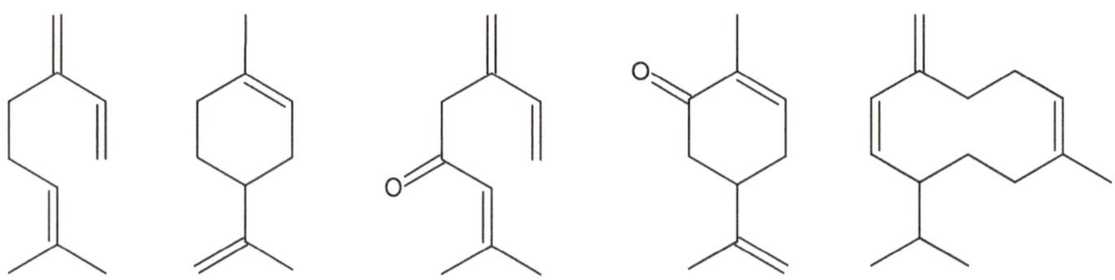

Myrcene Limonene Myrcenone Carvone Germacrene D

9.2 Non-volatile constituents

Several classes of non-volatile compounds have been identified in *L. javanica*, including organic acids and alcohols (Neidlein and Staehle, 1973), iridoid glycosides (Rimpler and Sauerbier, 1986), triterpenoids (Buckingham, 2006), flavones (Mujovo et al., 2008), phenolic compounds, caffeic acid derivatives (Olivier et al., 2010), phenolic glycosides, flavonoid alkaloids (Madzimure et al., 2011) and amino acids (Neidlein and Staehle, 1974). Some compounds isolated from the ethanolic extract of the aerial parts include 4-ethyl-nonacosane, (*E*)-2(3)-tagetenone epoxide, piperitenone, apigenin, cirsimaritin, 6-methoxyluteolin-4′-methyl ether, 6-methoxyluteolin and 3′,4′,7-trimethyl ether (Mujovo et al., 2008). Dlamini (2006) isolated the toxic triterpenoid saponin, icterogenin and Ludere et al. (2013) isolated lippialactone from the ethyl acetate extract. Rimpler and Sauerbier (1986) were the first to report the presence of the iridoid glycosides, theveside and theveridoside, currently used as marker molecules for *L. javanica*. Two additional phenylethanoid glycosides, verbascoside and isoverbascoside, were isolated and elucidated by Olivier et al. (2010). Other compounds present in the non-volatile fraction include crassifolioside, luteolin, diosmetin, chrysoeriol, tricin, isothymusin, eupatorin, 5-dimethyl noboletin, genkwanin, salvigenin and alkaloid xanthine amino acids (Neidlein and Staehle, 1974).

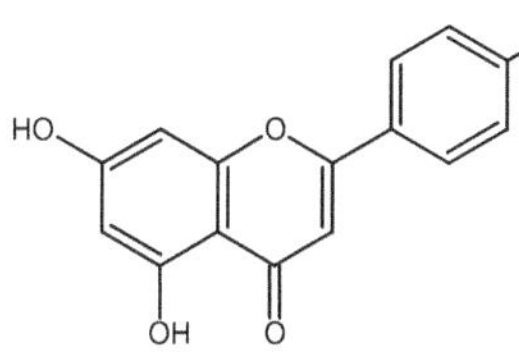

Apigenin

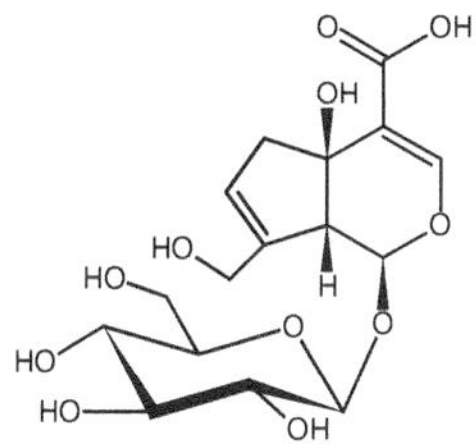

Theveside

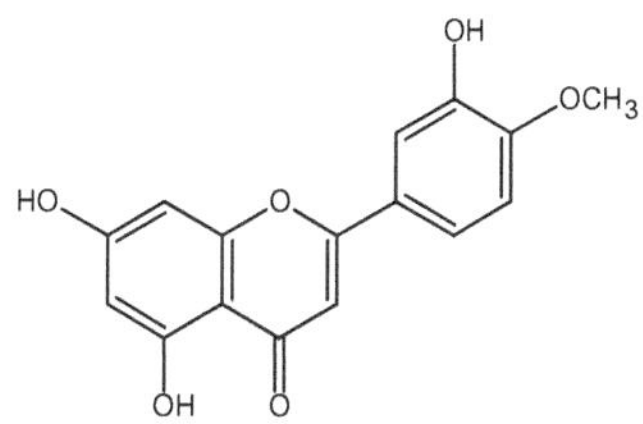

Diosmetin

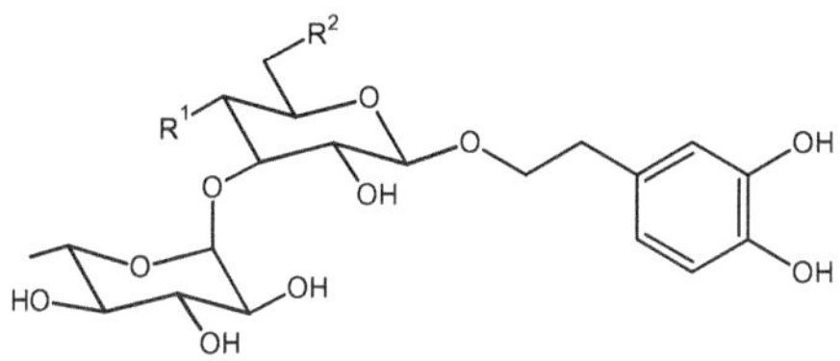

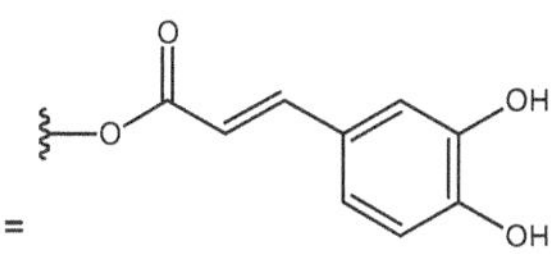

Isoverbascoside: R^1 = OH; R^2 =

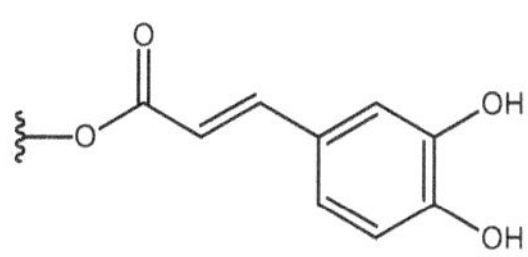

Verbascoside: R^2 = OH; R^1 =

Part B: Chemical profiling and quality control

10. Chromatography analysis

10.1 High-performance thin-layer chromatography (HPTLC) fingerprint analysis

General instrumentation: CAMAG HPTLC instrument consisting of an automatic TLC sampler (ATS 4), automatic developing chamber (ADC 2), CAMAG TLC visualiser 2, CAMAG immersion device and TLC plate heater. *HPTLC plates:* Silica gel glass plates 60 F_{254} (Merck).

10.1.1 Non-volatile fraction analysis

Plant part: Aerial parts, methanol extract. *Sample application:* Application volume of 10 μL methanol extract (10 mg/mL) spotted as 10 mm bands. Plates developed in a 20 × 10 × 4 cm glass twin-trough chamber to a migration distance of 85 mm. *Tank saturation:* 20 min at 25 °C and 47% RH, with 25 mL of mobile phase. *Mobile phase:* Ethyl acetate:formic acid:acetic acid:water (67:7.4:7.4:8 v/v/v/v). *Derivatisation: p*-Anisaldehyde reagent prepared by mixing 0.5 mL *p*-anisaldehyde with 85 mL methanol, 10 mL glacial acetic acid and 5 mL sulphuric acid, in that order. The plate was dipped in reagent and heated for 3 min at 100 °C on a TLC plate heater and visualised. *Visualisation:* The plate was viewed under white reflectance light.

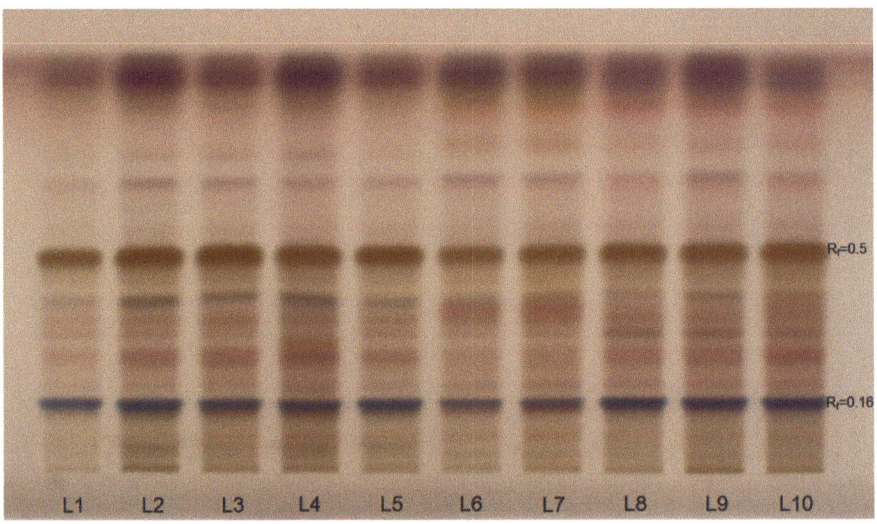

HPTLC plate of methanol extracts of *Lippia javanica* samples ($n = 10$) (L1–L10). The samples are characterised by a blue band for theveside ($R_f = 0.16$) and a brown band for verbascoside ($R_f = 0.5$).

10.1.2 Essential oil analysis

Plant part: Aerial parts, essential oil. *Sample application:* Application volume of 2 µL essential oil (25 µL/mL in toluene) spotted as 10 mm bands. Plates developed in a 20×10×4 cm glass twin-trough chamber to a migration distance of 70 mm. *Tank saturation:* 20 min at 15 °C and 45% RH, with 25 mL of mobile phase. *Mobile phase:* Toluene:ethyl acetate (95:5 v/v). *Derivatisation:* *p*-Anisaldehyde. The plate was sprayed with 3 mL of the reagent and heated for 3 min at 100 °C on a TLC plate heater and visualised. *Visualisation:* The plate was viewed under white reflectance light.

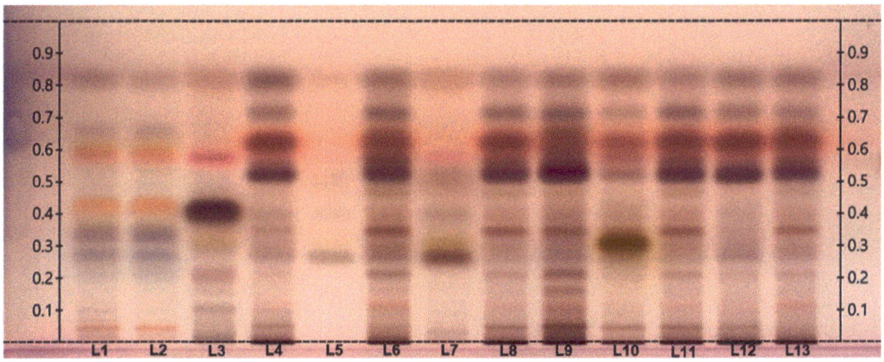

HPTLC plate of *Lippia javanica* essential oils ($n = 13$) (L1–L13) showing variation reflecting different chemotypes.

10.2 Ultra-performance liquid chromatography (UPLC) analysis

General instrumentation: Waters Acquity Ultra-Performance Liquid Chromatography system with photodiode array (PDA) detector combined with a Xevo G2QToF mass spectrometer (Waters, USA). *Plant part:* Aerial parts, methanol extract. *Sample application*: Injection volume: 2.0 µL (full-loop injection) at 1 mg/mL. *Column:* Acquity UPLC BEH C_{18} column (150 mm × 2.1 mm, i.d., 1.7 µm particle size, Waters). *Mobile phase:* 0.1% formic acid in water (solvent A) and acetonitrile (solvent B). *Analysis conditions:* Gradient elution at flow rate: 0.3 mL/min, changing as follows: 90% A: 10% B, held for 0.5 min, changed to 40% A: 60% B in 9.5 min, to 0% A: 100% B in 6 min, held for 1 min, back to initial ratio in 1 min, total run time 18 min. *Mass spectrometry:* ESI^- (negative ionisation mode), N_2 used as the desolvation gas, desolvation temperature 350 °C at a flow rate of 500 L/h, source temperature at 100 °C. Capillary and cone voltages, 2500 and 45 V, respectively. Data collected between *m/z* 100 and 1500.

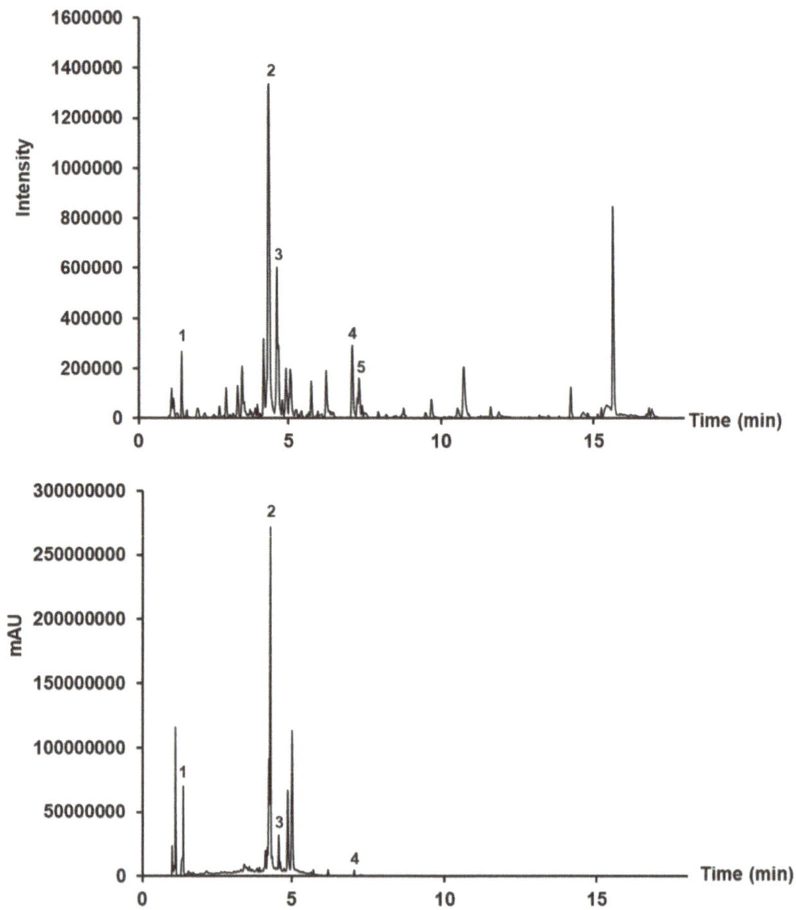

UPLC–ToF–MS ESI$^-$ (upper) and PDA (lower) chromatograms of *Lippia javanica* methanol extracts. [1] = theveside *m/z* 389.1160, [2] = verbascoside *m/z* 623.2047, [3] = isoverbascoside *m/z* 623.2047, [4] = apigenin *m/z* 269.0265, [5] = diosmetin *m/z* 299.0386.

10.3 Gas chromatography (GC) analysis

General instrumentation: An Agilent 6860 N chromatograph (Agilent Technologies, Hanova, USA) fitted with a flame ionisation detector and a mass spectrometer. *Plant part:* Aerial parts, essential oil. *Sample application:* Injection volume of 1 µL (split) at 20% (v/v) in hexane. *Column:* HP-Innowax, 60 m × 250 µm × 0.25 µm (polyethylene glycol column, Agilent Technologies, USA). *Analysis conditions:* Inlet temperature 250 °C, split ratio: 1:200, helium carrier gas, flow rate: 1.2 mL/min, pressure: 24.79 psi. Starting oven temperature at 60 °C and then rise to 220 °C at 4 °C/min, holding for 10 min and increase to 240 °C at 1 °C/min. *Mass spectrometry conditions:* Chromatograms obtained upon electron impact at 70 eV using an Agilent 5973 mass

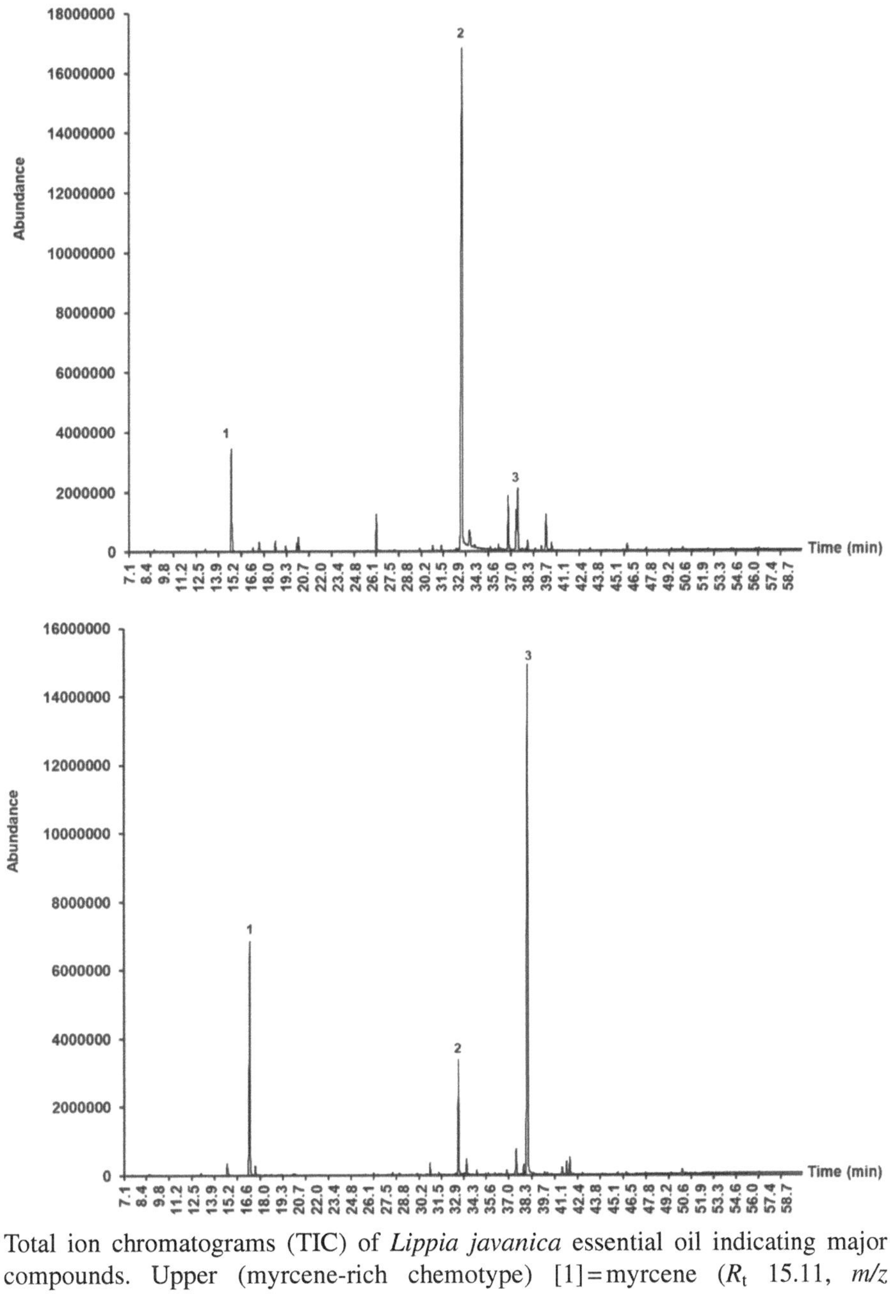

Total ion chromatograms (TIC) of *Lippia javanica* essential oil indicating major compounds. Upper (myrcene-rich chemotype) [1] = myrcene (R_t 15.11, *m/z* 136.1252), [2] = myrcenone <FA> (R_t 33.27, *m/z* 150.1044), [3] = germacrene D (R_t 37.64, *m/z* 204.1878) and lower (carvone-rich chemotype) [1] = limonene (R_t 16.85, *m/z* 136.1252), [2] = myrcenone (R_t 33.27, *m/z* 150.1044), [3] = carvone (R_t 38.48, *m/z* 150.44).

selective detector, scanning range: *m/z* 35 to 550 (Agilent Technologies, Hanova, United States). *Identification:* Authentic standards, NIST®, Mass Finder®.

11. Mid-infrared (MIR) spectroscopy analysis

General instrumentation: Alpha-P Bruker spectrometer, mounted with an attenuated total reflectance (ATR) diamond crystal. *Spectral acquisition:* Spectrum obtained in absorbance mode, with a spectral resolution of 4 cm^{-1} over the range 4000–550 cm^{-1} and captured using OPUS 6.5 software.

11.1 Powder analysis

Plant part: Aerial parts. *Sample preparation:* Aerial parts powdered, sieved (<500 μm), and placed directly onto the surface of the diamond crystal.

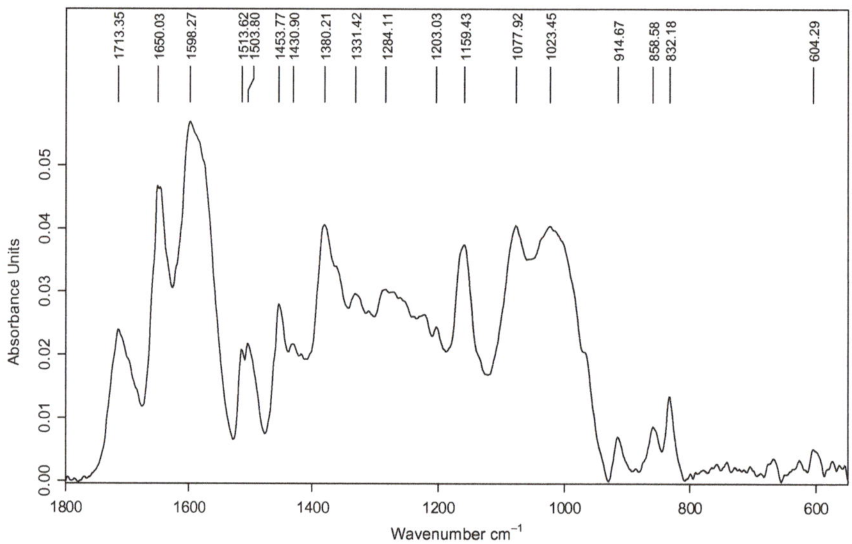

Mid-infrared spectrum of *Lippa javanica* powder displaying the fingerprint region (1800–550 cm^{-1}).

11.2 Essential oil analysis

Plant part: Aerial parts, essential oil. *Sample preparation:* Aerial parts, hydro-distillation to obtain essential oil, placed directly onto the surface of the diamond crystal.

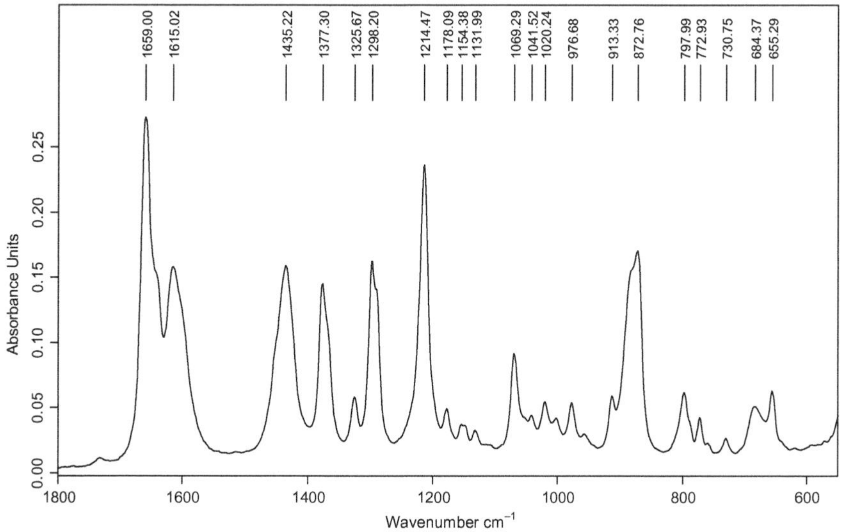

Mid-infrared spectrum of *Lippia javanica* essential oil displaying the fingerprint region (1800–550 cm^{-1}).

References

Adeogun, O.O., Maroyi, A., Afolayan, A.J., 2018. Trop. J. Pharm. Res., 17:105–115.

Arika, W.M., Abdirahman, Y.A., Mawia, M.M., Wambua, K.F., Nyamai, D.M., Ogola, P.E., Kiboi, N.G., Nyandoro, H.O., Njagi, S.M., Agyirifo, D.S., Ngugi, M.P., Njagi, E.N.M., 2015. J. Diabetes Metab., 6:624–630.

Asowata-Ayodele, A.M., Afolayan, A.J., Otunola, G.A., 2016. Afr. J. Tradit. Complement. Altern. Med., 13:237–242.

Ayuko, T.A., Njau, R.N., Cornelius, W., Leah, N., Ndiege, I.O., 2009. Mem. Inst. Oswaldo Cruz, 104:689–694.

Buckingham, J., 2006. Dictionary of Natural Products on CD-ROM. Chapman and Hall, London, UK.

Chagonda, L.S., Makanda, C.D., Chalchat, J., 2000. J. Essent. Oil Res., 12:1–6.

Chagonda, L.S., Chalchat, J.C., 2015. J. Essent. Oil Bear. Plants, 18:482–485.

Clarkson, C., Maharaj, V.J., Crouch, N.R., Grace, O.M., Pillay, P., Matsabisa, M.G., Bhagwandin, N., Smith, P.J., Folb, P.I., 2004. J. Ethnopharmacol., 92:177–191.

Cock, I.E., Van Vuuren, S.F., 2014a. Inflammopharmacology, 23:21–35.

Cock, I.E., Van Vuuren, S.F., 2014b. Inflammopharmacology, 22:23–36.

De Wet, H., Nkwanyana, M.N., Van Vuuren, S.F., 2010. J. Ethnopharmacol., 130:284–289.

Dlamini, T.P., 2006. Isolation and Characterisation of Bioactive Compounds From *Lippia javanica*. MSc dissertation, University of Johannesburg, Johannesburg, South Africa.

Dzoyem, J.P., Eloff, J.N., 2015. J. Ethnopharmacol., 160:194–201.

Endris, A., Asfaw, N., Bisrat, D., 2016. J. Essent. Oil Res., 28:221–226.

Fouche, G., Cragg, G.M., Pillay, P., Kolesnikova, N., Maharaj, V.J., Senabe, J., 2008. J. Ethnopharmacol., 119:455–461.

Fujita, Y., 1965. Government Industrial Research Institute (Osaka), 306:21–25.
Germishuizen, G., Meyer, N.L., Steenkamp, Y., Keith, M. (Eds.), 2006. A Checklist of South African Plants. Southern African Botanical Diversity Network, vol. 41, Pretoria, South Africa.
Govere, J., Durrheim, D.N., Du Toit, N., Hunt, R.H., Coetzee, M., 2000. Cent. Afr. J. Med., 46:213–216.
Huffman, A., Klepser, D.M.E., Keele, D.J., Roling, E., 2002. J. Infect. Dis. Pharmacother., 5:43–50.
Hutchings, A., Van Staden, J., 1994. J. Ethnopharmacol., 43:89–124.
Hutchings, A., Scott, A.H., Lewis, G., Cunningham, A.B., 1996. Zulu Medicinal Plants: An Inventory. University of Natal Press, Pietermarizburg, South Africa.
Hutchings, A., 2003. Enhancing HIV/AIDS support therapy with indigenous herbal preparations—a clinic experience. Joint International Conference SAAB & ISE, University of Pretoria, Pretoria, South Africa.
Katerere, D.R., Graziani, G., Thembo, K.M., Nyazema, N.Z., Ritieni, A., 2012. Afr. J. Biotechnol., 11:4103–4108.
Kamanula, J.F., Belmain, S.R., Hall, D.R., Farman, D.I., Goyder, D.J., Mvumi, B.M., Masumbu, F.F., Stevenson, P.C., 2017. Ind. Crop. Prod., 110:75–82.
Lekganyane, M.A., Matsebatlela, T.M., Howard, R.L., Shai, L.J., Masoko, P., 2012. Afr. J. Biotechnol., 11:13210–13219.
Ludere, M.T., Van Ree, T., Vleggaar, R., 2013. Fitoterapia, 86:188–192.
Lukwa, N., 1994. Cent. Afr. J. Med., 40:306–309.
Lukwa, N., Mølgaard, P., Furu, P., Bøgh, C., 2009. Trop. Biomed., 26:85–91.
Mabogo, D.E.N., 1990. The Ethnobotany of VhaVenda. MSc dissertation, University of Pretoria, Pretoria, South Africa.
Madzimure, J., Nyahangare, E.T., Hamudikuwanda, H., Hove, T., Stevenson, P.C., Belmain, S.R., Mvumi, B.M., 2011. Trop. Anim. Health Prod., 43:481–489.
Magano, S.R., Nchu, F., Eloff, J.N., 2011. Afr. J. Biotechnol., 10:8970–8975.
Maharaj, V.J., Fouche, G., Senabe, J., Nthambeleni, R.N., Kotze, F., 1995. Agro-Processing Opportunities Identified Through a Novel Mosquito Repellent From a Medicinal Plant. http://researchspace.csir.co.za/dspace/bitstream/handle/10204/2744/Maharaj_P_2008.
Manenzhe, N.J., Potgieter, N., Van Ree, T., 2004. Phytochemistry, 65:2333–2336.
Maroyi, A., 2017. Evid. Based Complement. Alternat. Med., 2017:6746071.
Mashela, P.W., Mphosi, M.S., Shimelis, H., Mokgalong, N.M., 2007. J. Phytopathol., 155:690–693.
Masoko, P., Nxumalo, K.M., 2013. Evid. Based Complement. Alternat. Med., 2013:586247.
Mavundza, E.J., Maharaj, R., Finnie, J.F., Kabera, G., Van Staden, J., 2011. J. Ethnopharmacol., 137:1516–1520.
Mavundza, E.J., Maharaj, R., Chukwujekwu, J.C., Finnie, J.F., Van Staden, J., 2013. S. Afr. J. Bot., 88:86–89.
Mavundza, E.J., Maharaj, R., Chukwujekwu, J.C., Finnie, J.F., Van Staden, J., 2014. Malar. J., 13:173–177.
McGaw, L.J., Jäger, A.K., Van Staden, J., 2000. J. Ethnopharmacol., 72:247–263.
Mkenda, P., Mwanauta, R., Stevenson, P.C., Ndakidemi, P., Mtei, K., Belmain, S.R., 2015. PLoS One, 10:e0143530.
Mpofu, D.A., Marume, U., Mlambo, V., Hugo, A., 2016. Anim. Nutr., 2:160–167.
Mnisi, C.M., Matshogo, T.B., Van Niekerk, R., Mlambo, V., 2017. S. Afri. J. Anim. Sci., 47:661–671.

Mujovo, S.F., Hussein, A.A., Meyer, J.J.M., Fourie, B., Muthivhi, T., Lall, N., 2008. Nat. Prod. Res., 22:1047–1054.

Mwangi, J.W., Addae-Mensah, I., Munavu, R.M., Lwande, W., 1991. Flavour Fragr. J., 6:221–224.

Mwangi, J.W., Addae-Mensah, I., Muriuki, G., Munavu, R.H., Lwande, W., Hassawnali, A., 1992. Int. J. Pharmacogn., 30:9–16.

Narzary, H., Islary, A., Basumatary, S., 2016. Mediterr. J. Nutr. Metab., 9:91–201.

Neidlein, R., Staehle, R., 1973. Dtsch. Apoth. Ztg., 113:993–997.

Neidlein, R., Staehle, R., 1974. Dtsch. Apoth. Ztg., 40:1588–1592.

Ngassapa, O., Runyoro, D.K.B., Harvala, E., Chinou, I.B., 2003. Flavour Fragr. J., 18:221–224.

Nkomo, L.P., Green, E., Ndip, R.N., 2011. Afr. J. Pharm. Pharmacol., 5:2184–2192.

Oketch-Rabah, H.A., Dossaji, S.F., Mberu, E.K., 1999. Pharm. Biol., 37:329–334.

Olivier, D.K., Shikanga, E.A., Combrinck, S., Krause, R.W.M., Regnier, T., Dlamini, T.P., 2010. S. Afr. J. Bot., 76:58–63.

Osée Muyima, N.Y., Nziweni, S., Mabinya, L.V., 2004. J. Essent. Oil Bear. Plants, 7:68–78.

Pascual, M.E., Slowing, K., Carretero, E., Sánchez Mata, D., Villar, A., 2001. J. Ethnopharmacol., 76:201–214.

Philemon, Y.K., Matasyoh, J.C., Wagara, I.N., 2015. Int. J. Biotechnol. Food Sci., 4:1–6.

Prozesky, E.A., Meyer, J.J.M., Louw, A.I., 2001. J. Ethnopharmacol., 76:239–245.

Retief, E., Herman, P.P.J., 1997. Plants of the Northern Provinces of South Africa: Keys and Diagnostic Characters. National Botanical Institute, Pretoria, South Africa.

Rimpler, H., Sauerbier, H., 1986. Biochem. Syst. Ecol., 14:307–310.

Samie, A., Obi, C.L., Bessong, P.O., Lall, N., 2005. Afr. J. Biotechnol., 4:1443–1451.

Samie, A., Obi, C.L., Lall, N., Meyer, J.J.M., 2009. Ann. Trop. Med. Parasitol., 103:159–170.

Samie, A., Tambani, T., Harshfield, E., Green, E., Ramalivhana, J.N., Bessong, P.O., 2010. Afr. J. Biotechnol., 9:2965–2976.

Shikanga, E., Regnier, T., Combrinck, S., Botha, B., 2009. Fruits, 64:75–82.

Shikanga, E.A., Combrinck, S., Regnier, T., 2010. S. Afr. J. Bot., 76:567–571.

Swargiary, A., Daimari, A., Daimari, M., Basumatary, N., Narzary, E., 2016. Indian J. Pharmacol., 48:418–423.

Terblanché, F.C., Kornelius, G., 1996. J. Essent. Oil Res., 8:471–485.

Thembo, K.M., Vismer, H.F., Nyazema, N.Z., Gelderblom, W.C.A., Katerere, D.R., 2010. J. Appl. Microbiol., 109:1479–1486.

Van Vuuren, S., Muhlarhi, T., 2017. S. Afr. J. Bot., 112:186–192.

Van Wyk, B.-E., Gericke, N., 2000. People's Plants. A Guide to Useful Plants of Southern Africa. Briza Publications, Pretoria, South Africa.

Van Wyk, B.-E., 2008. J. Ethnopharmacol., 119:342–355.

Van Wyk, B.-E., Van Heerden, F., Van Oudtshoorn, B., 2009. Poisonous Plants of South Africa. Briza Publications, Pretoria, South Africa.

Van Wyk, B.-E., 2011. S. Afr. J. Bot., 77:812–829.

Velasco-Negeureula, A., Perez-Alonso, M.J., Guzman, C.A., Zygadlo, J.A., Ariza-Espinar, L., Sanz, J., Garcıa-Vallejo, M.C., 1993. J. Essent. Oil Res., 5:513–524.

Viljoen, A.M., Subramoney, S., Vuuren, S.F.V., Başer, K.H.C., Demirci, B., 2005. J. Ethnopharmacol., 96:271–277.

Watt, J.M., Breyer-Brandwijk, M.G., 1962. The Medicinal and Poisonous Plants of Southern and Eastern Africa, second ed. E. & S. Livingstone Ltd, Edinburgh and London, UK.

Yang, C.S., Landau, J.M., Huang, M.-T., Newmark, H.L., 2001. Annu. Rev. Nutr., 21: 381–406.

York, T., De Wet, H., Van Vuuren, S.F., 2011. J. Ethnopharmacol., 135:696–710.

CHAPTER

Mesembryanthemum tortuosum 17

Alvaro Viljoen[a,b], Weiyang Chen[a] and Sandra Combrinck[a]

[a]*Department of Pharmaceutical Sciences, Tshwane University of Technology, Pretoria, South Africa*

[b]*SAMRC Herbal Drugs Research Unit, Faculty of Science, Tshwane University of Technology, Pretoria, South Africa*

Abstract

Mesembryanthemum tortuosum L. (Aizoaceae) was previously classified as Sceletium tortuosum and is still widely referred to under that name in literature. Locally, the plant is known as 'kanna'. The small scrambling succulent is endemic to South Africa and is found in the arid areas of the Western, Eastern and Northern Cape provinces. For centuries, the Khoi and San people used the aerial parts in the form of a masticant or infusion, as a mood enhancer, to promote sleep and to soothe digestive conditions. After traditional fermentation to boost its psychoactive properties, the remedy is referred to as 'kougoed'. The plant has been fully commercialised and selected chemotypes are cultivated as a source of raw material. Products are used for the management of mild depression, anxiety, insomnia, weak appetite, stress, bulimia, obsessive compulsive disorder and to alleviate drug-dependence. The psychoactive properties of the plant are attributed to the presence of mesembrine-type alkaloids. This monograph is a record of the ethnobotany, and the extensive research carried out to study the phytochemistry, in vitro and in vivo biological and pharmacological properties of M. tortuosum, as well as its toxicity profile. High-performance thin-layer chromatography (HPTLC) and ultra-performance liquid chromatography coupled to mass spectrometry (UPLC–MS) were used to establish typical chemical fingerprints of the plant. The marker compounds, mesembrenol, mesembranol, mesembrenone and mesembrine, were identified after both HPTLC and UPLC–MS analyses.

Keywords: *Mesembryanthemum tortuosum*, *Sceletium tortuosum*, Kanna, Psychoactive, Mesembrenol, Mesembrenone, Mesembrine, UPLC–MS, HPTLC, MIR spectroscopy

The South African Herbal Pharmacopoeia. https://doi.org/10.1016/B978-0-323-99794-2.00005-2

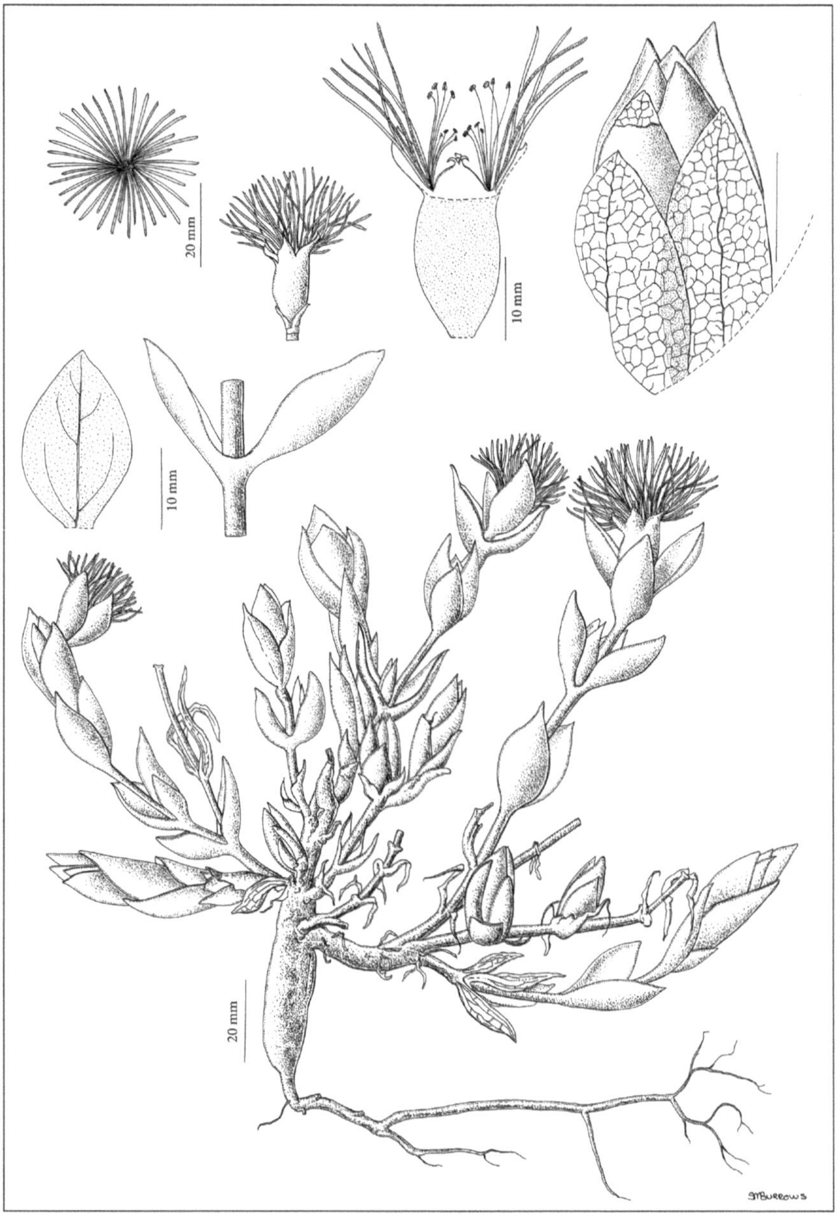
20 mm
10 mm
10 mm
20 mm

Part A: General overview

1. Synonyms

Sceletium tortuosum (L.) N.E.Br., *Mesembryanthemum aridum* Moench, *Mesembryanthemum concavum* Haw., *Pentacoilanthus tortuosus* (L.) Rappa & Camorrone, *Phyllobolus tortuosus* (L.) Bittrich, *Sceletium boreale* L.Bolus, *Sceletium compactum* L.Bolus, *Sceletium concavum* (Haw.) Schwantes, *Sceletium framesii* L.Bolus, *Sceletium gracile* L.Bolus, *Sceletium joubertii* L.Bolus, *Sceletium namaquense* L.Bolus, *Sceletium namaquense* L.Bolus var. *namaquense*, *Sceletium namaquense* L.Bolus var. *subglobosum* L.Bolus, *Sceletium ovatum* L.Bolus, *Sceletium tugwelliae* L.Bolus, *Tetracoilanthus concavus* (Haw.) Rappa & Camarrone.[a]

2. Common name(s)

Sceletium (English, French and German), ice plant (English), '*kanna*', '*channa*' (Khoi), '*iqina*' (isiXhosa), '*kougoed*', '*Hotnotskougoed*', '*Hottentotskougoed*' (Afrikaans).

3. Conservation status

Least concern[a].

4. Botany

Mesembryanthemum tortuosum (Aizoaceae), formerly known and still widely referred to as *Sceletium tortuosum*, is one of several recognised *Mesembryanthemum* species endemic to South Africa. It is the only species currently used commercially. *Mesembryanthemum tortuosum* is a small, scrambling or decumbent shrub that prefers to grow beneath other larger shrubs (A). The genus name is derived from the Latin word '*mesembria*' (which means midday), referring to the belief that the plants only flower at midday. The prominent vein-like lines of the plant are conspicuous in the old, dry and withered leaves (C) (Jackson, 1990). Flowers (2–3 cm in diameter) appear in spring and summer, and range in colour from white to different shades of yellow and light pink (A). They are characterised by four or five sepals and by a multitude of 1 mm wide petaloid staminoids with pointed tips. The stigmas are obtuse and are shorter than 2 mm. The leaves consist of large, planar idioblasts (B) and are about 4 cm in length, flat, imbricate and curved towards the tips (Gerbaulet, 1996).

[a] Red List of South African Plants (http://redlist.sanbi.org).

Small fruit, which have valve wings, precede the formation of crested brown seeds. The dried aerial parts (D) have a range of applications in African traditional medicine and complementary medicine systems.

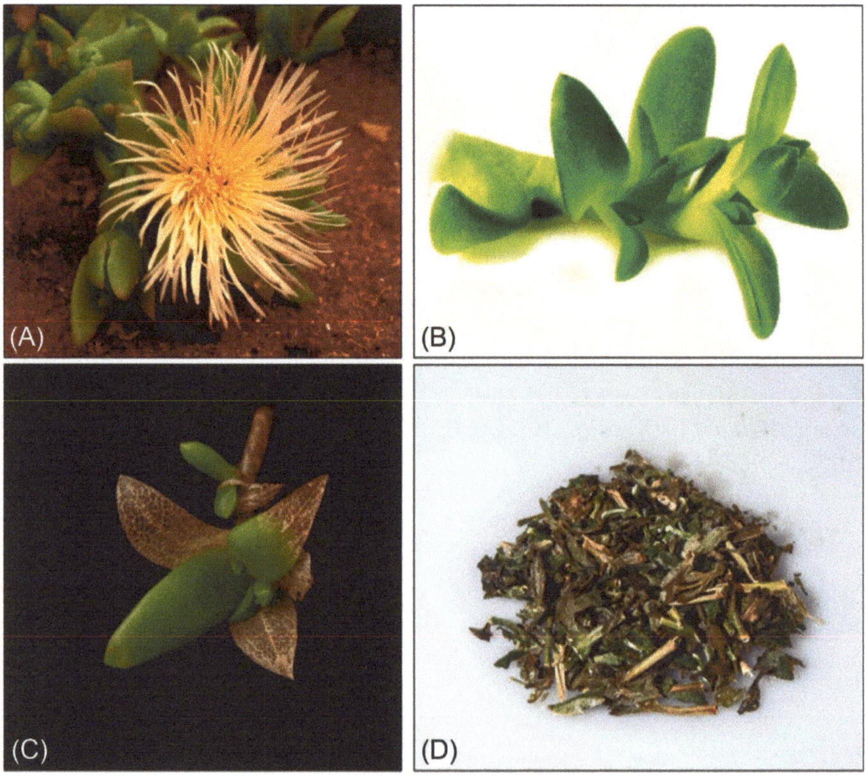

The creeping *Mesembryanthemum tortuosum* displaying yellowish-white flowers (A), large imbricate leaves (B), conspicuous vein-like lines on dried leaves (C) and crushed aerial parts used for medicinal purposes (D).

5. Geographical distribution

Mesembryanthemum tortuosum is endemic to South Africa and occurs in the Western, Eastern and Northern Cape provinces. The species is particularly abundant in arid regions, including the Little, Great and Upper Karoo, the Namaqualand Rocky Hills, Knersvlakte and Ceres Karoo, but it also grows in the more moist parts of the Western Cape Province (Patnala and Kanfer, 2008). The plants prefer rocky, inland habitats to coastal sites (Smith et al., 1998). Wild populations of *Mesembryanthemum* have been over-exploited through harvesting and have become scarce due to poor management of the veld.

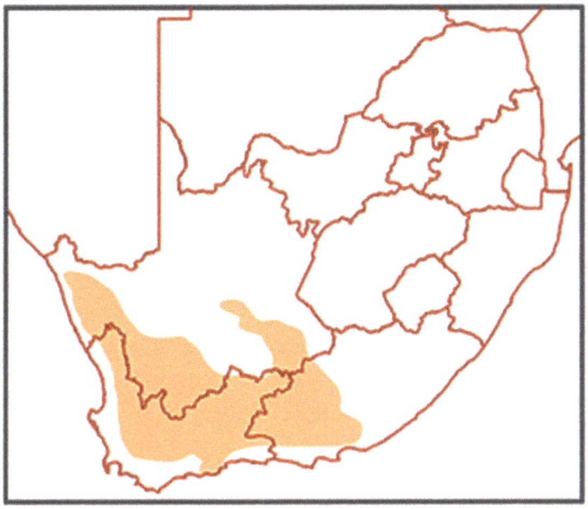

Geographical distribution of *Mesembryanthemum tortuosum* in South Africa.

6. Ethnopharmacology

Mesembryanthemum tortuosum has been used for several centuries by the Khoi and San people in Bushmanland, Namaqualand and the Karoo to increase their resilience during hunting expeditions, as a mood enhancer for relaxation, and for coping with stressful situations posed by their harsh living environment. It is one of the oldest recognised medicinal plants in South Africa and was first documented in 1685 by Simon van der Stel, one of the early governors of the Dutch Colony proclaimed in South Africa (Smith et al., 1996). He noted that the plant uplifted the spirits of those who used it. Tinctures (hydro-ethanolic extracts) prepared from the plant were popular among the colonisers of the Cape of Good Hope (Pappe, 1868). Traditionally, the whole plant material of *M. tortuosum* is used mainly by mastication, and also as a decoction, to induce weak narcotic, intoxicating and psychoactive effects, often as a form of recreation. A portion of leaves steeped in boiling water is administered as an emetic by the Zulu to combat heart weakness, thought to be associated with experiencing nightmares (Bryant, 1966). The traditional remedy prepared from *M. tortuosum* and used as a stimulant is referred to as '*kougoed*'. A whole plant, including the roots, is pulverised using stones. The pulp is then left to ferment in a sealed container for eight days. After fermentation, it is spread out in the sun to dry, whereafter it is ready to be chewed, smoked, or powdered and inhaled as snuff (Smith et al., 1996, 1998; Van Wyk and Gericke, 2003). The plant is used as a sedative to promote sleep in adults, children and babies, and to relieve digestive conditions (Smith et al., 1996; Van Wyk and Gericke, 2003).

7. Commercialisation

The trading of kanna has been ongoing for centuries and was recorded as early as 1682 (Smith et al., 1996). Shops in Namaqualand still keep supplies of the material when it is available (Gericke and Viljoen, 2008). At the beginning of the 18th century, an attempt was made to cultivate the plant in England and, later, in the United States (Smith et al., 1996). Grassroots Natural Products was the first company to undertake commercial cultivation of *S. tortuosum* (now *M. tortuosum*). This was started in 1996 under contract to Pharmacare Ltd., a South African pharmaceutical company. The bio-active mesembrine alkaloids present in *M. tortuosum* were patented in the United States by South African researchers (Gericke and Van Wyk, 1999). In 2009, a South African company HG&H Pharmaceuticals (Pty) Ltd. was granted an export and bioprospecting permit to export *Sceletium* products under the trade name Zembrin® (Patnala and Kanfer, 2009). Phyto Nova launched the first tablets containing powdered whole plant in the year 2000 (Van Wyk, 2011). HG&H Pharmaceuticals and the South African San Council signed an historic agreement, which involved the sharing of any financial benefits emanating from commercialisation with the Nama communities of Kamiesberg in Namaqualand. The cultivation of selected clones has since expanded to regions of the Northern, Western and Eastern Cape provinces and Namibia. Only *M. tortuosum* is used for commercial purposes, and products are indicated for the management of depression, anxiety, insomnia, weak appetite, stress, bulimia, obsessive compulsive disorder, and to alleviate drug-dependence, including aiding in stopping smoking. Several other products containing *M. tortuosum* (labelled as *S. tortuosum)* are available from pharmacies, health and wellness stores, and on the internet. These products include capsules, tablets, tea blends, sprays, extracts, drops, tinctures and powdered material.

Several specialised analytical techniques have been used to determine the alkaloid content of commercial samples. The variability in the mesembrine-type alkaloid content within wild specimens of *M. tortuosum* from the south-western region of South Africa was investigated by Shikanga et al. (2012a). The study included 151 specimens sampled from 31 localities. Analysis by gas chromatography–mass spectrometry (GC–MS) revealed that the total alkaloid content of the wild plants varied between 0.11% and 1.99% dry weight (dw). Five main chemotypes (labelled A, B, C, D and E) could be distinguished, following principal component analysis and hierarchical cluster analysis. Samples categorised as Chemotype A contained no mesembrine-type alkaloids, while high relative concentrations of mesembrenol (64.96%–95.55%), mesembrine (51.25%–92.50%) and mesembrenone (50.86%–72.51%) were found in samples from Chemotypes B, C and E, respectively. Chemotype D was described as an intermediate cluster, since all four alkaloids were present in these samples in moderate concentrations. The intra- and interpopulation differences were therefore found to be qualitative. In addition, eight commercial products were analysed and found to differ substantially in their alkaloid content, although mesembrine was identified as the main alkaloid constituent in most of them. Three of the alkaloids, namely mesembrenol, mesembrine and mesembrenone, were identified as appropriate marker compounds for monitoring the quality of *M. tortuosum* raw materials and products. A comprehensive study by Zhao et al. (2018) involving 289 samples of *S. tortuosum (M. tortuosum)* and using both proton nuclear magnetic resonance (^{1}H NMR) spectroscopy and ultra-performance liquid chromatography-mass spectrometry (UPLC–MS) metabolomics, revealed that specimens from the Northern Cape Province of South Africa produced considerably higher levels of sceletium alkaloids (population averages 4940–9380 mg/kg dw) than their counterparts from the Western Cape Province (population averages 16–4140 mg/kg). Mesembrine was the major alkaloid constituent in all the samples from the Northern Cape Province. In addition to the sceletium alkaloids, pinitol and two alkylamines were identified for the first time as markers for *M. tortuosum*, using chemometric analysis of the ^{1}H NMR data. These were quantified using quantitative-NMR (qNMR) and the results corresponded to those obtained using gas chromatography.

The use of high-throughput direct analysis in real-time-high-resolution-time-of-flight mass spectrometry (DART-HRToFMS) was demonstrated by Lesiak et al. (2016) as a powerful tool to screen commercially available *Sceletium* products for psychotropic alkaloids, but also to reveal the presence of scheduled substances and adulterants. Herbal tea blends often consist of two or more different species that are combined to enhance the taste and improve on the health benefits. Roscher et al. (2012) used a non-aqueous capillary electrophoresis coupled to mass spectrometry (NACE-MS) method that they developed and validated to determine the alkaloid composition of *S. tortuosum* and products prepared from the plant. It provided good resolution of isobaric compounds, indicated as diastereomers, double-bond isomers or structurally similar compounds. Quality control of herbal tea is vital to ensure consistency, safety and efficacy. In this regard, Sandasi et al. (2018) applied hyperspectral imaging (HSI) for the quality control of such blends. The technique is rapid and non-destructive and can be described as a combination of conventional spectroscopy and digital imaging. It provides chemical information of constituents in a sample and a visual pattern of their spatial distribution within a matrix. Hyperspectral images of certified raw materials (*M. tortuosum* and *Cyclopia genistoides*) and herbal tea blends, provided by Parceval Pty (Ltd), were captured on a SisuChema® SWIR (short-wave infrared) hyperspectral pushbroom imaging system using ChemaDAQ® software. Principal component analysis (PCA) of the data indicated that the chemical variation between the raw materials of *M. tortuosum* and *C. genistoides*, as described by the model, was 54.2%. The accuracy of the predictions indicated that HSI could be implemented as a visual tool in the quality monitoring of herbal tea blends.

8. Pharmacological evaluation

8.1 *In vitro* studies

8.1.1 Central nervous system effects

United States Patent 6,288,104 (Gericke and Van Wyk, 1997, 1999) disclosed the use of mesembrine and related compounds, including novel compounds, as serotonin-uptake inhibitors, and the use of standardised amounts of these compounds in pharmaceutical formulations in the management of psychiatric and psychological conditions, including depression, anxiety, drug-dependence, bulimia and obsessive compulsive disorder. Mesembrine-HCl was confirmed to act as a phosphodiesterase-4 (PDE4) inhibitor, as reflected by a half maximal inhibitory concentration (IC_{50}) value of 29 μM (Napoletano et al., 2001). Such PDE4 inhibitors are regarded as drug targets in the development of treatments for depression and a range of conditions associated with inflammation, including asthma, chronic obstructive pulmonary disease and psoriasis (Houslay et al., 2005). Mesembrenone has been reported to have cytotoxic effects towards a murine non-tumoural fibroblast cell line, as well as a human tumoural cell line (Molt4). The alkaloid was the only one of 25 isolated from Amaryllidaceae that was specific towards Molt4 cells in comparison to the fibroblast cells (Weniger et al., 1995). In 2011, a commercial product, Zembrin®, consisting of a standardised extract of *M. tortuosum*, was screened at 0.75 mg/mL, using 77 radioligand binding assays and a panel of PDEs. The extract comprised 0.35%–0.45% total alkaloids, with more than 60% contributed by mesembrenone and mesembrenol, while mesembrine represented less than 20% of the total alkaloids (Murbach et al., 2014). More than 80% inhibition of GABA receptors (non-selective), serotonin (5-HT) transporter, δ2- and μ-opioid receptors, the cholecystokinin-1 receptor, and PDEs 3 and 4 was recorded (Krstenansky, 2017). The IC_{50} value of the standardised extract towards 5-HT and PDE4 was reported as 4.3 and 8.5 μg/mL, respectively (Harvey et al., 2011). Mesembrine was the most potent of the tested alkaloids as a 5-HT inhibitor (K_i 1.4 nM), while mesembrenone was active against both the 5-HT transporter and PDE4 (IC_{50}'s < 1 μM).

Fermented and unfermented extracts of *M. tortuosum* were evaluated in the cannabinoid CB1 receptor binding assay (Lubbe et al., 2010). It was found that the unfermented alkaloid extract displayed a higher binding activity towards the CB1 receptor. The presence of higher alkaloid concentrations in the unfermented extract was confirmed by GC–MS analysis. The higher activity of the methanol extract, compared to the fermented one, indicated that non-alkaloid compounds may be involved in the activity of the methanol extract. The standardised extract was also subjected to the acetylcholinesterase (AChE) inhibitory assay to determine whether it can improve cognitive ability and memory. Both fermented and unfermented alkaloid extracts inhibited the enzyme, with IC_{50} values of 0.303 and 0.330 mg/mL, respectively. Notably, mesembrine, the major alkaloid in the extract, was unable to effectively inhibit the enzyme. The effect of a mesembrine-rich extract from *M. tortuosum*, marketed as Trimesemine™ by Botanical Resource Holdings (Pty) Ltd., on the release of mono-amine and on serotonin reuptake into human astrocytes and mouse hippocampal neurons, was investigated (Coetzee et al., 2016). The potential inhibition of the associated enzymes was also explored. It was found that treatment with the standardised extract did not affect cell viability. However, it was found to downregulate the expression of serotonin, similar to the action of the positive control (citalopram), and to upregulate vesicular mono-amine transporter-2 (VAMT-2), in both human astrocytes and mouse hippocampal neurons. Mild inhibition of AChE and mono-amine oxidase-A (MAO-A) was reported following exposure to the extract.

8.1.2 Anti-inflammatory and immune modulating activity

Although *M. tortuosum* was found to display moderate anti-inflammatory activity when assessed in cytokines, it was unable to effectively combat the surge of the immune response following an acute immune challenge (Bennett and Smith, 2018). Treatment with a *M. tortuosum* extract resulted in an increased mitochondrial viability, with a simultaneous upregulation of IL-10 release under basal conditions. Mitochondrial viability decreased significantly following exposure to lipopolysaccharide (LPS), but this was inhibited completely by treatment with the plant extract. In addition, the acute inflammatory response to LPS stimulation was not negatively affected. The most notable effects of the treatment were evident following treatment with a dose of 0.01 mg/mL. Excellent cytoprotection was afforded by *M. tortuosum* after endotoxin stimulation and it caused modulation of the basal inflammatory cytokine profile, but could not impede the acute response to the pathogenic challenge. A mesembrine-rich extract of *M. tortuosum* was reported to exhibit cytoprotective and moderate anti-inflammatory activities in monocytes, and to target specific P450 enzymes, resulting in reduced adrenal glucocorticoid synthesis (Bennett et al., 2018). It has been established that the development of both obesity and diabetes is closely linked to inflammation and the excessive production of glucocorticoid. The relationship between glucocorticoid action and inflammation prompted an investigation into the central immunomodulatory effects of two different *M. tortuosum* extracts. First, human astrocytes were treated for 30 min with each extract and then exposed to LPS from *Escherichia coli*. An assessment of the resulting cytotoxicity, mitotoxicity and cytokine responses (basally and in response to inflammatory stimulus) was made. In addition, the total polyphenol content, anti-oxidant capacity and selected neural enzyme inhibition capacity were determined for both extracts. Treatment with the extracts offered protection against both cytotoxicity and inflammation. The extract high in Δ^7-mesembrenone concentration, was found to be also rich in polyphenols, and displayed a strong anti-oxidant effect, but was regarded to pose a greater danger of adverse effects with overdose. Both *M. tortuosum* extracts were deemed to be appropriate as preventative supplements or complementary treatments for obesity and diabetes.

8.1.3 Pharmacokinetics

Since *M. tortuosum* is often masticated, but is also taken in the form of decoctions and infusions, the *in vitro* permeability of water and methanol crude *M. tortuosum* extracts, and an acid–base alkaloid-enriched extract, were compared to that of pure mesembrine, mesembrenone, mesembrenol and mesembranol, across porcine intestinal, sublingual and buccal tissues (Shikanga et al., 2012b). The permeability of mesembrine in its pure form, as well as in the form of crude extracts, across intestinal tissue was higher than that of caffeine, used as the positive control due to its high permeability. Mesembranol was found to have a similar intestinal permeability to caffeine, while mesembrenol and mesembrenone were less easily transported than caffeine, but were more permeable than atenolol, a poorly transported compound that served as the negative control. The alkaloids were generally more permeable across the intestinal tissue than across the sublingual and buccal tissues. Nevertheless, it was concluded from the results of the study that the overall bio-availability of the mesembrine alkaloids is increased through transport across the membranes of the oral cavity when the plant material is masticated and retained in the mouth for a long period.

8.1.4 Other activities

The effects of a '*Sceletium*' extract (Trimesemine™) containing a high concentration of mesembrine (1% of plant extract w/w) on adrenal steroid biosynthesis were investigated by Swart and Smith (2016). Steroidogenesis was assessed basally and in response to stimuli (forskolin, angiotensin II, KCl), in human adrenocortical carcinoma cells (H295R). Pregnenolone levels were increased and 16-hydroxyprogesterone levels decreased at the highest dose (1 mg/mL, 34.5 µM mesembrine), but only under forskolin-stimulated conditions. This finding implicated CYP17 enzyme inhibition, particularly since a significant reduction of forskolin-associated increases in cortisol levels, at the highest dose tested, and basal cortisol levels across all doses, were recorded. Independently of forskolin, Trimesemine™ inhibited the production of androstenedione and testosterone across all doses, indicating that 3βHSD and 17βHSD were inhibited, respectively. Both the angiotensin II- and forskolin-induced increases in aldosterone production were inhibited by the standardised extract (Swart and Smith, 2016). The anti-HIV and free radical scavenging activity of extracts of cultivated, commercially available *M. tortuosum* were investigated *in vitro*. Organic extracts prepared from the plants were tested for inhibitory activity against HIV-1 enzymes; protease, reverse transcriptase and integrase. An assay to determine HIV-1 reverse transcriptase inhibition yielded IC_{50} values of <50 for the ethanol and 121.7 ± 2.5 µg/mL for the ethyl acetate extract. Both extracts were found to inhibit HIV-1 protease with IC_{50} values <100 µg/mL. Dose-dependent radical scavenging ability was reported for 2,2-diphenyl-1-picryl-hydrazyl (DPPH) radicals, with corresponding IC_{50} values of 49.0 ± 0.2 and 64.7 ± 3.1 µg/mL for the ethanolic and ethyl acetate extracts of *M. tortuosum*, respectively (Kapewangolo et al., 2016).

8.2 *In vivo* studies and clinical trials

8.2.1 Central nervous system effects

The first *in vivo* study involving sceletium alkaloids was done as early as 1898 when Meiring (1898) injected an alkaloidal principle prepared from '*S. tortuosum*' into the skin of a frog and observed that it induced a pronounced hypnotic effect. This experiment was repeated by Meiring using an alkaloid mixture isolated from the plant. Within a few minutes of administering a subcutaneous injection comprising a few drops of the mixture to a frog, increases in the respiratory rate, moistness of the skin, and uneasiness were recorded. However, the respiratory rate slowed considerably after 10–12 min, but the frog remained unable to right itself when placed on its back. A 4–8 h period was necessary for a full recovery. Zwicky (1915) deduced from his experiments that mesembrine exerted a 'cocaine-like activity', although the activity was not as intense (Watt and Breyer-Brandwijk, 1962). From his research, he also concluded that the alkaloid mixture caused central nervous system depression in frogs, rabbits and humans, which is in direct contrast to the stimulation expected from a cocaine-like drug. A study on dogs was conducted by Hirabayashi et al. (2002) to determine the effects of *M. tortuosum* on canine dementia. Milled dry plant material was given daily at 10 mg/kg to seven affected dogs for six consecutive evenings. Night-time barking was decreased significantly, or stopped completely, for all the study animals, providing evidence of the efficacy of *M. tortuosum* in this regard. The study was later extended to cats, suffering from a range of conditions (Hirabayashi et al., 2004). Two cats in a cattery diagnosed with cage stress, one cat displaying travel stress when being transported by car, one cat that meowed excessively at night, and one cat unable to be administered with deep anaesthesia for a dental procedure (only given medetomidine as anaesthetic) were treated with *M. tortuosum* by veterinarians. Single doses or multiple daily doses of between 10 and 100 mg/kg were administered, for a period of up to 6 months. The cats with cage- and travel stress were notably calmer, for a period of 6–10 h following a single dose. The treatment controlled the excessive nocturnal meowing of the treated cat. In the last case, it was not necessary for physical restraint of the cat during teeth-scaling, since a single dose of *M. tortuosum* at 60 mg/kg, administered before the medetomidine, kept the cat resting quietly.

Treatment with *M. tortuosum* had a positive effect on anxiety induced by restraint in rats (Smith, 2011). A low dose had hardly any effect on stress-induced self-soothing behaviour or on stress-induced corticosterone levels. A possible suppressive effect on T helper 1 immune function was signalled by lower IL-2 and higher IL-10 levels in response to *M. tortuosum* treatment. Several rat models were used to evaluate the effects of *M. tortuosum* and mesembrine on nociception, depression, anxiety, ataxia and abuse liability. A study in male Sprague–Dawley rats revealed that *M. tortuosum* did not induce preference or aversion in conditioned place preference tests (Loria et al., 2014). Mesembrine displayed analgesic activity, but there was no sign of ataxis or the development of substance dependence. The metabolic fate of mesembrine and mesembrenone was studied *in vivo* in the rat, as well as *in vitro* using a human liver preparation (Meyer et al., 2015). Analysis by GC–MS and liquid chromatography coupled to linear ion trap high resolution-mass spectrometry (LC-HR-MS) was used to identify the metabolites. Both alkaloids were transformed through *O*- and *N*-demethylation, dehydration, and/or hydroxylation at different positions. The phenolic metabolites were partly excreted after conversion to glucuronides and/or sulphates. Many of the Phase I metabolites present in the rat urine were also identified in the human liver preparations. The acetylated demethyl-dihydro- and hydroxyl- metabolites were the most common metabolites of mesembrine, while the demethyl-dihydro forms of mesembrenone were the most abundant in rat liver. Electropharmacograms were constructed in the presence of three dosages of Zembrin® (2.5, 5.0 and 10.0 mg/kg) in adult Fischer rats (Dimpfel et al., 2016a). In addition, electropharmacograms were obtained for other herbal extracts, and for citicoline and rolipram, for comparative purposes and for discriminatory analysis. A significant reduction in alpha-2 and beta-1a waves was recorded, which corresponds to the activation of the dopaminergic and glutamatergic transmitter systems, respectively. A decrease in the delta and the theta frequency ranges were also noted, which corresponds to modifications of the cholinergic and norepinephrine systems, respectively. This pattern was found to be similar to those obtained for drugs used to treat neurodegenerative diseases. After administration of the highest dosage, an attenuation of alpha-1 waves was evident for all brain areas, corresponding to the effect of all antidepressants. The electropharmacogram obtained following treatment with citocoline, a synthetic compound developed to enhance cognitive function, was similar to that of Zembrin®. The electropharmacograms, reflecting treatment with the synthetic PDE4 inhibitor, rolipram and Zembrin®, were similar, suggesting that the latter has the potential to alleviate depression and improve cognitive function. When the results from the electropharmacograms were combined with the discriminatory analyses, it became apparent that Zembrin® has dose-dependent activity, with potential applications as an analgesic, antidepressant and cognitive function enhancer.

Using a chick anxiety-depression model, Carpenter et al. (2017) investigated the properties of *M. tortuosum*. This model is used for screening preclinical drug efficacy, because it has several features in common with clinical stress-related disorders. Dosages of 75 and 100 mg/kg of *M. tortuosum* reduced the open-circuit voltage (DVOC) rates during the anxiety phase, thereby reflecting anxiolytic activity. These results confirmed the stress-relieving properties of the plants. An ultra-high-performance liquid chromatography-quadrupole time-of-flight–mass spectrometry (UHPLC/QToF-MS) validated method was developed by Manda et al. (2017) and applied to evaluate the intravenous (i.v.) plasma pharmacokinetics of mesembrine and mesembrenone in mice. The compounds were extracted using protein precipitation with methanol (100%), with quinine as an internal standard, and the extracts were subsequently analysed. The lower limit of quantification for both the compounds was 10 ng/mL. The extraction recovery was between 87% and 93% for both compounds. Extracts of *M. tortuosum* have been investigated for safety, and their cognitive effects determined in several human trials, starting from 2009. The patented Zembrin® brand of *M. tortuosum* is backed by rigorous clinical trials and has self-affirmed Generally Regarded as Safe (GRAS) status in the United States. The dual PDE4 inhibition and 5-HT reuptake inhibition of Zembrin® were reported to be responsible for the pharmacological action of the herbal drug. This combinational mode of action provides therapeutic benefits. The first of these reports described a double-blind, placebo-controlled study that was completed in 2009. The aim was to determine the safety and tolerability of 8 and 25 mg doses taken once daily, over a period of 3 months (Nell et al., 2013). Adverse effects presented with the same or lower frequency than for the placebo group and both doses were well tolerated. In another study, the acute effects of Zembrin® in the brain were studied in 16 healthy volunteers using functional magnetic resonance imaging (fMRI). Anxiety-related activity in the amygdala and its connected neurocircuitry was of particular interest. The volunteers were scanned while taking part in a perceptual-load and an emotion-matching task. The response of the amygdala, after exposing participants to fearful faces under low perceptual load conditions, was attenuated after a single dose of the drug at 25 mg. A subsequent connectivity analysis involving the emotion-matching task also indicated a reduction in amygdala–hypothalamus coupling. The study substantiated the previous deduction that the binary action of 5-HT reuptake inhibition and PDE4 inhibition of this extract induces anxiolytic activity by attenuating responses to subcortical challenges (Terburg et al., 2013). These results were consistent with those reported by Harvey et al. (2011), who demonstrated serotonin reuptake inhibition (SRI) and PDE4 inhibitory activity. The neurocognitive effects of a 25 mg daily dose of Zembrin® were evaluated in mentally healthy participants (Chiu et al., 2014). Compared to the placebo group, the treated subjects demonstrated improved cognitive set flexibility and executive function. Mood and sleep patterns were also positively affected. It was proposed by Chiu et al. (2014) that the promising cognitive-enhancing effects of the drug involve the PDE4-cAMP-CREB cascade, which has been identified as a drug target in the potential treatment of early Alzheimer's disease. A more extensive double-blind, randomised, placebo-controlled study in 60 healthy adults (40–75 years) was conducted by Dimpfel et al. (2016b). Quantitative 17-channel electroencephalogram (EEG) and eye-tracking were used to monitor the responses of the participants after exposure to cognitive and emotional challenges initiated 2 h after taking placebo, or 25 or 50 mg doses of Zembrin®. Only a small improvement in psychometric performance was determined in the test subjects, and it was not statistically significant. However, the study made a valuable contribution to future studies by recording consistent, dose-related changes in brain activity after intake of the drug.

8.3 Safety

Mesembryanthemum tortuosum has been used for centuries as a mood-altering drug to relieve anxiety and stress, with no toxic effects documented. A study to assess the safety of *M. tortuosum* was conducted on dogs (Hirabayashi et al., 2002). Ground dry plant material was incorporated into the food [10 mg/kg body weight (bw)] given to seven healthy beagles. They were fed twice a day for 6 days. A dog with symptoms of dementia was also included in the study. Before and after feeding, the animals were inspected and a battery of blood tests was done, including glucose, platelet count, white cell count, red cell count, blood urea nitrogen, haemoglobin, creatinine, haematocrit, glutamic pyruvic transaminase (GPT), total protein and total cholesterol. Holter monitoring of the electrocardiogram (ECG) was conducted throughout the experiment. No behavioural changes, vomiting or diarrhoea were observed. The blood chemistry and blood counts remained the same and reflected no abnormalities in liver and kidney functions, haematology, glucose or lipid metabolism over the duration of the study. In addition, no cardiac arrhythmia or adverse effects on cardiac function were recorded. The dog diagnosed with dementia was not affected, according to the test results. It was concluded that *M. tortuosum* can be administered to canines at this dose, without any safety concerns. The same research group (Hirabayashi et al., 2004) conducted a similar toxicological study using six healthy cats between 2 and 10 years of age. A dose of 100 mg/kg bw of powdered *M. tortuosum* was mixed with their food and they were fed once a day for 7 days. A baseline blood test was done before the start of the experiment and again after its conclusion. Before and after drug administration, body mass and temperature were recorded. Full blood count, platelets, urea, creatinine, glucose, total protein, total cholesterol, ALP (alkaline phosphatase), CPK (creatine phosphokinase), GPT and GOT (glutamic oxaloacetic transaminase) levels were monitored. The general behaviour of the cats, change in appetite, vitality, and frequency of excretion were noted. No changes in behaviour, diarrhoea or vomiting were observed throughout the experiment. A small increase in the duration of daytime sleep was observed. The only other changes recorded were a small reduction in GOT and an increase in ALP, but the changes were still within normal limits.

The safety of Zembrin® was evaluated in 37 healthy adults over a period of 3 months by Nell et al. (2013). The study evaluated the effects of two doses (8 and 25 mg) of Zembrin® and a placebo, administered once a day. No differences were evident between the three treatments with regard to body mass, vital signs or ECG, from the start to the end of the trial. The haematology and biochemistry parameters remained within the normal range. The drug was well tolerated at both doses. Some of the patients reported headache, abdominal pain and upper respiratory tract infections, but these adverse effects were more frequent in the placebo group than in the treatment groups. Some participants in the Zembrin® groups diarised several positive effects on their mental state, which included improvements in the ability to cope with stress, and improvements in sleep. A safety assessment in rats was also conducted on a hydro-ethanolic extract (Zembrin®) prepared from *M. tortuosum* (Murbach et al., 2014). It was standardised to contain 0.35%–0.45% of total alkaloids, with mesembrenone and mesembrenol comprising more than 60% and mesembrine less than 20% of the alkaloids present. A 14-day repeated oral toxicity study was conducted at four dosage levels (0, 250, 750, 2500 and 5000 mg/kg bw/day). In addition, a 90-day subchronic repeated oral toxicity study was conducted at 0, 100, 300, 450 and 600 mg/kg bw/day. The rats were monitored using a battery of functional observations that included spontaneous locomotor activity, which was measured using a LabMaster ActiMot light-beam frames system. The locomotion, rearing behaviour, spatial parameters, and turning behaviour of the animals were observed in the last week of the trial. No adverse effects of any nature were observed. The researchers established the no-observable-adverse-effects-level (NOAEL) as 5000 mg/kg bw/day, which is consistent with the highest dose tested. The safety of the *M. tortuosum* extracts was demonstrated, even at high dosage concentrations tested.

9. Phytochemistry

9.1 Non-volatile constituents

Preliminary studies on *M. tortuosum*, done by Meiring (1898), suggested the presence of alkaloids. This was verified by Zwicky (1915). He studied two species, '*S. tortuosum*' and *Sceletium expansum*, and isolated 'mesembrin' with the molecular formula, $C_{16}H_{19}NO_4$, which was non-crystalline in nature. Many years later, Popelak et al. (1960) correctly reported the structure of 'mesembrin' as *N*-methyl-3a-(3′,4′-dimethoxyphenyl)-6-oxo-*cis*-octahydroindole, now known as mesembrine. This initiated interest in further studies on this unique group of alkaloids. The psychoactive properties of *M. tortuosum* have been mainly associated with four of these mesembrine-type alkaloids: mesembrine, mesembrenone, mesembrenol and mesembranol. Another alkaloid, tortuosamine, was isolated from *M. tortuosum* and this compound bears a close structural relationship to sceletium alkaloid A4, isolated initially from the related species, *Sceletium namaquense* and *Sceletium strictum* (Jeffs et al., 1974). Sceletium alkaloid A4 and tortuosamine were subsequently isolated from *M. tortuosum* by scientists from South Africa (Snyckers et al., 1971). Arndt and Kruger (1970) reported four alkaloids from *Sceletium joubertii* (now reduced to synonymy under *M. tortuosum*). Three of these alkaloids, joubertiamine, dehydrojoubertiamine and dihydrojoubertiamine, represented a new structural class, named the seco-mesembranes, which are clearly apart from the known mesembranes. They also isolated the structurally unrelated alkaloid, hordenine.

Alkaloids isolated from *Mesembryanthemum* species are subdivided into four structural classes (Herbert and Kattah, 1990). The first contains the 3a-aryl-*cis*-octahydroindole skeleton, which is referred to as the mesembrine group. Both the Δ^4- and Δ^7-series form part of this group and are distinguished by the double bond at positions 4–5 and 7–7a, respectively. Sceletium alkaloid A4 is currently the only member of the second subgroup. The tortuosamine-type alkaloids, similar in structure to the second, form the third subgroup, while the joubertiamine-type makes up the fourth group. These members are closely related to the mesembrine series (Herbert and Kattah, 1990), which comprises about 15 alkaloids, and is the largest subgroup. The stereochemistry of these isolated alkaloids was studied, and the two stereogenic centres of the sceletium alkaloid, (−)-mesembrine, were established by Denmark and Marcin (1997) through a total synthesis of the natural product. Using an optically active form of D-glucose as starting material, Ferrier's carbocyclisation was applied to yield (−)-mesembranol, as described by Chida et al. (1997). The stereochemistry of the quaternary carbon was achieved by Claisen rearrangement of the cyclohexenol intermediate. Sceletium A4 was first synthesised in an enantio-controlled manner, starting from a chiral cyclohexadienone synthon (Kamikubo and Ogasawara, 1998). The chiral 2,3,4-trioxycyclopentanone was used as a building block and transformed enantioselectively into a 4,4-disubstituted cyclohexenone derivative (Hayashi et al., 2002), to give rise to the mesembrine alkaloids. The absolute stereochemistry of the mesembrine-type alkaloids was confirmed through X-ray crystallography of 6-epimesembranol methiodide and (−)-MHCl (mesembrine hydrochloride) (Krstenansky, 2017). The stereochemistry was in agreement with the assignment of mesembrine, based on investigations using NMR spectroscopy and circular dichroism. More recently, Veale et al. (2018) isolated and elucidated channaine from *M. tortuosum.* The unusual cage-like ring structure was confirmed by X-ray crystallographic analysis.

There has been some speculation in the literature on whether the traditional method of preparation, involving fermentation, changes the alkaloid profile. Smith et al. (1998) simulated the traditional fermentation process by bruising plant material in the presence of some soil and sealing this in a plastic bag for a few days. The alkaloid content of plant samples, before and after fermentation under controlled conditions, was determined by Patnala and Kanfer (2009). Pure MHCl was treated in the same way. Results indicated that mesembrine was converted to Δ^7-mesembrenone, since the mesembrine content (1.33%) decreased to 0.05% after fermentation, whilst the concentration of Δ^7-mesembrenone (below the limit of quantification) increased to 0.11% on the 10th day. A similar transformation of pure MHCl took place in aqueous solutions, but it was not affected when dissolved in methanol. Sunlight and exposure to water seemed to enhance transformation. Solutions of MHCl that were kept in the dark remained stable, thereby confirming the findings. Chen and Viljoen (2019) compared the effect of fermenting *M. tortuosum* on the alkaloid composition using a validated UPLC–MS method. They reported that the mesembrenol and mesembranol concentrations remained unchanged after fermentation, while mesembrenone decreased from 8.0–33.0 to 1.3–32.7 μg/mL. In direct contrast to results reported by Patnala and Kanfer (2009), Roscher et al. (2012) and Smith et al. (1998). Chen and Viljoen (2019) reported an increase in mesembrine concentration after fermentation (from not detected-1.6 μg/mL to 7.4–20.8 μg/mL). The study of Chen and Viljoen was the only one of the four studies that analysed a fermented and unfermented portion of the same plant, used genetically similar plant material for triplicate analysis, in addition to using a validated quantitative method.

Characteristic markers for fingerprinting by high-performance liquid chromatography (HPLC) were isolated and identified by Patnala and Kanfer (2010). An HPLC method was validated for the determination of Δ^7-mesembrenone, mesembranol, mesembrenone, mesembrine and epimesembranol in '*Sceletium*' plant material. Other techniques were also used to develop quality control methods, such as a high-performance thin-layer chromatography (HPTLC) densitometric method developed by Shikanga et al. (2012c), for the simultaneous determination of mesembrenol, mesembranol, mesembrine and mesembrenone in raw materials and commercial products containing *M. tortuosum.* Good resolution of the compounds of interest was achieved using a single mobile phase. The quantitative densitometric method was validated for linearity, accuracy and precision. The limits of detection and quantification were determined. A good correlation of the analytical results with those from gas chromatography–mass spectrometry (GC–MS) analysis was reported. Shikanga et al. (2012d) went on to develop and validate UPLC-PDA and GC–MS methods for the determination of mesembrine-type alkaloids. The developed methods were found to be acceptable for the routine quality control of the alkaloids in raw materials and products, as reflected by the recoveries, precision, and the limits of detection and quantification achieved. The same group established an HSI technique to distinguish *Sceletium* species (Shikanga et al., 2013). Ultra-performance liquid chromatography (UPLC) and HSI, in combination with chemometric analysis, were successfully applied to not only distinguish species, but also to predict the identity of an unknown specimen, using the chemometric model, with high accuracy.

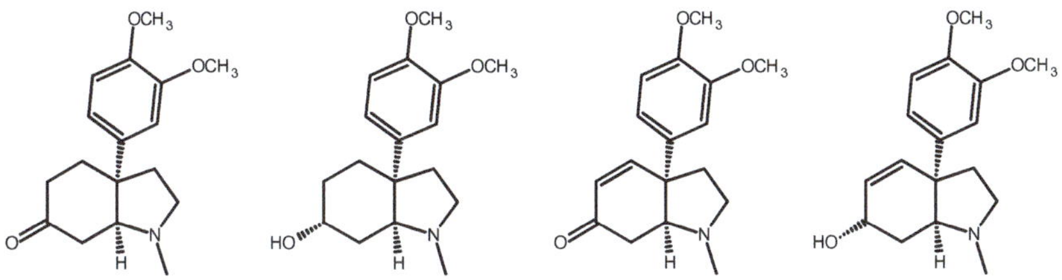

(-)-Mesembrine (-)-Mesembranol (-)-Mesembrenone (-)-Mesembrenol

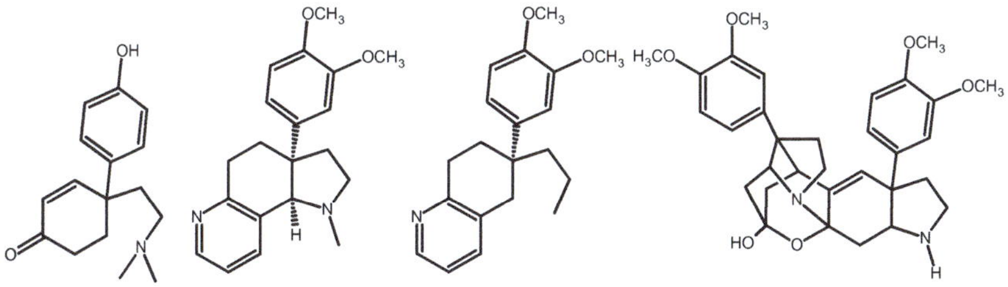

Joubertiamine (+)-Sceletium A4 alkaloid (+)-Tortuosamine Channaine

Part B: Chemical profiling and quality control

10. Chromatography analysis

10.1 High-performance thin-layer chromatography (HPTLC) fingerprint analysis

General instrumentation: CAMAG HPTLC instrument consisting of an automatic TLC sampler (ATS 4), automatic developing chamber (ADC 2), a Digistore Reprostar 3 (digital imaging device), chromatogram immersion device, and TLC plate heater. *HPTLC plates:* Silica gel glass plates 60 F_{254} (Merck). *Plant part:* Leaves and twigs, acid/base extract. *Sample application:* Application volume of 10 μL extract (20 mg/mL in methanol) and standards (1 mg/mL) spotted as 10 mm bands. Plates developed in a 20×10×4cm glass twin-trough chamber to a migration distance of 70mm. *Tank saturation:* 20min at 15°C and 33% RH, with 25mL of the mobile phase. *Mobile phase:* Toluene:ethyl acetate:methanol:ammonia (30:30:15:1, v/v/v/v). *Derivatisation:* Dragendorff reagent. The plate is sprayed with 3mL of Dragendorff reagent, followed by cooling for 3min at room temperature and then visualised. *Visualisation:* The plate was viewed under white reflectance light.

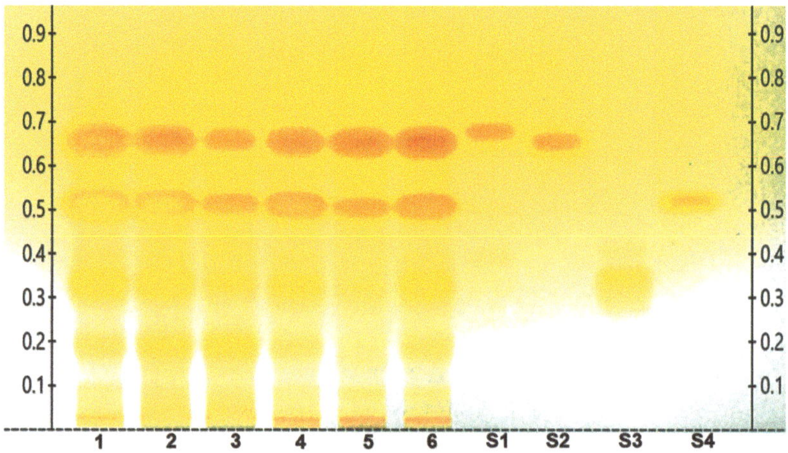

HPTLC plate of *Mesembryanthemum tortuosum* acid/base extracts (n=6) (1–6) and the standards (S1–S4). The samples are characterised by mesembrine (S1) (R_f=0.68), mesembrenone (S2) (R_f=0.66), mesembranol (S3) (R_f=0.34) and mesembrenol (S4) (R_f=0.52).

10.2 Ultra-performance liquid chromatography (UPLC) analysis

General instrumentation: Waters Acquity Ultra-Performance Liquid Chromatography system with photodiode array (PDA) detector combined with a Xevo G2QToF mass spectrometer (Waters, USA). *Plant part:* Leaves and twigs, acid/base extract. *Sample application:* Injection volume of 1.0 µL (full-loop injection) at 1mg/mL. *Column:* Acquity UPLC BEH C_{18} column (150mm×2.1mm, i.d., 1.7 µm particle size, Waters). *Mobile phase:* 0.1% ammonium hydroxide in water (solvent A) and 90% acetonitrile (solvent B). *Analysis conditions:* Gradient elution at a flow rate of 0.3mL/min, changing as follows: 80% A: 20% B, changed to 60% A: 40% B in 2min, to 50% B over 4.5min, back to initial ratio in 0.2min, equilibrating the system for 1.8min, total run time 8min. *Mass spectrometry*: ESI^+ (positive ionisation mode), N_2 used as desolvation gas, desolvation temperature 350°C at a flow rate of 500L/h, and source temperature at 100°C. Capillary and cone voltages, 3000 and 38V, respectively. Data collected between *m/z* 100 and 1200.

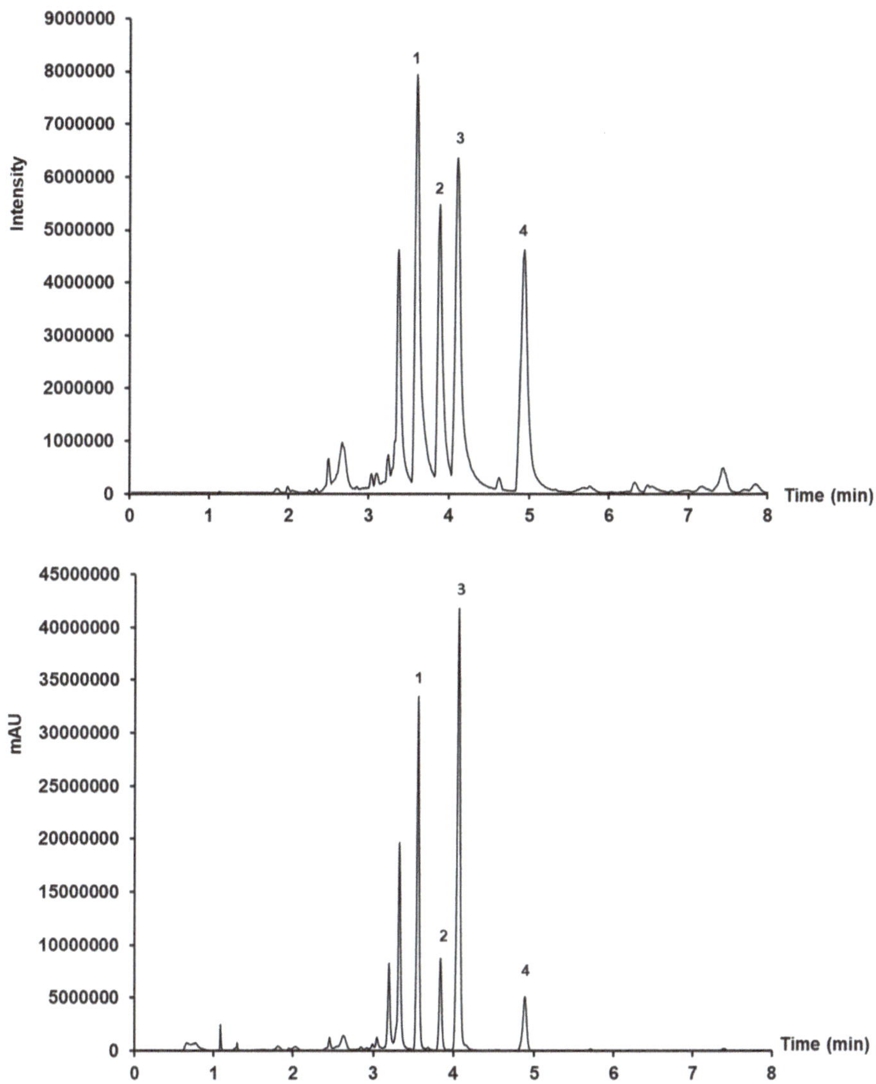

UPLC-ToF-MS ESI$^+$ (upper) and PDA (lower) chromatograms of *Mesembryanthemum tortuosum* acid/base extract: [1] = mesembrenol *m/z* 290.1678, [2] = mesembranol *m/z* 292.1834, [3] = mesembrenone *m/z* 288.1521, [4] = mesembrine *m/z* 290.1678.

11. Mid-infrared (MIR) spectroscopy analysis

General instrumentation: Alpha-P Bruker spectrometer, mounted with an attenuated total reflectance (ATR) diamond crystal. *Spectral acquisition:* Spectrum obtained in absorbance mode, with a spectral resolution of 4 cm^{-1} over the range 4000–550 cm^{-1} and captured using OPUS 6.5 software. *Plant part:* Leaves and twigs *Sample preparation:* Leaves and twigs powdered, sieved (< 500 µm), and placed directly onto the surface of the diamond crystal.

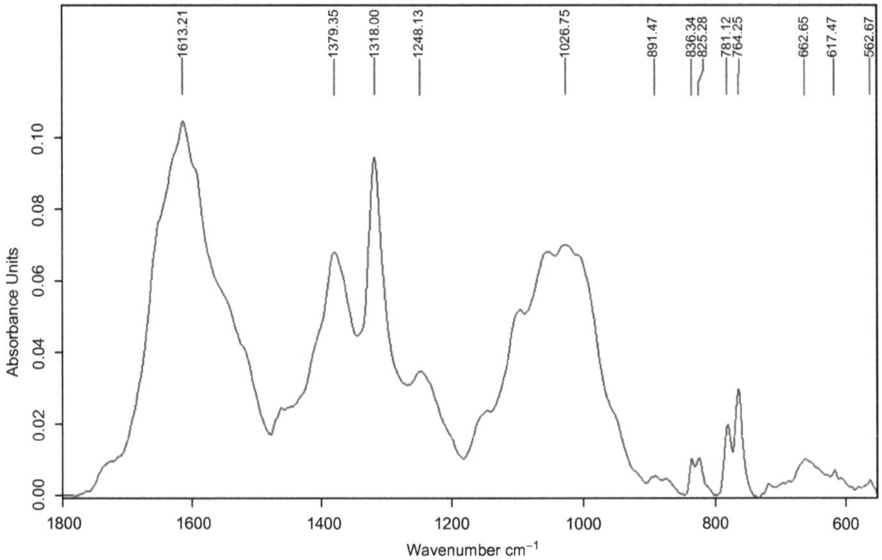

Mid-infrared spectrum of *Mesembryanthemum tortuosum* powder displaying the fingerprint region (1800–550 cm^{-1}).

References

Arndt, R.R., Kruger, P.E.J., 1970. Tetrahedron Lett., 37:3237–3240.

Bennett, A.C., Smith, C., 2018. J. Ethnopharmacol., 214:134–140.

Bennett, A.C., Van Camp, A., López, V., Smith, C., 2018. J. Physiol. Biochem., 74:539–547.

Bryant, A.T., 1966. Zulu Medicine and Medicine-Men. Struik, Cape Town, South Africa.

Carpenter, J.M., Jourdan, M.K., Fountain, E.M., Ali, Z., Abe, M., Khan, I.A., Sufta, K.J., 2017. J. Ethnopharmacol., 193:329–332.

Chen, W., Viljoen, A.M., 2019. S. Afr. J. Bot., 122:543–546.

Chida, N., Sugihara, K., Amano, S., Ogawa, S., 1997. J. Chem. Soc. Perkin Trans., 1(3):275–280.

Chiu, S., Cernovsky, Z., Gericke, N., Farina-Woodbury, M., Antongiorgi, J., Badmaev, V., Raheb, H., Terpstra, K., Bureau, Y., Hou, J., Sanchez, V., Williams, M., Goble, L., Copen, J., Husni, M., 2014. Evid. Based Complement. Alternat. Med., 2014, Art. No. 682014.

Coetzee, D.D., López, V., Smith, C., 2016. J. Ethnopharmacol., 177:111–116.

Denmark, S.E., Marcin, L.R., 1997. J. Org. Chem., 62:1675–1686.

Dimpfel, W., Schombert, L., Gericke, N., 2016a. J. Ethnopharmacol., 177:140–147.

Dimpfel, W., Gericke, N., Suliman, S., Dipah, G.N.C., 2016b. Neurosci. Med., 7:114–132.

Gerbaulet, M., 1996. Bot. Jahrb., 118:9–24.

Gericke, N., Van Wyk, B.-E., 1997. Pharmaceutical Compositions Containing Mesembrine and Related Compounds (Filed 3 June). PCT/GB97/ 01493.

Gericke, N., Van Wyk, B.-E., 1999. Pharmaceutical Compositions Containing Mesembrine and Related Compounds. US Patent 6,288,104.

Gericke, N., Viljoen, A., 2008. J. Ethnopharmacol., 119:653–663.
Harvey, A.L., Young, L.C., Viljoen, A.M., Gericke, N.P., 2011. J. Ethnopharmacol., 137:1124–1129.
Hayashi, M., Unno, T., Takahashi, M., Ogasawara, K., 2002. Tetrahedron Lett., 43:1461–1464.
Herbert, R.B., Kattah, A.E., 1990. Tetrahedron Lett., 46:7105–7118.
Hirabayashi, M., Ichikawa, K., Fukushima, R., Uchino, T., Shimada, H., 2002. J. Small Anim. Pract., 21:109–113.
Hirabayashi, M., Ichikawa, K., Yoshi, A., Uchino, T., Shimada, K., 2004. J. Small Anim. Pract., 23:85–89.
Houslay, M.D., Schafer, P., Zhang, K.Y., 2005. Drug Discov. Today, 15:11503–11519.
Jackson, W.P.U., 1990. Origins and Meanings of Names of South African Plant Genera. University of Cape Town, Ecolab, Cape Town, South Africa.
Jeffs, P.W., Capps, T., Johnson, D.B., Karle, J.M., Martin, N.H., Rauckman, B., 1974. J. Org. Chem., 39:2703–2710.
Kamikubo, T., Ogasawara, K., 1998. Chem. Commun., 7:783–784.
Kapewangolo, P., Tawha, T., Nawinda, T., Knott, M., Hans, R., 2016. S. Afr. J. Bot., 106:140–143.
Krstenansky, J.L., 2017. J. Ethnopharmacol., 195:10–19.
Lesiak, A.D., Cody, R.B., Ubukata, M., Musah, R.A., 2016. Forensic Sci. Int., 260:66–73.
Loria, M.J., Ali, Z., Abe, N., Sufka, K.J., Khan, I.A., 2014. J. Ethnopharmacol., 155:731–735.
Lubbe, A., Khatib, A., Yuliana, N.D., Jinap, S., Verpoorte, R., 2010. Int. Food Res. J., 17:349–355.
Manda, V.K., Avula, B., Ashfaq, M.K., Abe, N., Khan, I.A., Khan, S.I., 2017. Biomed. Chromatogr., 31 (3), Art. No. e3815.
Meiring, I., 1898. Trans. S. African Philos. Soc., 9:48–50.
Meyer, G.M.J., Wink, C.S.D., Zapp, J., Maurer, H.H., 2015. Anal. Bioanal. Chem., 407:761–778.
Murbach, T.S., Hirka, G., Szakonyine, I.P., Gericke, N., Endres, J.R., 2014. Food Chem. Toxicol., 74:190–199.
Napoletano, M., Fraire, C., Santangelo, F., Moriggi, E., 2001. Chemistry Preprint Archive. Cambridge University Press, Cambridge, UK, pp. 303–308.
Nell, H., Siebert, M., Chellan, P., Gericke, N., 2013. J. Altern. Complement. Med. (N.Y.), 19:898–904.
Pappe, L., 1868. *Mesembryanthemum tortuosum* Lin. In: Florae Capensis Medicae Prodromus; or, an Enumeration of South African Plants Used as Remedies by the Colonists of the Cape of Good Hope, third ed., Paragraph 39, page 17. W. Britain, Bureau Street, Cape Town, South Africa.
Patnala, S., Kanfer, I., 2008. J. Pharm. Biomed. Anal., 48:440–446.
Patnala, S., Kanfer, I., 2009. J. Ethnopharmacol., 121:86–91.
Patnala, S., Kanfer, I., 2010. J. Pharm. Pharm. Sci., 13:558–570.
Popelak, A., Lettenbauer, G., Haack, E., Spingler, H., 1960. Naturwissenschaften, 47:231–232.
Roscher, J., Posch, T.N., Pŭtz, M., Huhn, C., 2012. Electrophoresis, 33:1567–1570
Sandasi, M., Chen, W., Vermaak, I., Viljoen, A., 2018. Phytochem. Lett., 24:94–101.
Shikanga, E.A., Viljoen, A.M., Combrinck, S., Marston, A., Gericke, M., 2012a. Biochem. Syst. Ecol., 44:364–373.
Shikanga, E.A., Hamman, J.H., Chen, W., Combrinck, S., Gericke, N., Viljoen, A.M., 2012b. Planta Med., 78:260–268.

Shikanga, E.A., Vermaak, I., Viljoen, A.M., 2012c. J. Planar Chromatogr.–Mod. TLC, 25:283–289.

Shikanga, E.A., Kamatou, G.P.P., Chen, W., Combrinck, S., Viljoen, A.M., 2012d. S. Afr. J. Bot., 82:99–107.

Shikanga, E.A., Viljoen, A.M., Vermaak, I., Combrinck, S., 2013. Phytochem. Anal., 24:550–555.

Smith, C., 2011. J. Ethnopharmacol., 133:31–36.

Smith, M.T., Crouch, N.R., Gericke, N., Hirst, M., 1996. J. Ethnopharmacol., 150:119–130.

Smith, M.T., Field, C.R., Crouch, N.R., Hirst, M., 1998. Pharm. Biol., 36:173–179.

Snyckers, F.O., Strelow, F., Wiechers, A., 1971. J. Chem. Soc. D, 1467–1469.

Swart, A.C., Smith, C., 2016. J. Ethnopharmacol., 177:35–45.

Terburg, D., Syal, S., Rosenberger, L.A., Heany, S., Phillips, N., Gericke, N., Stein, D.J., Van Honk, J., 2013. Neuropsychopharmacology, 38:2708–2716.

Van Wyk, B.-E., 2011. S. Afr. J. Bot., 77:812–829.

Van Wyk, B.-E., Gericke, N., 2003. People's Plants. Briza Publications, Pretoria, South Africa.

Veale, C.G.L., Chen, W., Chaudhary, S., Kituyi, S.N., Isaacs, M., Hoppe, H., Edkins, A.L., Combrinck, S., Mehari, B., Viljoen, A., 2018. Phytochem. Lett., 23:189–193.

Watt, J.M., Breyer-Brandwijk, M.G., 1962. The Medicinal and Poisonous Plants of Southern and Eastern Africa, second ed. E. & S. Livingstone Ltd, Edinburgh and London, UK.

Weniger, B., Italiano, L., Beck, J.P., Bastida, J., Bergonon, S., Codina, C., Lobstein, A., Anton, R., 1995. Planta Med., 61:77–79.

Zhao, J., Khan, I.A., Combrinck, S., Sandasi, M., Chen, W., Viljoen, A.M., 2018. Phytochemistry, 152:191–203.

Zwicky, E., 1915. Vierteljahrsschr. Nat. Ges. Zur., 58:372–429.

CHAPTER

Pelargonium graveolens 18

Maxleene Sandasi[a,b], Guy Kamatou[a] and Nduvho Mulaudzi[a]

[a]*Department of Pharmaceutical Sciences, Tshwane University of Technology, Pretoria, South Africa*

[b]*SAMRC Herbal Drugs Research Unit, Faculty of Science, Tshwane University of Technology, Pretoria, South Africa*

Abstract

Pelargonium graveolens L'Her. (Geraniaceae), generally known as 'rose geranium', is an aromatic, erect plant that can reach a height of 1.3 m. The young plants have soft, succulent and hairy stems that become woody as the plant ages. The rose-scented leaves have deeply indented margins. The plant's distribution covers Mozambique, Zimbabwe, and the Limpopo and Eastern Cape provinces of South Africa. The aerial parts have been widely used in various traditional medicine systems to reduce general pain and inflammation, as well as for managing anxiety. The aromatic nature of the plant affords its various therapeutic properties that include relaxant, sedative, anxiolytic, antidepressant calming and tension-relieving effects. The plant aids to relieve premenstrual and menopausal problems, poor blood circulation, nausea, tonsilitis and gastro-intestinal disorders. Pelargonium graveolens produces a well-known commercialised essential oil, rose geranium. The global demand for rose geranium oil is high, as it a good substitute for the expensive rose oil in the fragrance industry. Pharmacological in vitro and in vivo studies of the oils and extracts of geranium have been conducted, including its anti-oxidant, antimicrobial and anti-inflammatory activities. Citronellol, geraniol, linalool, isomethone, citronellyl formate, geranyl formate and guaia-6,9-diene are marker constituents of the oils, and were identified by gas chromatography coupled to mass spectrometry (GC–MS). The presence of linalool and geraniol in the oil was also confirmed by semi-automated high-performance thin-layer chromatography (HPTLC).

Keywords: *Pelargonium graveolens*, Rose geranium, Essential oil, Geraniol, Citronellol, GC–MS, HPTLC, MIR spectroscopy

The South African Herbal Pharmacopoeia. https://doi.org/10.1016/B978-0-323-99794-2.00022-2

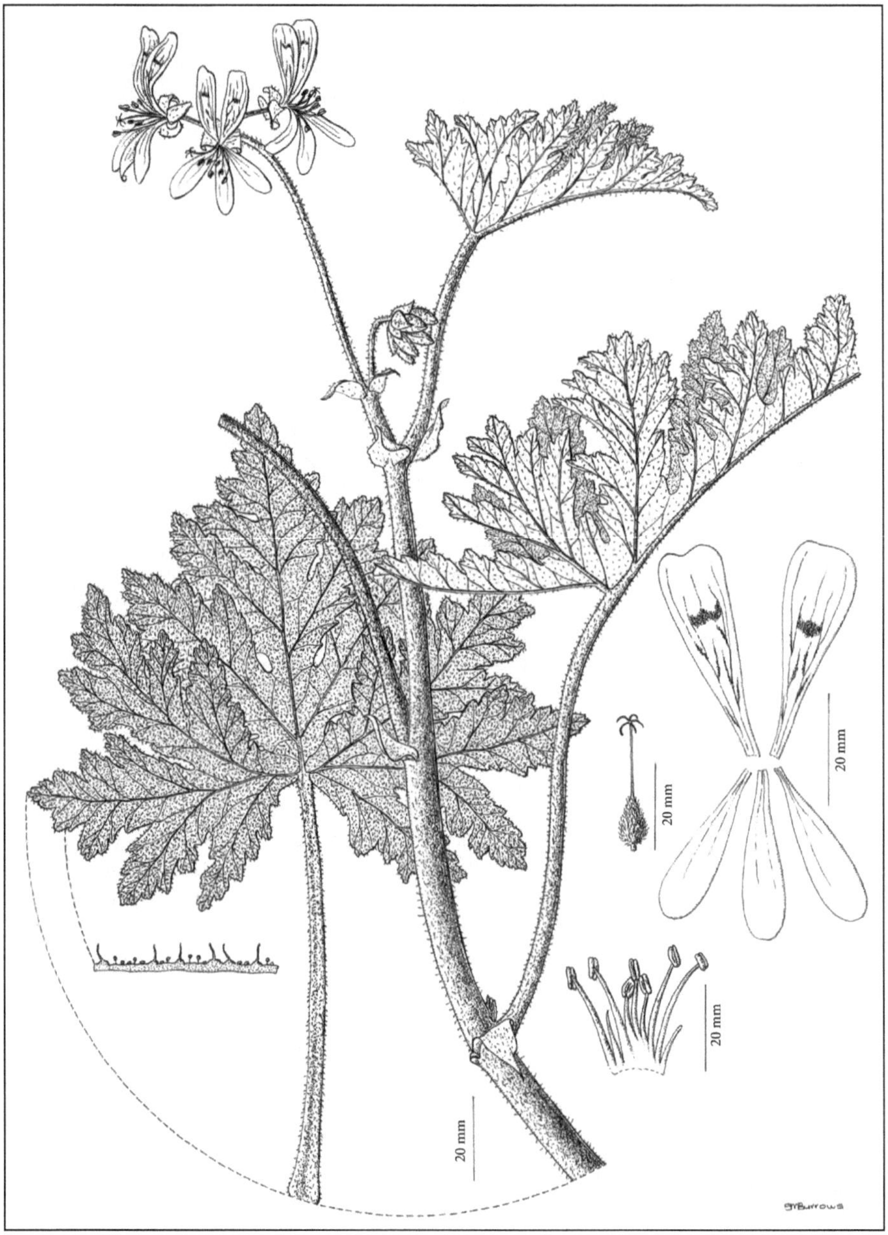
20 mm
20 mm
20 mm
20 mm

Part A: General overview

1. Synonyms

Pelargonium intermedium R.Knuth.[a]

2. Common name(s)

Rose-scented pelargonium, sweet-scented geranium, rose geranium (English), '*malva*', '*wildemalva*' (Afrikaans).

3. Conservation status

Least concern.[a]

4. Botany

Pelargonium graveolens (Geraniaceae) is one of over 200 natural species within the genus *Pelargonium*. The genus name is derived from the word '*pelargos*' (Greek) meaning stork, which refers to the similarities between the fruits of the plants and the beak of the bird. The species name '*graveolens*' (Latin) refers to the strong scent of the leaves. *Pelargonium graveolens* is an erect plant with multiple branches, which can reach a height of 1.3 m and 1 m in width (A). The young plants have soft, succulent and hairy stems that become woody as the plant ages. The rose-scented leaves have deeply indented margins (B), and are populated with numerous glandular hairs on the

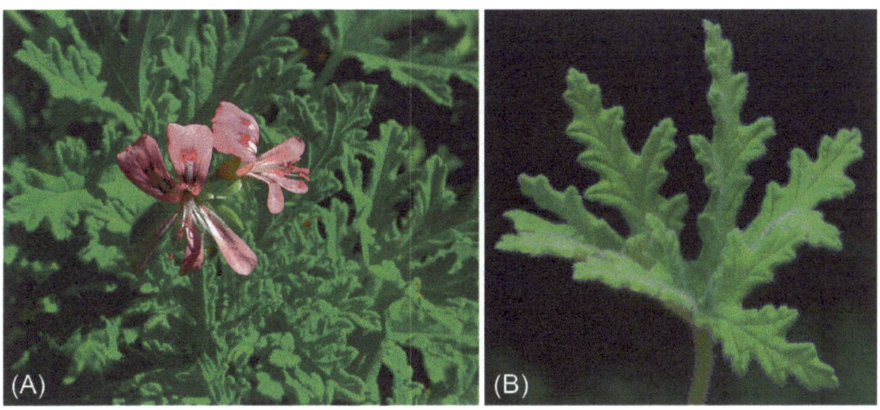

Pelargonium graveolens plant showing bright pink five-petalled flowers (A) and large, hairy leaves (B) that have deeply indented margins.

[a] Redlist of South African Plants (http://redlist.sanbi.org).

surface, giving them a velvety feel. The small five-petalled flowers are pinkish-white in colour and are borne in an umbel-like inflorescence (A) (Lis-Balchin, 2002).

5. Geographical distribution

Pelargonium species are native to southern Africa, where *P. graveolens* is disjunctly distributed in the northern and southern parts of the region. In the northern parts, its distribution covers Mozambique, Zimbabwe, and the Limpopo and Eastern Cape provinces of South Africa (Van der Walt and Demarne, 1988). The species, which is also located in the coastal areas, occurs in the south-eastern parts of the Western Cape Province (Lis-Balchin, 2002). The plant is also reported to occur in the Eastern Cape regions of Port Elizabeth (Gqeberha) and Grahamstown (Makhanda) (Van der Walt and Demarne, 1988). These areas receive an annual rainfall of ±700 mm. The plant grows in mountainous areas or semishaded areas, often close to water bodies.

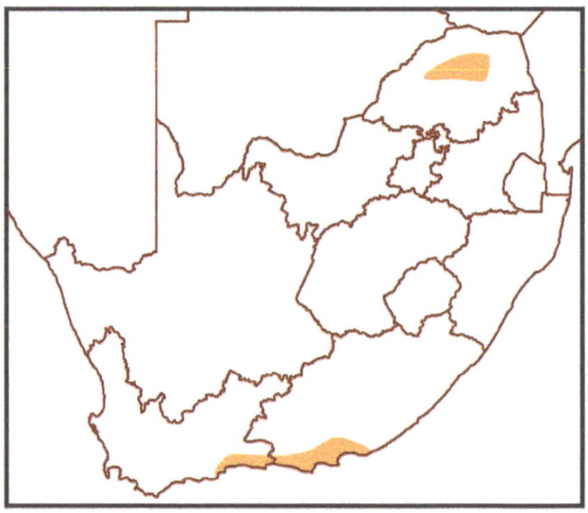

Geographical distribution of *Pelargonium graveolens* in South Africa.

6. Ethnopharmacology

The aerial parts of this aromatic plant have been widely used in various traditional medicine systems throughout the world. Steeping the leaves in hot water gives a tea that is used to reduce general pain and inflammation, as well as to manage anxiety (Asgarpanah and Ramezanloo, 2015). The aromatic nature of the plant affords it various therapeutic properties that include relaxant, sedative, anxiolytic, antidepressant, antistress, calming and tension-relieving effects. The plant aids to relieve premenstrual and menopausal problems, poor blood circulation, nausea, tonsilitis and gastro-intestinal disorders (Bown, 1995). Other topical applications include treatment of haemorrhoids, acne, eczema, bruises, ringworm, lice, wounds and nerve pain, and as an antiseptic or astringent (Bown, 1995). A report on the use of the plant to treat jaundice and gall stones, and to restrain nose bleeding, has been documented.

7. Commercialisation

France is the pioneer in the commercialisation of rose geranium, conducting the first distillation trials in 1819 in Lyon, and then establishing the first plantation in 1844 in Grasse (Gildemeister and Hoffmann, 1900). Production was then delocalised to Algeria in 1847 and the Reunion Island (1880), which became the largest producer with the most preferred Bourbon-type variety (citronellol:geraniol ratio ≈ 1:1). Reunion Island has since scaled down production, enabling other countries to enter the geranium oil market. Kenya, Spain, Egypt, Morocco, Belgium, the Democratic Republic of the Congo and Russia are among some of the countries that attempted commercial production of geranium oil. There are four major international competitors, namely South Africa, India, China and Egypt (DAFF, 2012). China is one of the main producers, with a rose-scented Chinese variety that is less preferred compared to the Bourbon type. The Kelkar (Egyptian) variety, produced in the Bani Sweif and Fayoum regions of Egypt, is equally accessible on the international market, with production now surpassing that of China. The K99 and Kelkar varieties have been produced by India; however, the domestic market absorbs most of India's production. This is also the case in Brazil and Russia. The Reunion Island, Madagascar, Israel, Morocco, Algeria and South Africa contribute a lower proportion to the international market (Blerot et al., 2016). The plant is also cultivated to a lesser extent in Central Africa, Japan, Central America and Europe. In South Africa, rose geranium is mostly grown commercially in the Mpumalanga, KwaZulu-Natal, Western Cape and the Free State provinces. The oil produced meets the 'Bourbon-type' standard and thus trades well on the international market (DAFF, 2012). The main importers of rose geranium oil are France and the United States, with France believed to import fine fragrance. The global demand for rose geranium essential oil is high, as it is a good substitute for the expensive rose oil in the fragrance industry.

8. Pharmacological evaluation

8.1 *In vitro* studies

8.1.1 Antimicrobial activity

The antimicrobial activity of *P. graveolens* essential oil and constituents is well documented. In one study, the effect of geranium oil and its constituent compounds on the growth of *Colletrotrichum gloesporoides,* a fruit fungus that causes anthracnose, was investigated (Chandravadana and Nidiry, 1994). Both geraniol and citronellol were highly active (100% growth inhibition) towards the fungus compared to the parent oil (60% inhibition) at 250 ppm. Linalool displayed the lowest activity (8% inhibition) towards the same plant pathogen. A synergistic antifungal interaction between geranium oil (or its major compounds) and ketoconazole against *Trichophyton schoenleinii* and *T. soudanense* was observed by Shin and Lim (2004). A similar synergistic or additive effect was reported when the oil or its major compounds (geraniol, citronellol, linalool and menthone) were combined with antibiotics (erythromycin, norfloxacin or oxacillin), and tested against antibiotic-resistant and -susceptible strains of *Streptococcus pneumoniae* (Choi et al., 2007). The best synergistic interaction was observed for the citronellol and norfloxacin combination, which recorded a fractional inhibitory concentration (FIC) of 0.16. Combining *P. graveolens* oil, geraniol, citronellol or linalool with oxacillin, norfloxacin or erythromycin, gave FIC values between 0.16 and 1.50, indicating enhanced antifungal activity in the presence of these natural compounds. Individually, geraniol and citronellol displayed moderate activity with minimum inhibitory concentrations (MICs) of 1 mg/mL, compared to geranium oil (1–2 mg/mL), linalool (4–8 mg/mL), and menthone (4–8 mg/mL) towards all the tested strains. A synergistic effect was also observed when *P. graveolens* oil was used in combination with ciprofloxacin against the uropathogens *Klebsiella pneumoniae* (fractional inhibitory concentration index, FICI = 0.375), *Proteus mirabilis* (FICI = 0.375) and *Staphylococcus aureus* (FICI = 0.5) (Malik et al., 2011).

Singh et al. (2008) reported the antifungal activity of *P. graveolens* essential oil towards two aflatoxigenic strains of *Aspergillus flavus*, with 100% growth inhibition at 1.0 mg/mL, an MIC of 0.75 mg/mL, and fungistatic activity (up to 1.0 mg/mL) against both strains. The results demonstrated that the oil was more efficacious as a fungitoxicant compared to other synthetic fungicides studied. When further evaluated for its ability to inhibit aflatoxin B1 production, the oil (at 0.50 mg/mL) inhibited aflatoxin B1 production completely. In a study by Sangeetha et al. (2010), the antifungal activity of geranium oil against the crown rot-causing pathogens, *Lasiodiplodia theobromae* and *Colletotrichum musae*, was confirmed, as the oil completely inhibited mycelial growth and cellulolytic and pectinolytic enzyme activities.

In a study to evaluate the effect of various essential oils on bacterial pathogenicity, geranium oil exhibited potent antiquorum sensing activity among other essential oils, towards selected *Chromobacterium violaceum* and *Escherichia coli* strains (Szabó et al., 2010). The oil also displayed good antimycotic activity against *Aspergillus flavus* (MIC = 0.1%), *A. niger* (MIC = 0.1%) and *Ascosphaera apis* (MIC = 0.025%) *in vitro* (Nardoni et al., 2018). When combined with three other oils, namely *Litsea cubeba*, *Cinnamomum zeylanicum* and *Cymbopogon flexuous* at 0.015% each, the mixture of four oils showed an additive effect (FICI = 0.6) towards all three pathogens. The antimicrobial effect of *P. graveolens* ethanolic extract was investigated against clinical isolates of *S. aureus* and the results displayed good antistaphylococcal activity, with MICs ranging from 0.2 to 0.8 mg/mL (Mahboubi et al., 2011). In another study, the antimicrobial and DNA cleavage effect of *P. graveolens* extract was investigated towards a range of pathogens, alone and in combination with Mn-Ni@Fe_3O_4 and Mn:$Fe(OH)_3$ nanoparticles (Dashamiri et al., 2018). The *P. graveolens* extract displayed good activity towards *Pseudomonas aeruginosa* and *S. aureus* (MIC = 0.78 mg/mL). When tested alone, and in combination with nanoparticles; good activity was observed towards *P. aeruginosa* with MICs = 0.78

and 0.39 mg/mL, for Mn-Ni@Fe_3O_4 and Mn:Fe$(OH)_3$ combinations, respectively. *Pelargonium graveolens*, in combination with Mn-Ni@Fe_3O_4, was able to degrade the DNA structure of *E. coli*. Szweda et al. (2018) reported satisfactory antistaphylococcal activity of geranium oil against a range of *S. aureus*, *S. epidermidis* and *S. xylosus* isolates with MICs ranging from 0.078% to 1.25% (v/v). The anti-*Malassezia* activity of *P. graveolens* essential oil was demonstrated against three *Malassezia* species of fungi, with a mean zone of inhibition of 26.1 mm, making the oil a potential natural candidate for the treatment of infections by *Pityriasis versicolor* (Naeini et al., 2011). Bigos et al. (2012) reported that geranium oil exhibited strong antistaphylococcal activity against 70 clinical isolates, including methicillin-resistant *S. aureus* (MRSA) strains, with an MIC range of 0.25–2.50 μL/mL. Bouzenna and Krichen (2013) investigated the antifungal and insecticidal activities of *P. graveolens* oil against *Rhizoctonia solani* and *Rhysoperta dominica*, respectively. The oil displayed 74.41% growth inhibition towards the fungus at 12.5 μL/mL, while a dose-dependent insecticidal effect was observed, with 100% mortality recorded after 15, 17 and 21 days, following exposure to 50, 12 and 3 μL/20 mL of the essential oil, respectively.

The efficacy of five essential oils was investigated against *Acinetobacter baumannii* isolated from patients. Essential oil isolated from *P. graveolens* was not as effective (MIC = 1.1 μL/mL) as the other oils used individually (MICs 0.7 μL/mL). However, when combined with amikacin, the *P. graveolens* oil showed the best synergistic activity with FICI = 0.23 (Mahboubi et al., 2014). When evaluated for its ability to inhibit the swarming ability of the urinary *P. mirabilis* pathogen, the oil dose-dependently reduced the colony diameter of the pathogen at concentrations ranging from 1.12 to 8.96 mg/mL (Malik et al., 2015). Furthermore, when compared to the negative control, which showed five concentric rings, the oil was able to reduce the number of concentric rings to two at concentrations of 8.96 and 4.48 mg/mL.

In an effort to identify natural biocides for use against stored grain fungal pathogens, the effect of *P. graveolens* oil on 11 fungal isolates (four *Aspergillus* spp., five *Eurotium* spp., and two *Penicillium* spp.) was investigated (Juárez et al., 2016). The results demonstrated that the oil exhibits strong antifungal activity towards all the tested isolates, with MICs ranging from 0.3 to 50 μg/mL. Another study investigated the antifungal effects of various essential oils (15), including *P. graveolens*, on the planktonic and biofilm forms of *Candida tropicalis* (Souza et al., 2016). *Pelargonium graveolens* oils exhibited the strongest antifungal effect against the planktonic form with MIC = 125 μg/mL across all nine tested isolates. The results demonstrate the potential antibiofilm effects of the oil and its major constituents, geraniol and linalool, in preventing the growth and development of *C. tropicalis* biofilm. In a study where the antifungal effect of six essential oils was tested on two seed-borne pathogens of rice, namely *Fusarium moniliforme* and *Helminthosporium oryzae,* geranium oil displayed antifungal activity (MIC = 0.1%) against both pathogens, as did *Cymbopogon citratus* and *C. martinii* (Muthukumar et al., 2016).

As biofilms are linked to resistant microbial infections, geranium oil has been investigated for its ability to arrest biofilm growth and development in some clinical isolates of *Candida* species, growing on surfaces (Giongo et al., 2016). The oil, tested in both its free form and as a nano-emulsion formulation (NEG), displayed good antifungal activity against planktonic *C. albicans* (MICs of 1.82 and 3.64 µg/mL, respectively) and *C. tropicalis* (MICs of 1.82 and 7.29 µg/mL, respectively), compared to the other two strains. Both geranium oil and NEG significantly prevented biofilm formation on the polyethylene surface in all tested species; however, the NEG displayed better activity than the oil for *C. albicans, C. tropicalis* and *C. glabrata* (Giongo et al., 2016).

Essid et al. (2017) profiled the antifungal activities of selected essential oils and compounds against *Candida* species, individually, and in combination with conventional antifungal drugs. The authors further investigated the mechanisms of action, as well as the inhibitory potential towards aspartic proteases, believed to contribute to virulence and pathogenicity. Although *P. graveolens* oil displayed low activity (MIC range 250–1000 µg/mL) when compared to the other oils, a better interaction was observed when combined with *Thymus capitatus* (FIC = 0.5), while all the other oil combinations did not show synergy. *Pelargonium graveolens* oil combined with fluconazole showed the highest synergistic interaction with FIC = 0.37, and the osmoprotectant assay revealed that the possible mechanism of action for the oil/drug combination is the disruption of the permeability barrier of the fungal cell wall. Both the *P. graveolens* oil and its combination with fluconazole exhibited strong inhibitory effects (80.35% and 78.31%, respectively) against aspartic proteases.

A study evaluated the fungicidal activity of six essential oils, including *P. graveolens*, against the wood-rot fungi, *Trametes hirsuta* and *Laetiporus sulphureus* (Xie et al., 2017). The results indicated weaker antifungal activity for *P. graveolens* oil, requiring a dose of 400 µg/mL to reach a 100% antifungal index against both pathogens, compared to ≤200 µg/mL for the other oils. An investigation into the effect of compositional variation in geranium oil on its antifungal potential was conducted using six different geranium oils of varying geraniol and citronellol content (Mahboubi et al., 2018). The oil samples with citronellol ranging from 7.7% to 43.7% and geraniol at 19.3%–48.5% did not display significant differences in their anticandidal activity (zone of inhibition (ZOI) range = 19.3–24.1 mm and MICs and MFCs = 1.06–1.48 µL/mL and 1.5–1.72 µL/mL, respectively). Diánez et al. (2018) further confirmed the antifungal activity of *P. graveolens* when tested against six plant pathogens and two mushroom pathogens. The oil was highly effective against five of the tested pathogens, with higher activity towards *Phytophthora parasitica, Sclerotinia sclerotiorum* and *Cladobotryum mycophilum*. In a study to evaluate the antifungal activity of geranium oils from different countries against five *Candida* species, the oil sample from South Africa (Laszlo) displayed the best antifungal activity towards most of the strains tested, with MICs of 128–256 µg/mL (Dos Santos et al., 2020). The active oil was then formulated into a nano-emulsion (NPG) and a hydrogel-thickened nano-emulsion (HCNPG), and further evaluated for antifungal activity against the same strains. The results showed that the HCNPG produced with chitosan displayed much better antifungal activity, with MICs as low as 8 µg/mL for *C. albicans* and *C. glabrata*, compared to NPG that did not result in an improvement in antifungal activity from the original essential oil.

8.1.2 Anti-inflammatory and anticancer activity

Three plant species, known in Brazil as malva (*Malva sylvestris*, and the leaves of *Sida cordifolia* and *P. graveolens*), were investigated for their anti-inflammatory properties *in vitro* (Martins et al., 2017). Crude ethanolic extracts and fractions (hexane, chloroform, ethyl acetate and the residual) of the aerial parts were assessed for their ability to inhibit the release of inflammatory mediators (PGE_2, PGD_2, TXB_2 and $PGF_{2\alpha}$) in cell culture medium, following stimulation with lipopolysaccharide (LPS). Although *P. graveolens* showed a potential inhibitory effect against secretion of prostanoids at 50 µg/mL, the other two malva plants displayed superior activity. The essential oil of *P. graveolens* was investigated for its anti-inflammmatory properties, among nine other oils in a pre-inflammed human dermal fibroblast system (Han et al., 2017). The *P. graveolens* oil at 0.01% was found to be significantly antiproliferative against the cell line used. Simões et al. (2018) described the estrogenicity potential of *P. graveolens* essential oil using the *in vitro* cancer cell growth and oestrogen reporter assays. The oil, together with *Cymbopogon martinii,* displayed marked estrogenicity, stimulating ER+ cell growth and ERE-luciferase reporter activity. In another study by El-Garawani et al. (2019), a mixture of geranium and fennel oils exhibited anticancer potential by triggering cell cycle arrest and apoptosis in MCF-7 cells, but was non-toxic towards normal peripheral blood lymphocytes.

8.1.3 Anti-oxidant activity

Pelargonium graveolens essential oil distilled from the aerial parts harvested at different phenological stages was investigated for anti-oxidant activity using the 2,2-diphenyl-1-picrylhydrazyl (DPPH) and 2,2′-azino-*bis*(3-ethylbenzthiazoline-6-sulphonic acid (ABTS) assays (Boukhris et al., 2015). The results demonstrated that the free radical scavenging activity of the oil varied depending on the stage of development, with the flowering stage demonstrating the best activity. In another study, a water extract of *P. graveolens* was fractionated to yield diethyl ether and ethyl acetate fractions, and the phenolic and flavonoid contents were determined alongside the DPPH radical scavenging activity (El Ouadi et al., 2017). The ethyl acetate fraction exhibited better anti-oxidant activity (IC_{50} = 1.49 µg/mL) compared to the diethyl ether (IC_{50} = 1.54 µg/mL) fraction, and the activity was observed to be concentration-dependent (0.2–2.0 µg/mL). This could be due to the higher flavonoid and polyphenol contents in the ethyl acetate fraction (29 ± 1.6 µg equivalent of rutin/mg extract and 437 ± 25 µg gallic acid equivalents (GAE)/mg extract, respectively) compared to the diethyl ether (12 ± 0.2 µg equivalent of rutin/mg extract and 400 ± 29 µg GAE/mg extract, respectively).

The *in vitro* anti-oxidant activity of five essential oils, namely geranium, peppermint, lemongrass, rosemary and bergamot, was evaluated *in vitro* using the DPPH and ferric reducing anti-oxidant power (FRAP) assays (Zardo et al., 2019). Chemical profiling revealed a monoterpene content of 80.5%–95.0% for the oils, and varying profiles. The anti-oxidant potential of the oils followed the order: lemongrass > peppermint > geranium > bergamot > rosemary, with radical scavenging activity ranging from 68.55% to 3.53%, determined using the DPPH assay, and 94.61–1.28 mmol Trolox equivalents (TE)/g when determined by the FRAP assay.

Lohani et al. (2019) determined the anti-oxidant and *in vitro* sun protection factor (SPF) of geranium and calendula oils for potential cosmeceutical applications. The nitric oxide scavenging activity of geranium oil was higher at 250 μg/mL (85.15% ± 0.09%), compared to calendula oil (72.48% ± 0.12%), as was the case with DPPH radical scavenging activity (85.51% ± 0.020% and 78.06% ± 0.04% for geranium and calendula oil, respectively). The reduction in the stable DPPH radical was achieved with IC_{50} = 10.38, 18.02 and 28.68 μg/mL for ascorbic acid, geranium and calendula oils, respectively. Spectrophotometric determination of the SPF revealed that both oils have poor SPF values (6.45 and 8.36 for geranium and calendula oils, respectively).

8.1.4 Antiviral activity

Three essential oils (lemongrass, geranium and vetiver grass) with known mosquito repellent properties were investigated for their antiviral activity against a Ross River virus (RRV) transmitted by mosquitoes (Ralambondrainy et al., 2018). Pretreatment of Vero cells with essential oils did not affect virus entry, as determined by the plaque assay, indicating non-virucidal activity. However, viral replication was inhibited prior or during viral adsorption by *P. graveolens* and *C. citratus*, including posttreatment (*P. graveolens*). Geranium oil demonstrated high anti-infective potential against RRV, with inhibitory effects worth noting when present prior, during or after infection.

8.2 *In vivo* studies and clinical trials

8.2.1 Wound-healing properties

The *in vivo* wound-healing potential of *P. graveolens* flowers and *Quercus brantii* fruits was determined in male Wistar rats (Lavasanijou et al., 2016). The *Q. brantii* extract exercabated wound healing, by speeding up the wound-contraction velocity, and resulted in a lower amount of fibrous-tissue formation and deformed scars. Although *P. graveolens* increased the wound-contraction velocity during the first few days, the rats achieved complete wound healing only after day 18, compared to 12 and 15 days for *Q. brantii* and the positive control, respectively.

8.2.2 Anaesthetic properties

The anaesthetic potential of geranium oil was demonstrated in two species of ornamental hap fish at varying oil concentrations, with a dose-dependent reduction in induction time and a dose-dependent increase in recovery time (Can et al., 2018). Deep anaesthesia occurred between 61.19 ± 7.25 and 165.43 ± 6.78 s for *Sciaenochromis fryeri* (electric blue hap), and 73.32 ± 8.92–171.12 ± 10.74 s for *Labidochromis caeruleus* (blue streak hap), while recovery occurred after 96 ± 6.87 s and 291.45 ± 8.31 s for *L. caeruleus* and *S. fryeri*, respectively.

8.2.3 Cosmetic properties

Geranium oil is applied to the skin for cosmetic purposes, and studies to confirm its cosmetic value have been documented. Kozlowska et al. (2017) investigated the ability to reduce excessive sebum production of cosmetic tonics containing *P. graveolens* and *Junipers communis* fruit oils, in a clinical trial. Sebum production data were captured using a Sebumeter® SM 815 probe, placed on the forehead of the participants at 10, 60 and 120 min posttonic application. The tonic containing 0.25% *P. graveolens* oil displayed better sebum-reducing potential, which was maintained for up to 2 h posttreatment (32, 40 and 44 absorption units (au), after 10, 60 and 120 min, respectively), compared to *J. communis* oil (30, 48 and 101 au, after 10, 60 and 120 min, respectively). The results of geranium oil were comparable to a known sebostatic, 3% niacinamide (44 and 58 au, after 60 and 120 min, respectively).

8.2.4 Acaricidal and insecticidal properties

Many aromatic plants are used as insect repellents due to the presence of highly odorous and bio-active volatile organic compounds. The insecticidal activity of various essential oils, including geranium oil, was investigated against the house fly (*Musca domestica*) (Pavela, 2008). *Pelargonium graveolens* was lethal at a dose of 19 µg/fly, while eight other oils were also lethal within the range 10–20 µg/fly. The highly active *Pogostemon cablin* essential oil was lethal at 3 µg/fly. The acaricidal activity of geranium oil and its constituents was also documented by Jeon et al. (2008). In the study, *P. graveolens* and its constituents were tested against the food mite, *Tyrophagus putrescentiae*, and the activity was compared to that of benzyl benzoate. The mite-control activity was determined using a modified impregnated-fabric disk method, and the half-maximal lethal dose (LD_{50}) was determined for each test compound. The results showed that the essential oil, geraniol, nerol and citral, were highly toxic towards *T. putrescentiae* with LD_{50}=4.17, 1.95, 2.21 and 9.65 µg/cm^3, respectively, compared to benzyl benzoate (11.27 µg/cm^3) and β-citronellol (15.86 µg/cm^3). The insect-repellent activity of 13 commercial oils was evaluated against *Leptotrombidium imphalum* larvae, the scrub typhus vector (Eamsobhana et al., 2009). Insect-repellent activity was assessed based on the ability of larvae to climb upward. The essential oil of *P. graveolens* exhibited low activity compared to other oils, as it achieved only 57.1% repellency in the undiluted form.

In a tick-repellency study, the ability of geranium oil and its constituents to repel the lone star tick, *Amblyomma americanum*, was evaluated (Tabanca et al., 2013). Using the vertical filter paper bio-assay, high tick repellence was observed for one of the geranium oils, which repelled more than 90% of the ticks at 0.103 mg/cm^2. Of the isolated compounds tested, (−)-10-epi-γ-eudesmol displayed the best activity, repelling 90% and 73.3% ticks at 0.103 and 0.052 mg of compound/cm^2 of impregnated filter paper, respectively. The compound displayed the same repellent activity as the positive control *N,N*-diethyl-*m*-toluamide (DEET) at ≥0.052 mg of compound/cm^2 of filter paper. Fanela et al. (2016) demonstrated the inhibition and the oviposition of the silverleaf whitefly (*Bemisia tabaci*) on tomato leaflets, by *P. graveolens*,

Piper callosum, *Adenocalymma alliaceum* and *Plectranthus neochilus* essential oils at 0.5% concentration. *Pelargonium graveolens* oil, as well as *J. communis*, *Z. officinale* and *C. aurantium* oils, displayed acaricidal activity towards the cattle tick (*Rhipicephalus microplus*), with 73% to 95% concentration-dependent efficacy (Pazinato et al., 2016). The oil of *P. graveolens* exhibited acute toxicity towards *Spodoptera frugiperda* larvae in a topical-application assay with $LD_{50}=1.13\,\mu g/mg$ per insect and $LD_{90}=2.56\,\mu g/mg$ per insect (Niculau et al., 2013). The oil constituents displayed better activity compared to the positive control Azamax®, with mortality scores of 90%, 84%, 64% and 30% for linalool, carvone, citral and geraniol, respectively.

8.2.5 Anti-oxidant and anti-inflammatory effects

The *in vivo* anti-oxidant and anti-inflammatory activities of *P. graveolens* and *Syzygium aromaticum* essential oils, used individually and in combination, were investigated (Marmouzi et al., 2019). The results demonstrated good anti-oxidant activity for *P. graveolens* and the essential oil combination in the protozoa model (*Tetrahymena pyriformis*), and good anti-inflammatory activity in the carrageenan-induced oedema model (Marmouzi et al., 2019). Treatment of cells with the essential oils indicated that *S. aromaticum* oil afforded only a poor protective effect against hydrogen peroxide (H_2O_2), but that the mixture and *P. graveolens* oil alone protected cells against the harmful effects of H_2O_2.

8.2.6 Immunological effects

A study investigated the effect of geranium essential oil on the insecticide profenofos (PFF)-induced toxicity by monitoring liver and kidney parameters in the carp fish, *Cyprinus carpio* (Abdel Rahman et al., 2020). Geranium oil-treated fish displayed improved histological architecture of the liver and kidney tissues, and clinical symptoms of toxicity, including low mortality rate. There was a restoration of biochemical parameters, including hepatic enzyme activity for serum alanine and aspartate aminotransferases, alkaline phosphatase, lactate dehydrogenase, creatinine, urea, cholesterol, triglycerides and malondialdehyde, to almost the same level as the negative controls, following consumption of a diet supplemented with geranium oil in the presence of PFF. The results demonstrate the suitability of geranium oil for use as a dietary supplement in aquaculture, due to its potential anti-oxidant capacity (Abdel Rahman et al., 2020).

8.2.7 Antidiabetic properties

The potential antidiabetic and anti-oxidant effects of *P. graveolens* essential oil were demonstrated in an alloxan-induced diabetic rat model, following oral treatment with the oil for 4 weeks (Boukhris et al., 2012). The oil administered at 150 mg/kg body weight (bw), displayed a significant antidiabetic effect compared to the 75 mg/kg bw. dose and the drug glibenclamide (0.6 mg/kg bw). The groups receiving essential oil treatment showed higher hepatic glycogen levels compared to the normal and diabetic control groups. The diabetic control also displayed decreased anti-oxidant enzyme activity for catalase (CAT), superoxide dismutase (SOD) and glutathione peroxidase (GPX) in the liver and kidneys, which was restored following treatment with geranium oil, while the lipid peroxidation content was also reduced. The *P. graveolens* oil resulted in a reduction in oxidative stress through inhibiting the production of free radicals, and the subsequent development of diabetes. Overall, geranium oil significantly reduced serum glucose levels and restored anti-oxidant perturbations (Boukhris et al., 2012). In another study, geranium oil was also reported to exert protective effects towards oxidative damage in alloxan-induced diabetic rats (Hajri et al., 2016). In the study, a subacute intraperitoneal injection of 42.5 mg/kg bw essential oil for 3 weeks produced a significant reduction in blood glucose, lipid peroxidation, and restored anti-oxidant enzyme activities (Hajri et al., 2016).

8.2.8 Reproductive and spermatogenesis properties

Slima et al. (2013) established the *in vivo* protective effects of *P. graveolens* essential oil in male mice following adeltamethrin-induced reprotoxicity. The oil suppressed oxidative stress and lipid peroxidation, thereby promoting sperm quality, motility, viability and morphology, and preventing testicular oxidative damage. The positive effects of geranium essential oil on the reproductive system were similar to that of vitamin E (Slima et al., 2013). Another study by Mirazi (2016) confirmed the protective effects of the non-volatile fraction of *P. graveolens*. The hydro-ethanolic extract was effective in curbing testicular damage induced by lead acetate, thereby resulting in a significant increase in sperm count compared to the control.

8.2.9 Hepatoprotective effects

Pelargonium graveolens has been documented to exert hepatoprotective effects *in vivo*, following carbon tetrachloride (CCl_4)-induced liver injury (Al-Sayed et al., 2015). Treatment of mice with *P. graveolens* ethanol extract (PGE), orally for 6 weeks, reduced the enzyme activity of alanine aminotransferase, aspartate aminotransferase, and alkaline phosphatase by 37% and 43%, 33% and 35%, 26% and 33%, at 500 and 1000 mg/kg/day, respectively. The extract reduced SOD, GPX, glutathione reductase and glutathione-*S*-transferase activity, as well as reducing glutathione levels. In addition, the ethanol extract was equally effective as silymarin in reducing the fatty changes, Kupffer cell hyperplasia, and necrosis induced by CCl_4 intoxication. *Pelargonium graveolens* extract enhances anti-oxidant defence systems and reduces lipid peroxidation, thereby protecting against liver damage (Al-Sayed et al., 2015).

8.3 Safety

Pelargonium graveolens is listed as Generally Regarded As Safe (GRAS) at 1.6 to 200 ppm (FDA, 2006). Lalli et al. (2008) reported a fairly non-toxic profile for *P. graveolens* acetone extract (half-maximal inhibitory concentration (IC_{50}) = 83.31 ± 2.56 μg/mL), compared to the highly toxic *P. sublignosum* and *P. citronellum*, and the negative quinine control (IC_{50} = 11.89 ± 1.54 μg/mL, 19.14 ± 0.98 μg/mL, and 125.56 ± 5.04 μg/mL, respectively). The *in vitro* toxicity study of *Pelargonium* species was based on the 3-[4,5-dimethylthiazol-2-yl]-2,5-diphenyltetrazolium bromide (MTT) cellular viability assay towards transformed human kidney epithelial (Graham) cells.

9. Phytochemistry

9.1 Volatile constituents

The chemical profile of *P. graveolens* essential oil has been extensively studied due to commercialisation and the need to establish quality standards. In a study by Lalli et al. (2006), the chemical profiles of various *Pelargonium* species, including *P. graveolens*, were established. The two samples included in the study contained high levels of isomenthone, accounting for 65.8% and 83.3% of the total oil composition. Other minor compounds accounting for at least 0.5%, were listed as menthane (1.0%–5.1%), *p*-cymene (0.9%–1.1%), limonene (0.6%–0.8%) and 2-phenylethyl tiglate (0.8%–1.9%), while 2-decenoic acid (trace-3.9%) and decanoic acid (trace-12.9%) concentrations varied markedly between the samples. Low levels of citronellol (0.4%), citronellyl formate (<0.05%) and linalool (0.3%) were also detected. In similar profiling studies, isomenthone was reported as a major constituent of *P. graveolens* essential oil, accounting for 75.0%–83.0% (Van der Walt and Demarne, 1988) and 7.0%–81.5% (Lis-Balchin, 2002). These chemical profiles differed from a report by Lawrence (1975) that listed geraniol, linalool and β-caryophyllene as the major constituents at 23.0%, 11.5% and 18.2%, respectively. Rana et al. (2002) reported a chemical profile devoid of isomenthone; however, 30 other compounds constituting 99.1% of the oil composition were identified. In this study, citronellol (33.6%), geraniol (26.8%), linalool (10.5%), citronellyl formate (9.7%) and *p*-menthone (6.0%) were the major compounds, and represented 86.6% of the oil sample from India.

In a chemotaxonomy study involving 70 geranium oils from various cultivation sites in South Africa, Egypt, India, Reunion Island, China and Madagascar, gas chromatography–mass spectrometry (GC–MS) and vibrational spectroscopy were used to determine the oil compositions (Sandasi et al., 2011). Although the composition varied quantitatively between samples, seven major compounds were identified as follows: citronellol (19.5%–51.3%), geraniol (5.9%–32.1%), linalool (0.8%–10.3%), isomethone (0.6%–8.0%), citronellyl formate (3.5%–19.9%), geranyl formate (0.10%–8.99%) and guaia-6,9-diene (0.2%–9.6%) (Sandasi et al., 2011). Most of these compounds, including β-citronellol (21.9%), citronellyl formate (13.2%), geraniol (11.1%), 10-epi-γ-eudesmol (7.9%), geranyl formate (6.2%) and linalool (5.6%), were reported by Boukhris et al. (2013) to be major constituents of geranium oil. Epi-α-cadinol (15.49%) and isomenthol (6.5%) were recently reported, among other previously documented compounds, in geranium oil from Egypt (Fekri et al., 2019). Szutt et al. (2019) also reported geraniol and citronellol as major compounds, together with a range of other compounds.

The study by Fekri et al. (2019) compared the profiles of oil extracted by hydro-distillation and solvent extraction, which resulted in a concrete, referred to as an absolute, following the removal of pigments and waxes. Differences in the oil yield were observed, with solvent extraction yielding more compared to hydro-distillation (0.19:0.11). The major compounds in the absolute were identified as citronellol (29.3%), geraniol

(7.5%), geranial (12.9%), isomenthone (9.9%) and epi-α-cadinol (8.8%), which were also present in the oil. However, linalool was absent from the absolute. Changes in the citronellol to geraniol ratio were monitored in the absolute, using proton nuclear magnetic resonance (NMR) spectroscopy, at different stages of leaf development. The results indicated that the geraniol content was the highest in young leaves and that the citronellol concentrations increased with leaf age (Fekri et al., 2019).

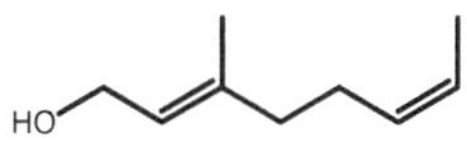

Geraniol

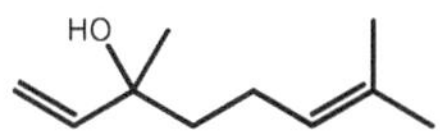

Linalool

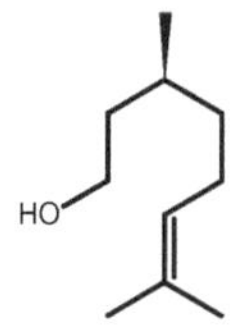

β-Citronellol

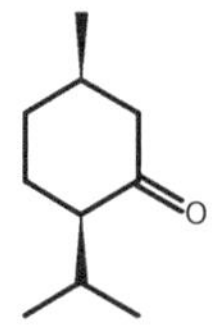

Isomenthone

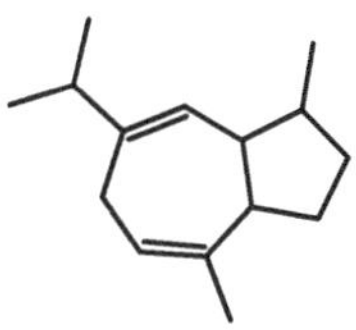

Guaia-6,9-diene

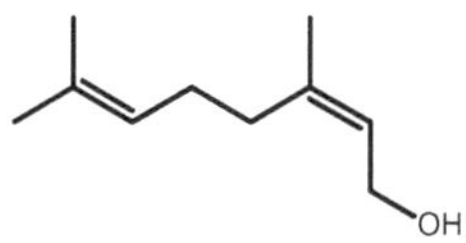

Nerol

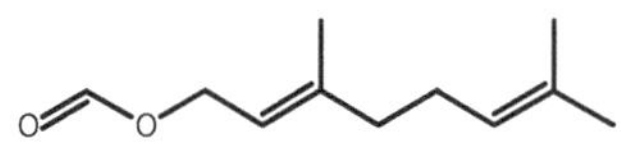

Geranyl formate

9.2 Non-volatile constituents

The chemical composition of *P. graveolens* methanol and water extracts was investigated by Boukhris et al. (2013), using high-performance liquid chromatography coupled to mass spectrometry (HPLC–MS). The HPLC analysis revealed the presence of nine flavonoids in total in the leaf and flower extracts. The water extract comprised kaempferol 3-*O*-rhamnoside-glucoside, isorhamnetin aglycone, quercetin 3-*O*-glucoside, kaempferol 3,7-di-*O*-glucoside, and quercetin 3-*O*-pentose, while kaempferol 3-*O*-glucoside, quercetin 3-*O*-rhamnoside-glucoside (rutin), quercetin 3-*O*-pentoside-glucoside and myricetin 3-*O*-glucoside-rhamnoside were detected in the methanol extracts. Furthermore, the total phenolic, flavonoid, and flavonol contents of the extracts were determined. The total phenolic content was higher in the methanol extracts of flowers and leaves (109.8 and 84.1 mg GAE/g of dry weight (dw) extracts, respectively) than in the water extracts (60.76 and 54.71 mg GAE/g dw, respectively). The flavonoid content of the methanol extracts for both plant parts was significantly higher (78.49 and 71.21 mg quercetin equivalent (QE)/g dw for flowers and leaves, respectively) than that of the water extracts (29.87 and 22.45 mg QE/g dw for flowers and leaves, respectively). The results also revealed that the methanol leaf extracts contained higher concentrations of flavonols (23.8 total flavonols mg rutin/g dw) than that of the flowers (23.8 total flavonols mg rutin/g dw).

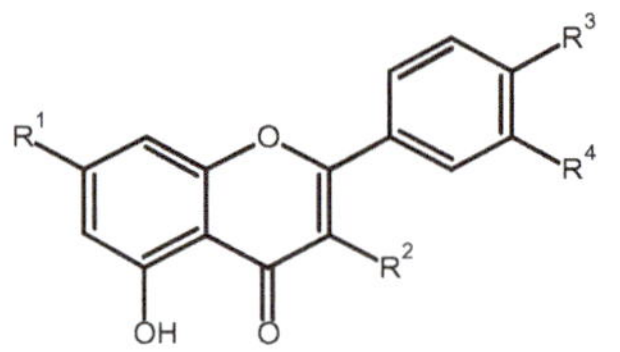

Rutin (quercetin-3-*O*-rhamnoside-glucoside):
R^1=OH, R^2=rutinoside, R^3=OH, R^4=OH
Kaempferol 3-*O*-glucoside: R^1=OH, R^2=glc, R^3=OH, R^4=H

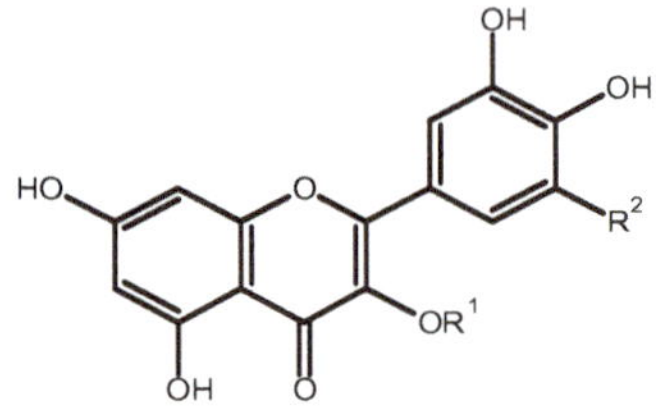

Quercetin 3-*O*-glucoside: R^1=glc; R^2=H

Part B: Chemical profiling and quality control

10. Chromatography analysis

10.1 High-performance thin-layer chromatography (HPTLC) fingerprint analysis

General instrumentation: A CAMAG HPTLC instrument consisting of an automatic TLC sampler (ATS 4), automatic developing chamber (ADC 2), CAMAG TLC Visualizer 2, CAMAG derivatiser, and TLC plate heater. *HPTLC plates:* Silica gel glass plates 60 F_{254} (Merck). *Plant part:* Aerial parts, essential oil. *Sample application:* Application volume of 2 μL essential oil (25 μL/mL in toluene) spotted as 10 mm bands. Plates developed in a 20×10×4 cm glass twin-trough chamber to a migration distance of 70 mm. *Tank saturation*: 20 min at 15 °C and 33% RH, with 25 mL of mobile phase. *Mobile phase:* Toluene: ethyl acetate (95:5 v/v). *Derivatisation: p*-Anisaldehyde. The plate was sprayed with 3 mL of *p*-anisaldehyde reagent and heated on a TLC plate heater at 100 °C until colour developed. *Visualisation:* The plate was viewed under white reflectance light.

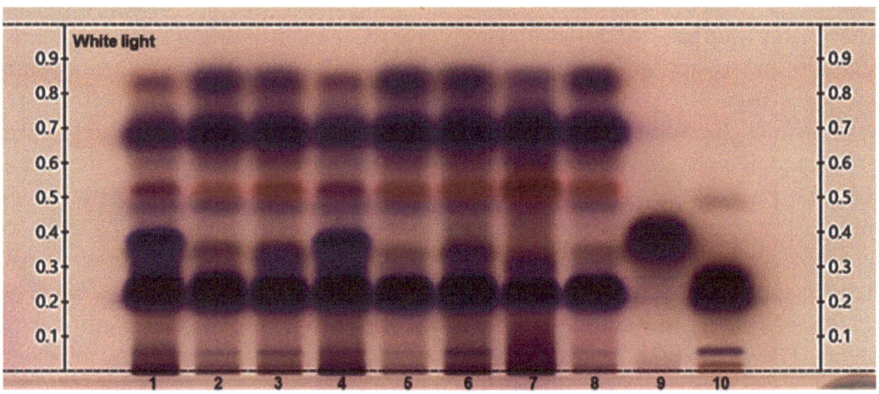

HPTLC plate of *Pelargonium graveolens* essential oils from various localities (1–8) and the standards (9–10). The samples are characterised by purple bands for geraniol (R_f=0.24) and linalool (R_f=0.37).

10.2 Gas chromatography (GC) analysis

General instrumentation: An Agilent 6860N chromatograph (Agilent Technologies, Hanova, USA) fitted with a flame ionisation detector (FID) and a mass spectrometer. *Plant part:* Aerial parts, essential oil. *Sample application:* Injection volume of 1 μL (split) prepared as 20% (v/v) in hexane, split ratio 1:200, and inlet temperature 250 °C. *Column:* HP-Innowax, 60 m × 250 μm × 0.25 μm (polye-thylene glycol stationary phase, Agilent Technologies, Hanova, USA). *Analysis conditions:* Helium carrier gas, flow rate: 1.2 mL/min, pressure: 24.79 psi. Starting oven temperature at 60 °C and then increased to 220 °C at 4 °C/min, held for 10 min and increased to 240 °C at 1 °C/min. *Mass spectrometry conditions:* Chromatograms obtained by applying electron impact ionisation at 70 eV using an Agilent 5973 mass selective detector, scanning range: *m/z* 35 to 550 (Agilent Technologies, Hanova, USA). *Identification:* Authentic standards, NIST®, Mass Finder®.

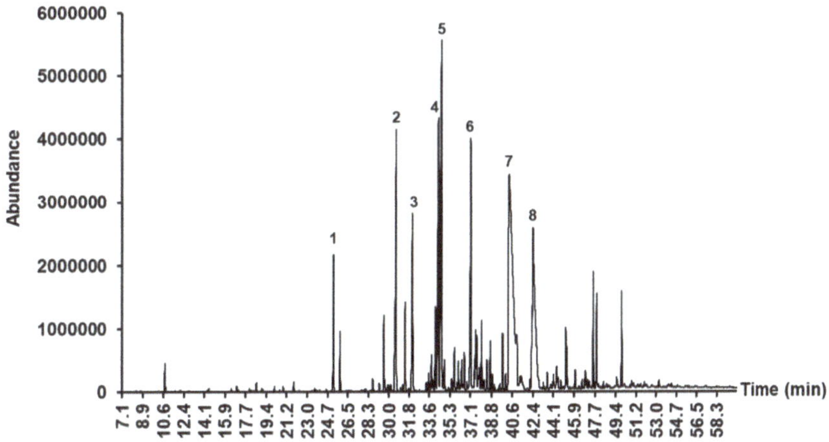

Total ion chromatogram (TIC) of *Pelargonium graveolens* essential oil indicating major compounds. [1] = menthone (R_t 29.61, *m/z* 154.1358), [2] = isomenthone (R_t 30.66, *m/z* 154.1358), [3] = linalool (R_t 32.07, *m/z* 154.1358), [4] = guaia-6,9-diene (R_t 34.30, *m/z* 204.3562), [5] = citronellyl formate (R_t 34.54, *m/z* 184.1463), [6] = geranyl formate (R_t 37.08, *m/z* 182.2628), [7] = citronellol (R_t 40.62, *m/z* 156.1514), [8] = geraniol (R_t 42.48, *m/z* 154.1358).

11. Mid-infrared (MIR) spectroscopy analysis

General instrumentation: Alpha-P Bruker spectrometer, mounted with an attenuated total reflectance (ATR) diamond crystal. *Spectral acquisition:* Spectrum obtained in the absorbance mode, with a spectral resolution of 4 cm^{-1} over the range 4000–550 cm^{-1} and captured using OPUS 6.5 software. *Plant part:* Aerial parts, essential oil. *Sample preparation:* Aerial parts, hydro-distillation to obtain essential oil, placed directly onto the surface of the diamond crystal.

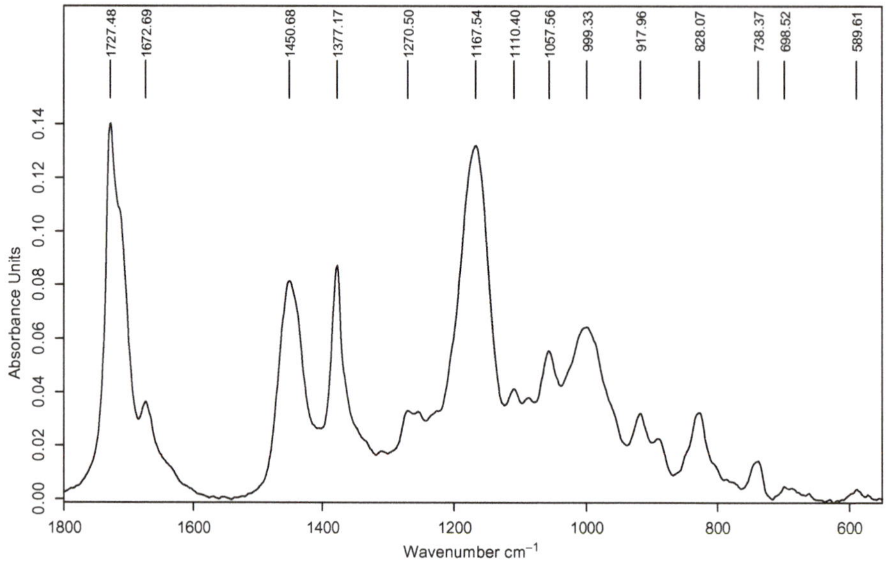

Mid-infrared spectrum of *Pelargonium graveolens* essential oil displaying the fingerprint region (1800–550 cm^{-1}).

References

Abdel Rahman, A.N., Mohamed, A.A.-R., Mohammed, H.H., Elseddawy, N.M., Salem, G.A., El-Ghareeb, W.R., 2020. Aquaculture, 517:734777.

Al-Sayed, E., Martiskainen, O., Seif El-Din, S.H., Sabra, A.-N.A., Hammam, O.A., El-Lakkany, N.M., 2015. Med. Chem. Res., 24:1438–1448.

Asgarpanah, J., Ramezanloo, F., 2015. Indian J. Tradit. Knowl., 14:558–563.

Bigos, M., Wasiela, M., Kalemba, D., Sienkiewicz, M., 2012. Molecules, 17:10276–10291.

Blerot, B., Baudino, S., Prunier, C., Demarne, F., Toulemonde, B., Caissard, J.-C., 2016. Phytochem. Rev., 15:935–960.

Boukhris, M., Bouaziz, M., Feki, I., Jemai, H., El Feki, A., Sayadi, S., 2012. Lipids Health Dis., 11:81.

Boukhris, M., Simmonds, M.S.J., Sayadi, S., Bouaziz, M., 2013. Phytother. Res., 27:1206–1213.

Boukhris, M., Hadrich, F., Chtourou, H., Dhouib, A., Bouaziz, M., Sayadi, S., 2015. Ind. Crop. Prod., 74:600–606.

Bouzenna, H., Krichen, L., 2013. Nat. Prod. Res., 27:841–846.

Bown, D., 1995. Encyclopaedia of Herbs and their Uses. Dorling Kindersley, London, UK.

Can, E., Kizak, V., Can, Ş.S., Özçiçek, E., 2018. Aquaculture, 491:59–64.

Chandravadana, M.V., Nidiry, E.S.J., 1994. Indian J. Exp. Biol., 32:908–909.

Choi, S.H., Lim, S., Shin, S., 2007. Nat. Prod. Sci., 13:342–346.

DAFF, 2012. Essential Oil Crops: Production Guidelines for Rose Geranium. Directorate Communication Services, Pretoria, South Africa.

Dashamiri, S., Ghaedi, M., Naghiha, R., Salehi, A., Jannesar, R., 2018. Braz. J. Pharm. Sci., 54 (4):e17724.

Diánez, F., Santos, M., Parra, C., Navarro, M., Blanco, R., Gea, F., 2018. Lett. Appl. Microbiol., 67:400–410.

Dos Santos, M.K., Kreutz, T., Danielli, L.J., De Marchi, J.G.B., Pippi, B., Koester, L.S., Fuentefria, A.M., Limberger, R.P., 2020. J. Drug Deliv. Sci. Technol., 56:101527.

Eamsobhana, P., Yoolek, A., Kongkaew, W., Lerdthusnee, K., Khlaimanee, N., Parsartvit, A., Malainual, N., Yong, H., 2009. Exp. Appl. Acarol., 47:257–262.

El Ouadi, Y., Bendaif, H., Mrabti, H.N., Elmsellem, H., Kadmi, Y., Shariati, M.A., Abdel-Rahman, I., Hammouti, B., Bouyanzer, A., 2017. J. Microbiol. Biotechnol. Food Sci., 6:1218–1220.

El-Garawani, I., El Nabi, S.H., Nafie, E., Almeldin, S., 2019. Anti Cancer Agents Med. Chem., 19:1103–1113.

Essid, R., Hammami, M., Gharbi, D., Karkouch, I., Hamouda, T.B., Elkahoui, S., Limam, F., Tabbene, O., 2017. Appl. Microbiol. Biotechnol., 101:6993–7006.

Fanela, T.L.M., Baldin, E.L.L., Pannuti, L.E.R., Cruz, P.L., Crotti, A.E.M., Takeara, R., Kato, M.J., 2016. Neotrop. Entomol., 45:201–210.

FDA, GRAS List, 2006. Herb Society of America *Pelargoniums*: An Herb Society of America Guide. Kirtland, Ohio, USA.

Fekri, N., El Amir, D., Owis, A., AbouZid, S., 2019. Nat. Prod. Res., 35:2593–2597.

Gildemeister, E., Hoffmann, F., 1900. In: Les Huiles essentielles (Ed.). Brockhaus & Tognol, Leipzig and Paris, Germany and France.

Giongo, J.L., De Almeida Vaucher, R., Fausto, V.P., Quatrin, P.M., Lopes, L.Q.S., Santos, R.C.V., Gündel, A., Gomes, P., Steppe, M., 2016. Microb. Pathog., 100:170–178.

Hajri, A., Selmi, S., Rtibi, K., Lamjed Marzouki, M., Sebai, H., 2016. J. Biol. Act. Prod. Nat., 6:299–314.

Han, X., Beaumont, C., Stevens, N., 2017. Biochim. Open, 5:1–7.

Jeon, J.-H., Kim, H.-W., Kim, M.-G., Lee, H.-S., 2008. J. Microbiol. Biotechnol., 18:1666–1671.

Juárez, Z.N., Bach, H., Sánchez-Arreola, E., Bach, H., Hernández, L.R., 2016. J. Appl. Microbiol., 120:1264–1270.

Kozlowska, J., Kaczmarkiewicz, A., Stachowiak, N., Sionkowska, A., 2017. Cosmetics, 4:36, https://doi.org/10.3390/cosmetics4030036.

Lalli, J.Y.Y., Viljoen, A.M., Baser, K.H.C., Demirci, B., Ozek, T., 2006. J. Essent. Oil Res., 18:89–105.

Lalli, J.Y., Van Zyl, R.L., Van Vuuren, S.F., 2008. S. Afr. J. Bot., 74:153–157.

Lavasanijou, M.R., Sohrabi, H.R., Karimi, M., Ashjazade, M.A., Salajeghe, M., Farzineejadizadeh, H., Parsaei, P., Elmamooz, A., 2016. Wounds, 28:369–375.

Lawrence, B.M., Hogg, J.W., Harney, P.M., 1975. Flavour, 42–44.

Lis-Balchin, M., 2002. Essential oils from different *Pelargonium* species and cultivars: their chemical composition (using GC, GC/MS) and appearance of trichomes (under EM). In: Lis-Balchin, M. (Ed.), *Geranium* and *Pelargonium*. Taylor and Francis, London, UK.

Lohani, A., Mishra, A.K., Verma, A., 2019. J. Cosmet. Dermatol., 18:550–557.

Mahboubi, M., Kazempour, N., Farzin, N., 2011. J. Biol. Act. Prod. Nat., 1:105–111.

Mahboubi, M., Kazempour, N., Taghizadeh, M., 2014. Songklanakarin J. Sci. Technol., 36:513–519.

Mahboubi, M., Mahdizadeh, E., HeidaryTabar, R., 2018. Infection, 22:9–12.

Malik, T., Singh, P., Pant, S., Chauhan, N., Lohani, H., 2011. Phytother. Res., 25:1225–1228.

Malik, T., Singh, P., Pant, S., Chauhan, N., Lohani, H., Kumar, V., Swarup, S., 2015. Bangladesh J. Med. Sci., 14:384–388.

Marmouzi, I., Karym, E.M., Alami, R., El Jemli, M., Kharbach, M., Mamouch, F., Attar, A., Faridi, B., Cherrah, Y., Faouzi, M.E.A., 2019. Orient. Pharm. Exp. Med., 19:201–210.

Martins, C.A.F., Campos, M.L., Irioda, A.C., Stremel, D.P., Trindade, A.C.L.B., Pontarolo, R., 2017. Molecules, 22:1883.
Mirazi, N., 2016. J. Zanjan Univ. Med. Sci. Health Serv., 24:58–70.
Muthukumar, A., Sangeetha, G., Naveenkumar, R., 2016. J. Environ. Biol., 37:1429–1436.
Naeini, A.R., Nazeri, M., Shokri, H., 2011. J. Mycol. Med., 21:87–91.
Nardoni, S., D'Ascenzi, C., Rocchigiani, G., Papini, R.A., Pistelli, L., Formato, G., Najar, B., Mancianti, F., 2018. Nat. Prod. Res., 32:385–390.
Niculau, E., Alves, P.B.D.L., Nogueira, P.C.D.S., Moraes, V.R., Matos, A.P., Bernardo, A.R., Volante, A.C., Fernandes, J.B., Da Silva, M.F.G.F., Correa, A.G., Blank, A.F., Silva, A.D.C., Ribeiro, L., 2013. Quim Nova, 36:1391–1394.
Pavela, R., 2008. Phytother. Res., 22:274–278.
Pazinato, R., Volpato, A., Baldissera, M.D., Santos, R.C.V., Baretta, D., Vaucher, R.A., Giongo, J.L., Boligon, A.A., Stefani, L.M., Da Silva, A.S., 2016. J. Adv. Res., 7:1029–1034.
Ralambondrainy, M., Belarbi, E., Viranaicken, W., Baranauskienė, R., Venskutonis, P.R., Desprès, P., Roques, P., El Kalamouni, C., Seâlambarom, J., 2018. PLoS One, 13:e0196757.
Rana, V.S., Juyal, J.P., Blazquez, M.A., 2002. Int. J. Aroma Ther., 12:216–218.
Sandasi, M., Kamatou, G.P.P., Gavaghan, C., Baranska, M., Viljoen, A.M., 2011. Vib. Spectrosc., 57:242–247.
Sangeetha, G., Thangavelu, R., Rani, S.U., 2010. Int. J. Food Sci. Technol., 45:1024–1032.
Shin, S., Lim, S., 2004. J. Appl. Microbiol., 97:1289–1296.
Simões, B.M., Kohler, B., Clarke, R.B., Stringer, J., Novak-Frazer, L., Young, K., Rautemaa-Richardson, R., Zucchini, G., Armstrong, A., Howell, S.J., 2018. Ther. Adv. Med. Oncol., 10:1–11.
Singh, P., Srivastava, B., Kumar, A., Kumar, R., Dubey, N.K., Gupta, R., 2008. J. Sci. Food Agric., 88:2421–2425.
Slima, A.B., Ali, M.B., Barkallah, M., Traore, A.I., Boudawara, T., Allouche, N., Gdoura, R., 2013. Lipids Health Dis., 12 (1):30.
Souza, C.M.C., Junior, S.A.P., Moraes, T.D.S., Damasceno, J.L., Mendes, S.A., Dias, H.J., Stefani, R., Tavares, D.C., Martins, C.H.G., Crotti, A.E.M., Mendes-Giannini, M.J.S., Pires, R.H., 2016. Med. Mycol., 54:515–523.
Szabó, M.Á., Varga, G.Z., Hohmann, J., Schelz, Z., Szegedi, E., Amaral, L., Molnár, J., 2010. Phytother. Res., 24:782–786.
Szutt, A., Dołhańczuk-Śródka, A., Sporek, M., 2019. Ecol. Chem. Eng. S, 26:807–816.
Szweda, P., Zalewska, M., Pilch, J., Kot, B., Milewski, S., 2018. Acta Vet. Scand., 68:95–107.
Tabanca, N., Wang, M., Avonto, C., Chittiboyina, A.G., Parcher, J.F., Carroll, J.F., Kramer, M., Khan, I.A., 2013. J. Agric. Food Chem., 61:4101–4107.
Van der Walt, J.J.A., Demarne, F.-E., 1988. S. Afr. J. Bot., 54:617–622.
Xie, O., Wang, Z., Huang, Q., Zhang, D., 2017. Ind. Crop. Prod., 108:278–285.
Zardo, D.M., Alvarez, L.V.H., Los, F.G.B., Ito, V.C., Travalini, A.P., Cardoso, T., Wojeicchoski, J.P., Alberti, A., Zielinski, A.A.F., Esmerino, L., Nogueira, A., 2019. Curr. Bioact. Compd., 15:592–599.

CHAPTER

Pelargonium sidoides

19

Alvaro Viljoen[a,b], Weiyang Chen[a], Nduvho Mulaudzi[a] and Thomas Brendler[c,d]

[a]*Department of Pharmaceutical Sciences, Tshwane University of Technology, Pretoria, South Africa*

[b]*SAMRC Herbal Drugs Research Unit, Faculty of Science, Tshwane University of Technology, Pretoria, South Africa*

[c]*Department of Botany and Plant Biotechnology, University of Johannesburg, Johannesburg, South Africa*

[d]*Plantaphile, Collingswood, New Jersey, United States*

Abstract

Pelargonium sidoides DC. (Geraniaceae), also known as 'African geranium', is a small perennial, rosette-like plant with crowded leaves and distinctive dark, reddish-purple flowers. The roots of the plant have long been used in South African traditional medicine for the treatment of sore throat, congestion, bronchitis, diarrhoea and dysentery. Pelargonium sidoides occurs in the Western Cape, throughout the Eastern Cape, parts of Gauteng, North West, Free State and Mpumalanga provinces of South Africa, and in Lesotho. A well-known commercial herbal tincture, known as Umckaloabo®, is available on the international market, among other P. sidoides products marketed for the management of upper respiratory tract infections. Both in vitro and in vivo activities have been extensively investigated and documented. Using a semi-automated high-performance thin-layer chromatography (HPTLC) system and ultra-performance liquid chromatography coupled to mass spectrometry and photodiode array detection (UPLC–MS–PDA), the chemical profiles of P. sidoides were obtained. The profiles of the methanol extracts viewed under 366 nm radiation, after derivatisation using potassium hydroxide reagent, revealed the presence of umckalin. In addition to umckalin, magnolioside was also identified in the UPLC–MS chromatogram.

Keywords: *Pelargonium sidoides*, African geranium, Bronchitis, Umckaloabo, Umckalin, Magnolioside, HPTLC, UPLC–MS, MIR spectroscopy

The South African Herbal Pharmacopoeia. https://doi.org/10.1016/B978-0-323-99794-2.00015-5

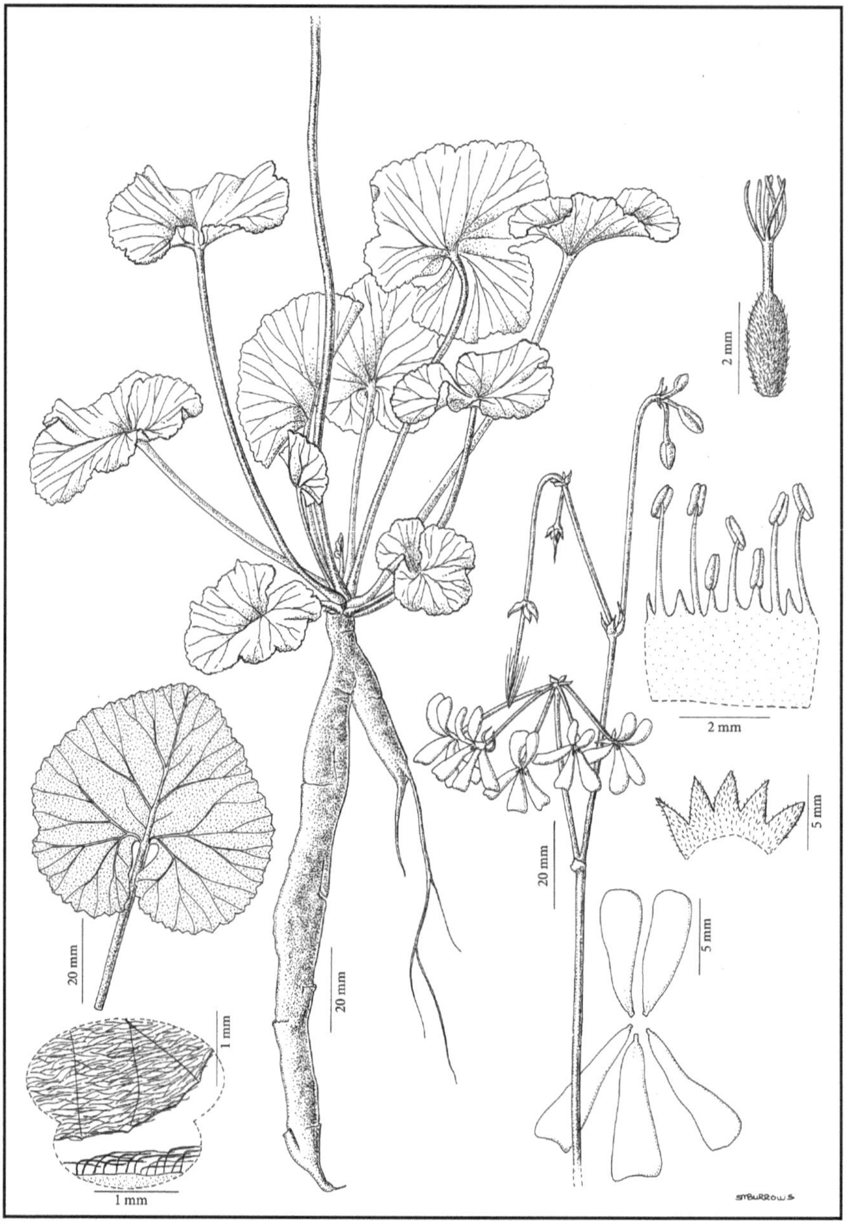
2 mm
2 mm
5 mm
20 mm
5 mm
20 mm
20 mm
1 mm
1 mm

Part A: General overview

1. Synonyms

Pelargonium reniforme Curtis var. *sidaefolium* (Thunb.) Harv., *Pelargonium sidaefolium* (Thunb.) R.Knuth.[a]

2. Common name(s)

African geranium, black pelargonium (English); '*rabassam*', '*kalwerbossie*' (Afrikaans); '*rabas*' (Khoi-Khoi), '*iyeza lesikhali*', '*ikubalo*' (isiXhosa); '*khoara-e-nyenyane*' (Southern Sotho), '*umckaloabo*' (German remedy).[a,b]

3. Conservation status

Least concern.[a]

4. Botany

Pelargonium sidoides belongs to the family Geraniaceae that comprises five genera, namely *Monsonia, Geranium, Sarcocaulon, Erodium* and *Pelargonium* (Van der Walt and Vorster, 1988). The genus *Pelargonium* includes more than 200 natural species of which the majority occurs in South Africa, with a few native to tropical Africa, Australia, Syria, and to some islands in the Indian Ocean. The genus name *'Pelargonium'* is derived from the Greek word '*Pelargos'* meaning stork. The rostrum of the seed capsule (schizocarp) resembles the bill of a stork. The species name *'sidoides'* mirrors the resemblance of the foliage to that of a European plant, *Sida rhombifolia*. *Pelargonium sidoides* is a small, perennial, rosette-like plant with crowded leaves (Van der Walt and Vorster, 1988). The long-stalked leaves are heart-shaped, velvety and mildly aromatic (A and C). The distinctive dark, reddish-purple flowers are seen almost throughout the year, and occur mostly from spring (October) to summer (January), with a peak in midsummer (December) (B). The thickened underground root-like branches of the plant are a special adaption that enables it to survive grass fires, which occur almost annually (D). When cultivated, the plant is an evergreen, but it dies back in nature in winter (May to August) and during droughts. The closely related species, *P. reniforme*, is morphologically similar, but has pink flowers (Van der Walt, 1977; Van Wyk and Wink, 2004).

[a] Redlist of South African Plants (http://redlist.sanbi.org).
[b] World Flora Online (www.worldfloraonline.org).

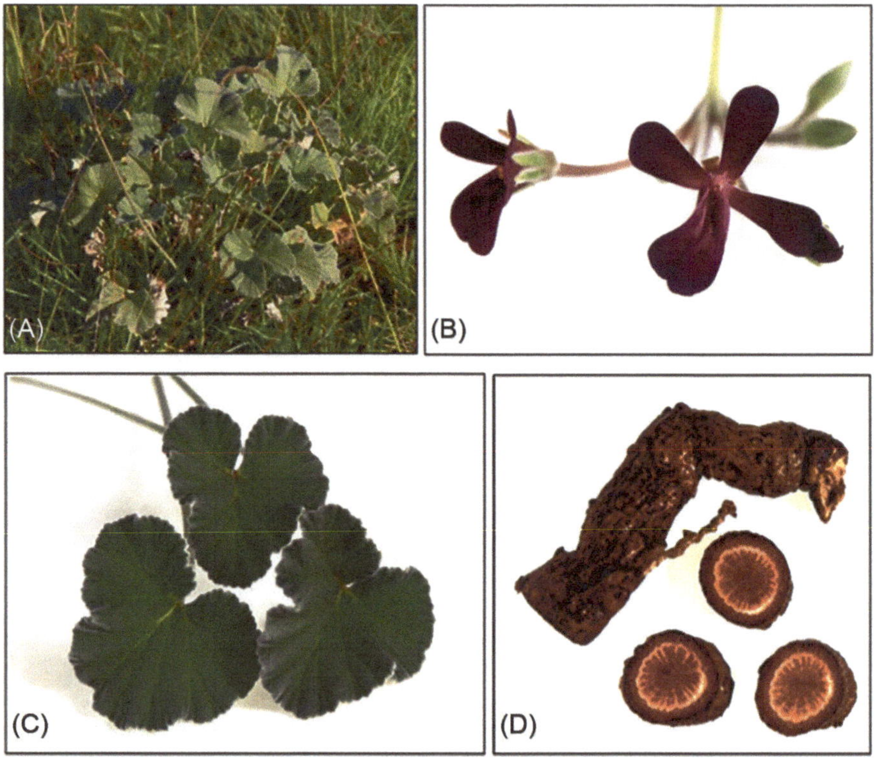

Pelargonium sidoides shrub in habitat (A), deep reddish-purple flowers on wiry stems (B), heart-shaped velvety leaves (C) and tuberous root, which is red inside (D).

5. Geographical distribution

Pelargonium sidoides is endemic to South Africa (Dreyer and Marais, 2000), where it grows along the extreme eastern boundary of the Western Cape, throughout the Eastern Cape, and in parts of the Gauteng, North West, Free State, KwaZulu-Natal and Mpumalanga provinces. The plant is usually found in open grassland, in rocky places, and in loamy to sandy soils derived from quartzite, basalt or shale. About 80% of South African plant species are confined to the south-western Cape, which is the only region with winter rainfall. *Pelargonium sidoides* occurs from near sea level to high altitudes, particularly in Lesotho, where it is found at more than 2300 m above sea level. The closely related species, *P. reniforme*, is restricted to the Eastern Cape Province of South Africa and has a much smaller distribution range.

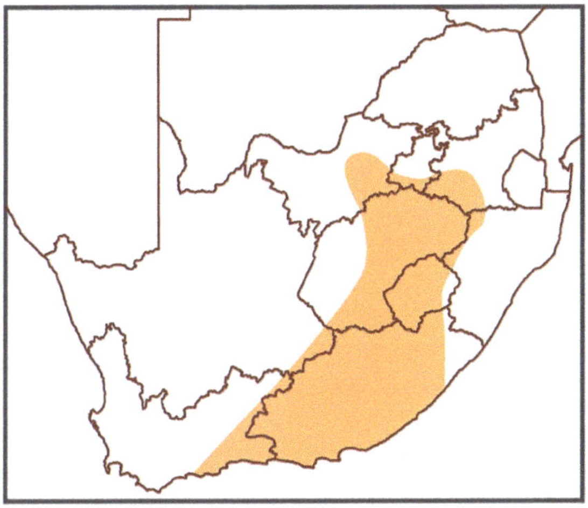

Geographical distribution of *Pelargonium sidoides* in South Africa.

6. Ethnopharmacology

The most detailed summary regarding the ethnobotany of the *P. sidoides*/*P. reniforme* complex is provided in Brendler and Van Wyk (2008). The earliest record of use likely stems from Carl Peter Thunberg, who noted in the diary of his travels at the Cape in 1773: *'Many gerania, with their red and pulpous roots, grew in the sandy plains near the town; and as these roots are of an astringent nature, the country people used them in the diarrhoea and dysentery'* (Forbes, 1986, p. 160). All early records focus on uses such as the treatment of diarrhoea and dysentery, owing to the astringent nature of their roots (Ecklon and Zeyher, 1837; Pappe 1847, 1850, 1857; Harvey and Sonder, 1860) (as *P. reniforme* Curtis var. *sidaefolium* (Thunb.) Harv.). The most detailed account of the value of *P. sidoides* is that of Smith (1895), stressing the exceptional uses of *P. sidoides* species (still regarded as a variety of *P. reniforme*), the one with *'flowers a dark port-wine colour'* in the treatment of dysentery where the usual course of medicine had failed. A record by Phillips (1917) reveals that the roots of *P. sidoides* were used in Lesotho to treat colic. From the Free State Province northwards, the name 'kalwerbossie' is used, because the plant was used as a dewormer for calves (Smith, 1966). Batten and Bokelman (1966) reported that the Xhosa people used the root of *Pelargonium* to treat liver conditions in calves and sheep and that Europeans used it to treat asthma. An ethnobotanical survey conducted by Matsiliza and Barker (2001) in the Grahamstown (Makhanda) region stated that *P. sidoides* is administered to infants with an upset stomach and air in the intestine, given as a gripe water. Water is added to the crushed root, mixed, and a teaspoonful of the red infusion is given orally. The traditional uses reported for *Pelargonium* species rarely include respiratory conditions. However, according to Smith (1895), *P. sidoides* should be regarded as a good tonic. The first record of use for respiratory conditions must be attributed to Charles Henry Stevens, an Englishman, who having contracted 'consumption' was sent to South

Africa and was treated and cured by a local healer, of unclear ethnicity, who prescribed the root of a local plant as a treatment. He took the root back to England and started to market it there as a patent medicine, never revealing its identity. However, a recent investigation (Brendler et al., 2021, unpublished data) proved it to have been *P. sidoides*.

7. Commercialisation

Stevens grew a veritable business in England, marketing the remedy as 'Stevens Consumption Cure' and 'Umckaloabo' as a cure for tuberculosis. Controversy developed as to the efficacy of the remedy, resulting in the British Medical Association accusing him of quackery and fraud and ordering him to pay substantial costs. Even so, Stevens continued to market the remedy with success, until his death in 1942. In that he received some help from Dr. Adrien Sechehaye of the University of Geneva. He had heard of Stevens' Cure, and started to treat patients using the concoction around 1920. He treated about 800 patients over a period of 9 years and reported successful cases to the Medical Society of Geneva, culminating in the publication of the case histories of 64 patients recorded in meticulous detail (Brendler, 2009). The identity of the plant used in the remedy remained a secret until 1974, when a doctoral study was commissioned by the German company ISO-Arzneimittel and the plant identified as either *P. reniforme* or *P. sidoides*, two closely related species (Bladt, 1974). This revelation prompted scientific research into the active constituents of the plant, with further clinical trials demonstrating the efficacy of the roots of the *Pelargonium* species for treating bronchial conditions (Brendler and van Wyk, 2008). In 1983, *P. sidoides* was marketed as 'Umckaloabo' by ISO-Arzneimittel as a liquid herbal (EP® 7630). Dr. Willmar Schwabe GmbH (hereafter referred to as 'Schwabe') acquired ISO-Arzneimittel in 1987, and *Pelargonium* then became one of Schwabe's top-selling plant-based remedies, with annual revenues in Germany rising from €4 million in 2000 to €50 million in 2005 (source, IMS). The Federal Institute for Drugs and Medical Devices (BfArM, Bonn) approved a licence in December 2005 for the use of Umckaloabo as a drug (Conrad et al., 2007a). The product thereby became a fully licensed herbal medicine on the German market. An extract of *P. sidoides* produced as a mother tincture, is marketed in Russia, Ukraine and Latvia as Umkalor. Solid and liquid products containing the plant are available as herbal supplements in Mexico and North America. In South Africa and neighbouring countries, a number of dry and liquid formulations are available, as well as herbal remedies that include *P. sidoides* e.g. Natura Pentagen, Phyto Nova Cough Syrup and Linctagon (Brendler and Van Wyk, 2008).

Modern trade focuses on *P. sidoides*, although both *P. sidoides* and *P. reniforme* have been investigated for their potential therapeutic value. The raw material of *P. sidoides* is collected from the wild in parts of Lesotho and the Eastern Cape Province of South Africa. Several hundred harvesters are involved in the collection of the plant's tuberous roots for the commercial market. Most wild-harvesting takes place on communal lands of the former 'homelands' of the Transkei and Ciskei regions that suffer high levels of poverty, inadequate provision of basic services, and widespread dependence on state welfare grants. Similar conditions are also present in Lesotho, one of the least developed countries in the region (Human Sciences Research Council, 2011). Harvesting communities in both Lesotho and South Africa are governed by traditional authorities, but these differ in the extent to which they are accepted by communities, and in their traditional involvement in *Pelargonium* management. Harvesters collect and sell the tubers to local and intermediary buyers. For example, Gowar Enterprises collects and transports plant material from the Eastern Cape to an intermediary buyer, BZH Export & Import, which is based in the Western Cape. Here, the tubers are dried, shredded and packaged. In Lesotho, Bophelo Natural Products collects the tubers, and the dried material is exported. Parceval, a South African pharmaceutical manufacturer, supplies the South African market with tinctures and other finished products based on *Pelargonium*, and also exports the plant material to Germany, where it is further processed into products. Schwabe, the world's main buyer of *Pelargonium* raw material, supplies markets in the United States, Germany and other European countries (Van Niekerk and Wynberg, 2012). Some initiatives were put in place in the Eastern Cape Province, where most material is collected from the wild, to cultivate significant quantities of raw material from seed-propagated, cultivated plants (Lewu et al., 2007).

The very similar-looking *P. reniforme* and *P. sidoides* often grow side by side. Although this may lead to the product being adulterated, the potential risks and impact on international trade seem relatively unimportant. However, chemical analysis of the raw material is required to check for adulteration, since the morphological distinction of the dried roots is very difficult. The chemical markers, umckalin and its 7-*O*-methylether (5,6,7-trimethoxycoumarin), can be used for the identification of *P. sidoides*, as these are low in concentration or absent in *P. reniforme*. Kayser and Kolodziej (1995) demonstrated that coumarins are appropriate for quality-control purposes, because they are detectable by thin layer chromatography (TLC) due to their strong UV fluorescence under 366 nm radiation. The long growth cycle of the tubers, roughly calculated to be 8–9 years, constrains cultivation, and has an influence on the commercially viable biomass (Wynberg et al., 2015), with further concerns about the potency of the cultivated plants. Clonal propagation was also investigated (Lewu et al., 2006) as a tool for cultivating *P. sidoides*, and conditions were determined that can be used for successful propagation to meet the high demand for *P. sidoides*.

Schwabe obtained several patents that were focused on methods of producing *Pelargonium* extracts (Willcox et al., 2015). Schwabe's patent on the process was challenged in 2008 by three of their competitors, as well as the Masakhane community and supporting non-governmental organisations (NGOs). The claims of the competitors were confirmed on grounds of lack of novelty, lack of inventive step, and insufficiency, whilst the various claims of the Masakhane community were rejected by the European Union (EU) patent court. The patent was indeed revoked in 2010. Subsequently, the brand owner announced that it would no longer pursue its four other *Pelargonium* patents. Demonstrating their social commitment, the brand owner donated 1 million Euros to the newly established 'Umckaloabo Stiftung' (Van Niekerk and Wynberg, 2012).

8. Pharmacological evaluation

8.1 *In vitro* studies

8.1.1 Antibacterial and antifungal activity

The antibacterial activity of the constituents of *P. sidoides* (umckalin, scopoletin, 6,8-dihydroxy-5,7-dimethoxycoumarin, 5,6,7-trimethoxycoumarin, gallic acid, methyl gallate and (+)-catechin), as well as that of extracts, was evaluated by Kayser and Kolodziej (1997) towards three Gram-positive (*Streptococcus pneumoniae, Staphylococcus aureus* and *Streptococcus* 1451) and five Gram-negative (*Klebsiella pneumoniae, Escherichia coli, Pseudomonas aeruginosa, Proteus mirabilis* and *Haemophilus influenzae*) bacteria. All compounds (except (+)-catechin) exhibited antibacterial activities, with minimum inhibitory concentrations (MICs) of 200–1000 μg/mL. Lewu et al. (2006) confirmed the findings of Kayser and Kolodziej (1997). An indirect antibacterial effect of an extract of *P. sidoides* was established by Daschner et al. (2004), through the induction of bacterial adhesion to buccal epithelial cells (BEC), as well as *via* inhibition of bacterial adhesion to human epithelial cells (HEp-2). The effect of Umckaloabo on the function of human phagocytes was investigated by Hansmann (2005). *Candida albicans* was selected as the test pathogen. Umckaloabo significantly stimulated oxidative burst and phagocytosis, but intracellular killing was hardly influenced. Bacterial adhesion to epithelial cells is an important step in infections, with subsequent colonisation, invasion and incorporation of pathogens into tissues. Therefore, anti-adhesive agents are important as prophylactic tools against bacterial infections. Flavan-3-ols (epicatechin, epigallocatechin-3-*O*-gallate and epigallocatechin), a pro-anthocyanidin and procyanidins from *P. sidoides*, based on catechin, epicatechin, combined flavanyl units, prodelphinidins containing epigallocatechin units, as well as oligomers possessing A-type units, were evaluated for anti-adhesive effects, using a model for mucosal pathogenesis with labelled group A-streptococci (GAS) and human laryngeal HEp-2 cells. Only prodelphinidins reduced microbial adherence, indicating that pyrogallol-type elements containing epigallocatechin units are structurally important for activity (Janecki and Kolodziej, 2010).

In vitro studies on cell surface receptor expression and cytokine production by Thäle et al. (2007) revealed that extracts of *Pelargonium* are potent modulators of macrophage activity. Their findings confirmed the hypothesis that an increase in adhesion of particles by Umckaloabo exhibited an increase in phagocytosis. Further studies by Dorfmüller et al. (2005) indicated that *P. sidoides* extract inhibited adhesion of GAS to HEp-2. Pre-incubation of GAS with *P. sidoides* also inhibited adhesion. The influence on adhesion of *Streptococcus pyogenes* on human BEC was further examined by Carrapatoso (2005), using a microscopic count of cells with bacteria and flow cytometry. Data indicated that Umckaloabo significantly increased adhesion of bacteria to BEC. Wittschier et al. (2007a) incubated intact human stomach tissue with fluorescent-labelled *Helicobacter pylori.* Pretreatment of the bacterium with the extract of *P. sidoides* displayed a dose-dependent anti-adhesive effect, with no direct cytotoxicity against *H. pylori*. It was also shown by Beil and Kilian (2007) that EPs® 7630 inhibited adhesion to gastric epithelial cells and *H. pylori* growth in a dose-dependent manner. The impact of therapeutic concentrations of EPs® 7630 (0–30 g/mL) on host–bacteria interaction and activity of human peripheral blood phagocytes (PBP) was investigated by Conrad et al. (2007b, c, 2008a, b, c). A flow cytometric assay was employed to investigate oxidative burst, phagocytosis, and adhesion of GAS to BEC and human HEp-2 (Wittschier et al., 2007b). A penicillin/gentamicin-protection assay was used to assess GAS invasion of HEp-2 cells. It was reported that EPs® 7630 increased the number of phagocytosing PBP in a concentration-dependent manner with enhanced intracellular killing. EPs® 7630 increased GAS adhesion to BEC, but reduced GAS adhesion to HEp-2 cells significantly, due to a difference in the types of epithelial cells. It was concluded that EPs® 7630 protect mucous membranes from micro-organisms invading the host defence mechanisms. The results showed the possible mechanisms of EPs® 7630 in the treatment of upper respiratory tract infections.

Another study (Janecki et al., 2011) investigated the anti-adhesive activity of an extract of *P. sidoides* using *S. pyogenes* as the micro-organism. An attempt was made to identify the active principle(s). *Pelargonium* extract, as well as a methanol-soluble fraction (MSF) and derivatives thereof, were investigated for their anti-adhesive properties. A number of purified pro-anthocyanidins, including homogenous catechin- and epicatechin-based polyflavones, an A-type pro-anthocyanidin mixture, a 'mixed' procyanidin sample, as well as a prodelphinidin test substance, were included in the anti-adherence study. After pretreatment of GAS with the extract and fractions [methanol insoluble fraction (MIF) or MSF] at concentrations of 30 μg/mL, inhibition of the pathogen to HEp-2 cells was observed at ca. 45%, ca. 35% and ca. 30%, respectively. However, no effects were evident after pre-incubation of cells with the extract and the fractions. The results indicated that the anti-adhesive effects are due to interactions with binding factors on the bacterial surface, and demonstrated that pro-anthocyanidins are associated with the anti-adhesive effect. Comparative studies revealed that the pyrogallol B-ring elements of constituent flavanyl units are an important structural feature of the anti-adhesive potential of this plant extract. From the study, it was concluded that *P. sidoides* extract exhibited potent anti-adhesion activity due to the presence of specific pro-anthocyanidins. Although specific interactions with bacterial binding sites were suggested, the adhesion molecules were not identified. These findings indicate that the anti-infective activity of EPs® 7630 may be due to its anti-adhesive properties at an early time point of bacterial infection (Janecki et al., 2011).

Other studies were conducted on *P. sidoides* extracts to determine their antibacterial activity and their effects on non-specific immune functions. Moderate antibacterial activities were recorded of aqueous acetone extracts of *P. sidoides* against a spectrum of bacteria, including *Mycobacteria* strains (Kolodziej, 2011). A large number of *in vitro* studies has provided strong evidence for an anti-infective principle associated with activation of the non-specific immune system (Conrad et al., 2007c; Uslu et al., 2009; Kolodziej, 2011). Kolodziej (2011) showed significant inhibition of interaction between host cells and bacteria, dominant to the pathogenesis of respiratory tract infections. Additionally, antiviral effects were reported, including inhibition of the enzymes haemagglutinin and neuraminidase, as well as replication of respiratory viruses. Furthermore, an increase in the ciliary beat frequency of respiratory cells can also contribute to the beneficial effects of *P. sidoides*. The extract EPs® 7630, used in Umckaloabo, was evaluated for its activity against GAS adhesion to human HEp-2 epithelial cells (Kolodziej, 2014). At a concentration of 30 µg/mL, the extract reduced microbial adherence by about 45%. This effect was only shown upon pretreatment of streptococci with EPs® 7630, and not by treatment of HEp-2 cells. These findings confirmed the fact that the prodelphinidins in the extract are responsible for the anti-adhesive activity and that these compounds reduce microbial adherence and protect the respiratory tract against bacterial colonisation and invasive superinfection following a viral infection.

The antimicrobial effects of different solvent extracts of *P. sidoides* towards food-borne diseases caused by pathogenic bacteria were investigated (Ibrahim et al., 2018). The highest phenolic content was present in the aqueous acetone extracts of calli prepared from roots, followed by calli from shoot tips (12.34 and 4.78 mg/g dry weight (dw), respectively). The highest values of pro-anthocyandins (0.290 $A_{550\ nm}$/mg) and flavonoid content (20.82 mg/g dw) were recorded for root calli extracted with aqueous acetone. The highest antimicrobial activity was displayed with callus from shoot tip explants extracted with aqueous acetone, against *Clostridium perfringens* ATCC 6538 (maximum inhibition zone diameter of 35 mm; oxytetracycline 30 µg/disc as control positive control—30 mm). Nowadays, bacterial resistance to antibiotics and the disruption caused by antibiotics to internal microflora are huge problems, resulting in greater interest in alternative medicine. Plant-derived preparations containing multicomponents are good alternatives, as they exhibit different simultaneous actions/mechanisms (Savickiene et al. 2018). Furthermore, plants with innate immune and regenerative capacity-stimulating properties, and displaying anti-inflammatory and antibacterial activities are good candidates to combat infections. Pro-anthocyanidins are among the most promising plant-derived compounds to address this problem. The pro-anthocyanidins isolated from the methanol root extract of *P. sidoides* were investigated by Savickiene et al. (2018), and active compounds were isolated and identified. The anti-oxidant and antibacterial activities of the pro-anthocyanidins were compared to those of the extract alone, and significant activities were reported for the pro-anthocyanidins with respect to anti-oxidant capacity, as well as antibacterial action. Selectivity was obtained for Gram-negative keystone peri-implant and periodontal pathogenic strains, such as *Porphyromonas gingivalis*, while preserving the viability of beneficial oral commensal *Streptococcus salivarius*. The data revealed that pro-anthocyanidins from *Pelargonium* are very good candidates for extended treatment of infectious diseases, specifically upper respiratory tract infections.

The roots of 50 *P. sidoides* plants were examined for the presence of fungi (Manganyi et al., 2018). The isolated fungi were subsequently screened to determine their antibacterial activity using a pathogenic *E. coli* strain, previously isolated from cattle. Among the isolates, the genus *Penicillium* was dominant (23%), when compared to *Fusarium* (12%), and *Aspergillus* and *Alternaria* species that were both present at 11%. *Penicillium expansum* (LC015096.1), *Aspergillus* sp. (KM458796.1), and *Aspergillus niger* (KP172477.1) produced the highest bactericidal activity against the *E. coli* strain with growth inhibition zone diameter measurements of 5, 11 and 4 mm, respectively (Manganyi et al., 2018). Fungal cultures were isolated from *P. sidoides* root material, and extracts prepared from plant material were tested separately, and in combination with the host plant, to determine interactions. The extract from the fungal isolate *Penicillium skrjabinii* showed antimicrobial activity against *E. coli* and *S. aureus* at 0.09 and 0.03 mg/mL, respectively (Aboobaker et al., 2019). Bio-assay-guided fractionation was used as a guide for the isolation of the active constituent, which was identified as dibutyl phthalate (known to be produced by micro-organisms). Synergistic interaction of some endophytes with the host plant was observed. Manganyi et al. (2019) investigated extracts from endophytic fungi (isolated from *P. sidoides*) in order to characterise the bio-active compounds for the control of bacteria of clinical importance. Extracts were isolated from 133 fungal strains and screened against Gram-negative and Gram-positive bacteria, namely *E. coli, Bacillus cereus, Enterococcus gallinarum* and *Enterococcus faecium*, using the disk diffusion assay. Twelve percent of the fungal extracts (16 from 133) displayed good antibacterial activity against selected bacteria. *Escherichia coli* was considered the most susceptible compared to *E. gallinarum* and *E. faecium*, which were the most resistant. *Alternaria* sp. (isolate MHE 68) exhibited a broad spectrum of antibacterial activities, affecting selected clinical bacterial strains, including resistant *E. gallinarum* and *E. faecium*. Cyclodecasiloxane and linoleic acid (9,12-octadecadienoic acid (Z,Z)) were identified from the extract of MHE 68, having antibacterial activity (Samie et al., 2019). Research work was conducted, aimed at evaluating *P. sidoides* plant parts for their antipathogenic properties and anticryptococcal activity towards selected virulence factors. Aerial and tuber tissue extracts exhibited fungicidal activity and constrained the development of antifungal resistance. The extracts did not target ergosterol biosynthesis and no haemolytic activity was displayed. However, the extracts displayed significant antipathogenic properties by inhibiting urease and laccase activity, as well as by reducing capsule size.

8.1.2 Antiproliferative, anticancer and anti-oxidant activity

Pereira et al. (2015) analysed an extract of *P. sidoides* using semipreparative high-performance liquid chromatography (HPLC), and its anticancer and anti-oxidant activities were determined. The results indicated that the hydrophilic fractions had strong reducing capacities and exhibited good radical scavenging activity. Significant cellular anti-oxidant activity in the human lung cell line, NCI-H460, was reported. Three fractions inhibited the cell growth of four cell lines in the National Cancer Institute (NCI, USA)-prescreen panel (NCI-H460, SF-268 and MCF-7) and the

Jurkat E6.1 cell line. Mass spectrometry analysis of the active fractions revealed that they contained polyphenolic compounds, such as pro-anthocyanidins, gallic acid, dihydroxycoumarin sulphates, trihydroxycoumarin and phenolic glycosides. *Pelargonium sidoides* calli were tested for anti-oxidant activity, employing the 2,2-diphenyl-1-picryl hydrazyl (DPPH) assay, oxygen radical absorbance capacity (ORAC) assay, as well as the β-carotene/linoleic acid assay (Kumar et al., 2015). Cultures supplemented with different combinations and concentrations of the plant growth inducer thidiazuron (TDZ) and picloram exhibited significantly higher callus induction compared to the control. Except for gallic acid, TDC/picloram combinations significantly increased the concentrations of hydroxybenzoic acid derivatives, namely *p*-hydroxybenzoic acid, protocatechuic acid, salicylic acid and vanillic acid (Kumar et al., 2015). Catechin was only detected in *P. sidoides* calli produced on plant growth regulator-free Murashige and Skoog medium, while the concentration of hydroxycinnamic acid derivatives in calli was variable, whereas caffeic acid was not detected in such calli. The strongest anti-oxidant activity, based on the β-carotene/linoleic acid and DPPH model systems, was obtained for plant growth regulator-free-produced calli, whereas TDZ/picloram combinations had a significant effect on ORAC. These findings imply that *P. sidoides* calli can be controlled on a large scale for the production of phenolic acids that exhibit potent anti-oxidant activity.

The antiproliferative activity of a *P. sidoides* radix mother tincture (PST) was evaluated by Pereira et al. (2016). Mass spectrometry was used to determine dihydroxycoumarin sulphates, gallocatechin dimers and trimers, as well as gallic acid in PST. The NCI prescreen panel was employed, and moderate antiproliferative effects were reported, with half-maximal inhibition of cell proliferation (GI_{50}) values between 80 and 40 µg/mL. Potent activity was recorded towards Jurkat cells, with a GI_{50} value of 6.2 µg/mL compared to the positive control 5-fluorouracil (GI_{50} value of 9.7 µg/mL). The PST arrested Jurkat cells at the G0/G1 phase of the cell cycle, dead cells increased from 4% to 17%, while the apoptotic cells increased from 9% to 21%. The antiproliferative mechanisms of *P. sidoides* were studied through *in silico* network pharmacology methodologies and target identification (Pereira et al., 2017). Twelve phenolic compounds were investigated and the protein targets identified using the server for predicting Drug Repositioning and Adverse Reactions *via* the Chemical–Protein Interactome (DRAR-CPI) and the target identification server PharmMapper. Protein–pathway and protein–protein interaction networks were constructed with Cytoscape 3.4.0 to investigate potential mechanisms of action. From a total of 142 potential human target proteins identified with the *in silico* target identification servers, 90 of these were related to cancer. The protein interaction network was created from 86 proteins involved in 209 interactions with each other, and two protein clusters were detected. Pereira et al. (2017) verified more than 80 Kyoto Encyclopaedia of Genes and Genomes (KEGG) pathways, enriched with the protein targets. Several pathways specifically linked to cancer were identified, as well as a number of signalling pathways discovered to be dysregulated in cancer. The data showed that the anti-proliferative activity of *P. sidoides* is multifactorial and can arise from the combined regulation of several interconnected cell signalling pathways.

A major pathway involved in tumour aggressiveness and inflammation in human cancers was identified as the transcriptional activation of NF-κB signalling pathway. Acetylsalicylic acid (ASA), dexamethasone, curcumin, celecoxib and EPs 7630 were evaluated in head-and-neck squamous cell carcinoma (HNSCC) lines (Meyer et al., 2011). The *P. sidoides* extract EPs® 7630 is a registered trademark of Dr. Willmar Schwabe GmbH & Co. KG, Karlsruhe, Germany. The inhibition of NF-κB led to an upstream regulation of a predominant receptor driving cell expansion, namely Toll-like-receptor 3 (TLR3). A noticeable downregulation of IKK and the TLR3 complex was found, affecting responses to NF-κB inhibition by all the agents tested. Furthermore, cytokine production, proliferation and alterations in the expression of downstream proteins, including c-Myc and cyclin D1, were shown. Results indicated decreased proliferation in response to incubation. The profile of relevant cytokines (IL-8 and IL-6) in HNSCC progression was altered with modulation of TLR3 and NF-κB expression, and proto-oncogenes cyclin c-myc and D1 were downregulated by all samples tested. Apart from the interplay of TLR3 and cytokines, *Pelargonium* was considered a new and natural NF-κB inhibitor. The root extracts of two *Pelargonium* species, namely *P. quercetorum* and *P. endlicherianum*, were studied for their anti-inflammatory effects on lipopolysaccharide (LPS)-stimulated macrophages (Cumaoğlu et al., 2018). Stimulation of the RAW 264.7 cells with LPS (0.5 μg/mL, 6 h treatment) resulted in an increased mRNA expression of inducible nitrogen oxide synthase and cyclooxygenase-2 (COX-2). The release of NO elevated the production of pro-inflammatory cytokines (tumour necrosis factor (TNF)-α and IL-6) and PGE2, activated MAPK (extracellular signal-regulated kinase, phosphorylation of c-Jun N-terminal kinase, P38) signalling pathway, and nuclear translocation of NF-κB (p65), which were noticeably inhibited by pretreatment with 70% methanol and 11% ethanol extracts *of P. endlicherianum*, indicating no cytotoxicity. *Pelargonium sidoides* root extract alleviated COX-2 mRNA expression with PGE2 production and P38/MAPK activation, while *P. quercetorum* extract only decreased TNF-α production.

8.1.3 Immunomodulating properties

Various assays were employed by Kayser et al. (1997, 2001, 2003) to determine the effects of extracts and compounds of *P. sidoides* on non-specific immune functions. All compounds and extracts displayed significant effects by reducing the intracellular survival of *Leishmania donovani*, but no activity was observed towards extracellular, promastigote *L. donovani*. The data indicated indirect activity, with a possible activation of leishmanicidal macrophage functions. Activation was verified through the presence of inorganic nitric oxides and TNF-α, which is a known mechanism against micro-organisms. Interferon-like activities in the supernatants of sample-activated bone marrow-derived macrophages, as well as TNF-inducing potencies, were observed for EPs® 7630 in several functional assays (Kolodziej and

Schulz, 2003; Janecki et al., 2007). It was further shown that EPs® 7630 induced significant TNF levels in GFP-transfected-*Leishmania* major-infected and non-infected macrophages. Subfractions of *Pelargonium* were also tested for TNF-, NO- and interleukin (IL)-12-inducing activity. Flow cytometry indicated a decrease in parasite numbers in cells treated with *Pelargonium*, with minor production of IL-12 and NO. The results indicated that efficient NO levels may be present in EPs® 7630, but low levels of radical scavengers. An investigation was conducted by Koch et al. (2002) to determine if EPs® 7630 interferes with interferon (IFN)-β synthesis in MG-63 human osteosarcoma cells. The data revealed the enhancement of natural killer cell-mediated cytotoxicity and an increase in IFN-β production in cells pre-incubated with *Pelargonium*. Polyphenol-containing extracts of *P. sidoides* and compounds, such as flavan-3-ols, pro-anthocyanidins, phenols and hydrolysable tannins, were studied for gene expressions (TNF-α, inducible nitrogen oxide synthase (iNOS), IL-1, IL-12, IL-10, IL-18 and IFN-α/γ) by Kolodziej et al. (1999, 2005). An increase in cytokine mRNA levels and iNOS was reported for extracts, and all compounds, in parasitised cells. Gene expression analyses, using the reverse transcription polymerase chain reaction for the cytokines iNOS, IL-1, IL-18, IL-12, IFN-α, TNF-α and IFN-γ were conducted by Trun et al. (2006) in major-infected and non-infected *Leishmania* RAW 264.7 cells. *Pelargonium* significantly upregulated transcript expressions in infected cells and induced low mRNA levels in non-infected cells with simultaneous stimulation of IFN-γ mRNA production. Similar results were obtained for gallic acid and the MIF, but the MIF and the bio-active compound umckalin did not show any gene-inducing capabilities worth noting. From the results, it was concluded that the inducing principle is located in the MIF.

The potential effects of EPs® 7630 were investigated on the release of antimicrobial peptides from neutrophils by Koch and Wohn (2007). A major cellular component of the immune response, namely the neutrophil granulocyte, contains proteins and antimicrobial peptides with a broad range of immunomodulating, chemotactic, antimicrobial and wound healing activities. The extract EPs® 7630, at concentrations of 0.3–30 g/mL, was added to heparinised whole human blood samples. Analysis of the plasma to determine human neutrophil peptide (HNP) 1–3 content and bactericidal/permeability-increasing protein (BPI) after 5 h of incubation, reflected a significant dose-dependent increase in the release of BPI and HNP 1–3. The extract seemed to stimulate host defence through enhancing the release of antimicrobial peptides. Mediators such as the molecular chaperones, Hsp72 and Hsp70, as well as neuropeptide Y (NPY), are known to play a key role in the immune response and regulation of the neuro-endocrine system. It was shown that extracts of *P. sidoides* had no influence on NPY release from neuroblastoma cells, yet significantly inhibited Hsp70 release. Asea et al. (2013) demonstrated, for the first time, that heat shock protein Hsp70 and neuropeptide Y can be used as molecular biomarkers for adaptogenic activity. Witte et al. (2015) demonstrated that the roots of *P. sidoides* induced a dose-dependent production of IL-6, IL-10 and TNF-α by human blood immune cells. Compared to the profile induced by viral or bacterial infection-mimicking agents, the

EPs® 7630-induced profile was more pro-inflammatory. They reported that T cells did not respond to *Pelargonium* stimulation by the production of IL-6, TNF-α or IL-10, and that pretreatment of T cells with *Pelargonium* did not modulate their IL-6, IL-10 and TNF-α secretion during activation. Monocytes displayed clear intracellular TNF-α staining after EPs® 7630 treatment, and the extract predominantly provoked activation of MAP kinases, while inhibition of p38 strongly reduced monocyte TNF-α production. Pretreatment of blood immune cells with *Pelargonium* lowered their secretion of IL-10 and TNF-α and caused an IL-6-dominant response during a second stimulation with bacterial or viral infection-mimicking agents. Witte et al. (2015) showed that mitogen-activated protein (MAP) kinase-dependent proinflammatory cytokines, induced by EPs® 7630, activated human monocytes, and specifically modulated the production capacity of mediators. These mediators are known to lead to an increase in acute phase protein production in the liver, the generation of adaptive Th17 and Th22 cells, and neutrophil generation in the bone marrow.

8.1.4 Antiviral activity

The antiviral effect of an aqueous extract of *P. sidoides* against herpes simplex virus (HSV) was examined in cell culture. The major constituents identified in the *Pelargonium* extract through liquid chromatography-mass spectrometry (LC-MS) analysis were catechin derivatives, coumarins and phenolic structures (Schnitzler et al., 2008). *In vitro* testing of the extract on RC-37 cells, using a plaque reduction assay, was consistent with potent antiviral activity against herpes simplex virus type 2 (HSV-2) and herpes simplex virus type 1 (HSV-1). The half-maximal inhibitory concentration (IC_{50}) values for the inhibition of HSV plaque formation for the aqueous extract of *P. sidoides* was determined at 0.000005% and 0.00006% for HSV-2 and HSV-1, respectively. Concentration-dependent antiviral activity against HSV was determined for the extract, and plaque formation was significantly reduced by >99.9% for HSV-2 and HSV-1 at maximum non-cytotoxic concentrations of the extract. An attempt was made to establish the mode of antiviral action. The extract was added at different time intervals to the viruses and cells during the infection period. When the extract was added during the adsorption phase, or when pretreated with the plant extract, both herpes viruses were significantly inhibited compared to acyclovir, which was only active during replication of HSV. Compared to the drug acyclovir, the extract of *P. sidoides* showed a different mode of action and affected the virus before penetration into the host cell. Schnitzler et al. (2008) demonstrated that an aqueous root extract of *P. sidoides* is capable of exerting an antiviral effect on HSC and can be used for topical therapeutic use, both in genital and in labial herpes infection. It was also shown that the extract of *P. sidoides* has a novel mode of action, since it protected macrophages and peripheral blood mononuclear cells from infection with various R5 and X4 tropic HIV-1 strains, including clinical isolates (Helfer et al., 2014). Data from the mode of action studies revealed that the extract interfered directly with viral infection by blocking the attachment of HIV-1 particles to target cells, and thereby protecting them from virus entry. Examination of the chemical footprint of anti-HIV activity indicated that HIV-1 inhibition is mediated by various polyphenolic compounds with low cytotoxicity. These compounds were separated selectively from the extract. The effects of EPs® 7630 on respiratory viruses (Michaelis et al., 2011), together with its excellent safety profile (Kamin et al., 2018; Schapowal et al., 2019), led to it being discussed as having potential to affect the human immune response in the context of COVID-19 (Brendler et al., 2020).

An extract of *P. sidoides* at concentrations up to 100 μg/mL, interfered with the replication of seasonal influenza A virus strains (H3N2,H1N1), human coronavirus, respiratory syncytial virus, coxsackie virus and para-influenza virus (Michaelis et al., 2011). It was concluded that these observed antiviral effects can contribute to the beneficial effects of *Pelargonium* in AB patients. However, determination of virus titres and virus-induced cytopathogenic effects indicated no effect on the replication of adenovirus, highly pathogenic avian influenza A virus (H5N1), or rhinovirus. *In vitro* effects of *P. sidoides* extract were investigated by Roth et al. (2019), using the expression of host defence supporting proteins and virus binding cell membrane on primary human bronchial epithelial cells (hBEC). Results showed that EPs® 7630 significantly increased hBEC survival in a concentration-dependent manner after rhinovirus infection, employing cells isolated from patients with moderate chronic obstructive pulmonary disease (COPD) ($n = 6$), severe asthma ($n = 6$) and non-diseased controls ($n = 6$). Other effects recorded were the decreased expression of inducible co-stimulator (ICOS), cell surface calreticulin (C1qR), and its ligand ICOSL, with upregulated expression of SOCS-1 and the host defence supporting proteins β-defensin-1, in rhinovirus infected and uninfected hBEC. Virus-interacting cell membrane proteins, such as TRL2/4, MyD88 and ICAM-1, were not affected by *Pelargonium*. It can be concluded that EPs® 7630 reduced rhinovirus infection of human primary BEC by upregulating host defence proteins and down-regulating cell membrane docking proteins.

8.1.5 Antimycobacterial activity

Seidel and Taylor (2004) and Taylor (2003a,b) investigated the antimycobacterial activity of the hexane extracts of the two species, *P. sidoides* and *P. reniforme*. The study showed several mono- and di-unsaturated fatty acids to be active, with linoleic and oleic acid exhibiting potent activity as reflected by the MICs of ± 2 g/mL. Gödecke (2005) tested the fractions and extracts of *P. sidoides* towards two strains of mycobacteria, but no significant effect on the bacterial growth was observed. It was concluded that the effectiveness of the plant under tubercular conditions could be due to the activation of the immune system. This conclusion was supported by Mativandlela et al. (2006, 2007), who investigated various compounds and extracts of *P. sidoides* for their antitubercular and antimycobacterial activities. Strains of *A. niger, Moraxella catarrhalis, Fusarium oxysporum, Rhizopus stolonifer, Mycobacterium tuberculosis, M. smegmatis* and *H. influenzae* were treated with ethanol and acetone extracts, as well as two flavonoids and four coumarins isolated from *P. sidoides*. None or poor activity was observed towards *M. tuberculosis* and

R. stolonifer, but significant activity was evident for the ethanol extract against *F. oxysporum* and *A. niger.* Another study (Kim et al., 2009) was conducted to determine the capacity of extracts of *P. reniforme* and *P. sidoides* to stimulate the killing and uptake of mycobacteria by murine macrophages, and to identify compounds responsible for the activity. They reported that compounds from the plant stimulated macrophage killing, but not uptake, of *M. fortuitum* and *M. tuberculosis* equally well, and that the kinetics of intracellular accumulation of *M. fortuitum* and *M. tuberculosis* by macrophages were similar. Therefore, *Pelargonium* extracts can be effective in the treatment of tuberculosis (Kim et al., 2009).

8.1.6 Other properties

In vitro evaluation of the capacity of EPs® 7630 to stimulate ciliary beat frequency in ciliated cell cultures of human nasal epithelium, a key defence mechanism of the mucociliary system, was carried out by Mickenhagen et al. (2004) and Neugebauer et al. (2005). A significantly increased ciliary beat frequency was observed that was dose-dependent, at concentrations of EPs® 7630 (1, 30 and 100 g/mL). Nöldner and Schötz (2007) and Nöldner and Koch (2004) studied the inhibition of sickness behaviour (listlessness, anorexia and reduced activity) by *Pelargonium* in male Naval Medical Research Institute (NMRI) mice induced by a LPS cytokine inducer. A dose-dependent antagonistic effect was seen after oral administration of EPs® 7630.

8.2 *In vivo* studies and clinical trials

8.2.1 Colds and influenza

The literature was accessed on herbal medicine used for cough, with a focus on upper respiratory tract infections and the common cold. Evidence was provided for *P. sidoides* being significantly superior in alleviating the severity and frequency of patients' cough symptoms compared to the placebo (Wagner et al., 2015). The common cold is one of the most widespread illnesses in the world, with symptoms including runny nose, sore throat and sneezing. It is a viral infection, and antibiotics are often prescribed, although colds are commonly caused by rhinoviruses. Lizogub et al. (2007) evaluated the efficacy of a liquid herbal drug preparation of *P. sidoides* (EPs® 7630) in adult patients infected with the common cold. A statistically significant difference was observed after 5 days and the mean sum of symptom intensity differences (SSID) improved by 14.6 ± 5.3 points in the treated group compared with the placebo group (7.6 ± 7.5 points). The mean cold intensity score (CIS) decreased by 5.6 ± 4.3 points and 10.4 ± 3.0 points in placebo and EP-treated patients, respectively. The placebo *vs* the EPs group (31.4% *vs* 78.8%) were clinically cured after 10 days with CIS equal to complete resolution of all or a maximum of one cold symptom. The mean duration of inability to work was significantly lower in the EPs treatment group (6.9 ± 1.8 days), than in the placebo group (8.2 ± 2.1 days). Treatment outcome [rates of major improvement from disease or complete recovery (integrative medicine outcomes scale)] was much better in the EPs treatment group than in the placebo group. Three of 103 patients (2.9%) showed adverse events (non-serious), with one of 51 (2.0%) and two of 52 (3.8%) patients in the placebo and EPs group, respectively. *Pelargonium* was considered an effective treatment for the common cold and all patients stated that the subjective tolerability of EPs was good or very good. It was concluded that *Pelargonium* significantly shortened the duration of the common cold and reduced the severity of symptoms compared to the placebo group.

An open, multicentre study investigated the change in subjective and objective symptoms and tolerability in patients (361) with acute exacerbation of chronic-recurrent sinusitis and acute sinusitis, under administration of EPs® 7630 from the roots of *P. sidoides* (Schapowal and Heger, 2007). After 4 weeks of treatment, 80.9% of the patients experienced a clear improvement in their symptoms or became symptom-free. Remission or improvement rates were more than 90% for every individual symptom, with 17 patients reporting minor adverse events, of which a causal relationship with the study medication could not be ruled out (mostly gastro-intestinal symptoms). In another study (Bachert et al., 2009), patients (103) were selected at inclusion with sinonasal symptoms of at least 7 days' duration, in addition to clinically and radiographically confirmed acute rhinosinusitis of presumably bacterial origin, with a Sinusitis Severity Score (SSS) of at least 12 out of 24 points. The mean decrease in the SSS was 5.5 points in the *P. sidoides* group, compared to 2.5 points in the placebo group, a difference of 3.0 points (95% confidence interval 2.0–3.9). All secondary parameters confirmed this and results indicated a faster recovery and a more favourable course of the disease in the EPs® 7630 group. Bachert et al. (2009) reported that the study was terminated after obtaining proof of efficacy for EPs® 7630, according to the prespecified decision rule. Renikan®, a herbal extract from the root of *P. sidoides*, has a three-fold mechanism of action: antiviral (it activates the natural antiviral mechanisms of defence), mucolytic (owing to its expectorant and secretomotory properties) and antibacterial (due to its indirect and direct bacteriostatic action) (Pérez et al., 2011). Of a total of 305 patients, 149 children and 156 adults were divided into three groups. In the first group, consisting of 97 rhinosinusitis patients, improvement of symptoms was shown in 80% of children and 86% of adults, with no antibiotic use in 91% of children and 86% of adults. In the second group of 108 tonsillitis patients, an improvement of symptoms was found in 89% of children and 92% of adults, with no antibiotic use in 93% of children and 86% of adults. In a third group consisting of 100 patients with bronchitis, improvement was reported in 73% of children and 98% of adults, with no antibiotic use in 96% of children and 88% of adults. The use of Renikan® was shown to be effective and safe in children over 6 years of age and in adults with upper respiratory tract infections, with decreased use of concomitant therapy in 50% of cases, and with only 0.02% of patients having adverse events. The use of Renikan® reduced the use of antibiotics, with fewer bacterial complications in upper respiratory tract infections (Pérez et al., 2011). In a placebo-controlled, monocentric pilot study, *P. sidoides* was given to 14 out of 28 patients with a diagnosed transient hypogammaglobulinaemia of infancy (THI)

(14 patients received the placebo) during upper respiratory tract infections (Patiroglu et al., 2012). The treatment was given for 1 week and serum alanine aminotransferase, complete blood count, gamma glutamyl transpeptidase, prothrombin time, activated prothromboplastin time, aspartate aminotransferase and bilirubin levels were measured. *Pelargonium sidoides* was found to be beneficial for recovery from daily and nocturnal cough, for nasal congestion, and increased appetite (Patiroglu et al., 2012).

A study evaluated the efficacy of an extract of *P. sidoides* for the treatment of the common cold. After treatment for 5 days, the mean cold intensity score (CIS) decreased by 11.2 ± 4.8 points for *Pelargonium*, compared to 6.3 ± 4.7 points for the control group (Riley et al., 2018). Results after 10 days indicated that 21.2% of the control group and 90.4% of the group receiving the active medication were clinically cured. Participants' inability to work was significantly lower in the treatment group, with a mean duration of 6.4 ± 1.6 days *vs* 8.3 ± 2.1 days for the control group. The treatment outcome (major improvement or complete recovery) was significantly better at day 5 for the *Pelargonium* treatment group compared to the control. The results showed that mild-to-moderate adverse events (all non-serious) occurred in only 15.4% of those receiving active treatment, *vs* 5.8% for the control group (Riley et al., 2018). *Pelargonium sidoides* can therefore be used as a well-tolerated, safe and effective treatment for colds, as it significantly shortened the duration of the condition and reduced the severity of symptoms. Another clinical trial showed similar results for the safety and efficacy of *P. sidoides* in the treatment of the common cold (Riley et al., 2019). On day 5, the mean SSID was significantly higher in the EPs® 7630 group compared with the placebo group (12.5 ± 4.4 *vs* 8.8 ± 6.8 points), and patients in the EPs® 7630 group (55%) rated the treatment outcome as 'major improvement' compared to patients in the placebo group (15%). After 10 days of treatment, 12% of patients of the placebo group and 45% of patients of the treated group had reached 0 points on the CIS (all, or all but one symptom, had completely resolved) in 74% (EPs® 7630) and 25% of patients (placebo), respectively. During the clinical trial, adverse events occurred in seven patients (13.5%) in the placebo and five patients (9.4%) in the EPs® 7630 group, with satisfaction higher in the *Pelargonium* group than in the placebo group (75% *vs* 37%).

8.2.2 Tonsillo-pharyngitis

Acute tonsillo-pharyngitis is one of the most common reasons for adolescents, children and young adults to consult a physician (Berezhnoi et al., 2016). Despite extensive prescription, antibiotic therapy is indicated in less than one-fifth of these cases. An extract of *P. sidoides* was investigated in patients (6–10 years old) with acute tonsillo-pharyngitis, who showed no evidence of group A β-hemolytic streptococcus, for a duration of 6 days. The change in the Tonsillitis Severity Score (TSS) was measured after 4 days for the *Pelargonium* (60 children) and the placebo (64 children) groups. The score decreased from 9.5 ± 1.3 to 6.1 ± 4.1 points in the placebo group and from 9.6 ± 1.2 to 2.8 ± 2.6 points in the active medication group.

The extract EPs® 7630 was found to be very well tolerated and efficacious in the treatment of acute tonsillo-pharyngitis in children. Clinical trial data suggest that antibiotics are not indicated for the treatment of acute non-group A β-hemolytic strep (non-GABHS) tonsillo-pharyngitis and effective alternatives are needed. A study showed that the extract of *P. sidoides* (EPs® 7630) was superior to placebo for the treatment of non-GABHS tonsillo-pharyngitis in children, with a decrease of the TSS from baseline (day 0) to day 4 [2.5 ± 3.6 points for placebo ($n=70$) and 7.1 ± 2.1 points for EPs® 7630 ($n=73$)]. The covariate adjusted decrease was 2.9 ± 2.4 points for the placebo group and 70 ± 2.4 points for the *Pelargonium*-treated group. The 95% Reliable Change Index (RCI) for the difference between the groups was [2.7;4.9] showing a significant difference in the efficacy of *Pelargonium vs* placebo. EPs® 7630 was considered superior to the placebo for the treatment of acute non-GABHS tonsillo-pharyngitis in children with low adverse events in 15 out of the 143 patients (EPs® 7630: 4/73 patients, placebo: 44/70). Treatment with EPs® 7630 shortened the duration of illness by at least 2 days, and reduced the severity of symptoms (Bereznoy et al., 2003). It was debated whether treatment with *P. sidoides* reduced the administration of paracetamol in children with AB or acute tonsillo-pharyngitis (ATP). The literature was scanned and six relevant trials were identified. The data included a total of 523 children, aged 6–10 years (EPs® 7630: 265; placebo: 258) and suffering from AB (three trials) or non-β-hemolytic streptococcal ATP (three trials) (Seifert et al., 2019). Compared to the placebo, *Pelargonium* reduced the cumulative dose of paracetamol in five of the six trials, by an average of 244 mg (95% confidence interval: [−0.53; −0.02]) in children receiving treatment for 7 days (AB) or six (ATP). In children aged 6–10 years with ATP or AB, treatment with *Pelargonium* accelerated recovery and the burden of symptoms. By the end of the treatment, 74.4% of the placebo group and only 30.2% of the EPs® 7630 group were still unable to attend school. The concomitant use of paracetamol was also reduced.

8.2.3 Bronchitis and influenza

The extract of *P. sidoides* (EPs® 7630; 30 drops three times daily) was evaluated in 468 patients with AB (present ≤48 h) and a Bronchitis Severity Score (BSS) ≥5 points (Matthys et al., 2003). The decrease in BSS after 7 days was 3.2 ± 4.1 points with the placebo group ($n=235$) and 5.9 ± 2.9 points with the EPs® 7630 group ($n=233$). The 95% confidence index for the difference of effects between the two groups was calculated, and *Pelargonium* exhibited significant superiority over the placebo group on day seven. The duration of illness was significantly shorter for patients treated with *Pelargonium* compared to the placebo, with a notable decrease in work inability (16%) in the EPs® 7630 group (43% in the placebo group). Within the first 4 days, the effect of the treatment was evident in 53.6% of patients compared to the placebo group (36.2%). All adverse events in 36 of the 468 patients were assessed as non-serious (placebo: 16/235 patients; EPs® 7630: 20/233 patients). The extract EPs® 7630 exhibited significant activity compared to the placebo in the treatment of adults with AB. A clear advantage was shown after EPs® 7630 treatment by a reduction in the severity of symptoms and shortened duration of work inability (nearly 2 days) (Matthys et al., 2003). Another study was conducted (Chuchalin et al., 2005) to investigate the safety and efficacy of the *P. sidoides* preparation EPs® 7630 in patients with AB. The 95% confidence index for the difference of effects between the two treatment groups (EPs® 7630 minus placebo) was calculated on day 7 as (1.21, 3.56) showing a significant improvement in the EPs® 7630 group compared to placebo: a decrease in BSS after 7 days of 4.9 ± 2.7 points with placebo ($n = 60$) and 7.2 ± 3.1 points with EPs® 7630 ($n = 64$). Rates of complete recovery were considerably higher in the EPs® 7630 group for each of the five individual symptoms. The onset of treatment effect was recognised in 33.3% of patients in the placebo group and 68.8% of patients in the EPs® 7630 group, within the first 4 days. Adverse events (all non-serious) occurred in 25 of 124 patients (placebo: 10/60 patients; EPs® 7630: 15/64 patients) with high rated improvement of quality of life in the EPs® 7630 group.

The tolerability and efficacy of a herbal extract of *P. sidoides* was demonstrated in a multicentric outcomes study including 205 patients, suffering from acute exacerbation of chronic bronchitis or AB (Matthys and Heger, 2007a). The score of five symptoms typical for bronchitis, namely wheezing/whistling on expiration, expectoration, cough, dyspnoea and chest pain during coughing, were assessed using a 5-point scale (from 4 = extremely pronounced to 0 = not present). A four-point scale (from 3 = very pronounced to 0 = not present) was used to assess other symptoms such as headache, hoarseness, fatigue and aching limbs. Matthys and Heger (2007a) recorded a total score of 6.1 ± 2.8 points on average, at the start of treatment, and the score decreased to 2.8 ± 2.6 points with the final examination on day seven. The patients (about 60.5%) stated that their health at the end of the study was much improved or symptom-free. Adverse events occurred in a total of 16 patients and all were considered non-serious, with onset of action typically occurring after 2 days. Most of the patients (78%) were satisfied or very satisfied with the *Pelargonium* treatment. The objective of another study (Matthys and Heger, 2007b) was focused on adults in the treatment of AB outside the restricted indication of antibiotic therapy. A dose of 30 drops of EPs® 7630 solution was given to 108 patients, three times daily with a similar dosage given to the placebo group (109 patients) for a period of 7 days. After this period, the BSS score decreased by 5.3 ± 3.2 points in the placebo group and by 7.6 ± 2.2 points in the EPs® 7630 group. The 95% confidence interval was calculated as 1.6–3.1, showing significant efficacy for the EPs® 7630 treatment group. There were also noticeable improvements in individual symptoms, such as sputum, cough, dyspnoea, chest pain upon coughing, and rales/rhonchi in the treatment group *vs* the placebo group. No serious adverse events (only transitory and minor events) were recorded with good patient satisfaction (Matthys and Heger, 2007b).

In Germany, a study site was located to evaluate the safety and efficacy of EPs® 7630 in patients with AB (Matthys et al., 2007). EPs® 7630 solution was given to 2099 patients (aged 0–93 years) with productive cough for <6 days, without indication for treatment with antibiotics in an age-dependent dosage for a period of 14 days. The mean change of the BSS score from baseline to last observation was considered as the primary outcome, with assessment criteria such as sputum, cough, chest pain at cough, rales/rhonchi, and dyspnoea. The mean BSS of all patients lowered to 1.0 ± 1.9 points by the patients' individual final visit, from 7.1 ± 2.9 points at baseline. A decrease in mean BSS was reported for children younger than 3 years from 5.2 ± 2.5 points to 1.2 ± 2.1 points, and for children from 6.3 ± 2.8 points to 0.9 ± 1.8 points. Adverse events (non-serious) occurred in 26 out of 2099 patients (1.2%). A randomised, multicentre, placebo-controlled clinical trial was conducted in adult outpatients (217), suffering from AB, using the roots of *P. sidoides* (EPs® 7630) (Matthys and Funk, 2008). The BSS score decreased by 5.3 ± 3.2 points for the placebo group and by 7.6 ± 2.2 (mean ± SD) points for the active treatment group. A marked improvement was demonstrated for EPs® 7630 for all disease symptoms associated with AB, such as pain on coughing, cough, rales, sputum, hoarseness, dyspnoea, fatigue, headache, limb pain and fever. Specifically, strong antifatigue and antitussive effects, with an early onset during treatment, were observed. In the treatment groups, the dosage of 3×30 drops/patient administered for 7 days was well-tolerated, and patients were able to go to work sooner in the EPs® 7630 group. The results showed that EPs® 7630 was superior in the treatment of AB, led to faster remission of bronchitis-related symptoms, and no serious adverse events were recorded.

Systematic literature searches were performed by Agbabiaka et al. (2008) using five electronic databases: Amed (1985—July 2007), Medline (1950—July 2007), Embase (1974—July 2007), The Cochrane Library (Issue 3, 2007) and CINAHL (1982—July 2007). Data were selected, extracted and validated by two researchers, independently. The methodological quality of most trials was rated good, with six randomised clinical trials meeting the inclusion criteria (of which four were suitable for statistical pooling). Five studies tested EPs® 7630 against a placebo, with one study comparing EPs® 7630 to acetylcysteine, a conventional non-antibiotic treatment. All of the trials reported positive results on the effectiveness of *P. sidoides* in treating AB. From the meta-analysis of the four placebo-controlled studies, it was concluded that EPs® 7630 significantly reduced bronchitis symptom scores after 7 days in patients with AB, with no serious adverse events reported. A study that was aimed at evaluating the tolerability and efficacy of an extract of *P. sidoides* in the treatment of patients (1–18 years) with AB, outside the strict indication for antibiotics, was conducted (Kamin et al., 2010a). Tolerability was shown to be good in both groups, and on day seven, the treatment with *Pelargonium* performed significantly better, with onset of effect faster, satisfaction with treatment more pronounced (77.6% *vs* 25.8%), and time of bed rest shorter than for the placebo group. No serious adverse events were observed and *Pelargonium* was shown to be safe and efficacious in the treatment of

AB in adolescents and children outside the strict indication for antibiotics. It was perceived that patients treated with EPs® 7630 experienced a more favourable course of the disease and good tolerability when compared to the placebo group.

A dose-finding study for an extract of *P. sidoides* was performed by Kamin et al. (2010b) in adolescents and children. The BSS total score was significantly higher in the 90 mg and 60 mg groups after 7 days of treatment, compared with the placebo group, and without many differences between the two dosages. There was a definite improvement related to sputum, coughing and rales at auscultation with EPs® 7630 treatment, and the onset of effect was faster, satisfaction with treatment better, and time of bed rest shorter. The EPs® 7630 extract was found to be effective in AB outside the strict indication for antibiotics in patients (6–18 years old), with a dose of 90 mg or 60 mg daily offering the best benefit and with good tolerability. It significantly reduced the severity of symptoms, led to a faster recovery from AB, and a more favourable course of the disease compared with the placebo. Tablets containing EPs® 7630 were evaluated for their ability to treat AB in adults, outside the strict indication for antibiotics (Matthys et al., 2010a). Data (0–7 days) revealed that the BSS score decreased by 4.3 ± 1.9 (30 mg group), 6.1 ± 2.1 (60 mg group), 6.3 ± 2.0 points (90 mg group) and 2.7 ± 2.3 (placebo), respectively, and the differences were statistically significant. The EPs® 7630 was well-tolerated, with secondary endpoints showing comparable results. All adverse events were considered mild to moderate, with no serious adverse events reported. All three tested dosages of EPs® 7630 were statistically superior and clinically more relevant than the placebo. Taking into account both safety and efficacy, the results of this study showed that a 20 mg tablet of EPs® 7630 taken three times daily constitutes the optimal dose with respect to the benefit–risk ratio, and is well-tolerated.

Health-related quality of life (HRQL) and patient-reported outcome (PRO) have become relevant outcome parameters for the assessment of medical treatment within clinical trials. Therefore, EPs® 7630 was tested for safety and efficacy in a clinical trial of AB in adolescents and children outside the strict indication for antibiotics (Huntley and Kamin, 2010). Patients treated with EPs® 7630 perceived a good tolerability and a more favourable course of the disease as compared with the placebo. Matthys et al. (2010b) conducted a study in 406 adults with four parallel treatment groups (30, 60 or 90 mg EPs® 7630 daily; placebo). At each study visit, PRO and HRQL were evaluated by questionnaires as secondary outcome measures. At day 7, the patient-reported outcome was significantly improved in all the three EPs® 7630 groups compared to placebo (patient-reported treatment outcome, EQ-5D and EQ VAS, impact of patient's sickness, SF-12, physical score, satisfaction with treatment, duration of activity limitation). A clinically relevant and statistically significant improvement in PRO/HRQL compared to placebo was demonstrated in all the three EPs® 7630 groups (Matthys et al., 2010b). EPs® 7630 showed dose-dependent anti-influenza activity at non-toxic concentrations against oseltamivir-sensitive and -resistant seasonal H1N1, pandemic H1N1, seasonal H3N2, and the laboratory H1N1 strain A/Puerto Rico/8/34, while no antiviral activity against measles virus or adenovirus was observed (Theisen and Muller, 2012). The extract impaired viral haemagglutination, as well as neuraminidase activity, and inhibited an early step of influenza infection. It is worth noting that EPs® 7630 did not show a direct virucidal effect, as *in vitro* virus pre-incubation (unlike cell pre-incubation) with the extract did not influence infectivity. An important observation was that EPs® 7630 showed no tendency to resistance development. Further analysis of the EPs® 7630 extract showed that the compounds responsible for activity were the prodelphinidins, and that chain length influenced antiviral activity, as oligo- and polymers were more effective than monomers and dimers. However, epigallocatechin and its stereoisomer, gallocatechin, exerted antiviral activity, also in their monomeric form. Furthermore, it was proven that EPs® 7630 taken by inhalation significantly enhanced survival, body temperature and body weight of influenza-infected mice, without observed toxicity, demonstrating the benefit of EPs® 7630 in the treatment of influenza.

Kamin et al. (2012) further investigated the tolerability and efficacy of *P. sidoides* in adolescents and children suffering from AB, without the strict indication for antibiotics. Patients (220) with AB were randomised and given either placebo or verum containing EPs® 7630 (>12–18/>6–12/1–6 years: 3×30/3×20/3×10 drops/day) for a period of 7 days. The decrease in the BSS total score was significantly higher for EPs® 7630 compared to placebo after 7 days (4.4 ± 1.6 *vs* 2.9 ± 1.4 points). Significant improvements were recorded for rales at auscultation and coughing. Tolerability was comparably good in both groups. Extract EPs® 7630 proved to be a well-tolerated and an efficacious option for the treatment of AB in adolescents and children outside the strict indication for antibiotics. A study by Ross (2012) also demonstrated tolerability and efficacy of *P. sidoides* in the treatment of AB outside the strict indication in children and adults. The BSS score of all patients studied lowered from a median of 7 points at baseline to a median of 0 points at the third-follow up visit, which related to an average decrease of 6 points. Significant improvement or complete recovery occurred in 94.2% of all patients. Bronchitis symptoms resolved in 80% of all cases, with the exception of cough symptoms, which showed a remission in 59.7% of cases with other symptoms, such as headache and hoarseness, at a remission rate of 80% in all patients. One-third of patients experienced complete resolution of symptoms prior to the third follow-up visit. In numerous systematic reviews and randomised controlled trials, such as those published by the Cochrane Collaboration, *P. sidoides* extract proved to be effective in acute respiratory tract infections (aRTI) in all the age groups investigated. Eight randomised control trials investigating the application of EPs® 7630 in acute tonsillo-pharyngitis, AB and aRTI in the context of chronic preconditions were identified. Results showed a statistically significant improvement of aRTI symptom severity for EPs® 7630 when compared to the control. The investigation of EPs® 7630 in asthmatic adolescents and children with aRTI showed a possible associated reduction of asthma attacks and a significant symptom-alleviating effect (Careddu and Pettenazzo, 2018). An alleviating effect of EPs® 7630 was reported in immune-compromised children with acute upper RTI, and all RCTs reported good tolerability and safety of EPs® 7630.

8.2.4 Asthma and chronic obstructive pulmonary disease (COPD)

There is no effective therapy for preventing an asthma attack during upper respiratory tract viral infection (Tahan and Yaman, 2013). *Pelargonium sidoides* therapy was investigated for preventing asthma attacks during upper respiratory tract viral infection over a period of 5 days. Asthmatic children (61) with upper respiratory tract viral infection were registered in a study, and the children were randomised to receive *P. sidoides* daily for 5 days (30 children) or not (31 children). Symptom scores were determined before and after treatment, and children were examined whether they had an asthma attack or not. *Pelargonium sidoides* treatment was not associated with statistically significant differences in muscle aches and fever. However, there were significant differences in nasal congestion and cough frequency between the groups. The *P. sidoides* group had fewer asthma attacks and the differences were statistically significant. It was subsequently concluded that *P. sidoides* prevented asthma attacks during upper respiratory tract viral infections.

Managing and preventing exacerbations is a major component of COPD treatment. An extract of *P. sidoides* (EPs® 7630) was investigated as an alternative treatment in patients with COPD stage II/III (Matthys et al., 2013). The superiority of EPs® 7630 was confirmed in secondary endpoints and included fewer exacerbations, fewer patients with antibiotic use, fewer days of inability to work, improved quality of life and higher patient satisfaction, with median time to exacerbation significantly extended, with EPs® 7630 compared to placebo (one-sided centre-stratified log-rank test, 57 *vs* 43 days). A lower number of gastro-intestinal adverse events were reported for the EPs® 7630 group. Data showed clinically relevant superiority and statistically significant effects for EPs® 7630 over the placebo group with good long-term tolerability in the treatment of COPD. Treatment with EPs® 7630 reduced antibiotic use and exacerbation frequency, and prolonged time to exacerbations (Matthys et al., 2013). Data of an already published clinical trial with EPs® 7630 in COPD patients, focusing on exacerbation frequency and antibiotic use, were further analysed by Matthys and Malek (2015). The number of patients with reported exacerbations was significantly higher in the placebo group (71.3%) *vs* the EPs® 7630 group (35.7%). Correspondingly, a significantly lower number of patients of the EPs® 7630 group needed antibiotic treatment (37.8% *vs* 72.5%) and the mean number of days off work due to exacerbations was significantly lower (5.5 ± 4.1 *vs* 7.5 ± 4.6 days). Treatment with EPs® 7630 resulted in a significant reduction in exacerbation frequency associated with reduced antibiotic use, and fewer days of inability to work in patients with COPD stage III or II. In another add-on therapy study with *P. sidoides,* adults (199) diagnosed with COPD stages III or II, receiving standard treatment according to the Global Initiative for Chronic Obstructive Lung Disease (GOLD), were investigated for a period of 24 weeks (Matthys and Funk, 2018). At week 24, all PRO and HRQoL measurements showed a pronounced improvement, with EPs® 7630 (SGRQ total score, EQ VAS, sputum production, IMOS, Symptom Severity Score of cough and sternal pain while coughing, IMPSS and duration of inability to work). Importantly, the difference seen for the SGRQ exceeded the minimal clinically important difference (MCID) threshold of 4 points. Therefore, therapy with EPs® 7630 led to a good long-term tolerability with improvement in HRQoL and other PROs in adult patients with COPD.

8.2.5 Anti-inflammatory effects

Animal experiments were conducted to access the secretolytic, antitussive and anti-inflammatory effects of the aqueous ethanolic extract of *P. sidoides*, following oral administration at human equivalent doses (Bao et al., 2015). A dose-dependent and significant reduction of cough frequency was observed, with a prolongation of cough latency time. In addition, the extract caused characteristic histopathological changes in lung tissue adjacent to bronchi and trachea in acute bacterial bronchitis with a marked secretolytic activity. The degree of lesions was significantly reduced in rats at doses of 60 and 30 mg/kg. A reduced serum level of malondialdehyde indicated an upregulation of superoxide dismutase and a subsequent protective effect against oxidative stress. In another study (Park et al., 2018), anti-inflammatory effects of a combination of *Coptis chinensis* root (CR) and *P. sidoides* (PS) extracts were evaluated *in vivo* and *in vitro*. The combination CR + PS significantly decreased the levels of COX-2 and iNOS and reduced the production of PGE 2, NO and three pro-inflammatory cytokines (interleukin (IL)-1β, TNF-α and IL-6). Treatment with CR + PS significantly reduced the phosphorylated inhibitor of NF-κB (p-I-κBα) and the protein expression levels of LPS-stimulated NF-κB. In addition, CR + PS significantly inhibited infiltrated inflammatory cells, increases in paw swelling, mast cell degranulation, skin thickness, iNOS-, TNF-α- and COX-2-immunoreactive cells in a rat model of carrageenan-induced acute oedematous paw. This combined therapy may therefore be a possible candidate for the treatment of inflammatory diseases.

8.2.6 Immunomodulatory effects

Exhaustive exercise can affect the immune response. Evidence for this is confirmed by upper respiratory tract infections that may be related to profile changes of systemic cytokines and local cytokines of the upper respiratory tract and/or the decrease in secretory immunoglobulin A in the upper airway mucosa (Luna et al., 2011). To evaluate the effect of an extract of *P. sidoides* on the immune response of athletes undergoing intense running training, Luna et al. (2011) determined cytokines, both systemically and locally, as well as the presence of immunoglobulin A in the saliva of the athletes. Data revealed that the *P. sidoides* extract regulated the production of secretory immunoglobulin A in saliva, both IL-6 and IL-15 in serum, and IL-15 in the nasal mucosa. Levels of IL-6 and IL-15 were decreased, while secretory immunoglobulin A levels were increased. They concluded from the study that *Pelargonium* exerted a significant modulating effect on the immune response associated with the upper airway mucosa in athletes undergoing extreme physical activity. Flow cytometry was employed to measure NO production of an extract of EPs® 7630-activated macrophages using *Leishmania* major GFP-infected murine bone marrow-derived macrophages (BMM), and the study was correlated with the reduction of the GFP signal measured at single cell levels (Thäle et al., 2011).

Results indicated that the anti-infectious effect of 310 µg/mL of EPs® 7630 (signal reduction: 2573%; NO production: 413 µM) was less eminent than that in combination with IFN standard (100 U/mL) (signal reduction: 3578%; NO production: 2027 µM). Furthermore, supernatants of 10 µg/mL of EPs® 7630-stimulated BMM significantly reduced the cytopathic effect of encephalomyocarditis virus (EMCV) on L929 fibroblasts, with an antiviral activity of 80 U/mL compared to 100 U/mL of an IFN standard. Mediation of cytoprotective effects was not observed with direct addition of EPs® 7630 to L929. The compounds responsible for the antiviral activity in *Pelargonium* have not been identified. Detection of IFNs by enzyme-linked immuno-assay (ELISA) was unsuccessful, and this may be due to their low concentrations in cell supernatants. The results strongly supported the induction of anti-infectious responses by EPs® 7630 (Thäle et al., 2011). *Pelargonium sidoides* was investigated for its immunomodulatory effects in calves by Seckin et al. (2018). Non-vaccinated calves (60, 25-day-old) were randomly selected and divided into five treatment groups (12 calves each); four treatment groups receiving different amounts and/or at different times of *Pelargonium*, and the placebo group (Seckin et al., 2018). Levels of IL-1-β, mRNAs for γ-interferon, total IgG, tumour necrosis factor-α genes and IL-4 were compared from days 0–9 posttreatment. Significant differences were found between untreated and treated calves, proving that *P. sidoides* is able to regulate immune functions in calves. A dose of 62.5 mg for 5 days was considered to be ideal.

8.2.7 Other properties

Caenorhabditis elegans was used to study the effect of an aqueous alcoholic root extract of *P. sidoides* on stress resistance *in vivo*. *Pelargonium* treatment reduced intracellular hsp-16.2:GFP expression (induced by the pro-oxidant juglone), reflecting anti-oxidant activity *in vivo* and proving that the secondary metabolites are bioavailable. A prominent role of DAF-16/FOXO in the daf-2 pathway was proven by Rezaizadehnajafi and Wink (2014) through the application of 50 µg/mL of the extract to the transgenic mutant TJ356. This resulted in the migration of the transcription factor DAF-16 from the cytosol to the nucleus. *Pelargonium sidoides* preparation was shown to be effective and safe in aRTIs through a reviewed clinical study (Kamin et al., 2018). This study included an overview of newly analysed data, as well as known data from children <6 years. In total, seven clinical studies involving 1067 children <6 years, exposed to EPs® 7630, were identified. The efficacy of EPs® 7630 was significantly superior to placebo, when considering time until complete recovery and symptom reduction intensity, in two randomised, double-blind trials in patients with AB. Similar results were also reported in two non-comparative observational studies of AB. In two other studies, which included an acute rhinosinusitis and a non-comparative, open-label study in acute tonsillo-pharyngitis, nearly all children showed major symptom improvements or complete recovery during the treatment trial. Similar changes were seen in controlled trials investigating older patient populations. The extract of EPs® 7630 was also proven to be well-tolerated and safe in an additional observational study including children with various diagnoses of aRTIs.

8.3 Safety

A very low incidence of side effects has been reported for the extracts of *P. sidoides*. The cytotoxicity of the coumarins present in the crude extract can be considered negligible (Kayser, 1997; Kolodziej, 2002). This was confirmed by Loew and Koch (2008), who established a no observable effect level (NOEL) of >750 mg/kg body weight in toxicological studies using rats and dogs, indicating a low risk linked to the coumarin content. A daily intake of 60 mg of extract is equivalent to a dose of 1 and 4 mg/kg body weight (60 kg for an adult or 15 kg for a child), respectively, converting to a safety factor of >100. The only coumarins present in EPs® 7630, namely 7-hydroxycoumarin derivatives, induced no hepatotoxic activity (Loew and Koch, 2008). Conrad et al. (2007c) and Schulz (2008) outlined the efficacy and safety findings for *Pelargonium* and to date, there are no reported drug interactions or contraindications for the plant. Furthermore, all controlled clinical trials indicated that EPs® 7630 is safe and well tolerated. When trials were conducted with over 7000 children and adults suffering from acute tonsillo-pharyngitis, AB or acute maxillary sinusitis, adverse events occurred in 1%–15% of patients. These adverse events were mainly mild, consisting of skin rashes and gastro-intestinal complaints. However, a total of 34 case reports of allergic hypersensitivity/allergic reactions have been documented through the World Health Organisation's (WHO) international pharmacovigilance programme. These reports may be linked to the use of *Pelargonium* extract. These case reports are limited to Germany (De Boer et al., 2007), but products containing *Pelargonium* are also marketed in other countries. No specific data on the effect of EPs® 7630 on pregnant or lactating women are available. Drug interactions of EPs® 7630 with penicillin V were investigated by Roots et al. (2004) in a double-blind, placebo-controlled trial with 28 healthy humans. This was done as antibiotics are often administered for the treatment of infections of the upper respiratory tract, particularly tonsillitis. Penicillin V and EPs® 7630 were administered for 7 and 8 days, respectively. No statistically significant difference of the target parameters was observed between verum and placebo. No adverse reactions were observed.

Other drug interactions with antiplatelet and -coagulant drugs were also investigated, with a particular focus on the coumarins in EPs® 7630. The extract was administered to rats and no changes in coagulation parameters or interactions with anticoagulants of the coumarin type, for example warfarin, were observed by Koch and Biber (2007). Extract EPs® 7630 was administered orally for a period of 2 weeks, with warfarin as a control. Treatment with warfarin resulted in a significant lowering of coagulation parameters. Cotreatment with warfarin and EPs® 7630 did not influence the pharmacokinetics of warfarin or affect the efficacy of the drug. The Drug Commission of the German Medical Association (DCGMA) has interpreted some spontaneous reports of assumed hepatoxicity linked to the use of *P. sidoides* to treat respiratory tract infections and the common cold (Teschke et al., 2012a). The assessment was done using the structured, liver-specific, quantitative, and updated scale of the Council for International Organisations of Medical Sciences (CIOMS). None of the 15 cases showed any probability of *Pelargonium* as the cause of hepatoxicity. However, the data from the analysis showed surprising factors unrelated to *Pelargonium*, such as poor quality and incorrect diagnoses in most cases. A minority of cases were linked to common other diseases of the liver. Data to exclude viral infections caused by hepatitis A–C were available in four cases and by cytomegalovirus (CMV) and Epstein–Barr virus (EBV) in one case; biliary tract imaging data were provided for only three patients; data to exclude virus infections by hepatitis A–C were shown in four cases, and by CMV and EBV in one case, while herpes simplex virus (HSV) and varicella zoster virus (VZV) infections remained unconsidered. Therefore, convincing evidence is lacking that *Pelargonium* was a potential hepatotoxin in the cases analysed.

Thirteen spontaneous cases with primarily suspected *P. sidoides* hepatotoxicity were included in a study (Teschke et al., 2012b). The data were submitted to an in-depth clinical evaluation with the use of the original and updated scale of CIOMS to assess causality levels. Causality for *P. sidoides* was evaluated using the liver-specific, quantitative, and structured updated scale of CIOMS. No safety concern was raised in any of the 13 cases and causality for *Pelargonium* could not be established after applying the CIOMS scales. Confounding variables included poor data quality, co-medication with synthetic drugs, major comorbidities, lack of appropriate consideration of differential diagnoses, and multiple alternative diagnoses. The study proved lack of hepatotoxicity by *Pelargonium* in all the cases. The antimutagenic effects of *P. sidoides* were investigated by Beceren et al. (2017) in two groups, with or without S9 metabolic activation. The data indicated that *P. sidoides* had antimutagenic effects towards TA 98 and TA 100, without S9 metabolic activation, but no antimutagenic effects were observed towards TA 98 and TA 100 with S9 metabolic activation. A literature review by Anheyer et al. (2018) was conducted to identify herbal therapy in the treatment of respiratory tract infections with efficacy and safety. Scopus, Medline/PubMed and the Cochrane Library were searched and 11 trials with 2181 participants were included. Meta-analysis revealed six trials with evidence for efficacy (confidence interval, risk ratio and safety of *P. sidoides* in treating respiratory tract infections compared with placebo). Furthermore, moderate evidence for efficacy and safety was found in the treatment of respiratory tract infections in children (Anheyer et al., 2018).

9. Phytochemistry

9.1 Volatile constituents

A large number (102) of compounds were identified using gas liquid chromatography (GLC) and gas chromatography coupled to mass spectrometry (GC–MS) analyses in the essential oil, obtained through hydro-distillation of the leaves of *P. sidoides* (Kayser et al., 1998). The largest fraction of the essential oil (approximately 60%) comprised sesquiterpenes, with caryophyllene (2.3%) and caryophyllene epoxide (13%) being the major compounds. The oil also contained phenylpropanoids (9%), monoterpenes (16%), elemicin (3.6%) and methyl eugenol (4.3%) as the most abundant compounds.

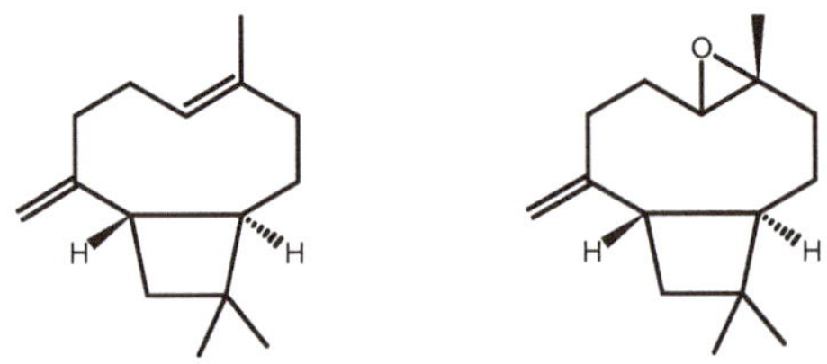

Caryophyllene Caryophyllene epoxide

9.2 Non-volatile constituents

Extraction of milled roots of *P. sidoides* with 11% (w/w) ethanol in water is commonly known as EPs® 7630 (active ingredient of Umckaloabo®, Iso Arzneimittel Ettlingen) (Schoetz et al., 2008). This polar solvent extracts a number of constituents that differ significantly from those extracted using non-polar solvents. The results revealed that EPs® 7630 is composed of six main groups of compounds, namely monomeric and oligomeric carbohydrates, unsubstituted and substituted oligomeric prodelphinidins, peptides, minerals, substituted benzopyranones and purine derivatives. The oligo-prodelphinidins have an uncommon diversity and consist of a large variety of connectivities and substructures, even at a low degree of polymerisation. Intermediates of DNA synthesis, second messengers, and three distinctive purine derivatives were characterised by phytochemical means. The major benzopyranones of EPs® 7630 are highly oxygenated at the phenyl unit (consisting of 3–4 oxygens) and sulphated at distinct positions. These constituents amount to about 70%–80% of the total weight of EPs® 7630. Schötz et al. (2008) and Schötz and Nöldner (2007) also reported the constituents of EPs® 7630, and six main constituent groups were identified, namely carbohydrates (oligomeric and monomeric, 12%), benzopyranones (2%), peptides (10%), purine derivatives (2%), unsubstituted and substituted oligomeric prodelphinidins (40%) and minerals (12%). The extensive use of *P. sidoides* in traditional medicine has led to an increase in scientific investigation of the chemical composition, as well as the active principles of this plant. This resulted in a considerable number of publications on the phytochemistry of *P. sidoides*. Theisen and Muller (2012) reported on the chemical compounds of the ethanolic extract of the roots, which contain mainly oligo- and polymeric pro-anthocyanidins, with gallocatechin and epigallocatechin moieties. The biological efficacy of

P. sidoides has been partly ascribed to the activity of oxygenated coumarins (6,8-dihydroxy-5,7-dimethoxycoumarin and 7-hydroxy-5,6-dimethoxycoumarin, also referred to as umckalin), phenolic and hydroxycinnamic acid derivatives, flavonoids and gallic acid derivatives (Moyo and Van Staden, 2014). A total of 15 benzopyranones were identified from the roots of *P. sidoides* with two of these, 6,8-bis(sulpho-oxy)-7-methoxy-2*H*-1-benzopyran-2-one and 6-methoxy-7-(sulpho-oxy)-2*H*-1-benzopyran-2-one, detected for the first time in *P. sidoides*. Hauer et al. (2010) also characterised two new compounds, namely 8-hydroxy-7-methoxy-6-(sulpho-oxy)-2*H*-1-benzopyran-2-one and 7-hydroxy-6-methoxy-8-(sulpho-oxy)-2*H*-1-benzopyran-2-one. Structure elucidation was done by both one-dimensional (1D)- and two-dimensional (2D) nuclear magnetic resonance (NMR) spectroscopy (Hauer et al., 2010).

The structures of the first identified pro-anthocyanidins from *P. sidoides* were disclosed by Janecki and Kolodziej (2010), showing prodelphinidins with A-type elements. Total phenolic content is currently used for the quality control of phytopreparations containing extracts of *P. sidoides*. Franco and de Oliveira (2010) reported the validation and development of a reversed phase (RP)-HPLC method for the analysis of commercial *P. sidoides* syrup and tincture phytopreparations (five batches) employing umckalin as a chemical marker. Several herbal products have been formulated using *P. sidoides*, of which Umckaloabo® is probably the most popular, and this has been successfully marketed in Germany. Methods using Fourier transform-infrared (FT-IR) spectroscopy were investigated by Maree and Viljoen (2011) in order to discriminate the closely related species, *P. reniforme* from *P. sidoides*. Spectroscopic data were interrogated using chemometric computations, including principal component analysis and orthogonal projections to latent structures-discriminant analysis. Phytochemical variation of 9.22% in the mid-infrared (MIR) dataset and 5.79% in the near-infrared (NIR) spectroscopy dataset was responsible for the separation of the two plant species. Seven absorption areas were identified as putative biomarkers and the data indicated that FT-MIR and FT-NIR spectroscopy can be used to distinguish between these two closely related species. Another method to distinguish between *Pelargonium* species was investigated by Viljoen et al. (2015) and untargeted ultra-high-performance liquid chromatography-mass spectrometry (UHPLC–MS) and proton-NMR (^1H NMR) metabolomic approaches were used for the plant species, *P. reniforme* and *P. sidoides*. A quantitative comparison of the marker constituents within both species was conducted using quantitative NMR (qNMR). The compound umckalin was identified as a marker for *P. sidoides* (0.0012%–0.2760% (w/w)) by UHPLC–MS, with only trace amounts occurring in *P. reniforme* (0%–0.0016% (w/w)). Distinctive chemical profiles were demonstrated between the two species by employing both UHPLC–MS and ^1H NMR, in combination with multivariate algorithms. The coumarins, scopoletin, isofraxoside and an isomer of scopoletin, were reported to occur in higher concentrations in *P. reniforme* when compared to *P. sidoides* (Viljoen et al., 2015). Hudaib et al. (2010) reported a rapid and simple HPLC method with ultraviolet (UV) detection for the quantitation of umckalin, as a chemical marker, in *Pelargonium* extract cough syrup. The method showed good linearity over the concentration range of 0.334–1.667 μg/mL, with a correlation co-efficient (r^2) of 0.9996. The limit of quantitation (LOQ) and limit of detection (LOD) for the marker umckalin were reported as 0.0344 and 0.1031 μg/mL, respectively (Hudaib et al., 2010).

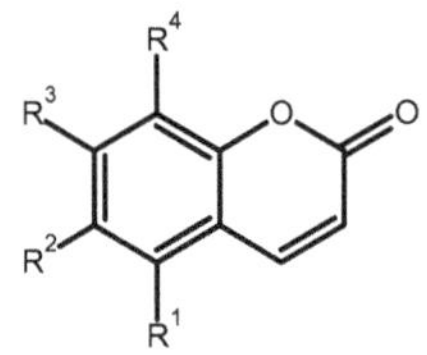

Umckalin: R^1, R^2=OCH_3, R^3=OH, R^4=H
Fraxidin: R^1=H, R^2, R^3=OCH_3, R^4=OH
Fraxinol: R^1, R^3=OCH_3, H, R^2=OH, R^4=H
Scopoletin: R^1=H, R^2=OCH_3, R^3=OH, R^4=H

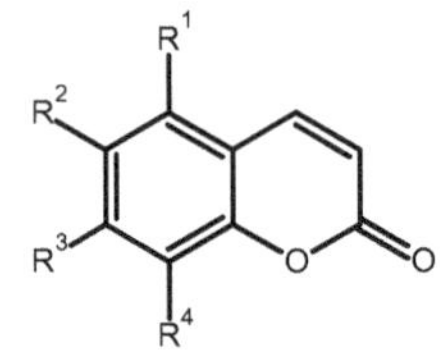

6-Methoxy-7-(sulpho-oxy)-2H-1-benzopyran-2-one:
R^2=OCH_3, R^3=OSO_3H
6,8-*Bis*(sulpho-oxy)-7-methoxy-2H-1-benzopyran-2-one:
R^2, R^4=OSO_3H, R^3=OCH_3
7-Hydroxy-6-methoxy-8-(sulpho-oxyl)-2H-1-benzopyran-2-one:
R^2=OCH_3, R^3=OH, R^4=OSO_3H
8-Hydroxy-7-methoxy-6-(sulpho-oxyl)-2H-1-benzopyran-2-one:
R^2=OSO_3H, R^3=OCH_3, R^4=OH

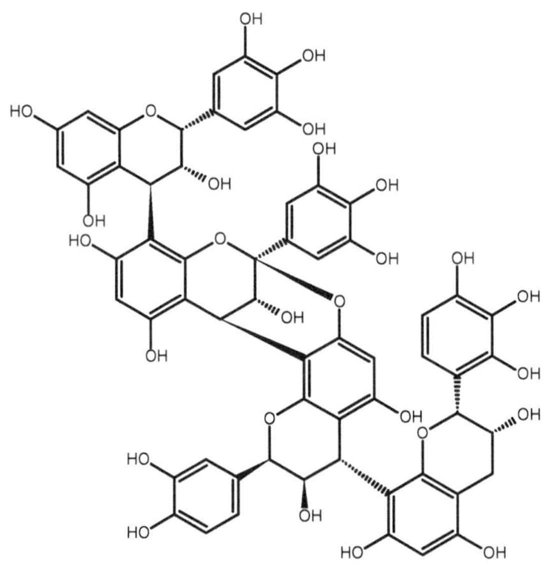

Prodelphinidin with A-type element

Part B: Chemical profiling and quality control

10. Chromatography analysis

10.1 High-performance thin-layer chromatography (HPTLC) fingerprint analysis

General instrumentation: A CAMAG HPTLC instrument consisting of an automatic TLC sampler (ATS 4), automatic developing chamber (ADC 2), CAMAG TLC Visualizer 2, CAMAG derivatiser, and TLC plate heater. *HPTLC plates:* Silica gel glass plates 60 F_{254} (Merck). *Plant part:* Rhizomes, methanol extract. *Sample application:* Application volume of 2 μL methanol extract (100 mg/mL) and 2 μL standard (1 mg/mL) spotted as 10 mm bands. Plates developed in a 20 × 10 × 4 cm glass twin-trough chamber to a migration distance of 70 mm. *Tank saturation:* 20 min at 25 °C and 47% RH, with 25 mL of mobile phase. *Mobile phase:* Ethyl acetate:acetonitrile:methanol:formic acid (64:4:4:1, v/v/v/v). *Derivatisation:* Methanolic potassium hydroxide (96%) reagent. The plate was derivatised with 3 mL of the methanolic potassium hydroxide reagent, and heated for 3 min at 100 °C on a TLC plate heater and then visualised. *Visualisation:* The plate was viewed under 366 nm radiation.

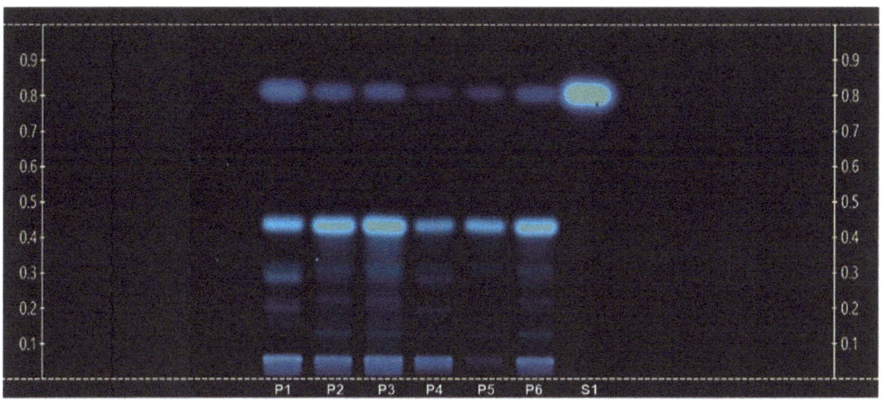

HPTLC plate of *Pelargonium sidoides* methanol extracts (n = 6) (P1–P6) and the standard S1. The samples are characterised by a blue band for umckalin (S1) (R_f = 0.82).

10.2 Ultra-performance liquid chromatography (UPLC) analysis

General instrumentation: A Waters Acquity Ultra-Performance Liquid Chromatography system with a photodiode array (PDA) detector combined with a Xevo G2QToF mass spectrometer (Waters, USA). *Plant part:* Rhizomes, methanol:water (8:2, v/v) extract. *Sample application:* Injection volume of 2.0 μL (full-loop injection) at 1 mg/mL. *Column:* Acquity UPLC BEH C_{18} column (150 mm × 2.1 mm, i.d., 1.7 μm particle size, Waters). *Mobile phase:* 0.1% formic acid in water (solvent A) and acetonitrile (solvent B). *Analysis conditions:* Gradient elution at flow rate: 0.35 mL/min, changing as follows: 95% A: 5% B to 50% A: 50% B in 3.5 min, to 0% A: 100% B in 3.5 min, held for 1 min, back to the initial ratio in 0.5 min, equilibrating the system for 1.5 min; total run time 10 min. *Mass spectrometry*: ESI^- (negative ionisation mode), N_2 used as desolvation gas, desolvation temperature 350 °C at a flow rate of 500 L/h and source temperature at 100 °C. Capillary and cone voltages 2900 and 45 V, respectively. Data collected between *m/z* 100 and 1000.

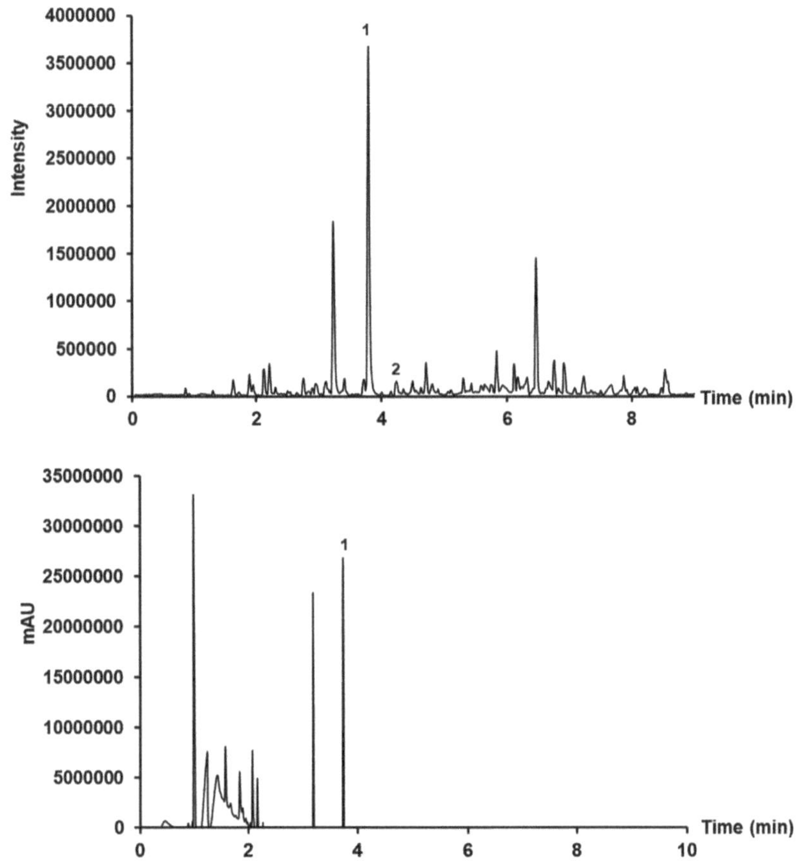

UPLC-ToF-MS ESI^- (upper) and PDA (lower) chromatograms of *Pelargonium sidoides* methanol: water (8:2, v/v) extract. [1] = umckalin *m/z* 221.0458, [2] = magnolioside *m/z* 399.0913.

11. Mid-infrared (MIR) spectroscopy analysis

General instrumentation: An Alpha-P Bruker spectrometer, mounted with an attenuated total reflectance (ATR) diamond crystal. *Spectral acquisition:* Spectrum obtained in the absorbance mode, with a spectral resolution of 4 cm^{-1} over the range 4000–550 cm^{-1} and captured using OPUS 6.5 software. *Plant part:* Rhizomes. *Sample preparation:* Rhizomes are sliced, powdered, sieved (< 500 μm) and placed directly onto the surface of the diamond crystal.

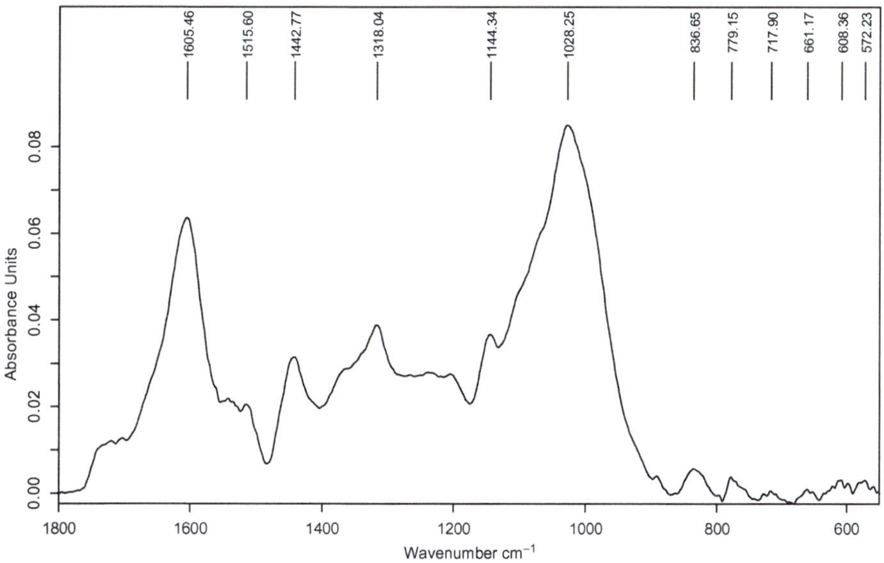

Mid-infrared spectrum of *Pelargonium sidoides* root powder displaying the fingerprint region (1800–550 cm^{1}).

References

Aboobaker, Z., Viljoen, A., Chen, W., Crous, P.W., Maharaj, V.J., Van Vuuren, S., 2019. S. Afr. J. Bot., 122:535–542.

Agbabiaka, T.B., Guo, R., Ernst, E., 2008. Phytomedicine, 15:378–385.

Anheyer, D., Cramer, H., Lauche, R., Saha, F.J., Dobos, G., 2018. Acad. Pediatr., 18:8–19.

Asea, A., Kaur, P., Panossian, A., Wikman, K.G., 2013. Phytomedicine, 20:1323–1329.

Bachert, C., Schapowal, A., Funk, P., Kieser, M., 2009. Rhinology, 47:51–58.

Bao, Y., Gao, Y., Koch, E., Pan, X., Jin, Y., Cui, X., 2015. Phytomed., 22:504–509.

Batten, A., Bokelman, H., 1966. Wild Flowers of the Eastern Cape Province. Books of Africa, Cape Town, South Africa.

Beceren, A., Sarikaya, B., Tatlipinar, E., Omurtag, G.Z., Şardaş, S., 2017. Marmara Pharm. J., 21:455–460.

Beil, W., Kilian, P., 2007. Phytomed., 14:5–8.

Berezhnoi, V.V., Heger, M., Lehmacher, W., Seifert, G., 2016. J. Compr. Pediatr., 7 (4):e42158.
Bereznoy, V.V., Riley, D.S., Wassmer, G., Heger, M., 2003. Altern. Ther. Health Med., 9:68–79.
Bladt, S., 1974. Zur Chemie der Inhaltsstoffe der *Pelargonium reniforme* Curt.—Wurzel (Umckaloabo). Ludwig-Maximilians-Universität, Munich, Germany.
Brendler, T., 2009. Umckaloabo: from a patent remedy to a modern herbal pharmaceutical based on *pelargonium sidoides* with clinically proven efficacy. In: Juliani, H.R., Simon, J.E., Ho, C.T. (Eds.), African Natural Plant Products: Discoveries and Challenges in Quality Control. American Chemical Society Symposium Series 1021. American Chemical Society, Washington, DC, USA.
Brendler, T., Van Wyk, B.E., 2008. J. Ethnopharmacol., 119:420–433.
Brendler, T., Al-Harrasi, A., Bauer, R., Gafner, S., Hardy, M.L., Heinrich, M., Hosseinzadeh, H., Izzo, A.A., Michaelis, M., Nassiri-Asl, M., Panossian, A., Wasser, S.P., Williamson, E.M., 2020. Phytother. Res., 35 (6):3013–3031.
Careddu, D., Pettenazzo, A., 2018. Int. J. Gen. Med., 11:91–98.
Carrapatoso, F.M.L., 2005. Adhäsionshemmung von bakteriellen Erregern oberer Atemwegsinfekte an buccalen Epithelzellen durch das Phytotherapeutikum Umckaloabo. Ph.D. thesis, University of Freiburg, Freiburg, Germany.
Chuchalin, A.G., Berman, B., Lehmacher, W., 2005. Explore: J. Sci. Heal., 1:437–445.
Conrad, A., Kolodziej, H., Schulz, V., 2007a. Wien. Med. Wochenschr., 157:331–336.
Conrad, A., Hansmann, C., Engels, I., Daschner, F.D., Frank, U., 2007b. Phytomedicine, 14:46–51.
Conrad, A., Jung, I., Tioua, D., Lallemand, C., Carrapatoso, F., Engels, I., Daschner, F.D., Frank, U., 2007c. Phytomedicine, 14:52–59.
Conrad, A., Engels, I., Frank, U., 2008a. Planta Med., 74 (6), 682–685.
Conrad, A., Bauer, D., Hansmann, C., Engels, I., Frank, U., 2008b. Z. Phytother., 29:15–18.
Conrad, A., Bauer, D., Jung, I., Lallemand, C., Carrapatoso, F., Engels, I., Frank, U., 2008c. Z. Phytother., 29:19–22.
Cumaoğlu, A., Karatoprak, G.Ş., Yerer, M.B., Koşar, M., 2018. Turk. J. Pharm. Sci., 15:107–115.
Daschner, F., Dorfmüller, A., Engels, I., Frank, U., 2004. Phytopharmaka und Phytotherapie, 2004, Abstracts 15.
De Boer, H.J., Hagemann, U., Bate, J., Meyboom, R.H., 2007. Drug Saf., 30:677–680.
Dorfmüller, A., Jung, I., Tioua, D.L., Engels, I., Daschner, F.D., Frank, U., 2005. Z. Phytother., 26:S6–S7.
Dreyer, L.L., Marais, E.M., 2000. S. Afr. J. Bot., 66:44–51.
Ecklon, C.F., Zeyher, K.L., 1837. Enumeratio Plantarum Africae Australis Extratropicae, vol. 1. Perthes & Besser, Hamburg, Germany.
Forbes, V.S. (Ed.), 1986. Carl Peter Thunberg Travels at the Cape of Good Hope 1772–1775. Van Riebeeck Society, Cape Town, South Africa, ISBN 0620109815.
Franco, L., de Oliveira, B.H., 2010. Talanta, 81:1368–1372.
Gödecke, T., Kaloga, M., Kolodziej, H., 2005. Z. Naturforsch., 60b:677–682.
Hansmann, C., 2005. Einfluss von Umckaloabo auf die Funktion humaner Phagozyten. Ph.D. thesis, University of Freiburg, Freiburg, Germany.
Harvey, W.H., Sonder, O.W., 1860. Flora Capensis: Being a Systematic Description of the Plants of the Cape Colony, Caffraria, & Port Natal, vol. 1. Hodges, Smith & Co., Dublin, Ireland.
Hauer, H., Germer, S., Elsäßer, J., Ritter, T., 2010. Planta Med., 76:350–352.
Helfer, M., Koppensteiner, H., Schneider, M., Rebensburg, S., Forcisi, S., Müller, C., Schmitt-Kopplin, P., Schindler, M., Brack-Werner, R., 2014. PLoS One, 9 (1):e87487.

Hudaib, M., Aldahasi, W.B., Khdair, A., Salah, R., Alkhatib, H.S., Bustanji, Y., Mohammad, M.K., 2010. Jordan J. Pharm. Sci., 3:109–116.

Human Sciences Research Council, 2011. Baseline Survey: Water, Health and Development—Three Site Rural Communities in the Amathole District Municipality. Human Sciences Research Council, Pretoria, South Africa.

Huntley, A., Kamin, W., 2010. Focus. Altern. Complement. Ther., 15:238–239.

Ibrahim, M.M., Ghani, S.A.E., El-Moez, S.I.A., 2018. J. Appl. Pharm. Sci., 8:109–118.

Janecki, A., Kolodziej, H., 2010. Molecules, 15:7139–7152.

Janecki, A.J., Kiderlen, A.F., Kolodziej, H., 2007. NO-, TNF-, and IL-12-inducing activity of fractions of EPs® 7630. In: Planta Medica 73, 55th International Congress and Annual Meeting of the Society for Medicinal Plant Research, Abstracts.

Janecki, A., Conrad, A., Engels, I., Frank, U., Kolodziej, H., 2011. J. Ethnopharmacol., 133:147–152.

Kamin, W., Maydannik, V., Malek, F.A., Kieser, M., 2010a. Int. J. Clin. Pharmacol. Ther., 48:184–191.

Kamin, W., Maydannik, V.G., Malek, F.A., Kieser, M., 2010b. Acta Paediatr., 99:537–543.

Kamin, W., Ilyenko, L.I., Malek, F.A., Kieser, M., 2012. Pediatr. Int., 54:219–226.

Kamin, W., Funk, P., Seifert, G., Zimmermann, A., Lehmacher, W., 2018. Curr. Med. Res. Opin., 34:475–485.

Kayser, O., 1997. Phenolische Inhaltsstoffe von *Pelargonium sidoides* DC. und Untersuchungen zur Wirksamkeit der Umcka-Droge (*Pelargonium sidoides* DC. und *Pelargonium reniforme* Curt.). Ph.D. thesis, University of Berlin, Berlin, Germany.

Kayser, O., Kolodziej, H., 1995. Phytochemistry, 39:1181–1185.

Kayser, O., Kolodziej, H., 1997. Planta Med., 63:508–510.

Kayser, O., Kolodziej, H., Kiderlen, A.F., 1997. Pharm. Pharmacol. Lett., 7:71–74.

Kayser, O., Latté, K., Kolodziej, H., Hammerschmidt, F.J., 1998. Flavour Fragr. J., 13:209–212.

Kayser, O., Kolodziej, H., Kiderlen, A.F., 2001. Phytother. Res., 15:122–126.

Kayser, O., Masihi, K.N.I., Kiderlen, A.F., 2003. Expert Rev. Anti-Infect. Ther., 1:319–335.

Kim, C.E., Griffiths, W.J., Taylor, P.W., 2009. J. Appl. Microbiol., 106:1184–1193.

Koch, E., Biber, A., 2007. Phytomedicine, 14:40–45.

Koch, E., Wohn, C., 2007. *Pelargonium sidoides* root extract EPs® 7630 stimulates release of antimicrobial peptides from neutrophil granulocytes in human whole blood. In: Planta Medica 73, 55th International Congress and Annual Meeting of the Society for Medicinal Plant Research, Abstracts.

Koch, E., Lanzendörfer-Goossens, H., Wohn, C., 2002. Naunyn Schmiedeberg's Arch. Pharmacol., 365:R75, 288.

Kolodziej, H., 2002. *Pelargonium reniforme* and *Pelargonium sidoides*: their botany, chemistry and medicinal use. In: Lis-Balchin, M. (Ed.), *Geranium* and *Pelargonium*. Taylor & Francis, London, UK, pp. 262–290.

Kolodziej, H., 2011. Pharmaceuticals, 4:1295–1314.

Kolodziej, H., 2014. Z. Phytother., 35:2–23.

Kolodziej, H., Schulz, V., 2003. Deutsche Apotheker Zeitung, 143:1303–1312.

Kolodziej, H., Kayser, O., Latte, K.P., Kiderlen, A.F., 1999. Basic Life Sci., 66:575–594.

Kolodziej, H., Burmeister, A., Trun, W., Radtke, O.A., Kiderlen, A.F., Ito, H., Hatano, T., Yoshida, T., Foo, L.Y., 2005. Bioorg. Med. Chem., 13:6470–6476.

Kumar, V., Moyo, M., Gruz, J., Šubrtová, M., Van Staden, J., 2015. Ind. Crop. Prod., 77:402–408.

Lewu, F.B., Grierson, D.S., Afolayan, A.J., 2006. Pharm. Biol., 44:279–282.

Lewu, F.B., Adebola, P.O., Afolayan, A.J., 2007. J. Arid Environ., 70:380–388.
Lizogub, V.G., Riley, D.S., Heger, M., 2007. Explore (N.Y.), 3:573–584.
Loew, D., Koch, E., 2008. Z. Phytother., 29:28–36.
Luna Jr., L.A., Bachi, A.L.L., Novaes e Brito, R.R., Eid, R.G., Suguri, V.M., Oliveira, P.W., Gregorio, L.C., Vaisberg, M., 2011. Phytomedicine, 18:303–308.
Manganyi, M.C., Regnier, T., Kumar, A., Bezuidenhout, C.C., Ateba, C.N., 2018. S. Afr. J. Bot., 116:192–199.
Manganyi, M.C., Tchatchouang, C.-D.K., Regnier, T., Bezuidenhout, C.C., Ateba, C.N., 2019. Mycobiology, 47:335–339.
Maree, J.E., Viljoen, A.M., 2011. Vib. Spectrosc., 55:146–152.
Mativandlela, S.P.N., Lall, N., Meyer, J.J.M., 2006. S. Afr. J. Bot., 72:232–237.
Mativandlela, S.P.N., Meyer, J.J.M., Hussein, A.A., Lall, N., 2007. Pharm. Biol., 45:645–650.
Matsiliza, B., Barker, N.P., 2001. S. Afr. J. Bot., 67:177–182.
Matthys, H., Funk, P., 2008. Planta Med., 74:686–692.
Matthys, H., Funk, P., 2018. Curr. Med. Res. Opin., 34:1245–1251.
Matthys, H., Heger, M., 2007a. Phytomedicine, 14:65–68.
Matthys, H., Heger, M., 2007b. Curr. Med. Res. Opin., 23:323–331.
Matthys, H., Malek, F.A., 2015. Atemwegs Lungenkr., 41:27–34.
Matthys, H., Eisebitt, R., Seith, B., Heger, M., 2003. Phytomedicine, 10:7–17.
Matthys, H., Kamin, W., Funk, P., Heger, M., 2007. Phytomedicine, 14:69–73.
Matthys, H., Lizogub, V.G., Malek, F.A., Kieser, M., 2010a. Curr. Med. Res. Opin., 26:1413–1422.
Matthys, H., Lizogub, V.G., Funk, P., Malek, F.A., 2010b. Wien. Med. Wochenschr., 160:564–570.
Matthys, H., Pliskevich, D.A., Bondarchuk, O.M., Malek, F.A., Tribanek, M., Kieser, M., 2013. Respir. Med., 107:691–701.
Meyer, C., Pries, R., Wollenberg, B., 2011. Oral Oncol., 47:818–826.
Michaelis, M., Doerr, H.W., Cinatl Jr., J., 2011. Phytomedicine, 18:384–386.
Mickenhagen, A., Walger, M., Neugebauer, P., 2004. Die pharmakologische Stimulation der Zilienschlagfrequenz nasaler Flimmerzellen in der Zellkultur. HNO Informationen, Abstract 22.25.
Moyo, M., Van Staden, J., 2014. J. Ethnopharmacol., 152:243–255.
Neugebauer, P., Mickenhagen, A., Siefer, O., Walger, M., 2005. Phytomedicine, 12:46–51.
Nöldner, M., Koch, E., 2004. Inhibition of endotoxin-induced sickness behaviour in mice by an extract from roots of *Pelargonium sidoides* (Umckaloabo). Focus on alternative and complementary therapies. In: Abstracts of the 11th Annual Symposium on Complementary Health Care, 17th–19th November 2004, Exeter, UK, vol. 9:20.
Nöldner, M., Schötz, K., 2007. Phytomedicine, 14:27–31.
Pappe, L., 1847. A list South African Indigenous Plants Used as Remedies by the Colonists of the Cape of Good Hope. Pike, Cape Town, South Africa.
Pappe, L., 1850. Florae Capensis Medicae Prodromus. Robertson, Cape Town, South Africa.
Pappe, L., 1857. Florae Capensis Medicae Prodromus, second ed. Robertson, Cape Town, South Africa.
Park, S.M., Min, B.-G., Jung, J.Y., Jegal, K.H., Lee, C.W., Kim, K.Y., Kim, Y.W., Choi, Y.-W., Cho, I.J., Ku, S.K., Kim, S.C., 2018. BMC Complement. Altern. Med., 18 (1):20, https://doi.org/10.1186/s12906-018-2088-x.
Patiroglu, T., Tunc, A., Eke Gungor, H., Unal, E., 2012. Phytomedicine, 19:958–961.
Pereira, A., Bester, M., Soundy, P., Apostolides, Z., 2015. Med. Chem. Res., 24:3838–3852.

Pereira, A., Bester, M., Soundy, P., Apostolides, Z., 2016. Pharm. Biol., 54:1831–1840.
Pereira, A.S.P., Bester, M.J., Apostolides, Z., 2017. Mol. Divers., 21:809–820.
Pérez, G., Rodríguez, N., Castro, H., Silva, O., Pabbou, D., Maestracci, F., Castillo, L., Sifontes, M., Alvarado, J., Rincón, A., Rojas, N., Quiroz, E., Milano, L., Petit, M., Soto, G., Gotera, A., Ríos, E., Chacín, B., Galué, H., Caraballo, T., Flores, D., Medina, Y., Villalobos, S., 2011. Arch. Venez. Farmacol. Ter., 30:79–85.
Phillips, E.P., 1917. Ann. S. Afr. Mus., 16:1–379.
Rezaizadehnajafi, L., Wink, M., 2014. Phytomedicine, 21:547–550.
Riley, D.S., Lizogub, V.G., Zimmermann, A., Funk, P., Lehmacher, W., 2018. Altern. Ther. Health Med., 24:16–26.
Riley, D.S., Lizogub, V.G., Heger, M., Funk, P., Mueller, H., Lehmacher, W., 2019. Integr. Med., 18:42–51.
Roots, I., Arold, G., Dienel, A., Meng, G., Wollny, A., Bauer, S., 2004. Kongressband Phytopharmaka Phytotherapie, 2004:22.
Ross, S.M., 2012. Holist. Nurs. Pract., 26:283–285.
Roth, M., Fang, L., Stolz, D., Tamm, M., 2019. PLoS One, 14 (2):e0210702.
Samie, S., Trollope, K.M., Joubert, L.-M., Makunga, N.P., Volschenk, H., 2019. J. Ethnopharmacol., 235:122–132.
Savickiene, N., Jekabsone, A., Raudone, L., Abdelgeliel, A.S., Cochis, A., Rimondini, L., Makarova, E., Grinberga, S., Pugovics, O., Dambrova, M., Pacauskiene, I.M., Basevičiene, N., Viškelis, P., 2018. Materials, 11 (9):1499.
Schapowal, A., Heger, M., 2007. Z. Phytother., 28:58–65.
Schapowal, A., Dobos, G., Cramer, H., Chung Ong, K., Adler, M., Zimmermann, A., Brandes-Schramm, J., Lehmacher, W., 2019. Heliyon, 5:11, e02904, https://doi.org/10.1016/j.heliyon.2019.e02904.
Schnitzler, P., Schneider, S., Stintzing, F.C., Carle, R., Reichling, J., 2008. Phytomedicine, 15:1108–1116.
Schoetz, K., Erdelmeier, C., Germer, S., Hauer, H., 2008. Planta Med., 74:667–674.
Schötz, K., Nöldner, M., 2007. Phytomedicine, 14:32–39.
Schötz, K., Erdelmeier, C., Germer, S., Hauer, H., 2008. Planta Med., 74:667–674.
Schulz, V., 2008. Z. Phytother., 29, 3–4.
Seckin, C., Kalayci, G.A., Turan, N., Yilmaz, A., Cizmecigil, U.Y., Aydin, O., Richt, J.A., Yilmaz, H., 2018. Food Agric. Immunol., 29:744–761.
Seidel, V., Taylor, P.W., 2004. Int. J. Antimicrob. Agents, 23:613–619.
Seifert, G., Brandes-Schramm, J., Zimmermann, A., Lehmacher, W., Kamin, W., 2019. BMC Pediatr., 19 (1):119.
Smith, A., 1895. A Contribution to the South African Materia Medica, third ed. Lovedale, South Africa.
Smith, C.A., 1966. Common Names of South African Plants. Memoirs of the Botanical Survey of South Africa 35. Department of Agricultural Technical Services, Pretoria, South Africa.
Tahan, F., Yaman, M., 2013. Phytomedicine, 20:148–150.
Taylor, P.W., 2003a. Umckaloabo—South African herbal remedy for tuberculosis. Antibiot. Chemother., 7:10.
Taylor, P.W., 2003b. S. Afr. Med. J., 93:904–907.
Teschke, R., Frenzel, C., Schulze, J., Eickhoff, A., 2012a. Regul. Toxicol. Pharmacol., 63:1–9.
Teschke, R., Frenzel, C., Wolff, A., Herzog, J., Glass, X., Schulze, J., Eickhoff, A., 2012b. Ann. Hepatol., 11:500–512.

Thäle, C., Kiderlen, A.F., Kolodziej, H., 2007. Antiinfective mode of action of EPs®7630 at the molecular level. In: Planta Medica 73, 55th International Congress and Annual Meeting of the Society for Medicinal Plant Research, Abstracts.

Thäle, C., Kiderlen, A.F., Kolodziej, H., 2011. Planta Med., 77:718–725.

Theisen, L.L., Muller, C.P., 2012. Antivir. Res., 94:147–156.

Trun, W., Kiderlen, A.F., Kolodziej, H., 2006. Phytomedicine, 13:570–575.

Uslu, H., Yoruk, O., Ayyildiz, A., Aktan, B., 2009. Eur. J. Gen. Med., 6:245–248.

Van der Walt, J.J.A., 1977. *Pelargoniums* of Southern Africa. Purnell, Cape Town, South Africa.

Van der Walt, J.J.A., Vorster, P.J., 1988. *Pelargoniums* of Southern Africa, vols. 1 and 3. National Botanic Gardens Kirstenbosch, Cape Town, South Africa.

Van Niekerk, J., Wynberg, R., 2012. Dev. South. Afr., 29:530–547.

Van Wyk, B.-E., Wink, M., 2004. Medicinal Plants of the World. Briza Publications, Pretoria, South Africa, p. 231.

Viljoen, A.M., Zhao, J., Sandasi, M., Chen, W., Khan, I.A., 2015. Metabolomics, 11:594–602.

Wagner, L., Cramer, H., Klose, P., Lauche, R., Gass, F., Dobos, G., Langhorst, J., 2015. Forsch. Komplementmed., 22:359–368.

Willcox, M., Diallo, D., Sanogo, R., Giani, S., Graz, B., Falquet, J., Bodeker, G., 2015. J. Ethnopharmacol., 176:281–285.

Witte, K., Koch, E., Volk, H.-D., Wolk, K., Sabat, R., 2015. PLoS One, 10 (9):e0138075.

Wittschier, N., Faller, G., Hensel, A., 2007a. Phytomedicine, 14:285–288.

Wittschier, N., Lengsfeld, C., Vorthems, S., Stratmann, U., Ernst, J.F., Verspohl, E.J., Hensel, A., 2007b. J. Pharm. Pharmacol., 59:777–786.

Wynberg, R., Laird, S., Van Niekerk, J., Kozanayi, W., 2015. Soc. Nat. Resour., 28:559–574.

CHAPTER

20

Prunus africana

Emmanuel Rubegeta, Felix Makolo, Weiyang Chen and Guy Kamatou
Department of Pharmaceutical Sciences, Tshwane University of Technology, Pretoria, South Africa

Abstract

Prunus africana (Hook.f.) Kalkman (Rosaceae), commonly known as 'African cherry', is an evergreen tree, which grows up to 40 m in height, has open branches and a mature stem diameter of up to 1 m, and bears a blackish-brown stem-bark. Prunus africana is distributed in Central Africa, sub-Saharan Africa and the Indian Ocean islands. The stem-bark is used traditionally to treat benign prostate hyperplasia, stomach complaints, chest pains, malaria and fever, hypertension, diabetes, gonorrhoea and kidney disease. Commercial harvesting and trade of P. africana bark was established in Cameroon many years ago, but has since expanded to other countries. Over 23 different pharmaceutical companies market products containing P. africana and formulated into tablets, capsules and liquid extracts as herbal medicine. Both in vitro and in vivo activities have been investigated for this important medicinal plant. The chemical profiles of P. africana were investigated using several analytical methods such as high-performance thin-layer chromatography (HPTLC), gas chromatography coupled to mass spectrometry (GC–MS), and ultra-performance liquid chromatography coupled to mass spectrometry (UPLC–MS). β-Sitosterol, friedelin, ferulic acid, atraric acid, N-butylbenzenesulphonamide, myristic acid, palmitic acid, linoleic acid and ursolic acid were identified in the extract of P. africana.

Keywords: *Prunus africana*, African cherry, Stem-bark, Benign prostate hyperplasia, β-Sitosterol, Maslinic acid, GC–MS, UPLC–MS, HPTLC, MIR spectroscopy

The South African Herbal Pharmacopoeia. https://doi.org/10.1016/B978-0-323-99794-2.00011-8

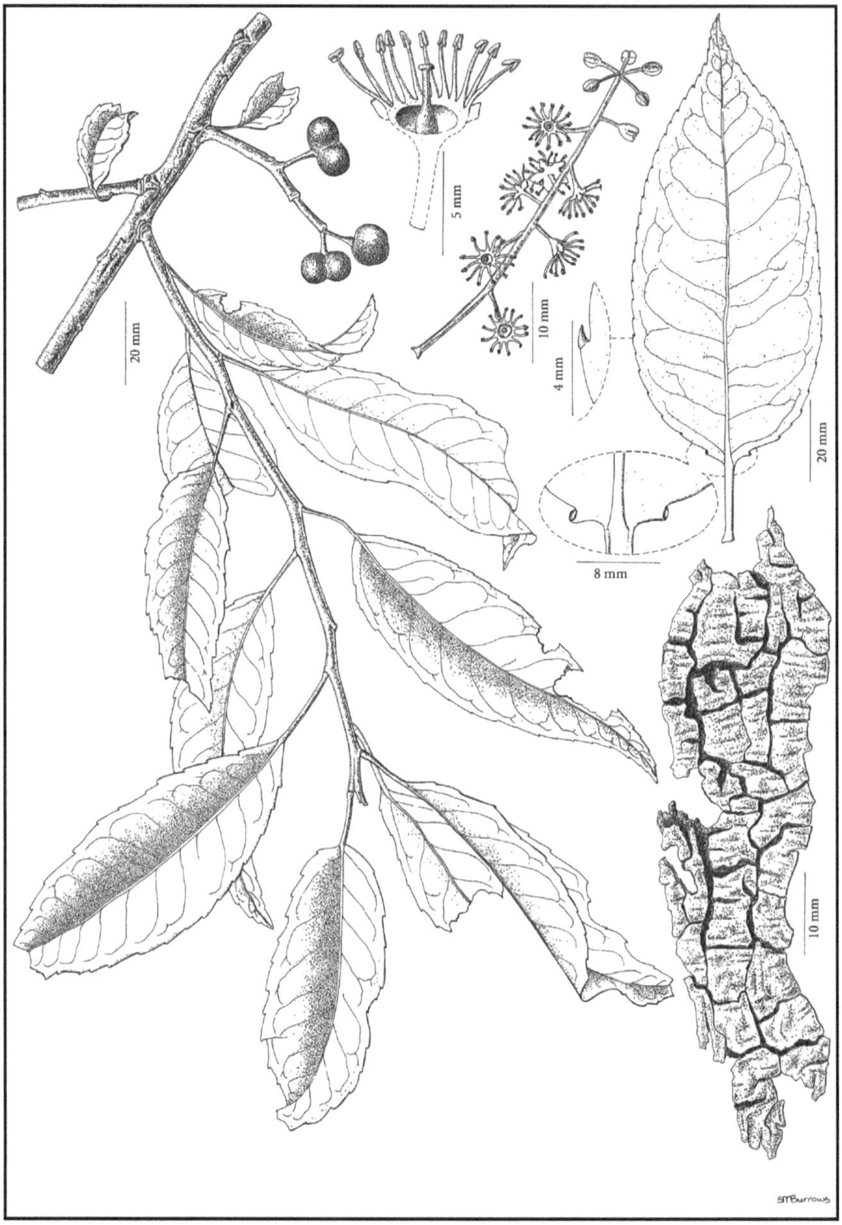
5 mm
10 mm
20 mm
4 mm
20 mm
8 mm
10 mm
SMBurrows

Part A: General overview

1. Synonyms

Pygeum africanum Hook.f.[a]

2. Common name(s)

African almond, bitter almond, bitter almond tree, red stinkwood, wild almond (English); *'Bitter-amandel'*, *'Afrika-amandel'*, *'Bitteramandelhout'*, *'Bitteramandelboom'*, *'Wilde-kersieboom'*, *'Rooi-stinkhout'*, *'Nuweamandelhout'* (Afrikaans); *'Umlalume'*, *'Inkokhokho'*, *'Ngubozinyeweni'*, *'Umdumezulu'*, *'Inyazangomelimnyama'*, *'Umkhakhazi'* (isiZulu); *'Mulala-maanga'* (Tshivenda); *'Mogohloro'* (Northern Sesotho); *'Umdumizulu'*, *'Inyazangoma'*, *'Umkhakhase'*, *'Itywina-elikhul'*, *'Umkhakhase'* (isiXhosa).[1]

3. Conservation status

Vulnerable.[a]

4. Botany

The genus *Prunus* (Rosaceae) is part of approximately 200 species that include almonds, plums, apricots, peaches and cherries (Kurtto, 2009). The name *Prunus africana* is derived from '*Prunus*', which refers to the plum-like shape of the fruit and '*africana*', which indicates the African origin of the species (SANBI, 2006). *Prunus africana* is an evergreen tree that grows up to 40 m in height. The plant has a cylindrical, straight, open-branched stem with a diameter of up to 1 m and a blackish-brown bark. The leaves are alternate, long (8–12 cm), oval-shaped and are a deep-shiny green colour on the top, and light green on the underside (A). The leaves give off an almond scent when bruised. Petioles are deep pink in colour and midribs are 5–15 cm long. The fruits are cherry-shaped, pinkish-brown in colour, and 8–12 mm in diameter (A). They are bilobed, with thin, reddish-brown to dark red pulp when ripe and have a very bitter flesh. The scented small flowers are white or greenish, with solitary inflorescences of 3–7 cm in length and corolla lobes up to 2 mm long (B). The hard wood is even-textured, pale red in colour, with a strong cyanide smell when freshly cut, darkening to mahogany brown or dark red when exposed to air (C) (Gachie et al., 2012; Allkanjari and Vitalone, 2015; Komakech et al., 2017).

[a] Red List of South African Plants (http://redlist.sanbi.org).

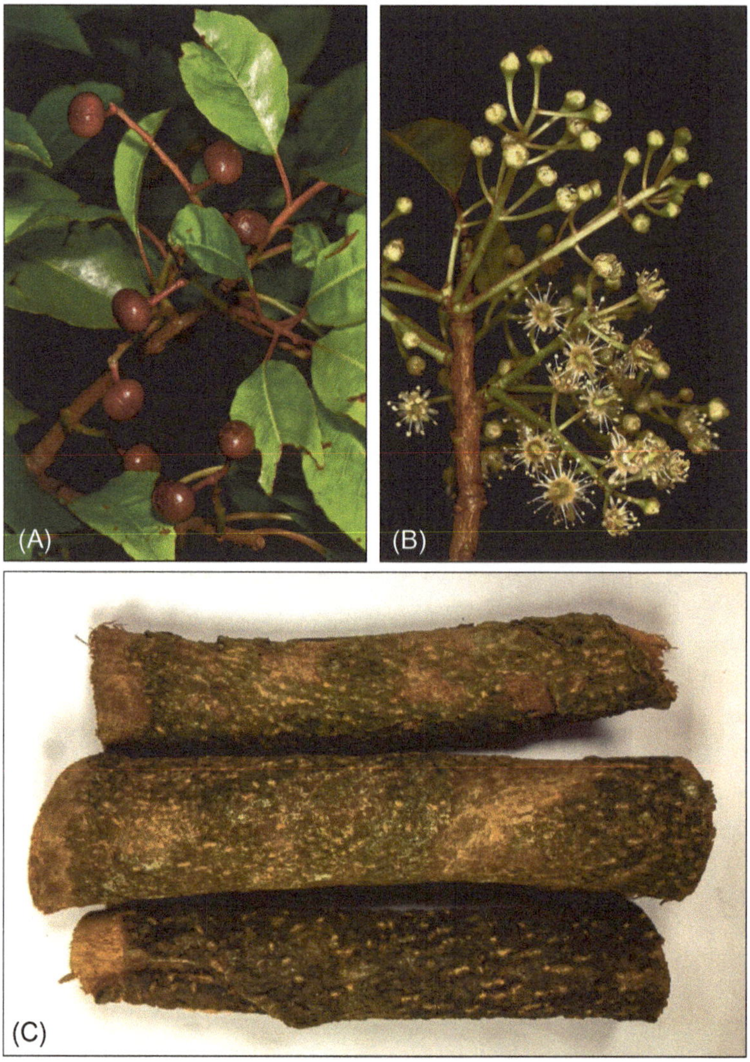

Prunus africana branchlet with shiny, oval-shaped leaves and red cherries (A), small white flowers (B) and even-textured bark (C).

5. Geographical distribution

Prunus africana is not endemic to South Africa and is geographically widespread. It is found in the Comoros, Madagascar, Central Africa and in sub-Saharan Africa, from the southern Cape, through KwaZulu-Natal and the Mpumalanga provinces of South Africa, and in neighbouring Swaziland (Eswatini) and Zimbabwe (SANBI,

2006). The plant is not shade tolerant and is most abundant along forest margins, in open areas, and often in riverine vegetation (Geldenhuys, 1981; Ewusi et al., 1992).

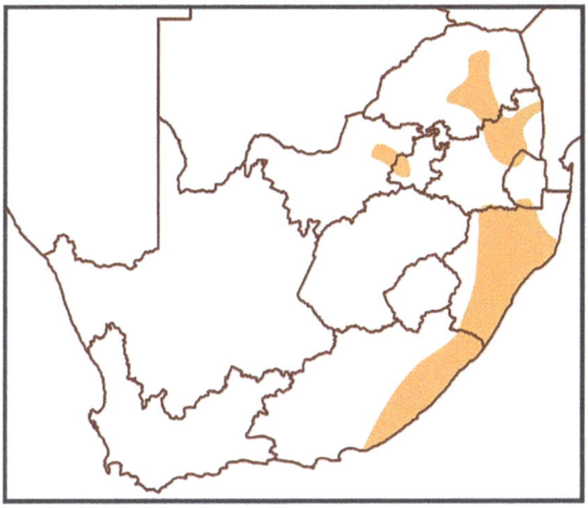

Geographical distribution of *Prunus africana* in South Africa.

6. Ethnopharmacology

In a survey conducted in Cameroon, it became apparent that *P. africana* is the fourth most popular medicinal plant species in the Mount Cameroon region, with 14% of households collecting the plant for use (Jeanrenaud, 1991). It is also an important medicine in the Kilum-Ijim area, where it is traditionally used to treat stomach ache, malaria and fever (Nsom and Dick, 1992). In East Africa, the bark is pounded and made into an infusion, which is used to soothe stomach pain and as a laxative for cattle (Kokwaro, 1976). The bark is administered as a treatment for pain in southern Africa (Pujol, 1990; Komakech et al., 2017). Zulu men in the Vryheid area of KwaZulu-Natal Province use the bark to improve the flow of urine. Roots and leaves of *P. africana* are used for the treatment of stomach aches, fever, gonorrhoea, urinary symptoms, heart infections and kidney disease (Sunderland and Nkefor, 1997; Stewart, 2003; Ingram et al., 2009). Stewart (2003) reported that the dry bark is crushed and taken as a tea for the treatment of various ailments. The Nandi community in Kenya use the plant to treat stomach problems, diabetes, high blood pressure, as a laxative, and for "old men's" disease (Pomatto, 2001; Abera, 2014; Ngule et al., 2014). In the Kakamega Forest, Kenya, the mantled guereza consumes the matured leaves of *P. africana* as part of its diet (Fashing, 2004). Bii et al. (2010) reported the use of the plant in Europe for malaria and chest pain, taken orally as an infusion. *Prunus africana* is used in Uganda to treat many diseases, but specifically for its analgesic and anti-inflammatory properties (Stewart, 2003). Emmanuel (2010) reported that the plant is considered a key ethnomedicine in the city of Foumban in Cameroon for the treatment of prostatic diseases.

7. Commercialisation

Cameroon has been the dominant producer and exporter of *P. africana* bark for many years. Stewart (2003) reported that smaller quantities of the plant are obtained from Kenya, Madagascar, Equatorial Guinea, the Democratic Republic of the Congo, Tanzania, Uganda, Burundi/Rwanda, South Africa and Asian countries with the majority of harvested bark exported to Europe. In 1972, commercial harvest and trade of *P. africana* bark was initiated in Cameroon with a small operation of only 10 tons, when Plantecam (previously Plantecam Medicam) started harvesting in the West and Northwest regions (Cunningham et al., 1997). Over 23 different Western pharmaceutical companies market products containing the plant species based on high demand, including Inverni Della Buffa and Indena Spa (Italy), Madaus (Germany), and Laboratoires Debat and Prosynthèse (France). In Africa, the traditional demand for bark is estimated to be around 500 tons per year, based on household surveys (Cunningham et al., 1997). In 1992, roughly 2000 tons of bark were harvested from Cameroon alone, with the majority sold to European markets (Cunningham and Mbenkum, 1993). By 1997, *P. africana* had an estimated annual value of close to US $220 million worldwide (Bii et al., 2010). According to the European Medicines Agency (2015), *P. africana* products are registered with relevant drug regulatory authorities and formulated into tablets, capsules and liquid extracts as herbal medicine in Greece, France, the Czech Republic and Poland. These are used for the treatment of micturition disorders associated with benign prostate hyperplasia (BHP) and lower urinary tract infections (European Medicines Agency, 2015). In Africa, the timber is locally marketed for axe handles, household purposes, construction and home appliances, and in Kenya, specifically, the hard wood is used to make railway sleepers (Cunningham and Mbenkum, 1993).

8. Pharmacological evaluation

8.1 *In vitro* studies

8.1.1 Anti-inflammatory and analgesic activities

The compound ursolic acid, isolated from the chloroform extract of *P. africana* bark, displayed anti-inflammatory activity by suppressing the expression of lipopolysaccharide (LPS)-induced pro-inflammatory mediators in RAW264.7 mouse macrophages (Nataraju et al., 2007; Amico et al., 2009). Ethanol and water extracts of *P. africana* (250 μg/mL) were investigated for anti-inflammatory effects using cyclooxygenase (COX-2 and COX-1) assays (Steenkamp et al., 2006). Both extracts inhibited COX-1-catalysed prostaglandin biosynthesis by 72% and 98%, respectively. Although the ethanolic extract was inactive towards COX-2, the water extract did exhibit a low inhibition of the enzyme (Steenkamp et al., 2006). Paubert-Braquet et al. (1994) demonstrated that *P. africana* extract inhibited the production of inflammatory cells by inhibiting the production of chemotactic leukotrienes, induced through 5-lipoxygenase (5-LOX) in human polymorphonuclear cells, stimulated by means of the calcium ionophore A23187.

8.1.2 Antimicrobial activity

Ethyl acetate and methanolic stem-bark extracts of *P. africana* exhibited poor and strong antimicrobial activity, with minimum inhibitory concentrations (MICs) of 12.5 and 0.78 mg/mL, respectively, against *Staphylococcus aureus* (Mwitari et al., 2013). Poor activity towards methicillin-resistant *S. aureus* (MRSA) were reflected by the reported MICs of 25 and 3.13 mg/mL, respectively. Bii et al. (2010) evaluated the antifungal and antibacterial properties of methanol and hexane stem-bark extracts of *P. africana* towards *Pseudomonas aeruginosa, S. aureus*, MRSA, *Streptococcus pneumoniae, Cryptococcus neoformans, Candida albicans, Trichophyton mentagrophyte* and *Microsporum gypseum*. The results indicated that the methanol extracts were active against *S. aureus, T. mentagrophyte, S. pneumoniae* and MRSA at 0.073 mg/mL, 0.039, 2.50 and 0.156 mg/mL, respectively. The methanol and hexane extracts did not display any activity towards the yeasts, *C. albicans* and *C. neoformans*. Different solvent extracts were prepared from the bark of *P. africana* (chloroform, petroleum ether, methanol and acetone) and tested against *Escherichia coli, S. aureus, Proteus mirabilis, Citrobacter freundii, Enterobacter cloacae, Enterobacter* spp., *Klebsiella pneumoniae, Enterobacter aerogenes, Citrobacter koseri* and *Staphyloccus pyogenes* (Gashe and Zeleke, 2017). The acetone extract of *P. africana* was the most effective, with a reported MIC of 0.65 mg/mL against *S. pyogenes* and *C. freundii*, while the methanol extract displayed the best activity towards the majority of strains. Ngule et al. (2014) examined the *in vitro* antibacterial activity of the bark hydro-methanolic extract of *P. africana* against *Proteus vulgaris, Bacillus cereus, Salmonella typhi, E. coli* and *Serratia marcescens*. The extract was active against all the micro-organisms tested. Penicillin, which was used as the positive control, inhibited the growth of all the micro-organisms tested, while the negative control (DMSO) did not inhibit growth of the tested micro-organisms. The largest zone of inhibition (ZI) was obtained for *S. typhi* (17.33 ± 0.88 *vs* 27.67 ± 1.20 mm), followed by *S. marcescens* (16.67 ± 0.33 *vs* 32.00 ± 0.58 mm), *P. vulgaris* (16.67 ± 0.33 *vs* 21.33 ± 0.33 mm), *E. coli* (12.33 ± 0.33 *vs* 20.33 ± 0.33 mm) and *B. cereus* (11.67 ± 0.33 *vs* 25.67 ± 0.33 mm). The methanol extracts of the bark and leaves of *P. africana* were investigated for anti-enzyme activity at 6 mg/mL (Gangoué-Piéboji et al., 2007). The percentage inhibition of β-lactamase-OXA-10, TEM-1, IMP-1 and P99 enzyme activity was 86.80%, 66.00%, 81.90% and 88.90%, respectively, for the leaf extract. The bark extract showed corresponding values of 48.60%, 73.90%, 85% and 75.20% inhibition. Dey et al. (2017) investigated the antimicrobial effect of an ethanolic extract of *P. africana* stem-bark towards *Shigella* species (*S. flexneri*—two strains, *S. dysenteriae* and *S. boydii*). The solvent, DMSO, was used as the negative control and chloramphenicol as the positive control. The results reflected antibacterial activity towards *S. boydii* (ZI = 10 mm) and an MIC of 2.625 mg/mL for all the tested strains.

8.1.3 Anti-oxidant activity

A chloroform extract of *P. africana* bark was fractionated using solvent-solvent partitioning and subsequent column chromatography for evaluation of inhibitory activity in microsomal preparations of rabbit livers against ferrous ion-induced stimulation of lipid peroxidation. The fractions and extract contained high concentrations of myristic acid (20 μg/mL), and strongly inhibited lipid peroxidation in the microsomal preparations by 97%, comparable to α-tocopherol (Hass et al., 1999). Many researchers have reported good anti-oxidant properties of *P. africana* extracts. The radical scavenging ability of the ethanol and water extracts of *P. africana* was determined at 4 mg/mL (Steenkamp et al., 2006). The ethanol extract displayed poor anti-oxidant activity < 50% at 4 mg/mL, while the aqueous extract exhibited good activity of 80% at the same concentration (Steenkamp et al., 2006). A chloroform bark extract of *P. africana*, coded as V-1326, together with its fractions, were tested for the inhibitory effects of ferrous ion (Fe^{2+})-stimulated lipid peroxidation in microsomal preparations from male New Zealand white rabbit livers (Hass et al., 1999). The half-maximal inhibitory concentration (IC_{50}) of the chloroform extract was calculated as 51 ± 3 μg/mL, with the percentage inhibition of one fraction (containing high concentrations of myristic acid) at 20 μg/mL reported as 97%.

8.1.4 Antiviral activity

Twenty-two plants popularly used in traditional remedies, including *P. africana,* were screened for activity against human immunodeficiency virus type 1 (HIV-1). Rukunga et al. (2002) reported that eight of the plants inhibited reverse transcriptase activity by 50% at different concentrations. Another study conducted by Tolo et al. (2006) demonstrated notable antiviral activity of a water extract of *P. africana* stem-bark against human cytomegalovirus (HCMV) and herpes simplex virus (HSV). Data obtained in the experiments showed that the extract inhibited effective plaque formation by 50% (EC_{50}) at a concentration of 80 μg/mL, and a safe therapeutic index was shown for the extract using the trypan blue exclusion test at the cell cytotoxic concentration (CC_{50}) (Tolo et al., 2007).

8.1.5 Antimutagenic activity

In vitro mutagenicity studies of the *P. africana* extract indicated a complete absence of clastogenic and mutagenic potential (ESCOP, 2009). Methanol (90%) and dichloromethane extracts of *P. africana* were tested for mutagenic activity in micronucleus and microsome/Salmonella assays. *Prunus africana* extracts did not change the effect of the mutagen 4-nitroquinoline-oxide (4NQO), and no mutagenicity was observed in the *S. typhimurium* TA98 strain (Elgorashi et al., 2003; Verschaeve et al., 2004). Extracts of *P. africana* significantly reduced the effect of the mutagen, mitomycin C (MMC) in the micronucleus test in human lymphocytes, *in vitro,* and the extract did not induce any genotoxicity (Verschaeve et al., 2004).

8.1.6 Antiproliferative and apoptotic activities

Extracts of *P. africana* (bark) exhibited antiproliferative and apoptotic activity on the prostate, thus improving urologic symptoms in patients with prostate cancer (Nyamai et al., 2015). *In vitro* testing in LNCaP and PC-3 cells demonstrated the anticancer effect of an ethanolic bark extract of *Pygeum africanum* (*P. africana*) (Shenouda et al., 2007). The results demonstrated that, in tissue culture, a 30% ethanolic extract of *P. africana* inhibited the growth of LNCaP and PC-3 cell lines; downregulated PKC-α and ERα protein; induced cell death (apoptosis); changed cell kinetics; and exhibited good binding ability to both LNCaP human androgen receptors and mouse uterine oestrogen receptors. It was concluded that at a concentration of 2.5 μL/mL, *P. africana* induced accumulation of the cells in the S phase of the cell cycle for both LNCaP and PC-3 cells. The activity of the *P. africana* extract on the proliferation of cultured human prostatic fibroblasts and myofibroblasts was investigated (Boulbès et al., 2006). Primary cultures of prostatic stromal cells were acquired from histologically confirmed human benign prostate hypertrophy (BPH) by enzymatic digestion (Boulbès et al., 2006). 5-Bromo-2′-deoxy-uridine (BrdU) incorporation assays were employed for cell proliferation measurements, and cytotoxicity was determined using the luminescent quantification of adenylate kinase activity. The results from the incorporation tests demonstrated that proliferation of cultured human stromal cells, stimulated by a basic fibroblast growth factor, by both foetal calf serum and epidermal growth factor, was inhibited by *P. africana* extracts (5–100 μg/mL) in a dose-dependent manner. No acute cytotoxicity of the extract was detected after 24 h of culture, except at a concentration of 100 μg/mL. In a similar manner, but to a lesser extent, the extract inhibited the proliferation of Madin–Darby canine kidney epithelial cells, dose-dependently, and no acute toxicity was observed in the cell line.

Reports have shown that a dimethyl sulphoxide extract of *P. africana* used in the treatment of BPH, exhibited inhibition of proliferation of prostate stromal cells from BPH tissues. In order to determine the mode of action, Quiles et al. (2010) investigated the apoptotic and proliferative responses of *P. africana* between non-BPH and BPH prostate stromal cells, focusing on the specific reaction displayed by stromal cell subsets. Primary prostate stromal cells obtained from patients not undergoing BPH cystectomy, as well as lower urinary tract symptoms (LUTS)/BPH patients undergoing open prostatectomy, were investigated using extracts of *P. africana*. The results on stromal cells demonstrated that apoptosis and antiproliferative potency induced by *P. africana* were increased in BPH *vs* non-BPH cells. It was shown that *P. africana* downregulated TGFB1 expression and that FGF2 increased cell sensitivity to *P. africana*. In contrast, incubation with mitogenic factors, such as DHT, VEGF and E2, decreased sensitivity to *P. africana*. Both E2 and TGFB1 stopped the antiproliferative activity of *P. africana*. *Pygeum africana* extract (Tadenan®) is used in the treatment of micturition disorders linked to BPH, and its effect on the proliferation of rat prostatic stromal cells stimulated by different growth factors was investigated (Yablonsky et al., 1997). *Pygeum africana* inhibited both stimulated and basal growth, with IC_{50} values of 7.7, 4.5 and 12.6 µg/mL for IGF-I, EGF and bFGF, respectively, in comparison to 14.4 µg/mL for untreated cells. Therefore, *P. africana* seems to be a potent inhibitor of rat prostatic fibroblast proliferation, in response to the defined growth factors EGF, bFGF and IGF-I, which are direct activators of protein kinase C and the complex mixture of mitogens in serum linked to the concentrations used (Yablonsky et al., 1997).

Prunus africana is used traditionally in Kenya, together with other plants that include *Warburgia ugandensis, Withania somnifera* and *Plectrunthus barbatus*, for the treatment of cancer. A study was conducted to evaluate the mode of action and the safety of dichloromethane extracts of *P. africana* using the cell counting Kit 8 cell proliferation assay protocol (Mwitari et al., 2013). The cytokine, interleukin 7 (IL-7), was examined *in vitro,* using reverse transcription polymerase chain reaction (RT-PCR) techniques and IEC-6 cells. *Prunus africana* inhibited the expression of IL-7 mRNA at a concentration of 50 µg/mL. The mode of action was demonstrated to be attributed to gene silencing, cytotoxicity and immunopotentiation. The authors reported that the mechanism responsible for *P. africana* action in traditional medicine is through the silencing of certain genes.The plant extract yielded an IC_{50} cytotoxicity value greater than 100 µg/mL when tested in IEC-6 cells. Nabende et al. (2015) reported the antiproliferative activity of *W. stuhlmannii, P. africana* and *M. senegalensis* in colon cancer (CT26.WT-ATCC® CRL-2638™) and breast cancer (4T1 ATCC® CRL-2539™) cell lines, and determined the toxicity levels based on responses in Swiss albino mice and against Vero cells, *in vitro*. The results demonstrated that the methanol leaf extract of *P. africana* was effective, with an IC_{50} value of 21.33 ± 0.5 µg/mL in the colon and 164.64 ± 4.14 µg/mL in the breast cancer cell lines. The methanol extract was also indicated as safe in the murine model and exhibited antiproliferative activity in both colon and breast cancer cells, with no toxicity to Vero cells (Nabende et al., 2015).

8.1.7 Anti-androgenic activity

Papaioannou et al. (2009) demonstrated that androgens play a key role in promoting the development of prostate cancer and BPH. Atraric acid (AA) was isolated from *P. africana* (bark) and exhibited anti-androgenic activity, with inhibition of the transactivation, mediated by the ligand-activated human androgen receptor. It was proven that the androgen antagonistic activity was receptor specific and did not inhibit the closely related progesterone or glucocorticoid receptors. Data showed that AA at a concentration of 10 µM inhibited the expression of the endogenous prostate-specific antigen gene in both C4–2 and LNCaP cells, through inhibiting the invasiveness of LNCaP cells by the extracellular matrix. Schleich et al. (2006a) compared the dichloromethane extract of *P. africana* at 600 µg/mL and 300 µg/mL with other plant species, for their anti-androgenic activity using an AR-responsive reporter gene assay. Fractions from the dichloromethane extract (F7 and F8) of *P. africana* stem-bark were screened for anti-androgenic effects and exhibited good activities at 4 µL, corresponding to 60 µg/mL, and at 2 µL, corresponding to 30 µg/mL, respectively. Chromatographic purification of the combined active fractions led to the isolation and identification of *N*-butylbenzenesulphonamide as a possible androgen antagonistic agent. Further fractionation of the extract of *P. africana* led to the isolation of AA, an anti-androgenic compound (Schleich et al., 2006b). The activity was demonstrated by an androgen receptor-responsive reporter gene assay. *N*-butylbenzenesulphonamide and AA also exhibited activity of human AR at a concentration of 1.0 µM. Total inactivation of human AR was reported at 100 µM. Inhibition of hormone-activated AR was determined as 50% at a concentration of 10 µM of *N*-butylbenzenesulphonamide in concentration-dependent analyses. Both compounds were proven to be the first natural, specific and complete AR antagonists.

8.2 *In vivo* studies and clinical trials

8.2.1 Antiproliferative and apoptotic activities

The activity of *P. africana* extract for the treatment of BPH has been proven in a number of double-blind and open placebo-controlled clinical trials. Eighteen double-blind, placebo-controlled studies, including 717 men with moderate-to-mild BPH, examined the effects of an oral lipophilic extract of *P. africana* (Barth, 1981; Dufour et al., 1984). The dose of the stem-bark extract ranged from 200 to 75 mg daily over a period of 6 weeks to 3 months. The number of patients in each study varied from 255 to 14. Ten studies measured night-time and daytime polyuria, and eight studies determined the maximum urinary flow. A dosage of 1 capsule in the evening and 1 capsule in the morning was administered over a period of 60 days, with capsules containing placebo or *P. africana* extract (50 mg). Trials were conducted in France, Germany and Austria, in eight centres, involving 263 patients. Evaluation was focused on quantitative parameters such as uroflowmetry, residual urine and the accurate monitoring of nocturnal and diurnal pollakiuria. Significant improvement in maximum urinary flow was reported in seven of the trials after treatment with the extract, when compared to the placebo (Barth, 1981; Dufour et al., 1984). These results were in contrast to those reported for an earlier relatively small clinical trial, which indicated no significant difference between patients treated with a placebo and Tadenan® (Donkervoort et al., 1977). Doremieux et al. (1973) conducted a histological study of prostate tissue biopsies from patients with BPH, given 75 mg *P. africana* extract daily for 1–3 months and observed that the extract increased prostate secretion, without reduction in prostate size. This lipophilic extract of the trunk bark also restored normal levels of total protein secretion from the prostate in patients with abnormally low levels of secretion, and reinstalled the activity of prostate acid phosphatase (Luchetta et al., 1984). Wilt and Ishani (1998) examined whether extracts of *P. africana* are effective in the treatment of BPH, compared its effect to that of standard pharmacologic BPH treatments, and also compared side effects to that of standard BPH drugs. *Pygeum africana* demonstrated a large improvement in the combined outcome of flow measures and urologic symptoms as evaluated by an effect size, defined by the difference of the mean change for each outcome divided by the pooled standard deviation for each outcome. Men using *P. africana* were more than twice as likely to report an improvement in overall symptoms (relative risk (RR) = 2.1, 95% confidence interval (CI) = 1.4 to 3.1). Residual urine volume was reduced by 24%, nocturia by 19%, and peak urine flow was increased by 23%. Mild adverse effects were observed for *P. africana* when compared to the placebo. The overall dropout rate was 12% and was similar for placebo (11%), *P. africana* (13%) and other controls (8%).

Several researchers conducted clinical trials on *P. africana*, and 14 of these trials indicated an improvement of global outcome assessments following oral treatment with a chloroform extract of the stem-bark in 461 men with stage II or I BPH (Lhez and Leguevague 1970; Robineau and Pelissier, 1976). In 10 of these studies, a total of 281 patients were given 100 mg extract daily for 21 days to 3 months and in four studies, a total of 180 patients received 75 mg extract daily for 21 days to 3 months. In all but three studies, the overall outcome was assessed as either excellent, very good, good, or improved in over 50% of the patients. Data from 19 other clinical trials involving 849 men with BPH, without controls (59–18 patients per study), revealed a significant improvement in their symptoms after treatment with a lipophilic extract of *P. africana* (stem-bark) (Andro and Riffaud, 1995). Patients were administered the extract daily, with either 200 mg extract (148 patients), 150 mg (42 patients), 100 mg (523 patients), 75–100 mg (20 patients), or 75 mg (116 patients) for 20–160 days. Improvements in daytime polyuria, nocturia, mean maximum urinary flow rate and postvoid residual volume were demonstrated in over 50% of patients in different studies. Symptoms such as urgency and hesitancy of micturition and dysuria were also improved. A large open-label study in 500 men with BPH evaluated improvements in urodynamic parameters after daily treatment with a lipophilic extract of the bark for over 5 years (Andro and Riffaud, 1995). Improvements in daytime nocturia and polyuria dysuria, were observed in over 68% of patients, and improvements in urinary volume and flow rate were reported in more than 61%. The best improvements were seen in patients with moderate symptoms, with baseline postvoid residual volume less than 100 mL and no prominent median lobe of the prostate. In the absence of prostate infection, an improvement in prostate secretion was also reported (Clavert et al., 1986).

Another multicentre study (no controls) determined the safety and efficacy of treatment with a stem-bark extract of *P. africana* (50 mg), administered twice daily for 2 months in 85 men with symptoms of BPH (the stage of BPH was not stated). Subjective evaluation of the outcomes was made using the Quality of Life (QL) score and the International Prostate Symptom Score (IPSS), and the urine flowmetry was used for objective evaluation (Breza et al., 1998). After administration, the QL and IPSS improved significantly by 31% and 40%, respectively. The nocturnal frequency was also significantly (32%) reduced. Levin et al. (2005) conducted a study to assess whether pretreating rabbits with a clinically relevant dose of Tadenan® (*P. africana*) could stop the bladder from developing contractile dysfunctions that are induced by bilateral ischemia followed by reperfusion, therefore possibly protecting the bladder from ischemic injury. New Zealand white rabbits were divided into two groups, of which Group I was pretreated with Tadenan® (3.0 mg/kg/day) by oral gavage for 3 weeks, while group II was given peanut oil (vehicle). The data demonstrated that Tadenan® pretreatment at the clinically relevant dose of 3.0 mg/kg/day protected the bladder from contractile dysfunctions induced by bilateral ischemia followed by reperfusion. The receptor-related apoptosis-mediating protein (TRAMP) mouse model was used to evaluate the anticancer effect of an ethanolic extract of the bark (Shenouda et al., 2007). The *in vivo* results demonstrated that TRAMP mice fed *P. africana* exhibited a significant reduction in prostate cancer incidence (35%), compared to casein diet-fed mice (62.5%). The TRAMP mice fed with the extract at a dose of 0.128 mg/kg of the diet exhibited a marked and significant reduction of differentiated carcinoma tumour incidence.

8.2.2 Anti-asthmatic activity

Karani et al. (2013) investigated the *in vivo* anti-asthmatic activity, as well as the safety of extracts of *P. africana* (stem-bark) and *W. ugandensis* in asthma-induced BALB/c mice. They determined the efficacy by quantification of eosinophil proportion in bronchoalveolar lavage fluid (BALF) and by assaying heart blood serum for ovalbumin-specific immunoglobulin E (IgE) antibodies. The results indicated that treatment with extracts of *P. africana* (500 mg/kg body weight) significantly reduced the BALF and IgE eosinophil to 2.80 ± 0.20 and 0.100 ± 0.0001, respectively. The results confirmed that stem-bark extracts of *P. africana* exhibited anti-asthmatic properties although the mechanism of action was not investigated.

8.2.3 Anti-inflammatory and analgesic activities

Anti-inflammatory activity in the treatment of symptoms associated with moderate-to-mild BPH has been demonstrated in chloroform bark extracts of

P. africana. It was reported that phytosterols, mainly β-sitostenone and β-sitosterol, isolated from *P. africana* induced anti-inflammatory effects and inhibited the synthesis of 5-α-reductase and prostaglandin activity, which is primarily responsible for the pathogenesis of BPH and prostate development (Steers, 2001). This activity has also been examined by a number of other research groups, showing the efficacy of dichloromethane bark extracts of *P. africana* in suppressing lower urinary tract symptoms, by decreasing inflammation through the inhibition of 5-α-reductase in patients with BPH (Andro and Riffaud, 1995; Ishani et al., 2000; Capasso et al., 2003). Furthermore, it was demonstrated that β-sitosterol reduced the elevated levels of prostaglandins in patients with BPH, while the pentacyclic triterpenoids inhibited enzymatic activity and therefore inhibited inflammation and swelling in the prostate (Bauer and Bach, 1986; Carbin et al., 1990; Holm and Meyhoff, 1997; Wasson and Watts, 1998; Quilez et al., 2003). Friedelin, a triterpenoid constituent present in *P. africana* extract, was shown to have anti-inflammatory effects through the inhibition of acetic acid-induced vascular permeability in mice (54.5%) using carrageenan-induced hind paw oedema (Catalano et al., 1984; Antonisamy et al., 2011). It was reported that a lipophilic extract of the bark significantly inhibited the synthesis of 5-LOX metabolites in human polymorphonuclear cells stimulated with the calcium ionophore A23187, *in vivo*: leukotriene B4 (LTB4) at 3 ng/mL, 5-hydroxyeicosatetraenoic acid (5-HETE) at 1 ng/mL, 20-carboxy-LTB4 at 3 ng/mL, and 20-hydroxy-LTB4 at 10 ng/mL (ESCOP, 2009). The lipophilic extract administered intragastrically at a dose of 400 mg/kg, significantly reduced carrageenan-induced paw oedema in rats. Inhibition of the increased vascular permeability caused by histamine was observed when the extract was administered intraperitoneally at dosages of 100 and 10 mg/kg (ESCOP, 2009).

8.3 Safety

After intragastric administration of a single dose of a lipophilic stem-bark extract of *P. africana* (1–8 g/kg in rats and 1–6 g/kg in mice), no fatalities or side effects were reported in both chronic and acute toxicity studies in rats and mice (Bombardelli and Morazzoni, 1997). Additionally, no adverse reactions were seen in rats and mice when the extract was administered intragastrically, daily at 600 and 60 mg/kg body weight, respectively, over a period of 11 months. Gathumbi et al. (2002) evaluated the safety of *P. africana*, after a reported increase in body weight at dosages of 1000, 100 and 10 mg/kg given daily for a period of 8 weeks. Sprague Dawley male rats were used (aged 8–10 weeks, weighing 200–250 g) and it was shown that the chloroform extract of *P. africana* did not cause pathology or clinical signs at daily oral doses of up to 1000 mg/kg for a period of 8 weeks. In another study, five groups of mice were administered with one dose of an aqueous extract of *P. africana*, varying from 5000 to 500 mg/kg body weight (Karani et al., 2013). Adverse reactions were reported in mice treated with *P. africana* at high dose levels (1582–5000 mg/kg) and these include pilo-erection, hypo-activity, hyperventilation and poor appetite. Mortality was observed within 24 h after administration of the extracts at 5000 mg/kg (100%), while 60% mortality was recorded at 2812 mg/kg, 20% mortality at 1582 mg/kg, and no mortality at 890 and 500 mg/kg.

9. Phytochemistry

Phytosterols were the first constituents isolated from the chloroform extract of *P. africana.* These were identified as 3-β-sitosterone, 3-β-sitosterol and 3-β-sitosterol-glucoside (Longo and Tira, 1981; Hass et al., 1999; Jimu, 2011; Nyamai et al., 2015). Catalano et al. (1984) reported other compounds from the chloroform extract of *P. africana* (bark), namely ursolic acid, friedelin, epi-maslinic acid, maslinic acid and 2α-hydroxyursolic acid. Scarpato et al. (1998) identified 4-*O*-β-D-glucopyranosyl-(7,8)-dimethoxyisolariciresinol from the butanolic extract *n*-Docosanol and ferulic acid were isolated by Fourneau et al. (1996), and detected by Kadu et al. (2012) in the bark extract of *P. africana* using gas chromatography-mass selective detection (GC-MSD). Bio-activity-guided fractionation of the dichloromethane and ethanolic extracts of *P. africana* (stem-bark) yielded *N*-butylbenzenesulphonamide (NBBS), atraric acid (methyl-2,4-dihydroxy-3,6-dimethylbenzoate) and phenolic compounds (Schleich et al. 2006a, b). Pentacyclic triterpenoid compounds, including oleanolic and ursolic acids, were isolated and identified from the aqueous methanolic and chloroform extracts of *P. africana* (Longo and Tira, 1981). Nine triterpenic acids were reported by Fourneau et al. (1996), isolated from the chloroform bark extract, namely 2α,3-β-dihydroxyurs-12-en-28-oic acid, 2α,3α-dihydroxyurs-12-en-28-oic acid, 3-β,24-dihydroxyurs-12-en-28-oic acid, 2α,3-β-dihydroxyolean-12-en-28-oic acid, 2α,3α,24-trihydroxyurs-12-en-28-oic acid, 2α,3α,23-trihydroxyurs-12-en-28-oic acid, 24-*O*-*cis*-feruly-3β-hydroxy-urs-12-en-28-oic acid, 24-*O*-*trans*-ferulyl-3β-hydroxy-urs-12-en-28-oic acid and 24-*O*-*trans*-ferulyl-2a,3a-dihydroxy-urs-12-en-28-oic acid. Ngule et al. (2014) demonstrated the presence of saponins, tannins, terpenoids, flavonoids, alkaloids, glycosides and phenols in the aqueous methanolic bark extract. Hass et al. (1999) and Ganzera et al. (1999) identified fatty acids such as palmitic acid, myristic acid, oleic acid, linoleic acid, arachidonic acid, stearic acid, lignoceric acid, behenic acid, and linolenic acid in the chloroform bark extract. The presence of hentriacontane and nonacosane were also reported from the chloroform bark extract of *P. africana* by Longo and Tira (1981). A HPLC method was employed for the identification and quantification of *n*-docosyl ferulate in soft gelatin capsules containing *P. africana* extract and also in *P. africana* extracts, at concentrations ranging from 100 to 10 mg/mL (Uberti et al., 1990; You and Cheng, 1997).

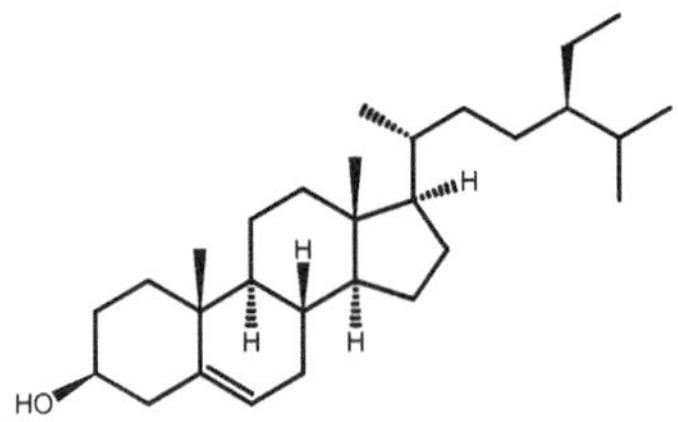

β-Sitosterol

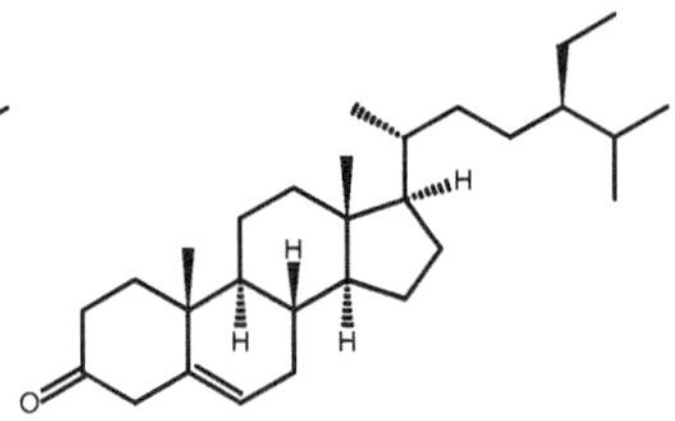

Sitostenone

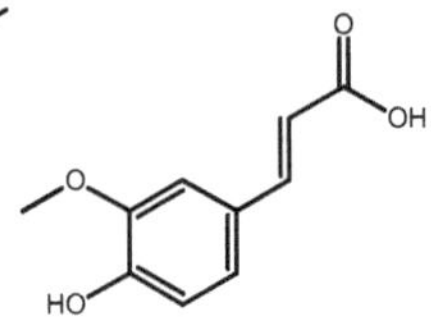

Ferulic acid

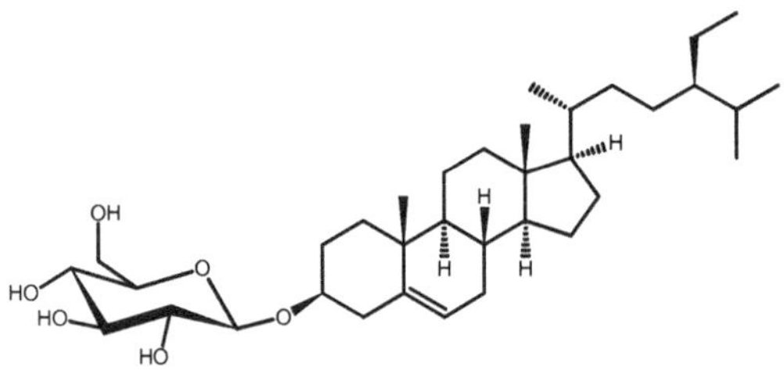

β-Sitosterol-D-glucopyranoside

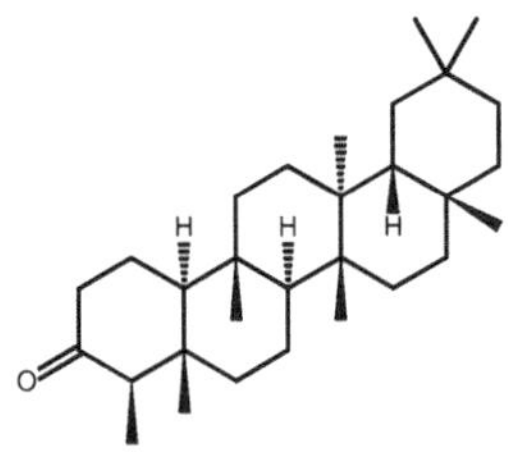

Friedelin

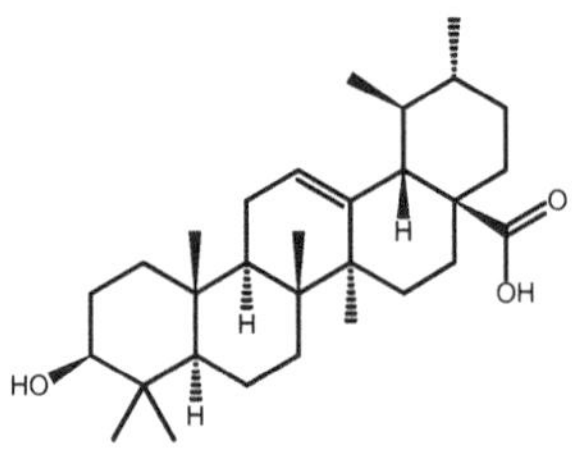

Ursolic acid

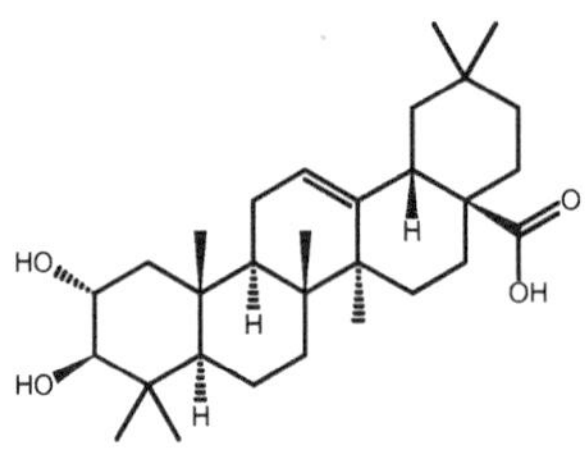

Maslinic acid

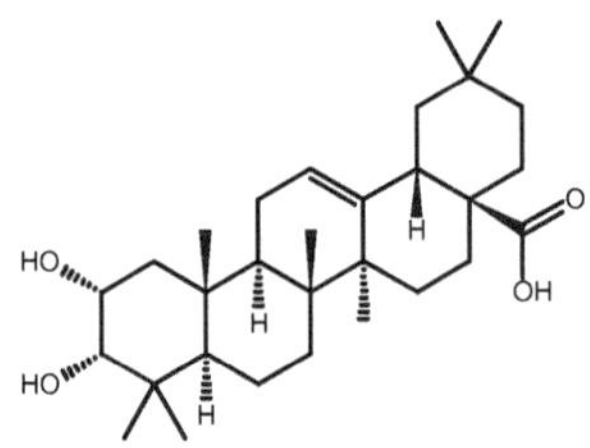

Epimaslinic acid

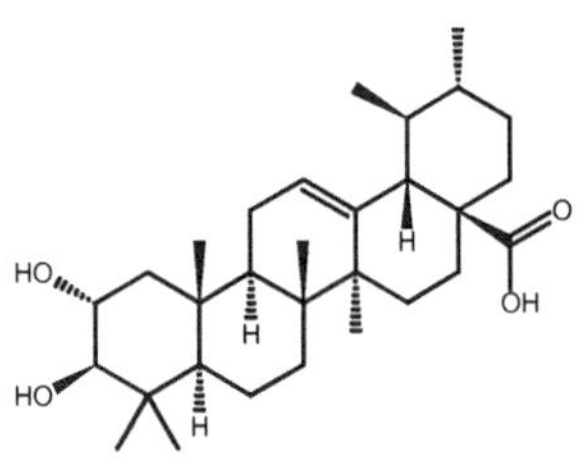

2α-Hydroxyursolic acid

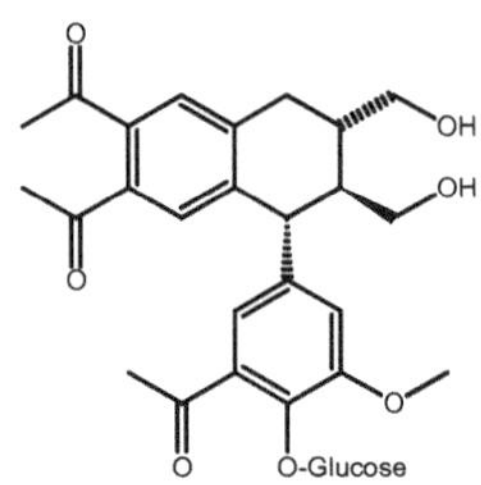

4-*O*-β-Glucopyranosyl-(7,8)-dimethoxyisolariciresinol

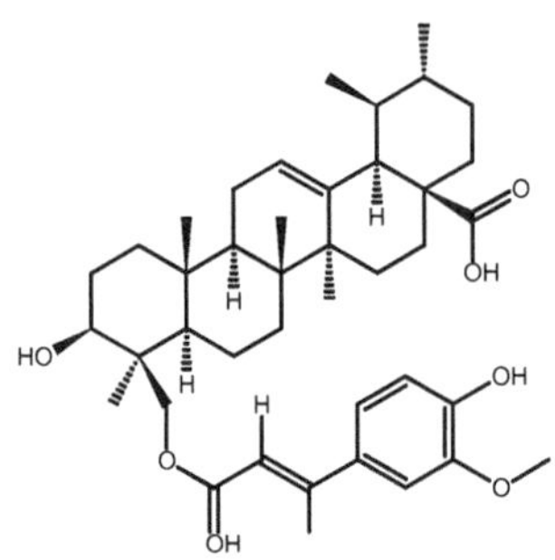

24-*O*-*trans*-Ferulyl-3β-hydroxy-urs-12-en-28-oic acid

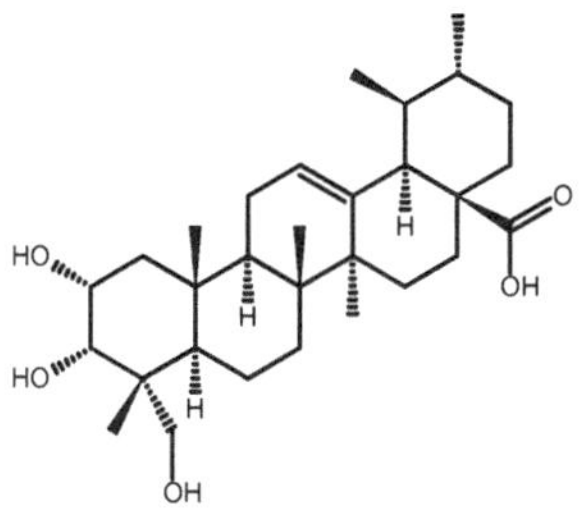

2α,3α,23-Trihydroxyurs-12-en-28-oic acid

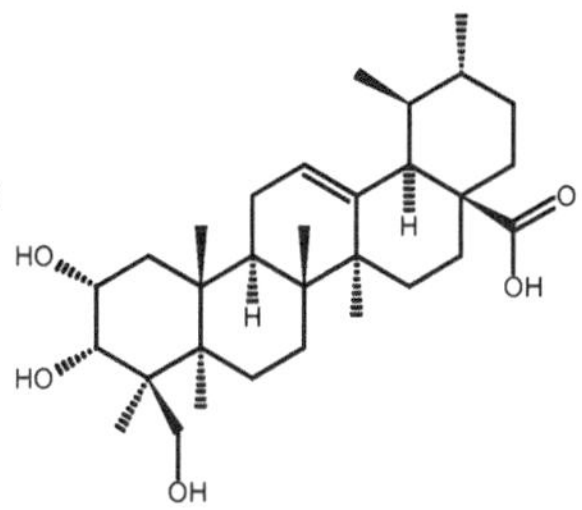

2α,3α,24-Trihydroxyurs-12-12-en-28-oic acid

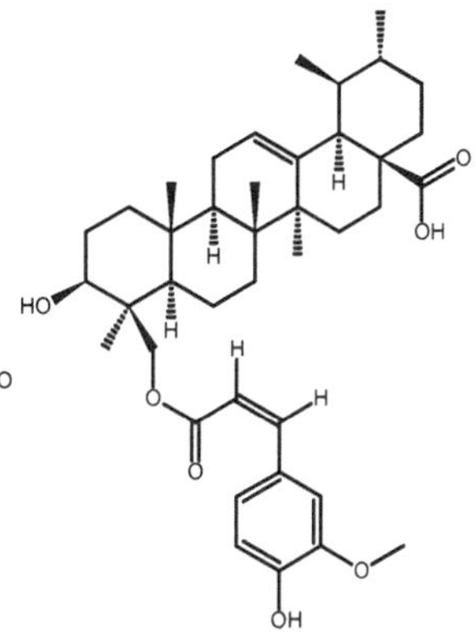

24-*O*-*cis*-Feruly-3β-hydroxy-urs-en-28-oic acid

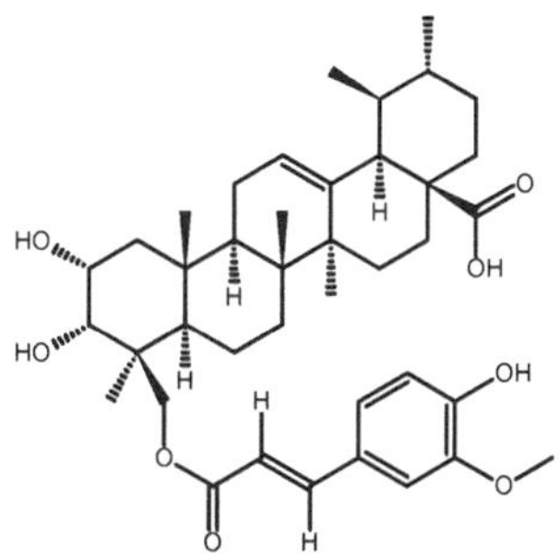

24-*O*-*trans*-Ferulyl-2α,3α-dihydroxy-urs-12-en-28-oic acid

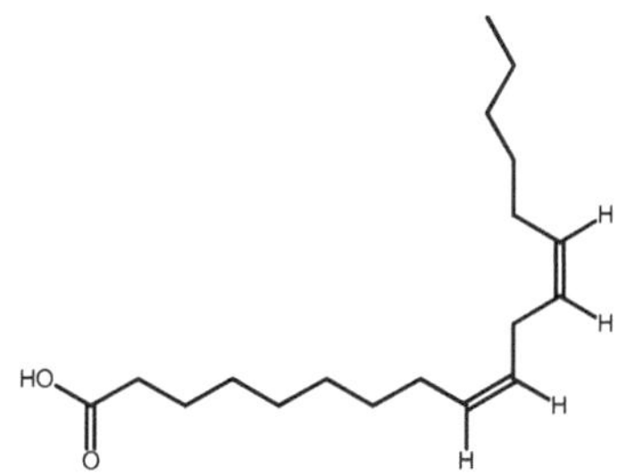

Linoleic acid

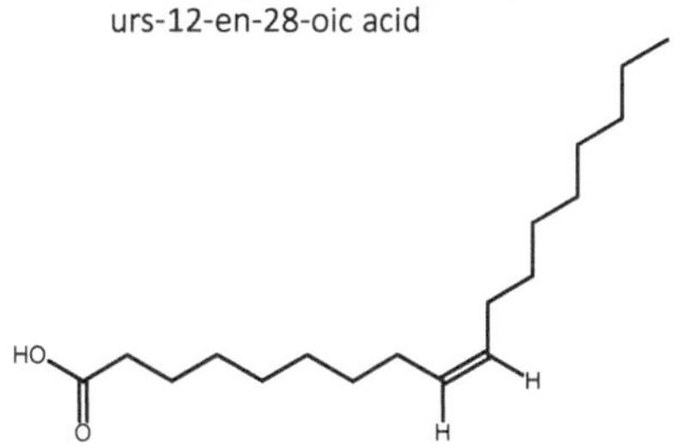

Oleic acid

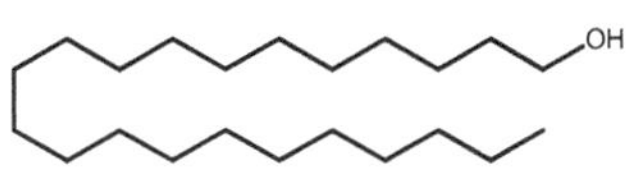

n-Docosanol

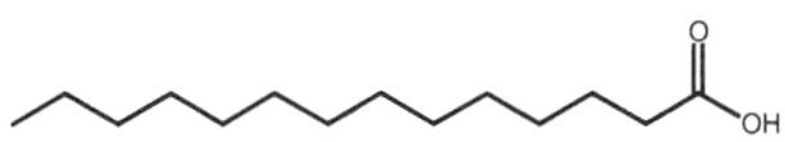

Myristic acid

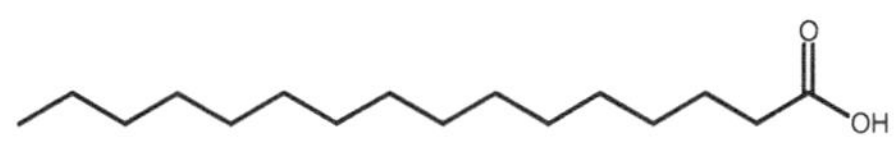

Palmitic acid

Part B: Chemical profiling and quality control

10. Chromatography analysis

10.1 High-performance thin-layer chromatography (HPTLC) fingerprint analysis

General instrumentation: A CAMAG HPTLC instrument consisting of an automatic TLC sampler (ATS 4), automatic developing chamber (ADC 2), CAMAG TLC Visualizer 2, CAMAG derivatiser, and TLC plate heater. *HPTLC plates:* Silica gel glass plates 60 F_{254} (Merck). *Plant part:* Stem-bark, extracted with ethyl acetate. *Sample application:* Application volume of 25 μL ethyl acetate extract (10 mg/mL) and 2 μL standard (1 mg/mL) spotted as 10 mm bands. Plates developed in a 20 × 10 × 4 cm glass twin-trough chamber to a migration distance of 70 mm. *Tank saturation*: 20 min at 15 °C and 45% RH, with 25 mL of mobile phase. *Mobile phase:* Toluene:ethyl acetate:methanol:formic acid:acetic acid (90:20:20:1:1, v/v/v/v/v). *Derivatisation:* A spraying reagent (10% sulphuric acid) prepared by diluting 10 mL of concentrated sulphuric acid in 90 mL of methanol under cooling. The plate was sprayed with 3 mL of the reagent and heated for 3 min at 100 °C on a TLC plate heater and visualised. *Visualisation:* The plate was viewed under white reflectance and under 366 nm fluorescent light.

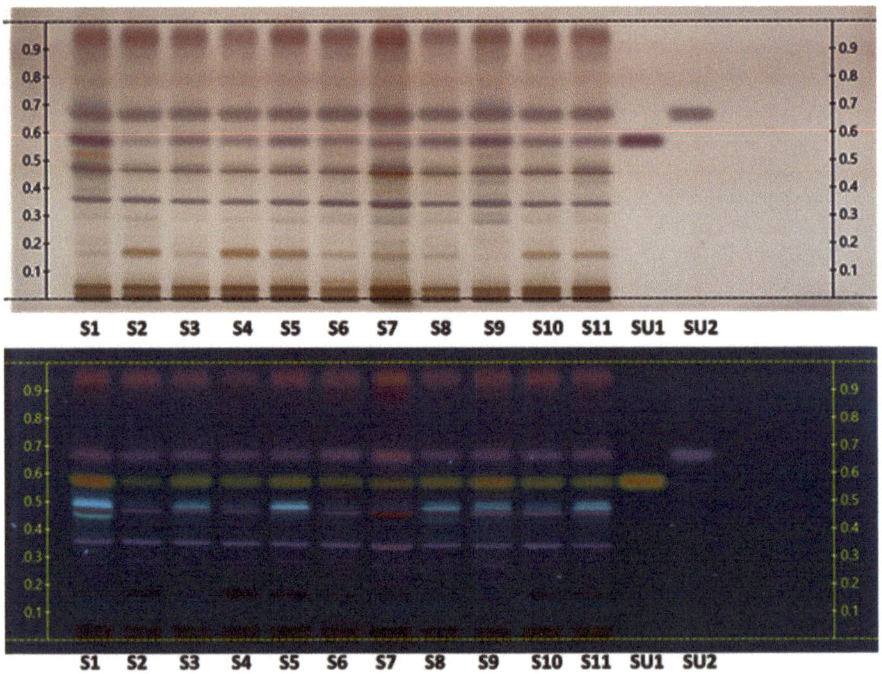

HPTLC plate of *Prunus africana* ethyl acetate extracts (n = 11) (S1–S11) and the standards, SU1 and SU2. The samples are characterised by a yellow-orange band for ursolic acid (R_f = 0.58) and a purple band for β-sitosterol (R_f = 0.67) under 366 nm radiation.

10.2 Ultra-performance liquid chromatography (UPLC) analysis

General instrumentation: A Waters Acquity Ultra-Performance Liquid Chromatography system with a photodiode array (PDA) detector combined with a Xevo G2QToF mass spectrometer (Waters, USA). *Plant part:* Stem-bark, extracted with ethyl acetate. *Sample application:* Injection volume of 2.0 µL at 1 mg/mL (full-loop

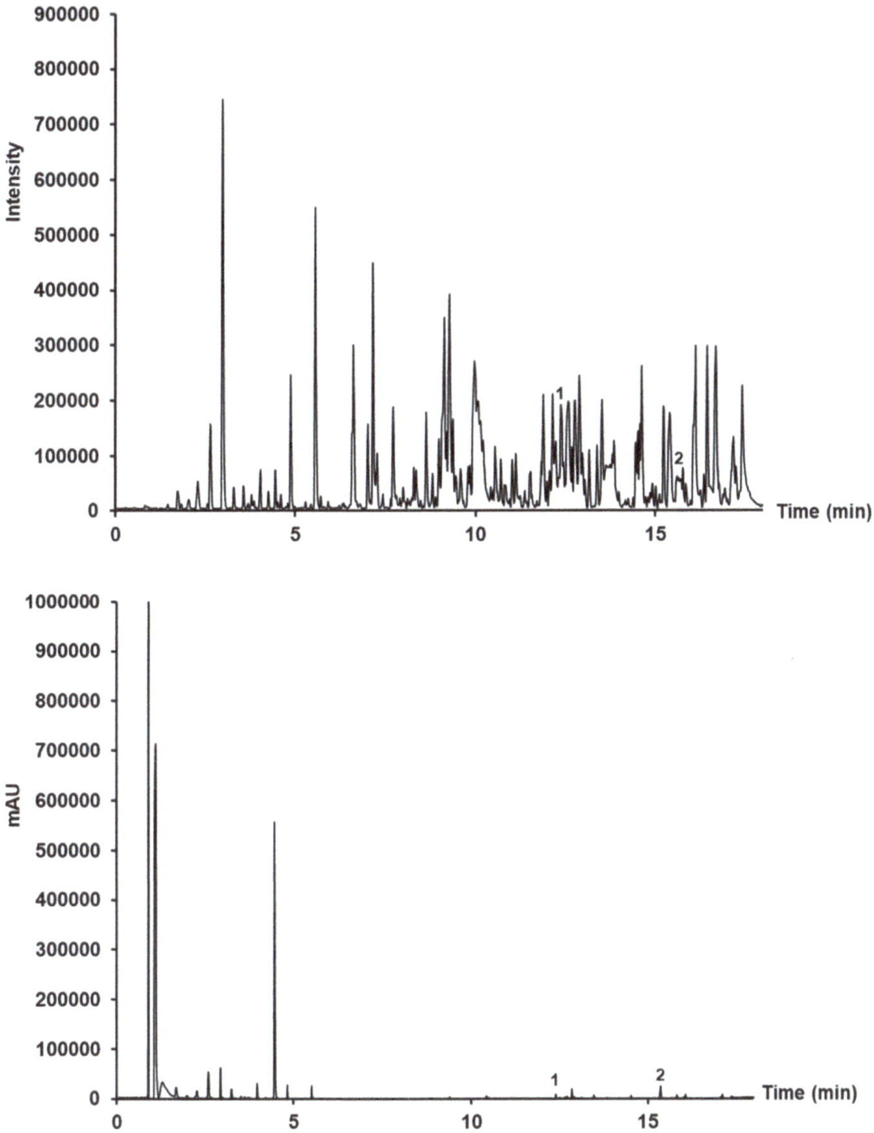

UPLC-ToF-MS ESI$^-$ (upper) and PDA (lower) chromatograms of *Prunus africana* ethyl acetate extract. [1] = maslinic acid *m/z* 471.3367, [2] = ursolic acid *m/z* 455.3266.

injection). *Column:* CORTECS UPLC C_{18} column (150 mm × 2.1 mm, i.d., 1.6 μm particle size, Waters). *Mobile phase:* 0.1% formic acid in water (solvent A) and acetonitrile (solvent B). *Analysis conditions:* Gradient elution at a flow rate: 0.3 mL/min, changing as follows: 90% A: 10% B, changed to 15% A: 85% B in 15 min, to 10% A: 90% B in 1 min, and back to initial ratio in 0.5 min, equilibrating the system for 1.5 min, total run time 18 min. *Mass spectrometry*: ESI^- (negative ionisation mode), N_2 used as desolvation gas, desolvation temperature 350 °C at a flow rate of 500 L/h and source temperature at 100 °C. Capillary and cone voltages, 2500 and 46 V, respectively. Data collected between *m/z* 100 and 1200.

11. Mid-infrared (MIR) spectroscopy analysis

General instrumentation: An Alpha-P Bruker spectrometer, mounted with an attenuated total reflectance (ATR) diamond crystal. *Spectral acquisition:* Spectrum obtained in the absorbance mode, with a spectral resolution of 4 cm^{-1} over the range 4000–550 cm^{-1} and captured using OPUS 6.5 software. *Plant part:* Stem-bark. *Sample preparation:* Stem-bark powdered, sieved (< 500 μm), and placed directly onto the surface of the diamond crystal.

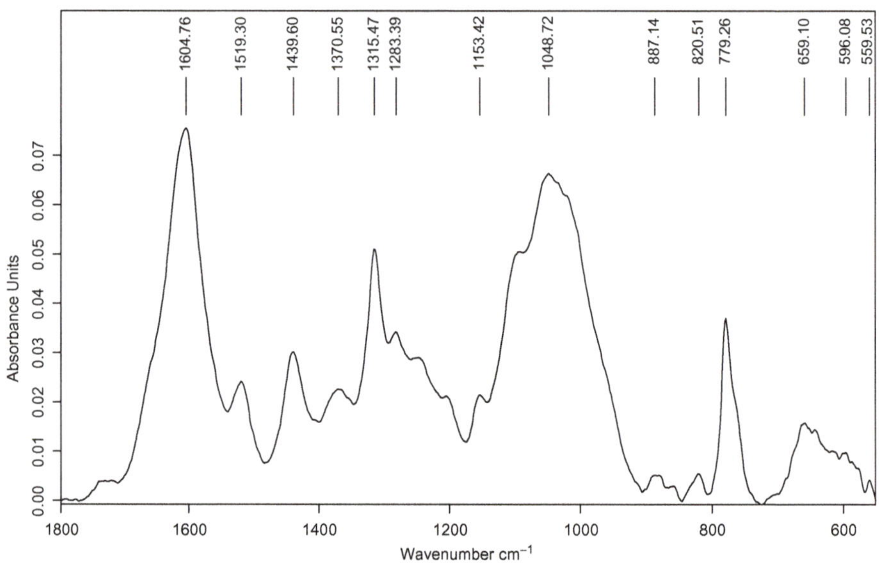

Mid-infrared spectrum of powdered *Prunus africana* stem-bark displaying the fingerprint region (1800–550 cm^{-1}).

References

Abera, B., 2014. J. Ethnobiol. Ethnomed., 10:1–15.
Allkanjari, O., Vitalone, A., 2015. Life Sci., 126:42–56.
Amico, V., Barresi, V., Chillemi, R., 2009. Nat. Prod. Commun., 4:27–34.
Andro, M.C., Riffaud, J.P., 1995. Curr. Ther. Res., 56:796–817.
Antonisamy, P., Duraipandiyan, V., Ignacimuthu, S., 2011. J. Pharm. Pharmacol., 63:1070–1077.
Barth, H., 1981. Non-hormonal treatment of benign prostatic hypertrophy. Clinical evaluation of the active extract of *Pygeum africanum*. In: Proceedings of the Symposium on Benign Prostatic Hypertrophy, Paris, France, pp. 45–51.
Bauer, H.W., Bach, D., 1986. Urol. Int., 41:139–144.
Bii, C., Korir, K.R., Rugutt, J., Mutai, C., 2010. J. Med. Plant Res., 4:995–998.
Bombardelli, E., Morazzoni, P., 1997. Fitoterapia, 68:205–218.
Boulbès, D., Soustelle, L., Costa, P., Haddoum, M., Bali, J., Hollande, F., Magous, R., 2006. BJU Int., 98:1106–1113.
Breza, J., Dzurny, O., Borowka, A., Hanus, T., Petrik, R., Blane, G., Chadha-Boreham, H., 1998. Curr. Med. Res. Opin., 14:127–139.
Capasso, F., Gaginella, T.S., Grandolini, G., Izzo, A.A., 2003. Phytotherapy, A Quick Reference to Herbal Medicine, Springer-Verlag, Berlin, Germany.
Carbin, B.E., Larsson, B., Lindahl, O., 1990. Br. J. Urol., 66:639–641.
Catalano, S., Ferretti, M., Marsili, A., Morelli, I., 1984. J. Nat. Prod., 47:910.
Clavert, A., Cranz, C., Riffaud, J.P., Marquer, C., Lacolle, J.Y., Bollack, C., 1986. Ann. Urol., 20:341–343.
Cunningham, A.B., Mbenkum, F.T., 1993. Sustainability of Harvesting *Prunus africana* Bark in Cameroon: A Medicinal Plant in International Trade. People and Plants Working Paper 2. UNESCO, Paris, France.
Cunningham, M., Cunningham, A.B., Schippmann, U., 1997. Trade in *Prunus africana* and the Implementation of CITES. German Federal Agency for Nature Conservation, Germany. ISBN 3-89624-608-9.
Dey, N., Chatterjee, D., Choudhury, M.C., Das, S., 2017. World J. Pharm. Pharm. Sci., 6:1155–1160.
Donkervoort, T., Sterling, A., Van Ness, J., Donker, P.J., 1977. Eur. Urol., 3:218–225.
Doremieux, J., Masson, J., Bollack, C., 1973. J. Méd. Strasbourg, 4:252–257.
Dufour, B., Choquenet, C., Revol, M., Faure, G., Jorest, R., 1984. Urol. Ann., 18:193–195.
ElgorashI, E.E., Taylor, J.L.S., Maes, A., Van Staden, J., De Kimpe, N., Verschaeve, L., 2003. Toxicol. Lett., 143:195–207.
Emmanuel, N., 2010. Afr. J. Pharm. Pharmacol., 4:793–805.
ESCOP, 2009. European Scientific Cooperative on Phytotherapy. Georg Thieme Verlag, Stuttgart, Germany.
European Medicines Agency, 2015. http://www.ema.europa.eu/docs/en_GB/document_library/Herbal_HMPC_assessment_report/2015/12/WC500198934.pdf.
Ewusi, B.N., Eben-Ebai, S., Asanga, C.A., Nkongo, J.B.N., 1992. Unpublished Report Prepared for Plantecam-Medicam. Douala.
Fashing, P.J., 2004. Biol. Conserv., 120:449–459.
Fourneau, C., Hocquemiller, R., Cavé, A., 1996. Phytochemistry, 42:1387–1389.
Gachie, P.K., Koech, E.K., Njunge, J.T., Simons, A.J., Ndalut, K., Avenue, U.N., Campus, C., 2012. For. Trees Livelihoods, 21:37–41.

Gangoué-Piéboji, J., Baurin, S., Frère, J.M., Ngassam, P., Ngameni, B., Azebaze, A., Pegnyemb, D.E., Watchueng, J., Goffin, C., Galleni, M., 2007. Phytother. Res., 21:284–287.
Ganzera, M., Croom, E.M., Khan, I.A., 1999. J. Med. Food, 2:21–27.
Gashe, F., Zeleke, G., 2017. Res. J. Med. Plants, 11:142–147.
Gathumbi, P.K., Mwangi, J.W., Mugera, G.M., Njiro, S.M., 2002. Phytother. Res., 16:244–247.
Geldenhuys, C.J., 1981. South. Afr. For. J., 118:61–66.
Hass, M.A., Nowak, D.M., Leonova, E., Levin, R.M., Longhurst, P.A., 1999. Phytomedicine, 6:379–388.
Holm, M., Meyhoff, H.H., 1997. Scand. J. Urol. Nephrol., 31:213–215.
Ingram, V.J., Awono, A., Schure, J., Ndam, N., 2009. Guidance for a National *Prunus africana* Management Plan, Cameroon, edited by CIFOR. Yaoundé, Cameroun: FAO-CIFOR-SNV-World Agroforestry Center-COMIFAC-GTZ. https://pure.uva.nl/ws/files/4205179/76923_ingram01.pdf.
Ishani, A., Macdonald, R., Nelson, D., Rutkis, I., Wilt, T.J., 2000. Am. J. Med., 109:564–664.
Jeanrenaud, S., 1991. The conservation-development interface: a study of forest use, agricultural practices, and perceptions of the rainforest. Etinde forest, South West Cameroon. Report submitted to the Overseas Development Administration.
Jimu, L., 2011. J. Ecol. Nat. Environ., 3:118–130.
Kadu, C.A., Parich, A., Schueler, S., Konrad, H., Muluvi, G.M., Eyog-Matig, O., Geburek, T., 2012. Phytochemistry, 83:70–78.
Karani, L.W., Tolo, F.M., Karanja, S.M., Khayeka, C.W., 2013. Eur. J. Med. Plants, 3:345–368.
Kokwaro, J.O., 1976. Medicinal Plants of East Africa. General Printers Ltd., Nairobi, Kenya.
Komakech, R., Kang, Y., Lee, J., Omujal, F., 2017. Evid. Based Complement. Alternat. Med., 2017:3014019.
Kurtto, A., 2009. Rosaceae (pro parte majore). Euro + Med Plant Base—the information resource for Euro-Mediterranean plant diversity. Published on the Internet, http://www2.,bgbm.,org/EuroPlusMed.
Levin, R.M., Whitbeck, C., Horan, P., Bellamy, F., 2005. Phytomedicine, 12:17–24.
Lhez, A., Leguevague, G., 1970. Vie Med., 2:1–4.
Longo, R., Tira, S., 1981. Planta Med., 42:195–203.
Luchetta, G., Weill, A., Becker, N., Clavert, A., Bollack, C., 1984. Urol. Int., 39:222–224.
Mwitari, P.G., Ayeka, P.A., Ondicho, J., Matu, E.N., Bii, C.C., 2013. PLoS One, 8:1–9.
Nabende, P.N., Karanja, S.M., Mwatha, J.K., Wachira, S.W., 2015. Eur. J. Med. Plants, 5:366–376.
Nataraju, A., Raghavendra, C.D., Rajesh, R., Vishwanath, B.S., 2007. Curr. Top. Med. Chem., 7:801–809.
Ngule, M.C., Ndiku, M.H., Ramesh, F., 2014. J. Nat. Sci. Res., 4:85–90.
Nsom, C.L., Dick, J., 1992. Unpublished Report Prepared for the Ijim Mountain Forest Project.
Nyamai, D.W., Mawia, A.M., Wambua, F.K., Njoroge, A., Matheri, F., Lagat, R., Kiambi J., Ogola, P., Arika, W., Cheseto, X., King'ori, E., Ramni, J., Ngugi, M.P., Muchugi, A., Ng'ang'a, M., Burugu, M.W., 2015. Pharmacol. Nat. Prod., 110:1–8.
Papaioannou, M., Schleich, S., Prade, I., Degen, S., Roell, D., Schubert, U., Tanner, T., Claessens, F., Matusch, R., Baniahmad, A., 2009. J. Cell. Mol. Med., 13:2210–2223.
Paubert-Braquet, M., Cave, A., Hocquemiller, R., Delacroix, D., Dupont, C., Hedef, N., Borgeat, P., 1994. J. Lipid Mediat. Cell Signal., 9:285–290.
Pomatto, V., 2001. Etude de marché de *Pygeum africanum* en Europe. GTZ. MINEF. Yaoundé, Cameroun, p. 59.

Pujol, J., 1990. Natur Africa: The Herbalist Handbook. Jean Pujol Natural Healers Foundation, Durban, South Africa.

Quiles, M.T., Arbós, M.A., Fraga, A., De Torres, I.M., Reventós, J., Morote, J., 2010. Prostate, 70:1044–1053.

Quilez, J., Garcia-Lorda, P., Salas-Salvado, J., 2003. Clin. Nutr., 22:343–351.

Robineau, Y., Pelissier, E., 1976. Diagnostics, 175:115–120.

Rukunga, G.M., Mawuli, W.T., Masahiko, K., Seiji, K., Mungai, G.M., Muli, J.M., Tolo, F.M., Kibaya, R.M., Muthaura, C.N., Kanyara, J.N., Tukei, P.M., Shiraku, K., 2002. Afr. J. Health Sci., 9:81–90.

SANBI, South African National Biodiversity Institute, 2006. Siyabulela Nonjinge. KwaZulu-Natal National Botanical Garden. Available from: http://pza.sanbi.org/prunus-africana.

Scarpato, R., Pistelli, L., Bertoli, A., Nieri, E., Migliore, L., 1998. Toxicol. *in vitro*, 12:153–161.

Schleich, S., Papaioannou, M., Baniahmad, A., Matusch, R., 2006a. Planta Med., 72:807–813.

Schleich, S., Papaioannou, M., Baniahmad, A., Matusch, R., 2006b. Planta Med., 72:547–551.

Shenouda, N.S., Sakla, M.S., Newton, L.G., 2007. Endocrine, 31:72–81.

Steenkamp, V., Gouws, M.C., Gulumian, M., Elgorashi, E.E., Van Staden, J., 2006. J. Ethnopharmacol., 103:71–75.

Steers, W.D., 2001. Urology, 58:17–24.

Stewart, K.M., 2003. J. Ethnopharmacol., 89:3–13.

Sunderland, T.C.H., Nkefor, J.P., 1997. Tropical Agriculture Association Newsletter, December.

Tolo, F.M., Rukunga, G.M., Faith, W.M., Eliud, N.M., Wilson, N., Kazuko, K., Geoffrey, M., Charles, N., Joseph, M., Lucia, K., Oishi, E., Mawuli, W.K., 2006. J. Ethnopharmacol., 104:92–99.

Tolo, F.M., Rukunga, G.M., Muli, F.W., Ochora, J., Eizuru, Y., Muthaura, C.N., Kimani, C.W., Mungai, G.M., Kofi-Tsekpo, M.W., 2007. Afr. J. Health Sci., 14:143–148.

Uberti, E., Martinelli, E.M., Pifferi, G., Gagliardi, L., 1990. Fitoterapia, 61:342–347.

Verschaeve, L., Kestensa, V., Taylora, J.L.S., Elgorashi, E.E., Maesa, A., Van Puyveldec, L., De Kimpe, N., Van Staden, J., 2004. Toxicol. *in vitro*, 18:29–35.

Wasson, K.M., Watts, S.A., 1998. Toxicol. Endocrinol., 120:425–431.

Wilt, T.J., Ishani, A., 1998. Cochrane Database Syst. Rev., 1–26.

Yablonsky, F., Nicolas, V., Riffaud, J., Bellamy, F., 1997. J. Urol., 157:2381–2387.

You, Y., Cheng, G., 1997. Se Pu, 3:259–260.

CHAPTER

Sclerocarya birrea

21

Baatile Komane[a], Guy Kamatou[a], Nduvho Mulaudzi[a], Ilze Vermaak[a,b] and Gerda Fouche[c]

[a]*Department of Pharmaceutical Sciences, Tshwane University of Technology, Pretoria, South Africa*

[b]*SAMRC Herbal Drugs Research Unit, Faculty of Science, Tshwane University of Technology, Pretoria, South Africa*

[c]*Chemistry Department, University of Pretoria, Pretoria, South Africa*

Abstract

Sclerocarya birrea (A. Rich.) Hochst. (Anacardiaceae) commonly known as "marula" is a deciduous tree that can reach up to 17 m in height. It is commonly distributed in southern Africa including South Africa, Zimbabwe, Botswana, Mozambique, Zambia and Namibia. Traditionally, the stem bark is used medicinally to treat several ailments such as general gastrointestinal complaints, indigestion, diarrhoea, dysentery, haemorrhoids, malaria, as well as fever and ulcers. Marula seed oil is used in southern Africa as a shampoo for damaged, fragile and dry hair, and as a base oil for soap. Seed oil is popularly included in cosmetic products, and ethnobotanical literature states that the oil is used in skincare. The fruit are eaten fresh or fermented to distill spirits and to brew beer. Marula fruit with its exotic flavour boasts a high nutritive value and a vitamin C content three times the equivalent weight of oranges. In vitro and in vivo pharmacological activities of marula bark and leaf extracts, as well as seed oils, have been investigated, and antidiarrhoeal, antidiabetic, antimicrobial, antiplasmodial, anti-inflammatory, anti-oxidant and anti-ageing properties documented. Semi-automated high-performance thin-layer chromatography (HPTLC), gas chromatography coupled to mass spectrometry and flame ionisation detection (GC-MS/FID), ultra-performance liquid chromatography coupled to mass spectrometry (UPLC–MS) and mid-infrared (MIR) spectroscopy were used to determine the chemical profiles of marula bark and seed oil. Oleic acid, palmitic acid, linoleic acid and stearic acid were the major fatty acid methyl esters detected in the seed oil. The presence of linoleic acid in the oil was confirmed by HPTLC when the plate was viewed under 366 nm radiation. The UPLC–MS analysis revealed the presence of catechin, epigallocatechin gallate and epicatechin in the methanol extract of the bark.

Keywords: *Sclerocarya birrea*, Marula, Seed oil, Stem bark, Fatty acids, HPTLC, UPLC–MS, GC–MS, MIR spectroscopy

The South African Herbal Pharmacopoeia. https://doi.org/10.1016/B978-0-323-99794-2.00027-1

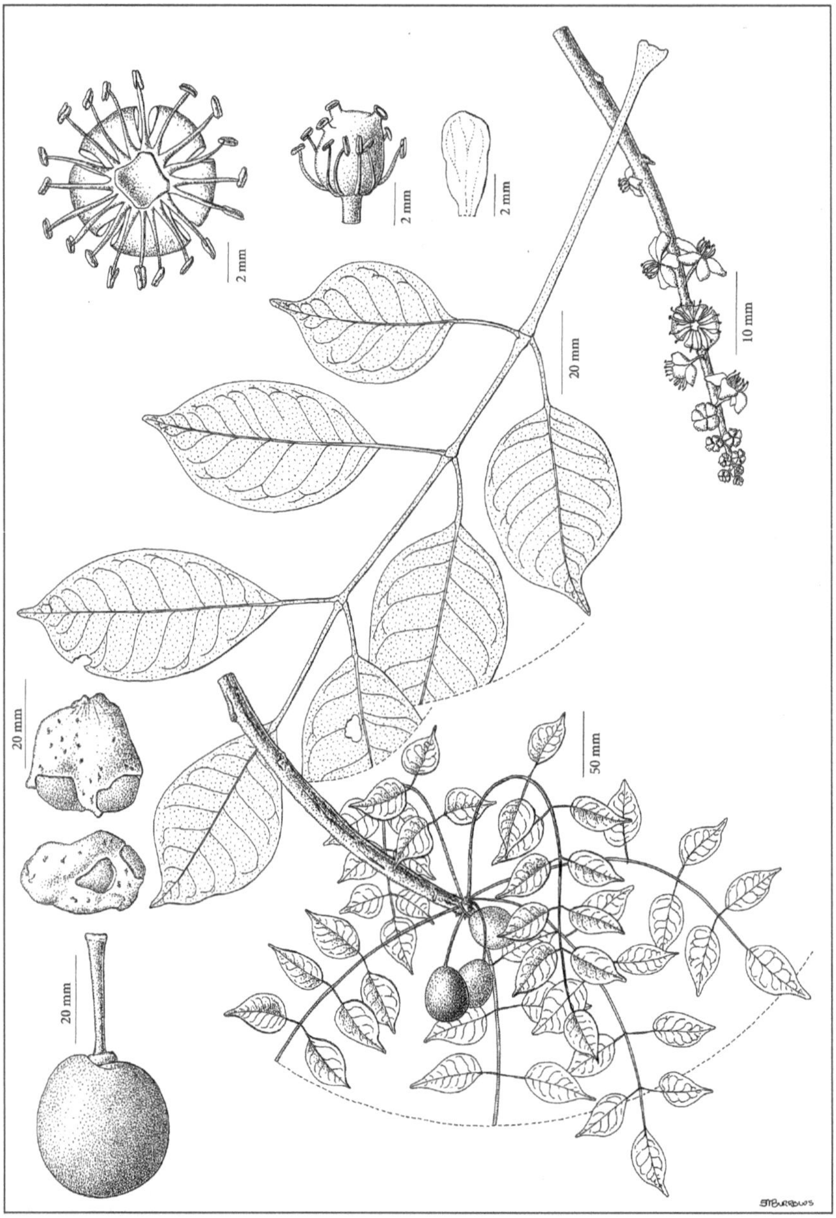
2 mm
2 mm
2 mm
10 mm
20 mm
20 mm
50 mm
20 mm

Part A: General overview

1. Synonyms

Sclerocarya birrea subsp. *caffra* (Sond.) Kokwaro, *S. birrea* subsp. *multifoliolata* (Engl.) Kokwaro, *Commiphora subglauca* Engl., *S. birrea* in sense of Van der Veken, not of (A.Rich.) Hochst., *Sclerocarya caffra* Sond., *Sclerocarya schweinfurthiana* Schinz.[a,b]

2. Common name(s)

Marula, maroola, cider, elephant tree (English); '*maroela*', '*maeroola*', '*maroela-boom*', '*moroelaboom*' (Afrikaans); '*morula*' (Sesotho sa Leboa/Setswana); '*ukanyi*' (Xitsonga); '*mufula*' (Tshivenda); '*umganu*' (isNdebele/isiZulu); '*mupfura*' (Shona).[b]

3. Conservation status

Least concern.[b]

4. Botany

Sclerocarya birrea (A. Rich.) Hochst. belongs to the Anacardiaceae family, which consists of 70 genera and 650 species. *Sclerocarya* is derived from the Greek words '*skleros*' (hard) and '*karyon*' (walnut), whereas the epithet '*birrea*' is derived from '*birr*', the Senegalese word for tree (Palmer and Pitman, 1972). *Sclerocarya birrea* is a medium- to large-sized deciduous tree that reaches heights of up to 17 m. The tree has an erect trunk, a rounded crown, grey-fissured bark, and stout branchlets with pale foliage (A). The rough stem bark is flakey, with a motley surface due to the distinct pale-brown and grey patches. The leaves are dark-green on the upper surfaces and are divided into pairs of ten or more leaflets, each roughly 60 mm long, with a sharp point above (C). The flowers are borne in small, oblong clusters (B), whereby female and male flowers are produced on separate trees. Male flowers produce pollen and female flowers produce fruit (Ogbobe, 1992). The green fruit (C) turns creamy-yellow when ripe (D), reaching 30 mm in diameter, and are borne in abundance in late summer to mid-winter in Africa. The sweet-sour, translucent white flesh of the fruit clings to the woody nuts that hold the kernels. The outer coating of the fruit has a strong, apple-like odour reminiscent of a mango fruit. The seeds are enclosed in locules embedded in lignified material of the drupe and comprise 10% of the drupe's dry weight.

[a] World Flora Online (www.worldfloraonline.org).
[b] Red List of South African Plants (http://redlist.sanbi.org).

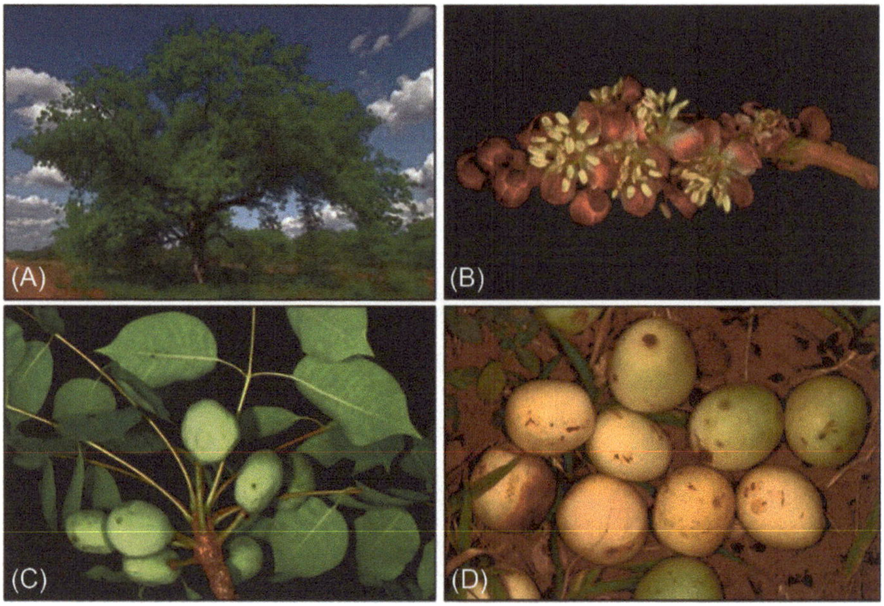

Sclerocarya birrea tree (A), an oblong cluster of its small red flowers (B), dark-green leaves with pointed tips (C), and ripened creamy-yellow fruits (D).

5. Geographical distribution

Sclerocarya birrea is distributed throughout Africa, extending to the north through tropical Africa into Sudan and Ethiopia. In southern Africa, it grows in Swaziland (Eswatini), Angola, Zimbabwe, Botswana, Namibia and Malawi (Ngorima, 2006). In West Africa, marula is found in Nigeria, Cameroon, Gambia and the Central African Republic. In South Africa, it occurs mainly in the Limpopo, KwaZulu-Natal and Mpumalanga provinces. The tree grows on sandy loam soils and in various woodland habitats, but is predominately found in savannah and semi-arid areas of sub-Saharan Africa. It thrives in the dry, hot environments of southern Africa, in regions at altitudes of up to 1800 m and down to sea level, with an annual average rainfall of 200–1500 mm.

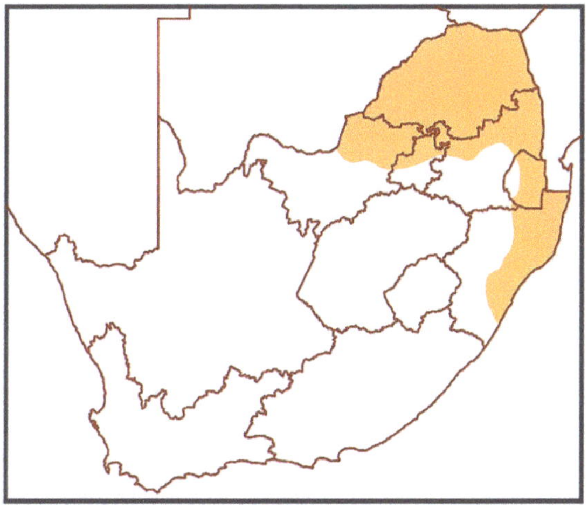

Geographical distribution of *Sclerocarya birrea* in South Africa.

6. Ethnopharmacology

Stem bark decoctions of *S. birrea* are used by the Zulu in South Africa as an enema to treat diarrhoea (Mathabe et al., 2006). The decoctions are taken in as 300 mL doses for the treatment of diarrhoea and dysentery (Watt and Breyer-Brandwijk, 1962; Mathabe et al., 2006). A decoction of the bark treats rheumatism and it has a prophylactic effect against malaria (Mariod and Abdelwahab, 2012). The Zulu traditional practitioners in South Africa use *S. birrea* stem bark decoctions as a wash prior to treating patients infected with gangrenous rectitis and also use the decoctions to treat the patient. Palgrave (1972) reported that the Zulu people crush marula nuts and boil them in water to separate the oil from the nuts, and use the oil as a massage medium. The Tsonga of Mozambique and South Africa use marula oil for hydrating and moisturising the skin (Botelle, 2001). The rural communities in Africa chew and swallow the astringent fresh marula leaf juice as a remedy for indigestion (Van Wyk et al., 2000). Ojewole et al. (2010) reported that the stem bark of *S. birrea* is used to treat proctitis. The Venda people use the stem bark for the treatment of stomach ailments, fever and ulcers (Ojewole et al., 2010). The roots are popularly used for various ailments in Zimbabwe, including sore eyes. In East Africa, the bark is used for the treatment of stomach disorders, while the roots form part of an alcoholic decoction taken for an internal ailment known as 'kati' (Kokwaro, 1976).

Sclerocarya birrea is also used in South African ethnoveterinary medicine for treating fractures and diarrhoea (McGaw and Eloff, 2008).

The women in the Limpopo region of South Africa use the oil to massage babies and as a moisturiser for their dry feet, hands and face (Hein et al., 2009). The oil is also used in southern Africa as a shampoo for damaged, fragile and dry hair and as base oil for soap. The oil is administered as nasal drops to infants. The moisturising capacity of the oil makes it possible to preserve meat and treat leather (Mariod et al., 2004). Pregnant women use powdered bark to determine the gender of their unborn baby. If a pregnant woman desires a boy she takes a preparation from the male plant, and for a girl, she uses the female plant. Traditional healers make use of the hard nut in the divining dice. The combination of the bark and roots is used as a laxative and the bark is beneficial in the treatment of haemorrhoids. A drink made from the leaves of marula is consumed for the treatment of gonorrhoea. South African and Zimbabwean inhabitants profit from the customary practice of using *S. birrea* wood for the manufacture of dishes, mealie stamping mortars, toys, drums, divining bowls, curios and carvings (Watt and Breyer-Brandwijk, 1962). The wood is also used for panelling, furniture, flooring and household utensils. Drums and yokes of animal figurines are produced from the wood of marula. The inner layer of the bark is used as ropes. In Namibia, the wood is used for sledges and boats are made from the trunk. The fresh skin of the bark produces a red-brown gummy dye, high in tannin, which is mixed with soot and used as ink. The fruit is used to produce an alcoholic beer known as Mukumbi by the Vhavenda people and is also eaten fresh or used to make a delicious jelly. The white nut is eaten or mixed with vegetables and is very nutritious. Fruit-farming communities favour planting these trees to attract pollinators to their farms in early spring.

7. Commercialisation

Marula tree products that include nuts, fruits, juice, gums and oils have been extensively researched and characterised in South Africa. The nuts and fruits have considerable commercial value, and marula fruit has high nutritive value. Marula has an exotic flavour with a vitamin C content three times higher than the equivalent weight of oranges (Weinert et al., 1990). The main commercial applications of the marula fruit are for cosmetic production and alcoholic beverage manufacturing (Amarula Cream Liqueur). The fruit is used in southern Africa for distilling spirits and brewing beer and it is considered a refreshing drink when fermented. In South Africa, Mozambique and Zambia, the marula fruit is used as a liqueur flavourant (Ojewole et al., 2010). The peel of marula fruit is important in the manufacturing process of oil for cosmetic use (Hillman et al., 2008). Shackleton et al. (2003) reported that the value of annual harvests of marula products (raw fruits and kernels) reached R1.1 million for South African communities that supplied two large commercial enterprises. Distell Group Limited exports liqueur to more than 149 countries (Mander et al., 2003). A 25.3% increase in liqueur exports over the previous year's sales (2006) was reflected in the Annual Report (Mander et al., 2003). Distell markets around 75% of all alcoholic fruit beverages and ciders, 50% of all spirits, and 15 million cases of wine in southern Africa. PhytoTrade® Africa patented a cosmetic extract of marula in partnership with Aldivia® (France) (Komane et al., 2015). Currently, marula oil is supplied to The Body Shop® by community fair-trade companies for cosmetic purposes. During harvest, rural communities in the Limpopo Province collect the marula fruit and transport it to central sites in and around Phalaborwa. Distell requires only 30% of the harvest for its manufacturing facility (Molelekoa et al., 2018). Therefore, a large proportion of the harvested fruit was not utilised and substandard fruit became waste. The study investigated the use of waste by-products to make vinegar through fermentation, and yields of acetic acid ranging between 41,000 and 57,000 mg/L (surface culture method) and between 41,000 and 54,000 mg/L (submerged culture method) were obtained. Physicochemical profiling data showed marula vinegar to be a possible source of bio-active compounds: total flavonoids 0.146–0.153 mg/L caffeic acid equivalents and total phenolics 0.289–0.356 mg/L gallic acid equivalents, with high activity against the 2,2-diphenylpicrylhydrazyl (DPPH) radical, 73.03% for the submerged culture and 78.85% for the surface culture (Molelekoa et al., 2018).

8. Pharmacological evaluation

8.1 *In vitro* studies

8.1.1 Anti-oxidant, anticancer and cytotoxic activity

Masoko et al. (2008) reported that extracts of *S. birrea* leaves and stem bark (hexane, dichloromethane and acetone) exhibited anti-oxidant activity. By comparing the different polyphenols in *S. birrea* it became evident that galloylate catechins and (−)-epicatechin 3-*O*-galloyl ester contributed considerably to the anti-oxidant activity of *S. birrea* (Braca et al., 2003). The Trolox equivalent anti-oxidant capacity (TEAC) assay showed that the galloylate catechins had TEAC values of 2.79 ± 0.01 mM ((−)-epicatechin 3-*O*-galloyl ester) and 3.01 ± 0.01 mM ((−)-epigallocatechin 3-*O*-galloyl ester), while the flavonoids, kaempferol 3-*O*-β-D-(6′-galloyl) glucopyranoside and quercetin 3–*O*-α-(5′-galloyl) arabinofuranoside, yielded TEAC values of 1.60 ± 0.01 and 0.68 ± 0.01 mM, respectively. *Sclerocarya birrea* methanolic extracts were investigated for anti-oxidant activity in an *in vitro* assay by Moyo et al. (2010). The EC_{50} values of the extracts in the DPPH free radical scavenging assay ranged from 6.92 to 4.26 μg/mL, in comparison to ascorbic acid (6.86 μg/mL). The methanolic extracts from *S. birrea* roots, barks, leaves and kernel oil cake were studied for anti-oxidant, as well as radical-scavenging activities (Mariod and Abdelwahab, 2012). The extracts constitute a large number of phenolic compounds and exhibited significant effects in preventing the oxidation of linoleic acid. The results indicated that the seedcake extract had the best anti-oxidant effect, followed by root, leaf, and bark extracts. Using the DPPH method, similar results were obtained and the seedcake extract showed the best anti-oxidant activity. The juice of *S. birrea* was found to be a potent anti-oxidant, due to the high concentration of polyphenolic compounds and flavonoids. The anticancer properties of acetone and water extracts of marula were investigated in three cell lines; HeLa, HT-29, and MCF-7, employing the cell titre blue viability assay in 96-well plates (Tanih and Ndip, 2013). The acetone extract displayed significant time- and dose-dependent antiproliferative activities towards MCF-7 cell lines after 48 and 24 h of incubation. The extract also induced apoptotic programmed cell death in MCF-7 cells with a noteworthy effect on the DNA.

Among four tested extracts prepared using different solvents, a methanolic root extract of marula exhibited the highest anti-oxidant activity when screened using nitric oxide (NO), superoxide, 2,2′-azino-bis(3-ethylbenzothiazoline-6-sulphonic acid (ABTS) and β-carotene bleaching assays (Armentano et al., 2015). The cytotoxic properties of the extract were also assessed towards the hepatocarcinoma cell line HepG2- and MRE-generated reactive oxygen species (ROS), and the extract induced apoptosis in a dose-dependent manner. The cytotoxic effect endorsed by the extract was inhibited by pretreatment of HepG2 cells with *N*-acetyl-L-cysteine (NAC), indicating that oxidative stress was essential for MRE-mediated cell death to occur. Furthermore, MRE treatment brought about mitochondrial membrane depolarisation and cytochrome C release from mitochondria into the cytosol. This result revealed that programmed cell death occurred in a mitochondrial-dependent pathway. It was proposed that the methanolic root extract of *S. birrea* can selectively enhance intracellular ROS levels in cancer cells and promote cell death (Armentano et al., 2015). The bark extract of *S. birrea* exhibited good anti-oxidant activities, with the water extract exhibiting significant activity against all the tested foodborne bacteria (Tabit et al., 2016). Russo et al. (2018) investigated marula for its *in vitro* anti-oxidant activity and reported that the methanol extracts of the bark have the highest tannin content (949.5 ± 29.7 mg of tannic acid equivalents/g) while the methanol leaf extracts were rich in flavonoids (132.7 ± 10.4 mg of quercetin equivalents/g). Four *in vitro* tests were used in the study: ABTS, β-carotene bleaching, nitric oxide and oxygen radical ($O_2\cdot^-$) assays. In all tests, the bark extract showed the best effect when compared to the leaf extract and the standards used (ascorbic acid and Trolox). The extracts were also evaluated for their activity in fibroblast and HepG2 cell lines. Higher cytotoxic activity was recorded for bark extract and this was verified by more pronounced alterations in cell morphology. The extract activated the intrinsic apoptotic pathway through ROS formation, and induced cell death, which triggered a loss of mitochondrial membrane potential with subsequent cytochrome C release from the mitochondria into the cytosol (Russo et al., 2018).

8.1.2 Antidiarrhoeal activity

Procyanidin (2.5–640 μg/mL) significantly inhibited contractile responses in guinea-pig isolated ileal preparations (Galvez et al., 1993). Pre-incubation of the ileal tissues with hexamethonium (10^{-4} M) remarkably reduced the inhibitory effects of procyanidin. In addition, procyanidin changed the biphasic mechanical response induced by acetylcholine (ACh, 10^{-7} M), with greater inhibition of the phasic response than the tonic response.

The antimotility activity of procyanidin was responsible for the antidiarrhoeal activity of the plant's stem bark extract, and the authors speculated that this effect may be linked to an interference with the succeeding events induced after muscarinic stimulus.

8.1.3 Antidiabetic and antihypertensive activity

It was demonstrated by Ojewole (2006a) that the stem bark water extract of *S. birrea* (12.5–200 mg/mL) caused relaxation (concentration-dependent) of the endothelium-intact rat isolated aortic rings, pre-contracted with noradrenaline. The vasorelaxant properties of the extract on endothelium-intact aortic rings were cancelled by the removal of the functional endothelium, suggesting that the vasorelaxant effects on vascular tissues are possibly facilitated to a high degree *via* endothelium-derived relaxing factor mechanisms and nitric oxide production. The inhibitory properties of *S. birrea* stem bark extracts against *Bacillus steatothermophilus* α-glucosidase and human urinary α-amylase were investigated (Mogale et al., 2011). Acetone and methanolic extracts blocked human urinary α-amylase more effectively than acarbose. The hexane extract inhibited α-glucosidase better than α-amylase. The extracts of *S. birrea* blocked the activities of α-glucosidase and α-amylase in a concentration-dependent manner, with values similar to that of the positive control, acarbose. Extracts of *S. birrea* caused a noteworthy improvement in glucose uptake in HepG2 and C2C12, 3T3-L1 cells, with the methanol extracts demonstrating potent free radical scavenging capacity (IC_{50} = 2.16 µg/mL) (Da Costa Mousinho et al., 2013). However, insulin secretion from RIN-m5F cells remained unchanged.

8.1.4 Anti-inflammatory activity

Fotio et al. (2010) evaluated TNF, nitrite, IL-6, IL-lP and IL-12p40 produced by bone marrow-derived macrophages (BMDM), pre-incubated without or with *S. birrea*, and infected with live *Mycobacterium bovis* Bacillus Calmette Guerin (BCG) or stimulated with lipopolysaccharide (LPS). Marula extract reduced, in a concentration-dependent manner, TNF, nitrite, IL-6, IL-lP and IL-12p40 formation by BMDM infected with live BCG or stimulated with LPS. The iNOS expression was inhibited by *S. birrea* after stimulus of BMDM with LPS. Furthermore, the nuclear factor kB (NF-kB) stimulation by both BCG and LPS was inhibited by marula. Extracts of *S. birrea* were tested for anti-inflammatory activity using the cyclooxygenase enzymes COX-1 and COX-2 (Moyo et al., 2011). Dichloromethane and petroleum ether extracts indicated potent COX-1 (90.7%–99.8%) and COX-2 (69.0%–92.6%) inhibitory activity at a concentration of 250 µg/mL.

8.1.5 Antimicrobial and antiparasitic activity

Sclerocarya birrea stem bark methanolic extract (0.5 mg/mL) exhibited good activity against nematodes (*Caenorhabditis elegans*) with 70% *in vitro* parasite chemo-suppression (McGaw et al., 2007). Both aqueous and hexane extracts of the plant's stem bark revealed poor anthelmintic activity, with parasite chemo-suppression evident only at a concentration of 2.0 mg/mL. Masoko et al. (2008) reported that non-polar *S. birrea* extracts did not exhibit activity towards the fungal organisms tested. However, the ethanol, acetone and methanol extracts of *S. birrea* reduced the growth of *Candida parapsilosis* and *Cryptococcus albidus*, with the acetone extract showing the best inhibitory activity on *C. albidus* (MIC value of 0.12 mg/mL). Runyoro et al. (2006) reported that the stem bark ethanolic extract of marula exhibited antifungal activity against *C. albicans*. An ethanolic root extract of *S. birrea* reduced the growth of *C. glabrata, C. albicans, C. parapsilosis, Candida kruseii, C. tropicalis* and *Cryptococcus neoformans*, with a minimum inhibitory concentration (MIC) of 0.5 mg/mL (Hamza et al., 2006). Microbiological experiments using *S. birrea* leaf, outer bark and inner bark acetone extracts, showed growth inhibition of *Pseudomonas aeruginosa, Staphylococcus aureus, Enterococcus faecalis* and *Escherichia coli* (Eloff, 2001). It was revealed that *S. birrea* stem bark, especially the inner bark, exhibited better activity than the leaves against the bacteria tested, with the highest activity recorded against *S. aureus* (MIC 0.15 mg/mL). A study by McGaw et al. (2007) using the methanol, hexane and water bark extracts, indicated activity for the methanol extract only, with MICs of 0.4 and 0.1 mg/mL against *E. faecalis* and *S. aureus*, respectively. The extracts did not exhibit any activity towards *P. aeruginosa* and *E. coli*.

The microdilution assay was employed to establish the antimicrobial activities of extracts of *S. birrea* (Moyo et al., 2010). A twig extract exhibited the highest overall activity of 1609.1 mL/g against *Bacillus subtilis* with an MIC value of 0.098 mg/mL. Ethanol extracts of *S. birrea* revealed high antibacterial activity (MIC < 1.0 mg/mL). Extracts of *S. birrea* were studied against 30 clinical strains of *Helicobacter pylori* (reference control strain, NCTC 11638) using standard microbiological methods (Njume et al., 2011a). The antibiotics, amoxicillin and metronidazole, were used in these investigations as positive controls. Anti-*H. pylori* activity was observed for the extracts with inhibition zones between 0 and 38 mm and MIC_{50} (half-maximal minimum inhibitory concentration) values ranging between 0.06 and 5.0 mg/mL. The MIC_{50} values for metronidazole and amoxicillin varied between 0.001 and 0.63 mg/mL, and 0.004–5.0 mg/mL, respectively. The acetone extracts of *S. birrea* showed significant bactericidal properties against *H. pylori*, inhibiting > 50% of the strains within 18 h at a concentration of 4 × MIC, and caused total removal of the organisms within a period of 24 h. The antimicrobial activity of marula fractions and extracts was investigated against five clarithromycin- and metronidazole-resistant strains of *H. pylori* (Njume et al., 2011b) with amoxicillin as positive control. Of the 18 fractions collected, 16 exhibited anti-*H. pylori* properties with MIC_{50} values of between 310 and 2500 μg/mL. The recorded MIC_{50} value ranges for terpinen-4-ol, amoxicillin and pyrrolidine were 0.004–0.06, 0.0003–0.06 and 0.005–6.3 μg/mL, respectively. It was found that the inhibitory properties of pyrrolidine and terpinen-4-ol were very similar to that of the positive control, amoxicillin. Ethanol extracts from 50 medicinal plants were evaluated *in vitro* against nematodes (*Heligmosomoides bakeri, Ancylostoma ceylanicum, Trichuris muris*) and trematodes (*Echinostoma caproni, Schistosoma mansoni*) (Koné et al., 2012). The best inhibition against *A. ceylanicum* was found for *S. birrea* at 2 mg/mL, which led to the inhibition of third-stage larvae and death of adult worms. The water and acetone extracts of the stem bark of *S. birrea* were evaluated for their antimicrobial activity towards selected fungal, yeast and bacterial species, including *Plesiomonas shigelloides, Aeromonas hydrophila, Streptococcus pyogenes, C. neoformans, Salmonella typhimurium, Trichosporon mucoides, Candida glabrata* and *C. krusei* employing both MIC and agar well-diffusion assays (Tanih and Ndip, 2012). All the fungi and bacteria were vulnerable to the plant extracts. The water extract exhibited the best activity towards the fungal species with MICs of 0.3125–1.25 mg/mL, while the acetone extract displayed the best activity towards the bacterial species with MICs of 0.156–0.625 mg/mL.

Mikail (2009) reported that the methanolic extract of stem bark and leaves from *S. birrea* caused 100% mortality of *Trypanosoma brucei in vitro*, but the mechanism of action was not elaborated on. Aqueous and ethanol extracts of marula revealed anti-amoebic activity (*Entamoeba histolytica*) when evaluated in a microtitre plate assay (Fennell et al., 2004). Plant parts of *S. birrea* were investigated for antimicrobial properties using a number of respiratory pathogens i.e. *Klebsiella pneumoniae, C. neoformans, Moraxella catarrhalis, S. aureus* and *Mycobacterium smegmatis* (York et al., 2012). The water extract displayed the best activity (0.10 mg/mL against *C. neoformans*). The acetone extracts (leaves and bark) were shown to be active against *S. aureus, P. aeruginosa, E. faecalis* and *E. coli,* with MICs ranging from 150 to 3000 μg/mL (Mativandlela et al., 2008). An organic extract of *S. birrea* exhibited a broad spectrum of activity against the pathogens tested with a mean broad-spectrum MIC of 0.45 mg/mL (Van Vuuren et al., 2015). It was also shown that the organic extract exhibited better antimicrobial effects compared to the water extract (Nciki et al., 2016). The organic extract revealed remarkable activity against 10 of the 12 pathogens tested (average MIC value of 370 μg/mL). Lediga et al. (2018) assessed the antimicrobial activities of *S. birrea* when incorporated into silver nanoparticles (AgNPs). The AgNPs and plant extracts were evaluated against fever-related pathogens i.e. two Gram-negative pathogens, *K. pneumoniae* (ATCC 13883) and *Acinetobacter baumannii* (ATCC 19606), as well as two Gram-positive pathogens, *E. faecalis* (ATCC 29212) and *Listeria monocytogenes* (ATCC 19111), using the broth microdilution method. *Sclerocarya birrea*-containing AgNPs showed a significant increase in antimicrobial activity against the four test pathogens compared to the respective water plant extracts.

8.1.6 Antiplasmodial activity

Gathirwa et al. (2008) reported that the methanol stem bark *S. birrea* extract exhibited fairly high activity in an *in vitro* study (IC_{50} 5.91 ± 0.36 μg/mL) against *Sierra Leonean* chloroquine (CQ)-sensitive D6 *Plasmodium falciparum*, while an aqueous extract of the stem bark exhibited moderate activity (IC_{50} of 18.96 ± 5.32 μg/mL). The activity of both extracts was remarkably lower against chloroquine-sensitive resistant clone isolates, indicating that the extracts and chloroquine might show similar antimalarial mechanism of action. Nundkumar and Ojewole (2002) investigated marula water stem bark and leaf extract activity against a chloroquine-sensitive D10 strain of *P. falciparum*. The IC_{50} values of the stem bark and leaf extracts were remarkably high (30–40 μg/mL, chloroquine, 6 μg/mL), revealing poor antiplasmodial properties for the extracts. The antiplasmodial activity of the crude extract of *S. birrea* was determined against chloroquine-resistant (W2) and -sensitive (D6) *P. falciparum* (Muthaura et al., 2015). The antiplasmodial activity of the extract exhibited good activity (IC_{50} 5.9 μg/mL) against D6.

8.1.7 Skin and anti-ageing properties

Shoko et al. (2018) reported on the anti-ageing properties of *S. birrea* extracts *in vitro*. The stem extracts of *S. birrea* exhibited potent anti-elastase properties similar to that of elafin (> 88%), as well as anticollagenase activity, similar to, and as potent as that of ethylenediaminetetraacetic acid (EDTA >76%). In contrast, the extract of the leaves showed moderate anti-elastase effects (54%) and had no activity against collagenase. Marula oil and fruit extract showed slight activity in both assays. The ethanol extract of the stems was the most appropriate, based on its suitability as solvent, to the cosmetic industry and also its anticollagenase properties (99%). The anti-ageing property of the ethanol extract was improved and this process also lowered the intensity of the colour of the extract. Epicatechin gallate and epigallocatechin gallate demonstrated similar activity as the standard, EDTA, at 5 μg/mL in the anticollagenase screen.

8.1.8 Other activities

The activity of the *S. birrea* leaf water extract on rat and rabbit vascular smooth muscles was accessed (Mawoza et al., 2012). The extract (50–400 mg/mL) exhibited a noteworthy, concentration-dependent increase in baseline tone in the aortic ring compositions. Indomethacin (20 μM) significantly reduced the contractile effects of the extract in both the endothelium-denuded and -intact aortic rings. The extract also elicited remarkable increases in the amplitude of the myogenic narrowing of the portal veins. It was concluded that marula possesses spasmogenic properties on vascular smooth muscle. An *in vitro* mammalian research investigation revealed that a *S. birrea* extract demonstrated spasmogenic activity on mammalian isolated uterine horns. The uterine contractile activity observed could be due to the effects of the extract on acetylcholine, oxytocin and serotonin receptors (Mawoza et al., 2015). A standardised extract of *S. birrea* significantly inhibited the swarming ability of the cells and also disturbed the quorum-sensing mediated production of biofilm construction. Sarkar et al. (2014) reported that the extract played a controlling role on the excretion of pyoverdin and protease, two quorum-sensing (QS)-dependent pathogenic factors present in *P. aeruginosa*. The methanol extract of marula was assayed for molluscicidal activity against *Helisoma duryi* and *Lymnaea natalensis* and (at 48 h) an LC_{50} of 50 mg/L was recorded for *L. natalensis* (Ndabambi et al., 2015).

8.2 *In vivo* studies and clinical trials

8.2.1 Antidiarrhoeal activity

A freeze-dried decoction of the stem bark extract of *S. birrea* (10–500 mg/mL) showed significant and dose-dependent protection of animals in experimental models against sodium picosulphate- and magnesium sulphate-induced diarrhoea (Galvez et al., 1991). It was reported that the antidiarrhoeal effects of the stem bark extract were possibly facilitated, *via* reduction of intestinal transit, by procyanidin (a condensed tannin found in the extract of the stem bark). This was verified by an additional study where the antidiarrhoeal effect of procyanidin (isolated from the stem bark) was evaluated. It was proven that procyanidin (150 mg/kg) demonstrated the protection of animals in this study against castor oil-, magnesium sulphate-, prostaglandin E2- and arachidonic acid-induced diarrhoea (Galvez et al., 1991).

8.2.2 Antidiabetic and antihypertensive activity

Trovato et al. (1995) reported that a decoction of *S. birroea* demonstrated hypoglycaemic effects, an incremented oral-glucose tolerance, as well as increased levels of plasma immunoreactive insulin (IRI), in normal rats. The decoction also displayed activity against diet-induced hyper-cholesterolaemia. At a dose of 0.5 g/kg, the decoction lowered glucose levels in blood in normoglycaemic rats, with noteworthy results evident 120 min after treatment, with the maximum reduction observed after 180 min. The effect continued as noteworthy for a period of up to 4 h after termination of treatment. Ojewole (2004) investigated the antidiabetic effect of *S. birrea* in rats. In the experiment involving antidiabetic/hypoglycaemic assessment, selected doses of the aqueous stem bark extract (25–800 mg/kg p.o.) were separately administered to groups of fasted diabetic, as well as fasted normal rats. Another experiment used a single dose of the water extract (SBE, 800 mg/kg p.o.) (Ojewole, 2004). The hypoglycaemic activity of this single dose was evaluated using chlorpropamide (250 mg/kg p.o.) as a control in both fasted streptozotocin (STZ)-treated diabetic and fasted normal rats. High to moderate doses of stem bark water extract (25–800 mg/kg p.o.) showed significant, dose-dependent lowering of the glucose concentrations in the blood of both fasted diabetic and fasted normal rats, following acute treatment. Chlorpropamide (250 mg/kg p.o.) also caused a substantial reduction in the blood glucose levels of the two experimental groups. Administration of a single dose of the stem bark water extract (800 mg/kg p.o.) remarkably lowered the blood glucose levels of both fasted STZ-treated, diabetic, and fasted normoglycaemic rats. The results revealed that the plant extract demonstrated hypoglycaemic properties. Belemtougri et al. (2007) conducted a study to investigate the hypotensive effects and the mechanisms of action of the water extract of the leaves in anaesthetised normotensive rats. Results revealed that the extract triggered a dose-dependent reduction in mean arterial pressure. Bilateral vagotomy did not stop the low blood pressure induced by *S. birrea*. Pretreatment of the rats with piperoxan, practolol or atropine did not abolish hypotension and the authors reported that muscarinic, β_2 and α_2 receptors are probably not involved in the initiation of hypotension. It was concluded that the hypotensive activity of the extract is probably facilitated through other routes that may include intracellular calcium decrease or nitric oxide release.

Sclerocarya birrea was assessed on its effect on insulin-secreting INS-1E cells and isolated rat islets (Ndifossap et al., 2010). The extract at 5 mg/mL (following 24 h treatment) significantly potentiated glucose-stimulated insulin secretion. Non-nutrient stimulation and basal insulin release were not affected. After 12 h of treatment, the potentiation of the secretory reaction at revitalising glucose became evident. At the active concentration, the extract was considered safe with respect to cell differentiation and integrity, since no acute effects were seen. After 24 h treatment, both ATP generation and glucose oxidation were enhanced, and it was concluded that the mode of action of marula was linked to glucose metabolism. In STZ-induced diabetic rats, extract administration restored glycaemia and corrected plasma insulin levels after 14 days of treatment. The results revealed the involvement of *S. birrea* in the activity of insulin-secreting cells, encouraging the use of the plant for managing diabetes (Ndifossap et al., 2010). Administration of the stem bark extract of *S. birrea* (oral; 60–240 mg/kg) to STZ-treated diabetic and non-diabetic rats (acute study) caused glucose reduction in the blood, dose-dependently (Gondwe et al., 2008). The hypoglycaemic activity of the extract was better in diabetic animals (4 h), relative to non-diabetic rats. However, when the stem bark extract (120 mg/kg) was given daily to the rats, blood glucose concentrations markedly lowered in STZ-treated diabetic rats in a chronic study, but was unsuccessful in lowering that of non-diabetic rats. When the animals were treated daily with stem bark extract and metformin, the extract produced a noteworthy increase in hepatic glycogen levels in diabetic and non-diabetic rats, over a period of 5 weeks. In the untreated groups, glycogen levels were much higher in non-diabetic, compared to diabetic rats. Based on the results, it was hypothesised that the mode of action of the stem bark extract is possibly similar to that of metformin. In a separate study, a methanol:dichloromethane (1:1) extract of the stem bark of marula increased plasma insulin concentrations and lowered blood glucose in STZ-treated diabetic rats (Dimo et al., 2007). Furthermore, administration of the extract (300 mg/kg) produced a remarkable decrease in water and food intake, as well as glucose plasma levels in STZ-treated diabetic rats. In addition, there was no noteworthy reduction in body weight at the end of the treatment period (3 weeks), indicating that the stem bark extract can possibly compensate for the energy provided from food intake, or improve the metabolism of the extract-treated diabetic animals. Plasma triglyceride, cholesterol and urea levels were partially decreased after treatment with 300 mg/kg of the stem bark extract for a period of 3 weeks. Nevertheless, the change between untreated and treated diabetic groups did not show statistical significance after the period. The results obtained by Dimo et al. (2007) are comparable to those described by Ojewole (2003a), in that the stem bark water extract (100–800 mg/kg) caused significant, dose-dependent reductions in glucose concentrations in the blood of diabetic rats. The hypoglycaemic activity of the stem bark extract reached significance 1 h after oral treatment, reaching its peak within 4 h, and the effect was still substantial 8 h after oral treatment. Ojewole (2003a) ascribed this effect to a mode of action similar to that of insulin and/or chlorpropamide excretion from pancreatic β-cells. Dimo et al. (2007) reported that the antidiabetic properties of *S. birrea* extract (stem bark) are probably linked to the stimulus of insulin secretion. Yet, in another study by Van de Venter et al. (2008), the stem bark extract of *S. birrea* [extracted with a mixture of cold methanol:dichloromethane (1:1) and purified water], showed a substantial increase in glucose utilisation in C2C12 muscle and Chang liver cells, demonstrating a different mode of action to that reported by Dimo et al. (2007) and Ojewole (2003a).

Ojewole (2006a) evaluated the activity of the stem bark extract (25–400 mg/kg) of *S. birrea via* bolus intravenous administrations *in vivo* and observed transient, significant dose-dependent reductions in heart rates and systemic arterial blood pressures of anaesthetised hypertensive and normotensive Dahl salt-sensitive rats. Acute intravenous administration of the extract (120 mg/kg) to STZ-treated diabetic and non-diabetic rats resulted in a brief vasodepressive effect, with peak activities showing within 1 h of the extract's infusion. Nevertheless, the mean arterial blood pressure increased slowly, reaching values similar to that of the control group (Gondwe et al., 2008). Long-term treatment of 120 mg/kg of the stem bark extract (5 weeks), in STZ-treated diabetic and non-diabetic rats, activated a substantial reduction in the mean arterial blood pressure. Blood pressure was lowered during the 5-week period when compared to the control group. Gondwe et al. (2008) reported that electrolyte and renal fluid handling in non-diabetic and diabetic rats were not affected after acute, short-term marula (120 mg/kg) treatment. However, chronic, long-term stem bark extract (120 mg/kg) administration markedly lowered plasma urea and creatinine concentrations in STZ-induced diabetic rats, and produced an increase in the glomerular filtration rate, indicating a positive effect of the plant. Hexane extracts of marula lowered postprandial glucose levels substantially after oral treatment with sucrose, but failed to induce comparable effects after oral treatment with glucose and starch in both diabetic and normal rats. It was concluded from the results that the hexane extract possibly blocked the increase in postprandial hyperglycaemia through inhibition of α-glucosidase *in vivo* (Mogale et al., 2011). Musabayane et al. (2006) researched the activity of the stem bark aqueous extract orally at different dosages (240, 120 and 60 mg/kg bw) on markers denoting cardiovascular and kidney mechanisms in diabetic rats. A significant decrease in blood glucose levels and the levels of K^+ and Na^+ ion elimination rates were seen, which did not change after prolonged or short-term treatment with the extract. Gondwe et al. (2008) investigated the ethanolic stem bark extract at similar doses and the results reflected an improvement in the glomerular filtration rate, blood glucose and mean arterial blood pressure using an STZ-induced T1D rat model.

Animals receiving a supplement of sucrose and oxidised palm oil demonstrated glucose intolerance, hyperglycaemia, and a noteworthy increase in body weight, insulin resistance and abdominal fat mass, when compared to normal rats (Ngueguim et al., 2015). A noteworthy decrease in the activities of the catalase and superoxide dismutase (SOD) in kidney and liver, and reduced glutathione (GSH) concentrations in the heart, were also reported. Concomitant administration of marula extract with sucrose and oxidised palm oil lowered the glycaemia and blood pressure to normal values, restored insulin sensitivity and glucose tolerance. The plant extract also reduced nitrites and malondialdehyde (MDA) levels.

8.2.3 Anticonvulsant activity

Ojewole (2006b) studied the stem bark extract (100–800 mg/kg) and observed a significant delay in the start of incidence of pentylenetetrazole (PTZ, 90 mg/kg)-induced seizures in mice. The extract also profoundly antagonised picrotoxin (PCT, 10 mg/kg bw)-induced seizures, but only partially antagonised bicuculline (BCL, 30 mg/kg bw)-induced seizures. The start of convulsions was shown to be delayed, while the mean duration of convulsion was significantly lowered. It was suggested that the marula extract probably produces its anticonvulsant activity *via* improvement of GABAergic neurotransmission in the brain.

8.2.4 Antiplasmodial properties

Administration of the stem bark aqueous and methanolic extracts of *S. birrea* at a dose of 100 mg/kg to male Balb C mice infected with *Plasmodium berghei*, resulted in more than 60% chemo-suppression (Gathirwa et al., 2008). There was a noteworthy parasite density decrease in the animals given the extracts, compared to the animals administered with placebo. Additionally, there was a reduction in peak parasitaemia on day four in the treated groups, compared to the negative control group, illustrating possible antimalarial effects of the extracts. The survival time of mice that were treated with the marula extracts with high chemo-suppression effects was extended, when compared to the animals that were given the extracts with low chemo-suppression activity.

8.2.5 Anti-inflammatory and analgesic properties

Methanolic and aqueous stem bark extracts of marula (500–50 mg/kg) administered to Wistar rats were reported to time-dependently, and progressively, reduce rat paw oedema induced by fresh egg albumin (0.5 mL/kg) (Ojewole, 2003b). The methanol extract exhibited a higher anti-inflammatory effect compared to the water extract. However, the anti-inflammatory activity of the two extracts was significantly lower when compared to the positive control, acetylsalicylic acid (100 mg/kg). It was further shown by Ojewole (2003a) that both extracts (methanol and water) at 500 mg/kg p.o., decreased rat paw oedema induced by subplantar inoculation of fresh egg albumin. This was attributed to the inhibition of the prostaglandin and histamine pathways in rats. Further investigations by Ojewole (2004) in rats revealed that the plant extract (25–800 mg/kg p.o.) exhibited time- and dose-related, substantial and a sustained decrease in the fresh egg albumin-induced acute swelling of the hind paw. These results scientifically support the reported folkloric practices of the stem bark in the management of and/or control of inflammatory diseases. Ojewole (2004) researched the analgesic activity of the stem bark water extract of marula in mice. Diclofenac (100 mg/kg p.o.) was employed as a positive control. *Sclerocarya birrea* stem bark water extract (10–800 mg/kg p.o.) demonstrated significant protection (dose-dependently) against electrical heat-induced pain. The analgesic activity of the extract was calculated to be about 10–15 times lower than that of diclofenac.

The activity of the methanol and aqueous stem bark extracts of marula (300 or 150 mg/kg) was investigated on histamine, serotonin- or carrageenan-induced paw oedema in rats (Fotio et al., 2009). The methanolic extract (300 mg/kg) displayed the best activity with a determined inhibition of 55.3% and 75.5% towards histamine- and carrageenan-induced inflammation, respectively. The methanol extract of marula exhibited 54.4% activity on the 21st day and an 80.7% effect on the 10th day in complete- or formalin Freund's adjuvant (CFA)-induced paw oedema. When treated with 300 mg/kg of the extract in rats, malondialdehyde (MDA) values were markedly lowered (31.2%) and GSH levels significantly increased (75.1%) in the liver of CFA rats administered with 300 mg/kg of marula. The data demonstrated that the anti-inflammatory property of the methanol and water extracts of marula is due to the effect on the prostaglandin and histamine pathways, together with its anti-oxidant effect (Fotio et al., 2009). The same group (Fotio et al., 2010) investigated the activity of the plant extract *in vivo* in an assay of liver injury induced by D-galactosamine/LPS (D-GaINILPS) in mice. *Sclerocarya birrea* lowered D-GaIN/LPS-liver injury as evaluated by a decrease in transaminases and IL-lP, TNF and IL-6 serum levels, as well as the translocation of NF-kB to the nucleus. The data revealed that the methanol stem bark extract exhibited anti-inflammatory effects through inhibition of cytokine release and NF-kB activation induced by infectious or inflammatory stimuli (Fotio et al., 2010).

8.2.6 Skin and anti-ageing properties

Marula oil was evaluated, with some success, in clinical tests (such as transepidermal water loss, skin hydration and occlusive properties) for its possible use as a component in cosmetic product formulations (Houghton, 1999). A high oleic acid absorption ability and the presence of linoleic acid (4%–7%) contributed to classifying the oil as suitable for topical application. The safety and efficacy of marula oil was assessed in healthy adult Caucasian female volunteers, who fulfilled the exclusion and inclusion criteria for the moisture efficacy, irritancy patch, occlusivity and hydrating tests (Komane et al., 2015). It was found that the oil is non-irritant when applied to the skin. When the oil was applied to a lipid-dry (xerosis) skin, hydrating and moisturising properties were noted. When applied to normal skin, occlusive effects were recorded. The oil is rich in fatty acids, with oleic acid as the major fatty acid, followed by palmitic acid. These fatty acids, are similar to those present in the epidermis and are well absorbed. The oil moderately prevents transepidermal water loss, and together with its noteworthy occlusive effects, its traditional use as skin moisturiser may be justified.

8.2.7 Aphrodisiac activity

Aphrodisiac activity was studied *in vivo* for an extract of *S. birrea* (Sewani-Rusike et al., 2015). Marula pulp extract and fruit juice were very effective in stimulating sexual performance in male rats. Although there was no change in sperm count and the number of ejaculations compared to the control, the treatment increased sperm motility.

8.2.8 Other effects

In a study by Garba et al. (2006), the activity of the water extract of marula was assessed towards alcohol-CCl_4-induced hepatocellular damage in rats, for a period of 21 days. Administration of the water extract was conducted orally at a dose of 2, 5 and 8 mg/kg body weight (bw) to the rats, respectively, from days 15 to 21, and a single dose of CCl_4 at 0.1 mL/kg bw in pure corn oil was given subcutaneously on day 20 for the induction of hepatotoxicity. Blood was collected after the experimental period and assessed for serum values of AST (aspartate aminotransferase), bilirubin, ALT (alanine aminotransferase), ALP (alkaline phosphatase), protein and albumin levels. Histopathological evaluation of liver damage was conducted and the concentrations of ALP, albumin and AST were markedly improved in the rats treated with 2 mg/kg, with an even greater increase in the 5 mg/kg groups. Results revealed several foci of cloudy hepatocyte swelling, vacuolar cytoplasmic degeneration, and central zones of hepatocyte necrosis with macrophage penetration, pointing to supportive indications for the biochemical study with higher toxicity in the groups given 2 and 5 mg/kg of extract. The data indicated that the water extract of the stem bark demonstrated probable antihepatotoxic and hepatotoxic effects at high and low doses, respectively (Garba et al., 2006). Marula leaf extract (1–10 mg/mL) antagonised caffeine-induced calcium release from the sarcoplasmic reticulum in a noteworthy manner (Belemtougri et al., 2001). The leaf extract of marula did not exhibit any effect on the latent calcium content, indicating that the extract probably does not have an effect on the fundamental mechanisms regulating resting inner Ca^{2+} homeostasis. *Sclerocarya birrea* fruit juice administered as a supplement to healthy persons for 3 weeks, markedly lowered the participants overall serum cholesterol (by 8%), triglycerides (by 7%), LDL (low-density lipopolysaccharide)-cholesterol (by 17%), and attenuated serum oxidative stress and improved their HDL (high-density lipopolysaccharide)-cholesterol levels (by 10%). Some of these effects continued, somewhat, after a 4-week washout period (Borochov-Neori et al., 2008).

8.3 Safety

Intraperitoneal treatment of different dosages of stem bark methanol and water extracts of marula yielded LD_{50} values of 1087 ± 41 and 1215 ± 38 mg/kg, respectively in mice, indicating that the plant is non-toxic to mice and relatively safe (Ojewole,

2003b). Methanol, hexane and water extracts (10–1000 mg/mL) of the stem bark did not reveal toxic effects in a brine shrimp assay (McGaw et al., 2007; McGaw and Eloff, 2008). The LD_{50} values of marula extracts were shown to be 5000 mg/kg bw in an acute toxicity assay, and no animals died after receiving the extracts in the suppressive test period of 4 days (Gathirwa et al., 2008). *Sclerocarya birrea* extracts exhibited no adverse effects in the Ames test, indicating that the extracts are lacking mutagenic effects (Verschaeve and Van Staden, 2008). Yet, in another toxicity test, concerns were raised over the chronic use of marula extracts (Van de Venter et al., 2008). The stem bark extract (600–1000 mg/mL) demonstrated a significant concentration-dependent decrease in cell viability after 48 and 72 h administrations in a renal epithelial cell culture study. It was reported that LLC-PK1 cells were more vulnerable to the stem bark extract treatment, compared to MDBK cells (Gondwe et al., 2008). In an MTT (3-(4,5-dimethylthiazol-2-yl)-2,5-diphenyltetrazolium bromide) cell viability screen, continued contact of kidney distal- and proximal tubule cell lines to marula stem bark extract (1000–600 mg/mL) lowered cell capability, with proximal cells showing vulnerability (Gondwe et al., 2008). It was reported that the reduction in cell viability was due to phenolic and weakly acidic components detected in the extract, which possibly lower the mitochondrial effect by producing mitochondrial depolarisation. In an *in vivo* model, phenolic and weakly acidic constituents are mostly expelled by the kidneys, while in the *in vitro* cultured model, the distal and proximal tubule cultured cells were constantly exposed to phenolic compounds for up to 72 h. This can explain why chronic, long-term marula stem bark extract (120 mg/kg) administration did not show any substantial effect on electrolyte handling and renal fluid in STZ-treated diabetic and non-diabetic rats (Gondwe et al., 2008).

9. Phytochemistry

9.1 Volatile constituents

Headspace volatiles of the fruit pulp and the whole fruits were investigated by Viljoen et al. (2008) and showed the presence of hydrocarbons and esters, namely β-caryophyllene (91.3%), benzyl 4-methylpentanoate (8.8%), heptadecene (16.1%), (Z)-3-decen-1-ol (8.4%), α-humulene (8.3%), benzyl butyrate (6.7%), cyclopentadecane (5.7%), (Z)-13-octadecenal (6.2%), 11-hexadecanal (4.4%), 6-dodecen-1-ol (3.8%) and germacrene D (0.1%). Essential oils were obtained from fresh leaves of *S. birrea* by steam distillation. The oil yield from plants collected in August was higher (0.24%), compared to that of plants collected in February (0.10%). Analysis by gas chromatography–mass spectrometry (GC–MS) and gas chromatography-flame ionisation detection (GC-FID) assisted in the identification of 49 compounds, representing 98% of the hydrodistillate. The essential oils consisted of approximately 96% sesquiterpenes.

The major constituents of the oil collected in February were 7-epi-α-selinene (38.3%), valencene (17%), β-caryophyllene (3.2%), β-selinene (4.3%), α-muurolene (2%), 14-hydroxy-α-humulene (1.5%) and *allo*-aromadendrene-epoxide (1.5%). The essential oil obtained in August was characterised by β-caryophyllene (1.8%), α-selinene (8.1%), valencene (12.9%), β-selinene (15.1%) and 7-epi-α-selinene (51.7%) (Kpoviessi et al., 2011). A marula extract was prepared and fractionated (Njume et al., 2011a). Two fractions containing 24 and 5 components, representing 86.6% and 40.5% of the overall composition, respectively, were obtained. The main components were identified as terpinen-4-ol (35.83%), aromadendrene (13.6%), pyrrolidine (32.2%) and α-gurjunene (8.8%). Most of these constituents were reported from marula for the first time. Analysis (GCxGC–ToF–MS) of marula oil indicated several unsaturated and saturated fatty acids (Komane et al., 2015). The main fatty acid constituent of the oil was oleic acid (69.0%), while linoleic acid (9.2%), palmitic acid (15.3%), stearic acid (1.5%) and palmitoleic acid (4.1%) were also identified. Matemu et al. (2017) investigated the overripe and ripe wild fruit of *S. birrea* using gas chromatography time-of-flight-mass spectrometry (GC-ToF-MS). Hexadecanoic acid was the most abundant compound in *S. birrea* (55.9%–71.3%). Octadecanoic acid was present at the second highest concentration (9.1%–17.0%). The major unsaturated fatty acids were identified as 9-octadecenoic acid (5.3%–18.8%) and 9,12,15-octadecatrienoic acid (2.8%). The amino acid and fatty acid composition of *S. birrea* was also determined (Magaia and Skog, 2017). The fat content of the kernels was ±49% and they are rich in unsaturated fatty acids. In marula kernels, the major fatty acid was reported as oleic acid (72.4%) and linoleic acid (around 7%).

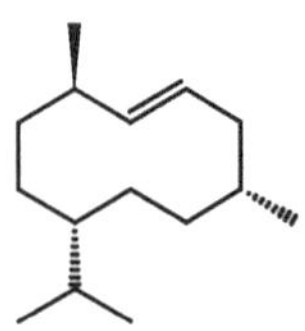

Germacrene D

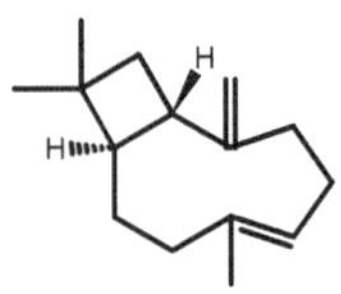

β-Caryophyllene

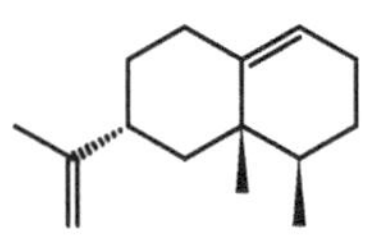

7-epi-α-Selinene

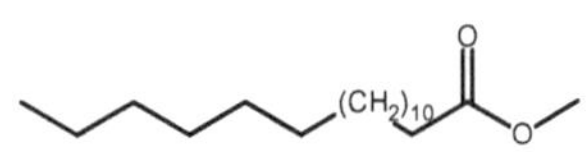

Stearic acid methyl ester

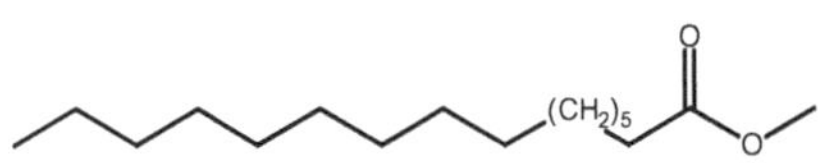

Palmitic acid methyl ester

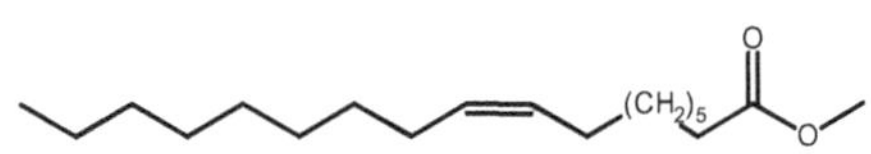

Oleic acid methyl ester

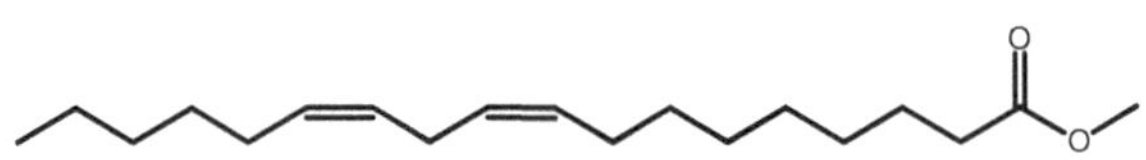

Linoleic acid methyl ester

9.2 Non-volatile constituents

Phytochemical studies undertaken by Galvez et al. (1993) on stem bark of *S. birrea* led to the isolation and identification of (−)-epicatechin-3-galloyl ester, procyanidin compounds (polyphenols) and catechin derivatives. Braca et al. (2003) reported the following flavonoids in the leaves: quercetin and its derivatives [quercetin 3-*O*-β-D-(6′-galloyl) glucopyranoside, quercetin 3-*O*-α-(5″-galloyl) arabinofuranoside, quercetin 3-*O*-α-L-rhamnopyranoside, quercetin 3-*O*-β-D-(6′-galloyl) galactopyranoside and quercetin 3-*O*-β-D-glucopyranoside], kaempferol and its derivatives [kaempferol 3-*O*-α-L-rhamnopyranoside, kaempferol 3-*O*-β-D-(6′-galloyl)glucopyranoside] and myricetin 3-*O*-α-L-rhamnopyranoside. The presence of (−)-epicatechin 3-*O*-galloyl ester, gallic acid and (−)-epigallocatechin 3-*O*-galloyl ester was also reported. The main phenolic constituents observed in the fruit are hydrolisable catechin derivatives, tannins and hydroxycinnamic acid (Borochov-Neori et al., 2008). Jiménez-Sánchez et al. (2015) used a reversed phase high-performance liquid chromatography-electrospray ionisation-quadrupole time-of-flight-mass spectrometry (RP–HPLC–ESI–QToF–MS) method to investigate the chemical profiles of the extracts, and identified 95 components classified as polyphenols, fatty acid derivatives, organic acids, among others, with most of the compounds reported for the first time in marula extracts. The extracts contained high concentrations of polyphenols, especially pro-anthocyanidins. This method was used to detect monomers and dimers of (epi)gallocatechin, (epi)catechin, and (epi)afzelechin units with two or one galloyl residues. A high percentage of galloylation was observed in these extracts, which may be responsible for the bio-activity observed. In a study of *S. birrea* by Russo et al. (2018), the concentrations of flavonoids, tannins and polyphenols in the methanol extracts of the bark and leaves were determined. Reported results indicated that methanolic leaf extracts were rich in flavonoids (132.7 ± 10.4 mg of quercetin equivalents/g), whereas methanolic extracts of the bark had the highest concentration of tannins (949.5 ± 29.7 mg of tannic acid equivalents/g). Shoko et al. (2018) tentatively identified six compounds in the ethanolic extract of marula stems, of which four compounds (catechin, quinic acid, epicatechin gallate and epigallocatechin gallate) were identified by UPLC–QToF–MS analysis, using standards. Cádiz-Gurrea et al. (2019) compared various methods to extract bio-active constituents from the bark of marula. Supercritical fluid extraction (SFE), solid–liquid extraction and pressurised liquid extraction (PLE) were investigated, using only "food-grade" solvents and selected conditions. The different methodologies were assessed in terms of yield, and the phenolic configuration was determined using HPLC–ESI–ToF–MS analysis. A good extraction yield was obtained using PLE with all the experiments. With regard to bio-active constituents, a total of 71 compounds were distributed in five major categories, with a significant percentage in a galloyl form. The highest number of components was extracted by PLE, mostly flavonoid aglycones, and when extraction was conducted at low temperatures.

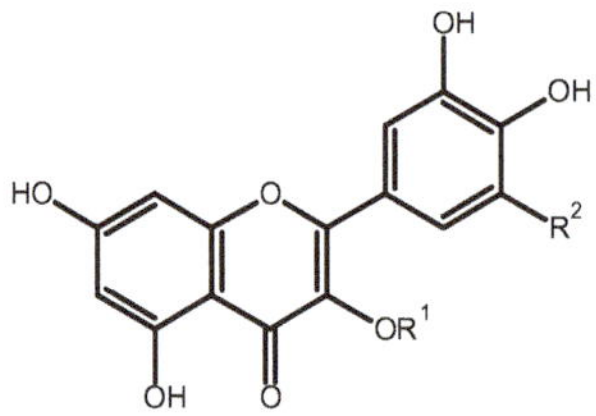

Quercetin 3-*O*-β-D-(6″-galloyl)glucopyranoside: R^1=(6″-galloyl)-glc; R^2=H
Quercetin 3-*O*- β-D-(6″-galloyl)galactopyranoside: R^1=(6″-galloyl)-gal; R^2=H
Quercetin 3-*O*-α-L-rhamnopyranoside: R^1=rha; R^2=H
Quercetin 3-*O*-β-D-glucopyranoside R^1=glc; R^2=H
Myricetin 3-*O*-α-L-rhamnopyranoside R^1=rha; R^2=OH

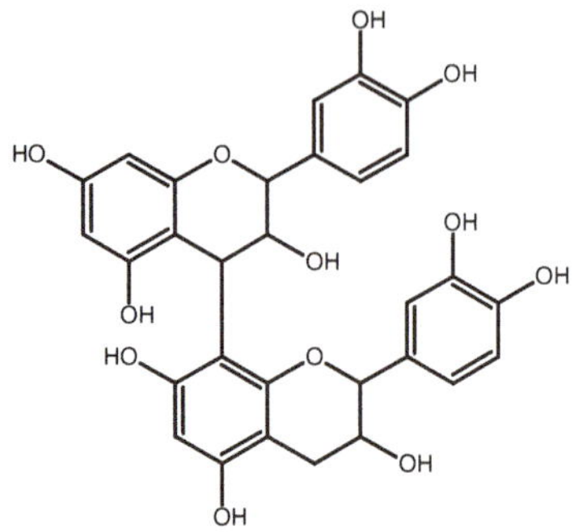

Procyanidin B2

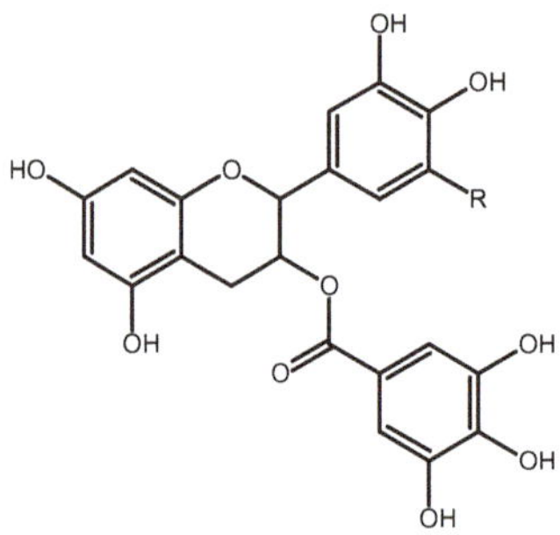

(-)-Epicatechin 3-*O*-galloyl ester: R=H
(-)-Epigallocatechin 3-*O*-galloyl ester: R=OH

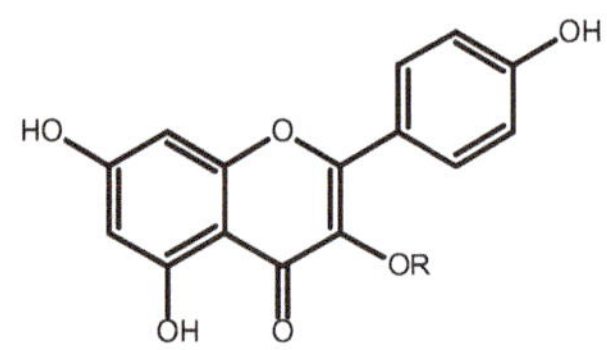

Kaempferol 3-*O*-α-L-rhamnopyranoside: R=rha
Kaempferol 3-*O*-β-D-(6″-galloyl)glucopyranoside: R=(6″ galloyl)-glc

Part B: Chemical profiling and quality control

10. Chromatography analysis

10.1 High-performance thin-layer chromatography (HPTLC) fingerprint analysis

General instrumentation: CAMAG HPTLC instrument consists of an automatic TLC sampler (ATS 4), automatic developing chamber (ADC 2), CAMAG TLC visualiser 2, CAMAG derivatiser, and TLC plate heater. *HPTLC plates:* Silica gel glass plates 60 F_{254} (Merck).

10.1.1 Non-volatile fraction analysis

Plant part: Bark, methanol extract. *Sample application:* Application volume of 2 μL methanol extract (100 mg/mL) and standards (1 mg/mL) spotted as 10 mm bands. Plates developed in a 20×10×4 cm glass twin-trough chamber to a migration distance of 70 mm. *Tank saturation:* 20 min at 15 °C and 33% RH, with 25 mL of mobile phase. *Mobile phase:* Toluene:acetone:formic acid (9:9:2, v/v/v). *Derivatisation:* *p*-Anisaldehyde sulphuric acid reagent. The plate was sprayed with 3 mL of anisaldehyde reagent, followed by heating for 3 min at 100 °C and then visualised. *Visualisation:* The plate was viewed under white reflectance light.

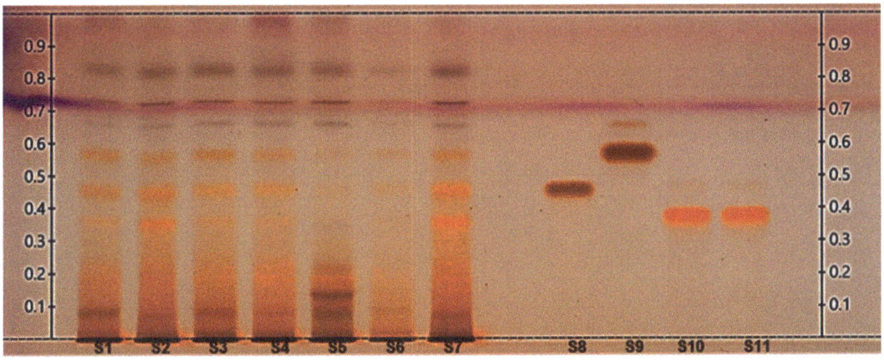

HPTLC plate of *Sclerocarya birrea* methanol extracts ($n = 7$) (S1–S7) and the standards (S8–S11). The samples are characterised by dark brown bands for epigallocatechin (S8) ($R_f = 0.47$) and catechin (S9) ($R_f = 0.58$) and light brown bands for epigallocatechin gallate (S10) ($R_f = 0.38$) and epigallocatechin saliace (S11) ($R_f = 0.38$).

10.1.2 Seed oil analysis

Plant part: Seed kernels, seed oil. *Sample application:* Application volume of 2 μL seed oil (25 μL/mL in toluene) and standards (25 μL/mL in hexane) spotted as 10 mm bands. Plates developed in a 20×10×4 cm glass twin-trough chamber to a migration distance of 70 mm. *Tank saturation:* 20 min at 15 °C and 33% RH, with 25 mL of mobile phase. *Mobile phase:* Toluene:ethyl acetate (95:5 v/v). *Derivatisation:* *p*-Anisaldehyde sulphuric acid reagent. The plate was sprayed with 3 mL of anisaldehyde reagent, followed by heating for 3 min at 100 °C and then visualised. *Visualisation:* The plate was viewed under white reflectance light.

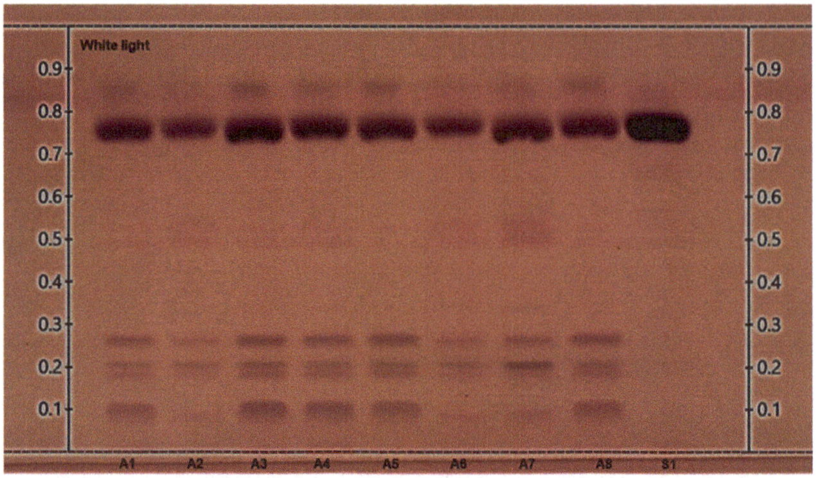

HPTLC plate of *S. birrea* seed oil ($n = 8$) (A1–A8) and the standard linoleic acid (S1) characterised by a bold black band at $R_f = 0.77$.

10.2 Ultra-performance liquid chromatography (UPLC) analysis

General instrumentation: Waters Acquity Ultra-Performance Liquid Chromatography system with photodiode array (PDA) detector combined with a Xevo G2QToF mass spectrometer (Waters, USA). *Plant part:* Bark, methanol extract. *Sample application:* Injection volume of 2.0 µL (full-loop injection) at 1 mg/mL. *Column:* Cortecs UPLC C_{18} column (150 mm × 2.1 mm, i.d., 1.6 µm particle size, Waters). *Mobile phase:* 0.1% formic acid in water (solvent A) and acetonitrile (solvent B). *Analysis conditions:* Gradient elution at a flow rate: 0.3 mL/min, changing as follows: 95% A: 5% B, held for 0.5 min, changed to 80% A: 20% B in 1.5 min, to 20% A: 80% B in 8 min, to 5% A: 95% B in 5 min and back to initial ratio in 0.5 min, equilibrating the system for 2.5 min, total run time 18 min. *Mass spectrometry*: ESI^- (negative ionisation mode), N_2 used as desolvation gas, desolvation temperature 350 °C at a flow rate of 500 L/h and source temperature at 100 °C. Capillary and cone voltages, 2500 and 45 V, respectively. Data collected between *m/z* 100 and 1200.

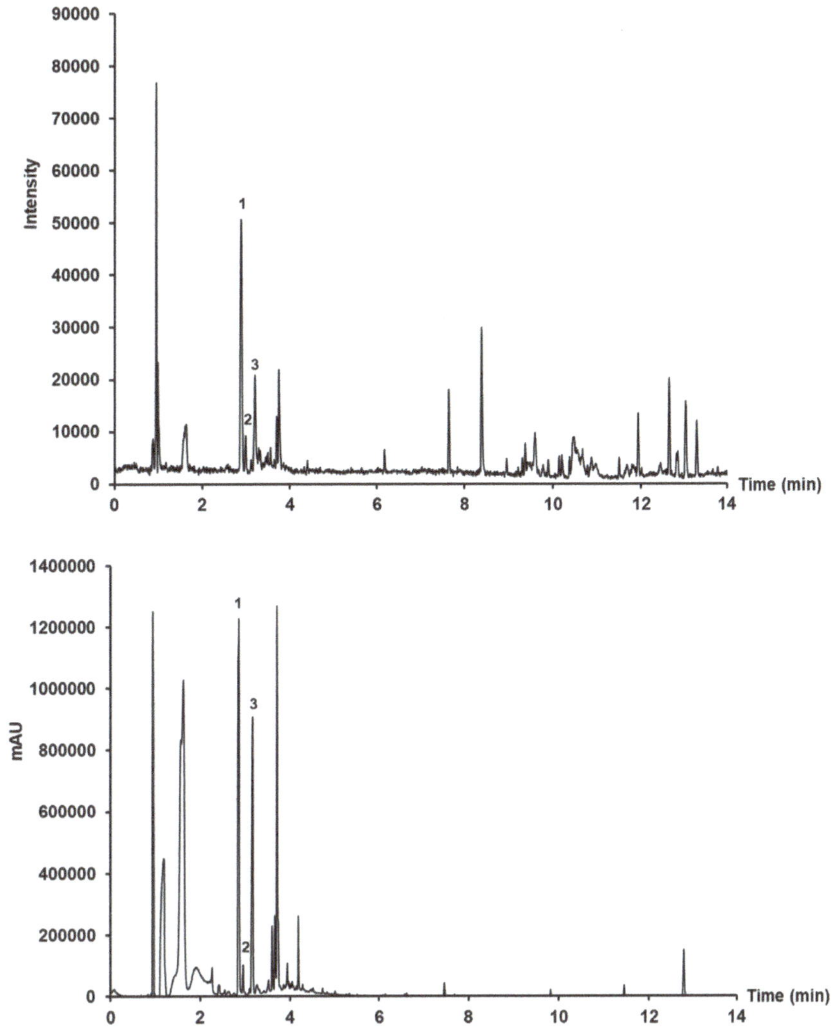

UPLC-ToF-MS ESI$^-$ (upper) and PDA (lower) chromatograms of *Sclerocarya birrea* methanol extract. [1]=catechin *m/z* 289.0812, [2]=epicatechin *m/z* 289.0769, [3]=epigallocatechin gallate *m/z* 457.1004.

10.3 Gas chromatography (GC) analysis

General instrumentation: An Agilent 6860N chromatograph (Agilent Technologies, Hanova, USA) fitted with a flame ionisation detector and a mass spectrometer. *Column:* HP-Innowax, 60 m × 250 µm × 0.25 µm (polyethylene glycol column, Agilent Technologies, Hanova, USA). *Plant part:* seed oil. *Sample application:* Injection volume of 1 µL (split) prepared at a concentration of 20% (v/v) in hexane. *Analysis conditions:* Inlet temperature 250 °C, split ratio: 1:200, helium carrier gas, flow rate: 1.2 mL/min, pressure: 24.79 psi. Starting oven temperature at 80 °C for 2 min, then increasing at a rate of 10 °C/min to 240 °C. *Mass spectrometry conditions:* Chromatograms obtained on electron impact at 70 eV on an Agilent 5973 mass selective detector, scanning range: *m/z* 35 to 550 (Agilent Technologies, Hanova, USA). Identification: Authentic standards, NIST®, Mass Finder®. *Identification:* Authentic standards, NIST®, Mass Finder®.

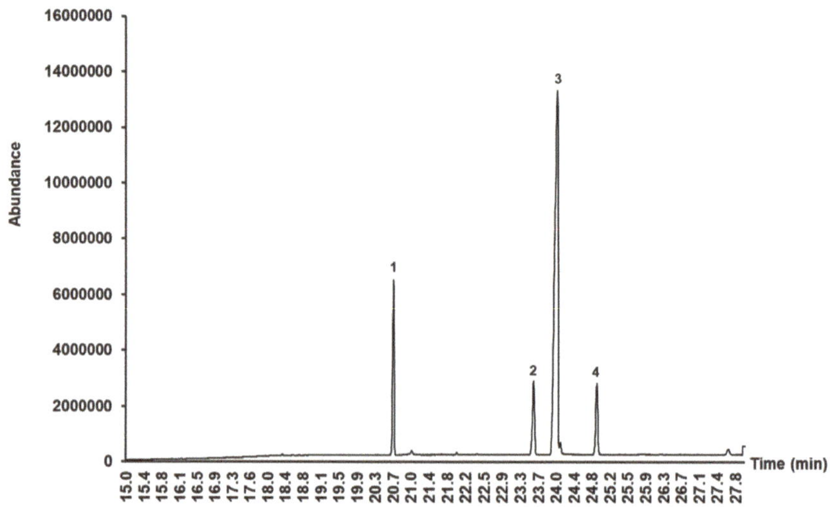

Total ion chromatograms (TIC) of *Sclerocarya birrea* seed oil indicating major compounds. [1] = Palmitic acid methyl ester (R_t 20.65, *m/z* 270.2559), [2] = stearic acid methyl ester (R_t 23.60, *m/z* 298.2872), [3] = oleic acid methyl ester (R_t 24.05, *m/z* 296.2715, and [4] = linoleic acid methyl ester (R_t 24.90, *m/z* 294.5959).

11. Mid-infrared (MIR) spectroscopy analysis

General instrumentation: Alpha-P Bruker spectrometer, mounted with an attenuated total reflectance (ATR) diamond crystal. *Spectral acquisition:* Spectrum obtained in absorbance mode, with a spectral resolution of 4 cm^{-1} over the range 4000–550 cm^{-1} and captured using OPUS 6.5 software.

11.1 Powder analysis

Plant part: Bark parts. *Sample preparation:* Bark powdered, sieved (< 500 μm), and placed directly onto the surface of the diamond crystal.

11.2 Seed oil analysis

Plant part: Seed kernel, oil. *Sample preparation:* Seed kernels, cold-pressed to obtain the oil, placed directly onto the surface of the diamond crystal.

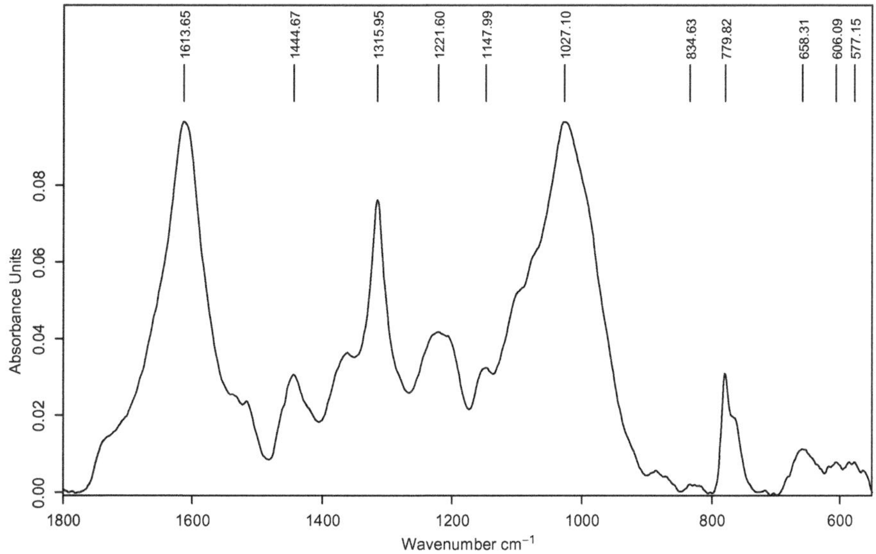

Mid-infrared spectrum of *Sclerocarya birrea* bark powder displaying the fingerprint region (1800–550 cm^{-1}).

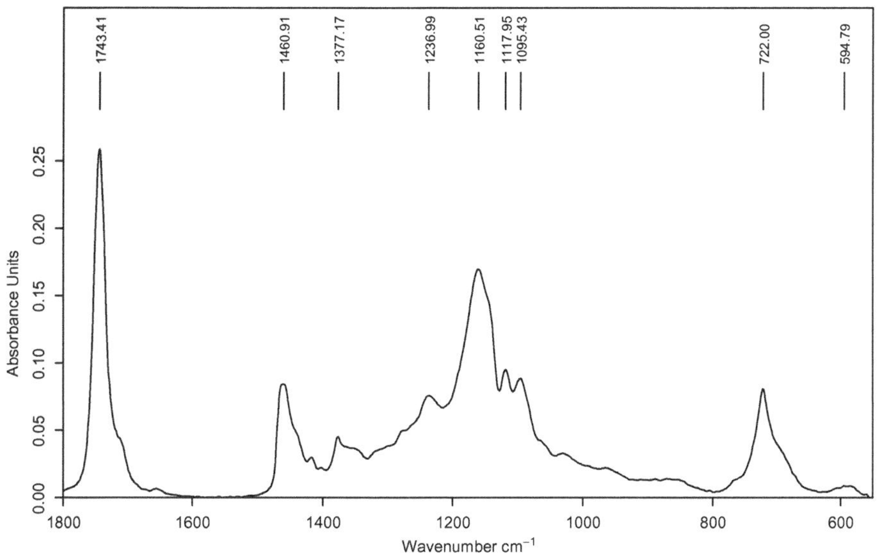

Mid-infrared spectrum of *Sclerocarya birrea* seed oil displaying the fingerprint region (1800–550 cm^{-1}).

References

Armentano, M.F., Bisaccia, F., Miglionico, R., Russo, D., Nolfi, N., Carmosino, M., Andrade, P.B., Valentã£o, P., Diop, M.S., Milella, L., 2015. Biomed Res. Int., Art. No. 561589.
Belemtougri, R.G., Constantin, B., Cognard, C., Raymond, G., Sawadogo, L., 2001. J. Ethnopharmacol., 76:247–252.
Belemtougri, R.G., Dzamitika, S.A., Ouedraogo, Y., Sawadogo, L., 2007. J. Biol. Sci., 7:570–574.
Borochov-Neori, H., Judeinstein, S., Greenberg, A., Fuhrman, B., Attias, J., Volkova, N., Hayek, T., Aviram, M., 2008. J. Agric. Food Chem., 56:9884–9891.
Botelle, A., 2001. A History of Marula Use in North-Central Namibia. Windhoek, Namibia.
Braca, A., Politi, M., Sanogo, R., Sanou, H., Morelli, I., Pizza, C., De Tommasi, N., 2003. J. Agric. Food Chem., 51:6689–6695.
Cádiz-Gurrea, M.D.L.L., Lozano-Sánchez, J., Fernández-Ochoa, Á., Segura-Carretero, A., 2019. Molecules, 24 (5):966.
Da Costa Mousinho, N.M.H., Van Tonder, J.J., Steenkamp, V., 2013. Nat. Prod. Commun., 8:1279–1284.
Dimo, T., Rakotonirina, S.V., Tan, P.V., Azay, J., Dongo, E., Kamtchouing, P., Cros, G., 2007. J. Ethnopharmacol., 110:434–438.
Eloff, J.N., 2001. J. Ethnopharmacol., 76:305–308.
Fennell, C.W., Lindsey, K.L., McGaw, L.J., Sparg, S.G., Stafford, G.I., Elgorashi, E.E., Grace, O.M., van Staden, J., 2004. J. Ethnopharmacol., 94:205–217.
Fotio, A.L., Dimo, T., Nguelefack, T.B., Dzeufiet, P.D.D., Ngo Lemba, E., Temdie, R.J., Ngueguim, F., Olleros, M.L., Vesin, D., Dongo, E., Kamtchouing, P., Garcia, I., 2009. Inflammopharmacology, 17:229–237.
Fotio, A.L., Olleros, M.L., Vesin, D., Tauzin, S., Bisig, R., Dimo, T., Nguelefack, T.B., Dongo, E., Kamtchouing, P., Garcia, I., 2010. Int. J. Immunopathol. Pharmacol., 23:61–72.
Galvez, J., Zarzuelo, A., Crespo, M.E., Utrilla, M.P., Jimenez, J., Spiessens, C., De Witte, P., 1991. Phytother. Res., 5:276–278.
Galvez, J., Crespo, M.E., Zarzuelo, A., 1993. Phytother. Res., 7:25–28.
Garba, S.H., Ahmadu, S., John, I.A., 2006. Pak. J. Biol. Sci., 9:2283–2287.
Gathirwa, J.W., Rukunga, G.M., Njagi, E.N.M., Omar, S.A., Mwitari, P.G., Guantai, A.N., Tolo, F.M., Kimani, C.W., Muthaura, C.N., Kirira, P.G., Ndunda, T.N., Amalemba, G., Mungai, G.M., Ndiege, I.O., 2008. J. Ethnopharmacol., 115:223–231.
Gondwe, M., Kamadyaapa, D.R., Tufts, M., Chuturgoon, A.A., Musabayane, C.T., 2008. Phytomedicine, 15:699–709.
Hamza, O.J.M., Van den Bout-Van den Beukel, C.J.P., Matee, M.I.N., Moshi, M.J., Mikx, F.H.M., Selemani, H.O., Mbwambo, Z.H., Van der Ven, J.A.M., Verweij, P.E., 2006. J. Ethnopharmacol., 108:124–132.
Hein, A.J., Wicker, C.M., Palmer, C.F., 2009. Natural Butters Reconstituted by Transesterification With Glycerine and Its Use in Cosmetic Applications. Patent US 2009/0285876 A1.
Hillman, Z., Mizrahi, Y., Beit-Yannai, E., 2008. Sci. Hortic., 117:321–328.
Houghton, C., 1999. New natural Oils and Their Properties. Anglia Oils Ltd., Bulk Speciality Division, Norfolk, UK.
Jiménez-Sánchez, C., Lozano-Sánchez, J., Gabaldón-Hernández, J.A., Segura-Carreteroa, A., Fernández-Gutiérrez, A., 2015. Ind. Crop. Prod., 71:214–234.

Kokwaro, J.O., 1976. Medicinal Plants of East Africa, third ed. University of Nairobi Press, Nairobi, Kenya.

Komane, B., Vermaak, I., Summers, B., Viljoen, A., 2015. J. Ethnopharmacol., 176:327–335.

Koné, W.M., Vargas, M., Keiser, J., 2012. Parasitol. Res., 110:2351–2362.

Kpoviessi, D.S.S., Gbaguidi, F.A., Kossouoh, C., Agbani, P., Yayi-Ladekan, E., Sinsin, B., Moudachirou, M., Accrombessi, G.C., Quetin-Leclercq, J., 2011. J. Med. Plant Res., 5:4640–4646.

Lediga, M.E., Malatjie, T.S., Olivier, D.K., Ndinteh, D.T., Van Vuuren, S.F., 2018. S. Afr. J. Bot., 119:172–180.

Magaia, T.L.J., Skog, K., 2017. Afr. J. Food Agric. Nutr. Dev., 17:12441–12454.

Mander, M., Cribbins, J., Shackleton, S.E., Lewis, F., 2003. The Commercial Marula Industry in South Africa: A Sub-Sector Analysis. Winners and Losers, Final Technical Report, Appendix 1.6. Centre for Ecology and Hydrology, Wallingford, UK, http://www.nerc-wallingford.ac.uk/research/winners/documents/Volume%202/R7795_FTR_App1.6.pdf.

Mariod, A.A., Abdelwahab, S.I., 2012. Food Rev. Int., 28:375–388.

Mariod, A., Matthaus, B., Eichner, K., 2004. J. Food Lipids, 11:179–189.

Masoko, P., Mmushi, T.J., Mogashoa, M.M., Mokgotho, M.P., Mampuru, L.J., Howard, R.L., 2008. Afr. J. Biotechnol., 7:3521–3526.

Matemu, A.O., Adeyemi, D., Nyoni, H., Mdee, L., Tshabalala, P., Mamba, B., Msagati, T.A.M., 2017. Int. J. Environ. Res. Public Health, 14 (11):1401, https://doi.org/10.3390/ijerph14111401.

Mathabe, M.C., Nikolova, R.V., Lall, N., Nyazema, N.Z., 2006. J. Ethnopharmacol., 105:286–293.

Mativandlela, S.P.N., Meyer, J.J.M., Hussein, A.A., Houghton, P.J., Hamilton, C.J., Lall, N., 2008. Phytother. Res., 22 (6):841–845.

Mawoza, T., Ojewole, J.A.O., Owira, P.M.O., 2012. Cardiovas. J. Afr., 23:12–17.

Mawoza, T., Tagwireyi, D., Nhachi, C., 2015. J. Ethnopharmacol., 164:129–135.

McGaw, L.J., Eloff, J.N., 2008. J. Ethnopharmacol., 119:559–574.

McGaw, L.J., Van der Merwe, D., Eloff, J.N., 2007. Vet. J., 173:366–372.

Mikail, H.G., 2009. Afr. J. Biotechnol., 8:2047–2049.

Mogale, A.M., Lebelo, L.S., Thovhogi, N., De Freitas, A.N., Shai, L.J., 2011. Afr. J. Biotechnol., 10:15033–15039.

Molelekoa, T.B.J., Regnier, T., Da Silva, L.S., Augustyn, W.A., 2018. S. Afr. J. Sci., 114 (11–12):a4874, https://doi.org/10.17159/sajs.2018/4874.

Moyo, M., Ndhlala, A.R., Finnie, J.F., Van Staden, J., 2010. Food Chem., 123:69–76.

Moyo, M., Finnie, J.F., Van Staden, J., 2011. S. Afr. J. Bot., 77:592–597.

Musabayane, C.T., Gondwe, M., Kamadyaapa, D.R., Moodley, K., Ojewole, J.A.O., 2006. Endocr. Abstr., 12:36.

Muthaura, C.N., Keriko, J.M., Mutai, C., Yenesew, A., Gathirwa, J.W., Irungu, B.N., Nyangacha, R., Mungai, G.M., Derese, S., 2015. J. Ethnopharmacol., 175:315–323.

Nciki, S., Van Vuuren, S., van Eyk, A., de Wet, H., 2016. Pharm. Biol., 54:2420–2436.

Ndabambi, M., Basopo, N., Nkiwane, L.C., Naik, Y.S., 2015. Afr. J. Aquat. Sci., 40:107–108.

Ndifossap, I.G.M., Frigerio, F., Casimir, M., Tsofack, F.N., Dongo, E., Kamtchouing, P., Dimo, T., Maechler, P., 2010. J. Endocrinol., 205:79–86.

Ngorima, G.T., 2006. Towards Sustainable use of Marula (*Sclerocarya birrea*) in the Savannah Woodlands of Zvishavane District, Zimbabwe. MSc dissertation, University of the Witwatersrand, Johannesburg, South Africa.

Ngueguim, F.T., Esse, E.C., Dzeufiet, P.D.D., Gounoue, R.K., Bilanda, D.C., Kamtchouing, P., Dimo, T., 2015. BMC Complement. Altern. Med., 16 (1):47.

Njume, C., Afolayan, A.J., Green, E., Ndip, R.N., 2011a. Int. J. Antimicrob. Agents, 38:319–324.

Njume, C., Jide, A.A., Ndip, R.N., 2011b. Int. J. Mol. Sci., 12:5652–5665.

Nundkumar, N., Ojewole, J.A.O., 2002. Methods Find. Exp. Clin. Pharmacol., 24:397–401.

Ogbobe, O., 1992. Plant Foods Hum. Nutr., 42:201–206.

Ojewole, J.A.O., 2003a. Phytomedicine, 10:675–681.

Ojewole, J.A.O., 2003b. J. Ethnopharmacol., 85:217–220.

Ojewole, J.A.O., 2004. Phytother. Res., 18:601–608.

Ojewole, J.A.O., 2006a. Cardiovasc. J. S. Afr., 17:117–123.

Ojewole, J.A.O., 2006b. J. Nat. Med., 61:67–72.

Ojewole, J.A.O., Mawoza, T., Chiwororo, W.D.H., Owira, P.M.O., 2010. Phytother. Res., 24:633–639.

Palgrave, K.C., 1972. Trees of Southern Africa. C. Struik Publishers, Cape Town, South Africa.

Palmer, E., Pitman, N., 1972. Trees of Southern Africa. Balkema, Cape Town, South Africa.

Runyoro, D.K.B., Ngassapa, O.D., Matee, M.I.N., Joseph, C.C., Moshi, M.J., 2006. J. Ethnopharmacol., 106:158–165.

Russo, D., Miglionico, R., Carmosino, M., Bisaccia, F., Andrade, P.B., Valentão, P., Milella, L., Armentano, M.F., 2018. Int. J. Mol. Sci., 19 (1):186.

Sarkar, R., Chaudhary, S.K., Sharma, A., Yadav, K.K., Nema, N.K., Sekhoacha, M., Karmakar, S., Braga, F.C., Matsabisa, M.G., Mukherjee, P.K., Sen, T., 2014. J. Ethnopharmacol., 154:170–175.

Sewani-Rusike, C.R., Iputo, J.E., Ndebia, E.J., Gondwe, M., Kamadyaapa, D.R., 2015. Afr. J. Tradit. Complement. Altern. Med., 12:22–26.

Shackleton, S.E., Wynberg, R.P., Sullivan, C.A., Shackleton, C.M., Leakey, R.R.B., Mander, M., McHardy, T., Den Adel, S., Botelle, A., Du Plessis, P., Lombard, C., Laird, S.A., Cunningham, A.B., Combrinck, A., O'Regan, D.P., 2003. Marula Commercialization for Sustainable and Equitable Livelihoods: Synthesis of a Southern African Case Study. Winners and Losers, Final Technical Report, DFID FRP R7795, Appendix 3.5. Centre for Ecology and Hydrology, Wallingford, UK.

Shoko, T., Maharaj, V.J., Naidoo, D., Tselanyane, M., Nthambeleni, R., Khorombi, E., Apostolides, Z., 2018. BMC Complement. Altern. Med., 18 (1):54, https://doi.org/10.1186/s12906-018-2112-1.

Tabit, F.T., Komolafe, N.T., Tshikalange, T.E., Nyila, M.A., 2016. J. Med. Food, 19:324–329.

Tanih, N.F., Ndip, R.N., 2012. Evid. Based Complement. Alternat. Med., 834156.

Tanih, N.F., Ndip, R.N., 2013. Sci. World J., 2013:956206.

Trovato, A., Kirjavainen, S., Galati, E.M., Forestieri, A.M., Iauk, L., 1995. Phytother. Res., 9:591–593.

Van de Venter, M., Roux, S., Bungu, L.C., Louw, J., Crouch, N.R., Grace, O.M., Maharaj, V., Pillay, P., Sewnarian, P., Bhagwandin, N., Folb, P., 2008. J. Ethnopharmacol., 119:81–86.

Van Wyk, B.E., Van Oudshoorn, B., Gericke, N., 2000. Medicinal Plants of South Africa, second ed. Briza Publications, Pretoria, South Africa.

Van Vuuren, S.F., Nkwanyana, M.N., de Wet, H., 2015. BMC Complement. Altern. Med., 15 (1):53.

Verschaeve, L., Van Staden, J., 2008. J. Ethnopharmacol., 119:575–587.

Viljoen, A.M., Kamatou, G.P.P., Başer, K.H.C., 2008. S. Afr. J. Bot., 74:325–326.

Watt, J.M., Breyer-Brandwijk, M.G., 1962. The Medicinal and Poisonous Plants of Southern and Eastern Africa, second ed. E. & S. Livingstone Ltd, Edinburgh and London, UK.

Weinert, I., Van Wyk, P.J., Hoitzhausen, L.C., 1990. Marula. In: Nagy, S., Shaw, P.E., Wardowski, W.F. (Eds.), Fruit of Tropical and Subtropical Origin. Florida Science Inc., Lake Alfred, Florida, USA, pp. 88–115.

York, T., Van Vuuren, S.F., De Wet, H., 2012. J. Ethnopharmacol., 144:118–127.

CHAPTER

Siphonochilus aethiopicus 22

Alvaro Viljoen[a,b], Guy Kamatou[a] and Gerda Fouche[c]

[a]*Department of Pharmaceutical Sciences, Tshwane University of Technology, Pretoria, South Africa*

[b]*SAMRC Herbal Drugs Research Unit, Faculty of Science, Tshwane University of Technology, Pretoria, South Africa*

[c]*Chemistry Department, University of Pretoria, Pretoria, South Africa*

Abstract

Siphonochilus aethiopicus (Schweinf.) B.L.Burtt (Zingiberaceae), commonly known as 'African ginger' or 'wild ginger', is a deciduous plant with large leaves that develop annually from a small cone-shaped rhizome. This aromatic plant, with spectacular pink flowers, can grow to a height of about 60 cm. The rhizomes have a distinct fragrance when crushed. Although the plant is critically endangered in South Africa, it is widely distributed in other African countries. The fresh or dried rhizomes have been used by native South African tribes for many years to treat fever, coughs, colds, influenza, hysteria, headache, toothache, stomach pain, asthma and menstrual cramps. The plant is one of the most traded medicinal plants in South Africa, and its first commercial product was produced two decades ago. In vitro and in vivo studies showed promising results, including antimalarial, anti-inflammatory, antimicrobial, anti-allergic, and bronchodilator effects. Gas chromatography coupled to mass spectrometry (GC–MS), semi-automated high-performance thin-layer chromatography (HPTLC) and ultra-performance liquid chromatography coupled to mass spectrometry (UPLC–MS) were used to determine the chemical profiles of the volatile and non-volatile constituents of the rhizomes. Siphonochilone, 1,8-cineole, cis-allo-ocimene and (E)-β-ocimene were identified as major compounds in the oil as determined by GC–MS, while 9aβ-hydroxy-4aαH-3,5α,8aβ-trimethyl-4,4a,8a,9-tetrahydronaphtho([2,3-b]-dihydrofuran-2-one)-8-one and 2-hydroxy-4aαH-3,5α,8aβ-trimethyl-4,4a,8a,9-tetrahydronaphtho-[2,3-b]furan-8-one were identified as major non-volatile constituents from the hydromethanolic extract using UPLC–MS.

Keywords: *Siphonochilus aethiopicus*, Wild ginger, Rhizome, Siphonochilone, 9aβ-hydroxy-4aαH-3,5α,8aβ-trimethyl-4,4a,8a,9-tetrahydronaphtho([2,3-*b*]-dihydrofuran-2-one)-8-one, GC–MS, UPLC–MS, HPTLC, MIR spectroscopy

The South African Herbal Pharmacopoeia. https://doi.org/10.1016/B978-0-323-99794-2.00009-X

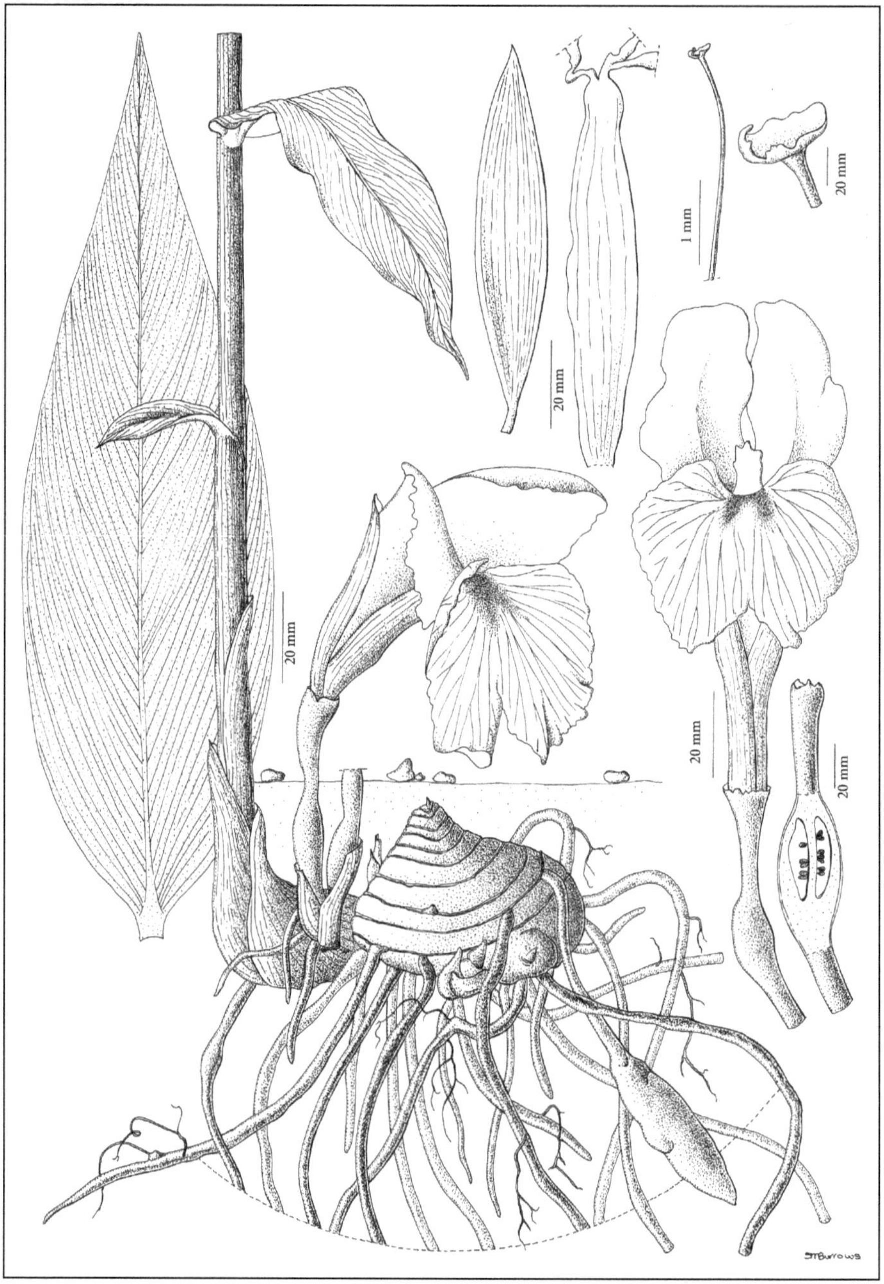
20 mm
1 mm
20 mm
20 mm
20 mm
20 mm

Part A: General overview

1. Synonyms

Kaempferia aethiopica (Schweinf.) Benth., *Kaempferia ethelae* J.M.Wood, *Kaempferia natalensis* Schltr. & K.Schum., *Siphonochilus natalensis* (Schltr. & K.Schum.) J.M.Wood & Franks.[a,b]

2. Common name(s)

Natal ginger, African ginger, wild ginger (English); '*gemmerhout*' (Afrikaans); '*indungulu*', '*isiphephetho*', '*sherungulu*' (isiZulu); '*serokolo*' (Northern Sotho).[a]

3. Conservation status

Critically endangered.[a] Overharvested from the wild to a point just short of total extinction.

4. Botany

Siphonochilus aethiopicus (Schweinf.) B.L.Burtt is a member of the family Zingiberaceae, which is the largest family in the order Zingiberales, with 53 genera and over 1200 species (Kress et al., 2002). The genus name '*Siphonochilus*' is derived from the Greek word, '*siphono*' for tube, and '*chilus*' for lip, referring to the floral tube and prominent floral lips. The specific name *aethiopicus* means 'from southern Africa'. It is an aromatic, deciduous plant that grows to a height of about 60cm, with leafy, pseudo-stems arising from conical rhizomes (A). The plants usually have five to ten large smooth leaves, with the leaf petioles sheathed in the false stem. The large parallel-veined leaves are up to 30cm long and 12cm broad. The flowers are strikingly beautiful, arising from ground level, pink to mauve in colour, with a white throat that bears distinct yellow markings (A). Small berry-like fruits are produced at or near ground level, or sometimes below the ground (Van Wyk et al., 2009). During dormancy in winter, the leaves are shed to reveal characteristic erect conical rhizomes. Translucent, succulent, spindle-shaped tuberous roots fan out from the base of the rhizome (B). The crushed or cut rhizomes have a distinct, almost antiseptic fragrance and a fleshy, yellow centre (C) (Adebayo et al., 2021).

[a] Red List of South African Plants (http://redlist.sanbi.org).
[b] World Flora Online (www.worldfloraonline.org).

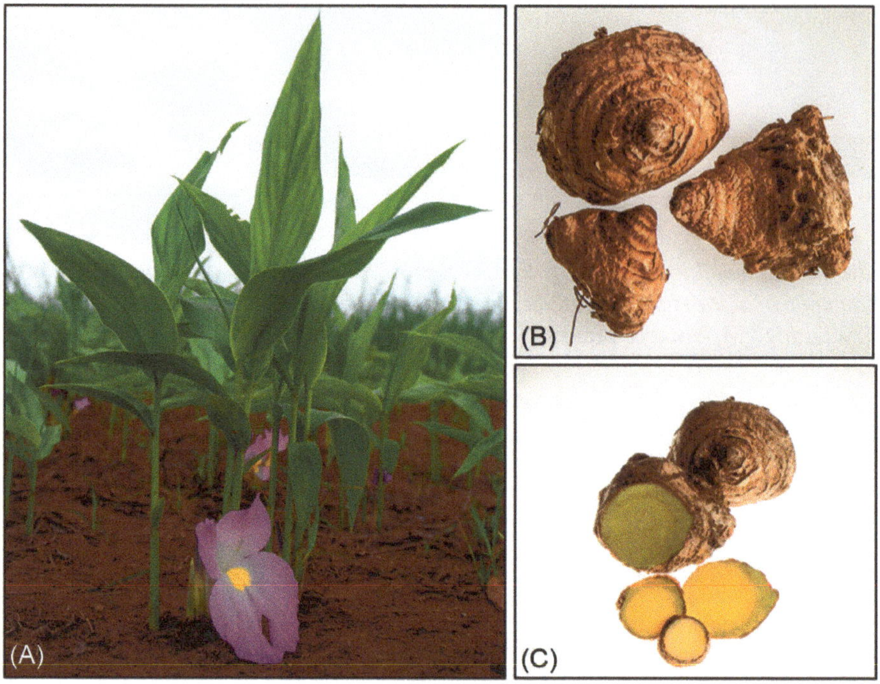

Siphonochilus aethiopicus plant with leafy pseudo-stems, pink to mauve flowers (A) and conical rhizomes (B) that are fleshy and yellow inside (C).

5. Geographical distribution

Siphonochilus aethiopicus currently covers a much smaller distribution area than before. It occurs sporadically from the Letaba catchment in the Limpopo Lowveld to Swaziland (Eswatini). It is extinct in KwaZulu-Natal, but the southern provenances represent a single clone thought to be an ancient Zulu crop plant of tropical African origin (Van Wyk et al., 2009). The plant is widespread in other African countries.

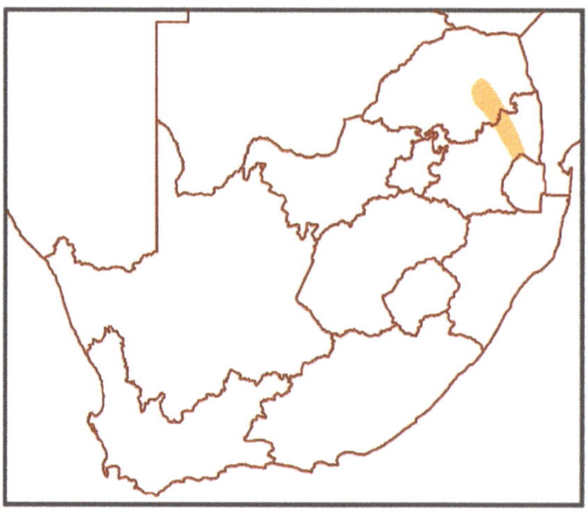

Geographical distribution of *Siphonochilus aethiopicus* in South Africa.

6. Ethnopharmacology

The highly aromatic roots of *S. aethiopicus* have a variety of medicinal and traditional uses. Native South African people have cultivated this plant for many years. In rural areas, people chew pieces of fresh or dried rhizomes to treat fever, coughs, colds, influenza, hysteria, asthma and menstrual cramps (Gerstner, 1939; Manzini, 2005). The plant sap expressed from crushed fresh rhizomes was traditionally prescribed by Zulu healers as a douche to treat vaginal thrush, and women chew the rhizomes during menstruation, probably to relieve pain (Watt and Breyer-Brandwijk, 1962). Zulu people used the plant for protection against lightning and snakes. Fresh rhizomes are chewed to treat headache and toothache (Manzini, 2005). The crushed root is taken in cold water for heart problems and the grated root is a remedy for stomach ache (Reynolds, 1966). A preparation of this plant is administered to horses as prevention against African horse sickness (Gerstner, 1939). *Siphonochilus aethiopicus* is used by the Swati people to treat malaria (Watt and Breyer-Brandwijk, 1962) and used as a spice to improve the flavour of food (Igoli, 2018). The plant has been incorporated into the *Materia Medica* of South African Rastafarian bush doctors, who use the rhizomes as a treatment for respiratory and circulatory problems (Philander, 2011).

7. Commercialisation

Siphonochilus aethiopicus is presently the most sought-after medicinal plant on the South African traditional medicine market (Lötter et al., 2006) and is one of the top 10 most traded medicinal plants in the South African provinces of Mpumalanga, KwaZulu-Natal and Limpopo (Mander, 1998; Moeng and Potgieter, 2011). Trade in dried rhizomes of *S. aethiopicus* was reported from Mpumalanga to Gauteng Province, mainly for sale to mine workers (Burtt-Davy, 1910; Goulding and Roberts, 1915). Based on the available quantitative information (Williams et al., 2007), the total annual consumption of *S. aethiopicus* rhizomes in South Africa alone could be in the range of 4–8 tons. Although cultivated plant material is now appearing on traditional '*muthi*' markets (Crouch et al., 2000), this represents only a very small fraction of the overall trade of the plant. Successful commercial production of *S. aethiopicus* by New Guelderland Sugar Estates in Stanger, KwaZulu-Natal Province was initiated in the early 1990s, and continued until 2013. The plant was grown in plastic tunnels and under shade cloth in Johannesburg at an elevation of 1753 m, outside of its natural locality range. The average rhizome fresh weight per plant was 90 g after 6 months, and 122 g after 9 months, demonstrating that the plant can be successfully grown at high altitudes, as community-based projects (Manzini, 2005). The first commercially manufactured product from *S. aethiopicus* was produced by the South African natural medicines company, Phyto Nova (Pty) Ltd. in 2000, which marketed the freeze-dried rhizomes as 'African Ginger' (Van Wyk, 2011) for treating colds, flu and candidiasis. Other products have since appeared on the South African market and the internet. Tablets produced from the dried rhizomes are used to treat sinusitis, sore throat, tension headache, asthma, premenstrual syndrome and menstrual cramps (Brendler et al., 2010).

8. Pharmacological evaluation

8.1 *In vitro* studies

8.1.1 Antimicrobial activity

The anticandidal activity of *S. aethiopicus* rhizome was tested against three strains of *Candida albicans*, two clinical isolates and a laboratory strain (ATCC 10231). The minimum inhibitory concentration (MIC) of the aqueous extract was found to be greater than 25 mg/mL, indicating no activity. The MICs determined for the ethanolic, ethyl acetate and hexane extracts were the same (1.03 mg/mL) for the clinical isolates and 2.09 mg/mL for the ATCC 10231 strain, reflecting poor activity (Motsei et al., 2003). Ethanolic extracts of *S. aethiopicus* have shown activity against *Bacillus subtilis, Staphylococcus aureus, Escherichia coli* and *Klebsiella pneumoniae.* The MIC value was lower for dry material stored for 90 days, compared to that of the fresh material against *B. subtilis, S. aureus* and *K. pneumoniae* (fresh 3.13 mg/mL, dry 1.56 mg/mL after 90 days) and unchanged for *E. coli* at 1.56 mg/mL (Stafford et al., 2005). Aqueous, ethyl acetate and acetone extracts were prepared from dried leaves and rhizomes of *S. aethiopicus*, and tested for activity against five strains of Gram-positive bacteria (*B. subtilis, Micrococcus kristinae, B. cereus, S. aureus* and *S. epidermidis*) and four strains of Gram-negative bacteria (*E. coli, Proteus vulgaris, Enterobacter aerogenes* and *Shigella sonnei*). All Gram-positive bacteria, except for *S. epidermis*, were inhibited by the ethyl acetate extracts from the rhizomes. The acetone extracts inhibited all of the Gram-positive bacteria. Both ethyl acetate and acetone extracts obtained from leaf samples showed inhibition against the Gram-positive bacteria, except for *S. aereus*, *S. epidermis*, *E. coli* and *P. vulgaris*. No inhibitory activity was recorded for the aqueous extracts. The highest activity reported was for the acetone extract against *S. epidermidis*, with a MIC of 2 mg/mL (Coopoosamy et al., 2010). Aqueous and ethanolic extracts of leaves and rhizomes were also tested for antifungal activity towards cultures of *Aspergillus flavus, Aspergillus glaucus, C. albicans, Candida tropicalis, Trichophyton mentagrophytes* and *T. rubrum.* The antifungal activity was greater for the ethanolic extract than for the aqueous extract. Strong to moderate activity against all the cultures was reported for the ethanolic extracts of the rhizomes. However, the leaf extracts displayed weaker activity (Coopoosamy et al., 2010). Water, ethanol and ethyl acetate extracts were prepared from the leaves, rhizomes and roots of *S. aethiopicus* plants (Light et al., 2002). The ethanol and ethyl acetate extracts tested showed greater antibacterial activity, with MICs ranging from 0.78 to 3.13 mg/mL, against the Gram-positive bacteria (*B. subtilis, S. aureus*) than towards the Gram-negative bacteria (*E. coli, K. pneumoniae*). *In vitro* testing of the three isolated compounds was done against cultures of *S. aureus, K. pneumoniae, Mycobacterium tuberculosis* and *C. albicans*. The obtained IC_{50} value of 250 μg/mL reflected the antimycobacterial activity of the compounds, but no activity against the bacteria or yeast was recorded for this concentration (Lategan et al., 2009).

8.1.2 Anti-inflammatory activity

Aqueous and ethanolic extracts of dried samples of *S. aethiopicus* demonstrated significant cyclooxygenase (COX-1) inhibitory activity, particularly for the ethanolic extracts of leaves and tubers. The COX-1 activity for *S. aethiopicus* was in the top three of the 10 plant species tested (Lindsey et al., 1998). The COX-1 activities of ethyl acetate extracts of *S. aethiopicus*, at a concentration of 250 µg/mL, were found to be the greatest for leaf and stem extracts, which had similar levels of activities to the rhizome extracts, which, in turn, had greater activity than that of the roots (Zschocke et al. 2000; Light et al., 2002). Attempts to isolate the compounds responsible for COX-1 inhibition from *S. aethiopicus* were unsuccessful, and the authors concluded that many compounds contributed to the activity (Jäger and Van Staden, 2005). Aqueous and ethanolic extracts of fresh *S. aethiopicus,* and material stored for 90 days, were assayed to compare the change in COX-1 activity of the extracts (Stafford et al., 2005). The aqueous extract of the plant material, stored for 90 days, lost activity, but an increase in the activity of the ethanolic extract was noted. A diethyl ether extract of rhizomes of *S. aethiopicus*, containing siphonochilone, was claimed to show significant inhibitory activity in the NF-kB transcription response cellular assay in a US patent application, with no associated cytotoxic effects (Horak et al., 2010).

8.1.3 Other activities

An ethyl acetate extract of *S. aethiopicus* rhizomes was tested for *in vitro* antiplasmodial activity and found to be active against both chloroquine-sensitive and chloroquine-resistant strains of *Plasmodium falciparum*, with IC_{50} values of 2.9 and 1.4 µg/mL, respectively. Bio-assay-guided fractionation led to the isolation of three furanoterpenoids with moderate *in vitro* antiplasmodial activity (Lategan et al., 2009). The anti-asthmatic properties of the plant extracts and the isolated siphonochilone were evaluated towards glucocorticoid and histamine receptors as mediators of inflammation in asthma, and on phosphodiesterase IV (PDE4), as a mediator of inflammation and smooth muscle contraction in asthma. The diethyl ether extract exhibited good activity towards the glucocorticoid receptor with an IC_{50} value of 12.9 µg/mL, and towards PDE4 with an IC_{50} value of 26.6 µg/mL. The purified compound induced a similar activity as the diethyl ether extract. The activity on the histamine receptor was weak. The results indicated that the diethyl ether extract and the isolated compound have significant *in vitro* activity (Fouche et al., 2011). Ethanolic extracts of *S. aethiopicus* were tested for smooth muscle-relaxing activity in a preparation of isolated guinea pig uterine tissue in the presence of oxytocin (Lindsey, 1999). However, the extracts did not relax or reduce the contractions of the precontracted uterine muscle.

Aqueous and methanolic extracts of the rhizomes of *S. aethiopicus* were tested for lipid peroxidation (Okimoto et al., 2000). The water extract showed potentiation of lipid peroxidation in the membranes of peripheral blood mononuclear cells. The methanolic extract of the plant showed similar protection against lipid peroxidation as the vitamin C (1 mM) positive control (Steenkamp et al., 2005). Aqueous and methanolic extracts of the rhizomes of *S. aethiopicus* were tested for their ability to scavenge the hydroxyl radical, generated *via* a Fenton-type reaction. The scavenging activity of the aqueous extract was the highest (84%) of 13 aqueous plant extracts tested, while that of the methanolic extract was 72% (Steenkamp et al., 2005). It was demonstrated that different *S. aethiopicus* parts can produce substantial amounts of anti-oxidants and carbohydrates after plants were subjected to nitrogen and reduced water supply during the phenological cycle (Mokgehle et al., 2017). Tests were done to determine the botryticidal efficacy of *S. aethiopicus* extracts, alone or combined with kresoxim-methyl, in decay inhibition studies on Granny Smith apples. Synergistic and additive effects were observed when tested against *Botrytis cinerea* (Fielding et al., 2015). *Siphonochilus aethiopicus* exerted potent synergistic interaction at the low extract dose of 62.5 mg/mL. PCT Patent Application PCT/IB2013/052215 disclosed the food, beverage, dietary supplement and medicinal applications of siphonochilone and related compounds as selective melatonin MT1 agonists (Gericke and Gericke, 2013).

8.2 *In vivo* studies and clinical trials

An ethyl acetate extract of *S. aethiopicus* rhizomes was tested *in vivo* for antimalarial activity in mice infected with chloroquine-resistant *Plasmodium yoelii*. The treated animals, given 400 mg/kg of extract orally, presented with significant suppression of parasitaemia on day 4 compared to the control (Lategan et al., 2009). In an allergic asthma study, mice sensitised and challenged with the allergen ovalbumin, were given extracts of *S. aethiopicus* or isolated siphonochilone. In a methacholine challenge, neither the extracts nor the dexamethasone control decreased airway hyperreactivity. Given intraperitoneally, the diethyl ether extract decreased the allergic inflammation and eosinophilia of the lung, while the isolated compound did not reduce the inflammation or eosinophilia, possibly due to problems with solubility (Fouche et al., 2011).

8.3 Safety

An ethyl acetate extract of *S. aethiopicus* rhizomes was tested for *in vitro* cytotoxicity towards the Chinese Hamster Ovarian cell-line using the 3-(4,5-dimethylthiazol-2-yl)-2, 5-diphenyltetrazolium bromide (MTT) assay, and no cytotoxicity was observed (Lategan et al., 2009). Aqueous and methanolic extracts of the rhizomes were tested for cytotoxicity *in vitro*, by incubating with peripheral blood mononuclear cells (PMNC), but no cytotoxicity was reported (Steenkamp et al., 2005). DNA damage was also assessed by visual scoring in 100 cells placed on each slide. The methanol extract of *S. aethiopicus* produced extensive damage. The leaf and root extracts of *S. aethiopicus* were considered non-toxic in the brine shrimp lethality assay (Akhalwaya et al., 2018). The mutagenicity of methanolic and dichloromethane extracts of dried rhizome was tested using the Ames bacterial test. Both extracts were negative in the Ames test, indicating that they are devoid of any mutagenic properties (Verschaeve and Van Staden, 2008). *Siphonochilus aethiopicus* rhizome extracts were tested for genotoxicity in a preliminary *in vitro* micronucleus test and in the alkaline comet assay. In the micronucleus test, the methanol:water extract was found not to be genotoxic in human lymphocytes. For the comet assay, only the methanolic extract was tested and found not to be toxic (Taylor et al., 2003).

9. Phytochemistry

9.1 Volatile constituents

The first report of distillation was in 1915, when it was reported that dried tubers yielded about 2% of volatile oil, which was pale yellowish-brown, with a pleasant odour resembling orange-flower oil (Watt and Breyer-Brandwijk, 1962). Two furanoterpenoid derivatives, namely 4aαH-3,5α,8aβ-trimethyl-4,4a,9-tetrahydro-naphtho[2,3-*b*]-furan-8-one and the 2-hydroxy-substituted compound, were isolated from the essential oil of *S. aethiopicus* (Holzapfel et al., 2002). The essential oil contains more than 70 monoterpenoids and sesquiterpenoids, with siphonochilone, 1,8-cineole, *cis*-allo-ocimene and (*E*)-β-ocimene identified as major compounds (Viljoen et al., 2002). Naudé et al. (2016) reported that 1,8-cineole was one of three major compounds present in the vapour phase of fresh rhizomes, concentrated by headspace solid phase micro-extraction (H/S-SPME), and analysed by gas chromatography-time-of-flight-mass spectrometry (GC–ToF–MS). The drying of rhizomes caused a significant loss of 1,8-cineole and other compounds (Naudé et al., 2016). The effects of operating parameters such as extraction duration, moisture content, particle size, and heating of the samples at temperatures between 80 °C and 100 °C, were studied to optimise oil recovery. A maximum yield of 0.61% (w/w) was achieved after 270 min of extraction time, with samples of particle size 2.4–4 mm, containing 6.37% moisture, and heating at 100 °C (Malaka et al., 2017).

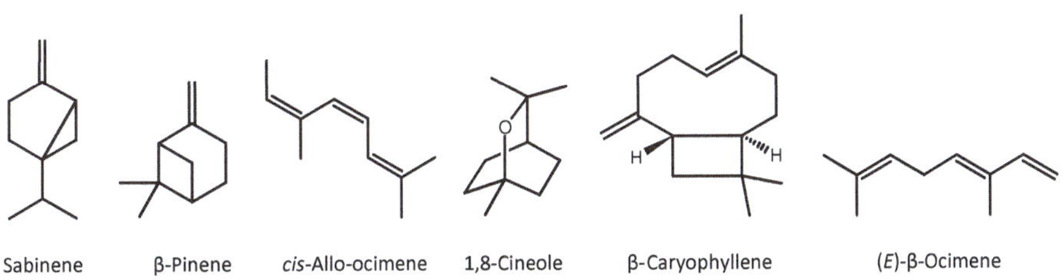

9.2 Non-volatile constituents

Bio-assay-guided fractionation of an ethyl acetate extract of the dried rhizomes of *S. aethiopicus*, led to the isolation of three furanoterpenoids with moderate *in vitro* antiplasmodial activity, namely 9aβ-hydroxy-4aαH-3,5α,8aβ-trimethyl-4,4a,8a,9-tetrahydronaphtho-([2,3-*b*]-dihydrofuran-2-one)-8-one, 4aαH-3,5α,8aβ-trimethyl-4,4a,8a,9-tetrahydronaphtho-([2,3-*b*]-dihydrofuran-2-one)-8-one and 4aαH-3,5α,8aβ-trimethyl-4,4a,8a-trihydronaphtho-([2,-3*b*]-dihydrofuran-2-one)-8-one (Lategan et al., 2009).

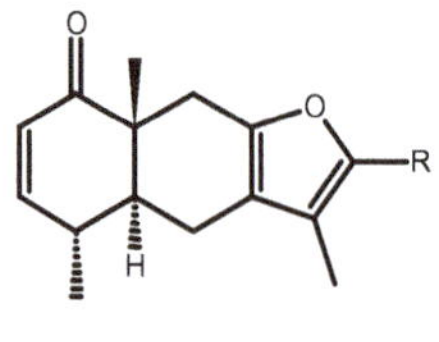

R=H: Siphonochilone, 4aαH-3,5α,8aβ-trimethyl-4,4a,9-tetrahydro-naphtho[2,3-*b*]-furan-8-one
R=OH: 2-hydroxy-4aαH-3,5a,8aβ-trimethyl-4,4a,9-tetrahydronaphtho[2,3-*b*]-furan-8-one

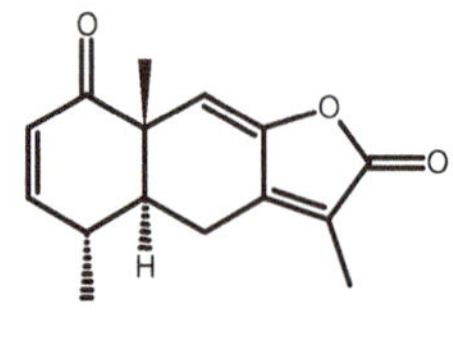

4aαH-3,5α,8aβ-trimethyl-4,4a,8a-trihydronaphtho-([2,3-*b*]-dihydrofuran-2-one)-8-one

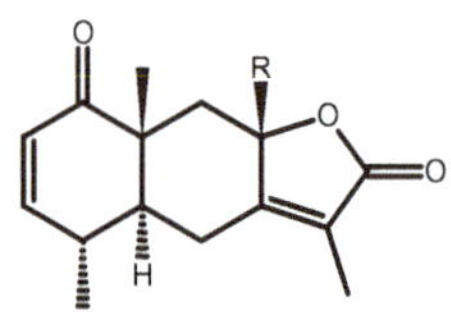

R=OH; 9aβ-hydroxy-4aαH-3,5α,8aβ-trimethyl-4,4a,8a,9-tetrahydronaphtho-([2,3-*b*]-dihydrofuran-2-one)-8-one
R=H; 4aαH-3,5α,8aβ-trimethyl-4,4a,8a,9-tetrahydronaphtho-([2,3-*b*]-dihydrofuran-2-one)-8-one

Part B: Chemical profiling and quality control

10. Chromatography analysis

10.1 High-performance thin-layer chromatography (HPTLC) fingerprint analysis

General instrumentation: CAMAG HPTLC instrument consisting of an automatic TLC sampler (ATS 4), automatic developing chamber (ADC 2), CAMAG Digistore Reprostar 3, CAMAG immersion device, and TLC plate heater. *HPTLC plates:* Silica gel glass plates 60F_{254} (Merck). *Plant part:* Rhizome, 70% aqueous methanol extract. *Sample application:* Application volume of 2 μL methanol extract (5 mg/mL) and standard (1 mg/mL) spotted as 6 mm bands. Plates were developed in a 20×10×4 cm glass twin-trough chamber to a migration distance of 70 mm. *Tank saturation:* 20 min at 25 °C and 47% RH, with 25 mL of the mobile phase. *Mobile phase:* Toluene: acetonitrile (93:7, v/v). *Derivatisation:* *p*-Anisaldehyde was prepared by mixing 0.5 mL *p*-anisaldehyde with 85 mL methanol, 10 mL glacial acetic acid and

5 mL sulphuric acid, in that order. The plate was dipped in the reagent and heated for 1 min at 100 °C on a TLC plate heater and then visualised. *Visualisation:* The plate was viewed under white reflectance light.

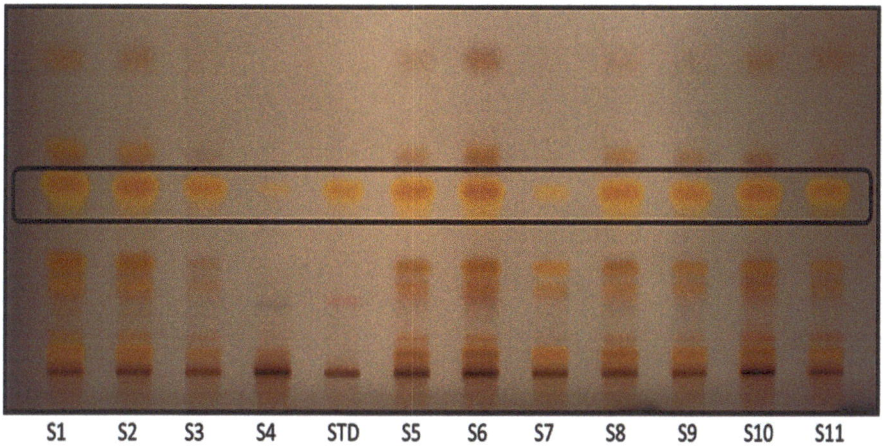

HPTLC plate of *Siphonochilus aethiopicus* hydromethanolic extracts ($n = 11$) (S1–S4; S5–S11), and the standard (STD). The samples are characterised by a yellow band for [4aαH-3,5α,8aβ-trimethyl-4,4a,8a,9-tetrahydronaphtho-([2,3-*b*]-dihydrofuran-2-one)-8-one] (STD) ($R_f = 0.57$).

10.2 Ultra-performance liquid chromatography (UPLC) analysis

General instrumentation: Waters Acquity Ultra-Performance Liquid Chromatography system with photodiode array (PDA) detector combined with a Xevo G2QToF mass spectrometer (Waters, USA). *Plant part:* Rhizomes, 70% aqueous methanol extract. *Sample application:* Injection volume: 2.0 µL (full-loop injection) at 1 mg/mL. *Column:* Acquity UPLC BEH C_{18} column (150 mm × 2.1 mm, i.d., 1.7 µm particle size, Waters). *Mobile phase:* 0.1% formic acid in water (solvent A) and acetonitrile (solvent B). *Analysis conditions:* Gradient elution at a flow rate of 0.3 mL/min, changing as follows: 85% A: 15% B, changed to 80% A: 20% B in 1 min, to 65% A: 35% B in 10 min, to 50% A: 50% B in 1 min, to 10% A: 90% B in 4 min, held for 1 min, back to initial ratio in 0.5 min, total run time 18 min. *Mass spectrometry:* ESI^+ (positive ionisation mode), N_2 used as the desolvation gas, desolvation temperature 400 °C at a flow rate of 500 L/h and source temperature 100 °C. Capillary and cone voltages, 3000 and 30 V, respectively. Data were collected between *m/z* 100 and 1000.

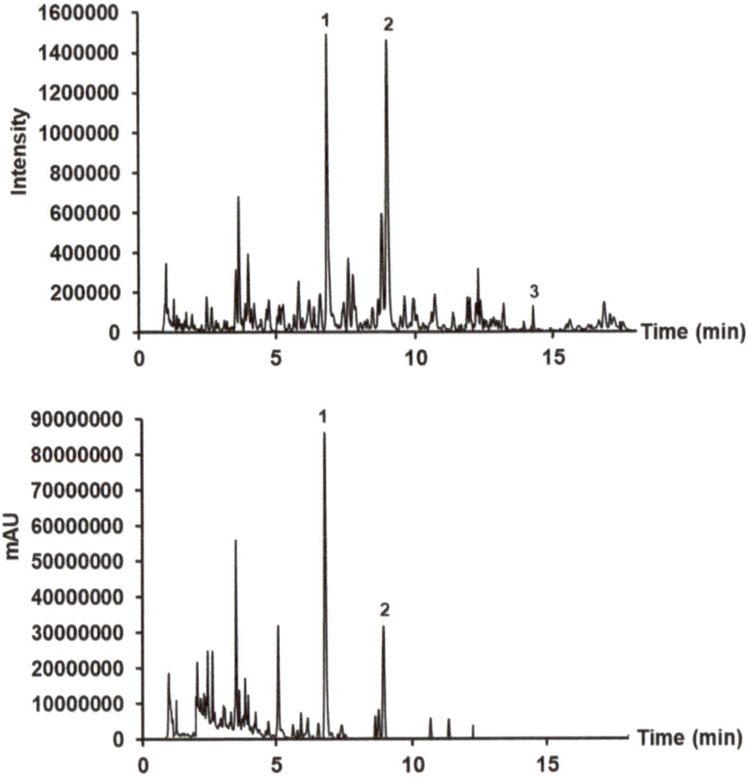

UPLC-ToF-MS ESI$^+$ (upper) and PDA (lower) chromatograms of *Siphonochilus aethiopicus* hydromethanolic extract. [1] = 9aβ-hydroxy-4aαH-3,5α,8aβ-trimethyl-4,4a,8a,9-tetrahydronaphtho ([2,3-*b*]-dihydrofuran-2-one)-8-one *m/z* 263.1282, [2] = 2-hydroxy-4aαH-3,5α,8aβ-trimethyl-4,4a,8a,9-tetrahydronaphtho-[2,3-*b*]furan-8-one *m/z* 247.1330, [3] = 4aαH-3,5α,8aβ-trimethyl-4,4a,8a,9-tetrahydronaphtho([2,3-*b*]-dihydrofuran-2-one)-8-one *m/z* 231.1292.

10.3 Gas chromatography (GC) analysis

General instrumentation: An Agilent 6860N chromatograph (Agilent Technologies, Hanova, USA) fitted with a flame ionisation detector and a mass spectrometer. *Column:* HP-Innowax, 60 m × 250 µm × 0.25 µm (polyethylene glycol column, Agilent Technologies, Hanova, USA). *Plant part:* Rhizomes, essential oil. *Sample application:* Injection volume of 1 µL (split) at 20% (v/v) in hexane. *Analysis conditions:* Inlet temperature 250 °C, split ratio: 1:200, helium carrier gas, flow rate: 1.2 mL/min, pressure: 24.79 psi. Starting oven temperature at 60 °C and then rise to 220 °C at 4 °C/min, holding for 10 min and increased to 240 °C at 1 °C/min. *Mass spectrometry conditions:* Chromatograms obtained upon electron impact at 70 eV using an Agilent 5973 mass selective detector, scanning range: *m/z* 35 to 550 (Agilent Technologies, Hanova, USA). *Identification:* Authentic standards, NIST®, Mass Finder®.

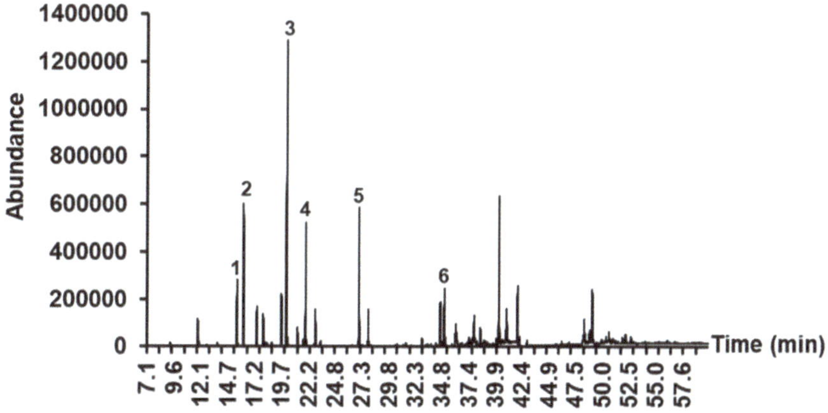

Total ion chromatogram (TIC) *of Siphonochilus aethiopus* essential oil indicating major compounds. [1] = β-pinene (R_t 15.56, *m/z* 136.1252), [2] = sabinene (R_t 16.19, *m/z* 136.1252), [3]=1,8-cineole (R_t 20.20, *m/z* 154.1358), [4]=*E*-β-ocimene (R_t 22.00, *m/z* 136.1252), [5]= allo-ocimene (R_t 26.99, *m/z* 136.1252), [6] = β-caryophyllene (R_t 35.06, *m/z* 204.1878).

11. Mid-infrared (MIR) spectroscopy analysis

General instrumentation: Alpha-P Bruker spectrometer, mounted with an attenuated total reflectance (ATR) diamond crystal. *Spectral acquisition:* Spectrum obtained in absorbance mode, with a spectral resolution of 4 cm^{-1} over the range 4000–550 cm^{-1} and captured using OPUS 6.5 software. *Plant part:* Rhizomes. *Sample preparation:*

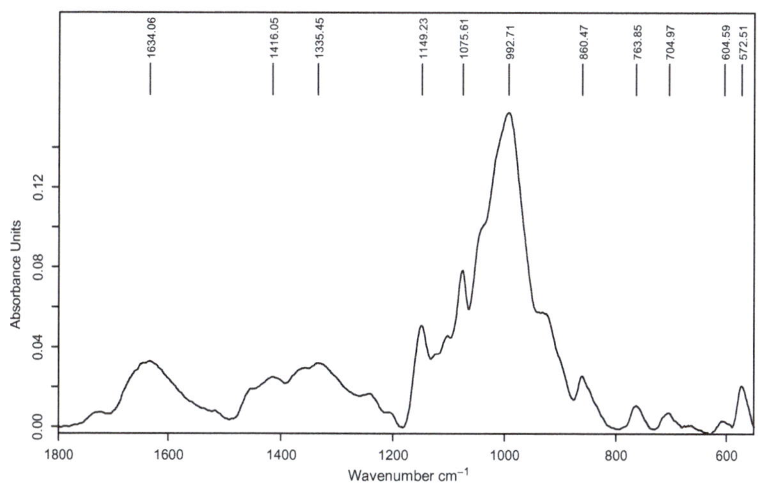

Mid-infrared spectrum of *Siphonochilus aethiopus* powder displaying the fingerprint region (1800–550 cm^{-1}).

Rhizomes were powdered, sieved (< 500 μm), and placed directly onto the surface of the diamond crystal.

References

Adebayo, S.A., Amoo, S.O., Mokgehle, S.N., Aremu, A.O., 2021. J. Ethnopharmacol., 266:113459.

Akhalwaya, S., Van Vuuren, S., Patel, M., 2018. J. Ethnopharmacol., 210:359–371.

Brendler, T., Eloff, J.N., Gurib-Fakim, A., Phillips, L.D., 2010. African Herbal Pharmacopoeia. Association for African Medicinal Plants Standards. Available from: http://www.aamps.org.

Burtt-Davy, J., 1910. Transvaal Agric. J., 9:45–46.

Coopoosamy, R.M., Naidoo, K.K., Buwa, L., Mayekiso, B., 2010. J. Med. Plant Res., 4:1228–1231.

Crouch, N.R., Lötter, M.C., Krynauw, S., Pottas-Bircher, C., 2000. Herbertia, 55:115–129.

Fielding, B.C., Knowles, C.-L., Vries, F.A., Klaasen, J.A., 2015. Agriculture, 5:400–411.

Fouche, G., Nieuwenhuizen, N., Maharaj, V., Van Rooyen, S., Harding, N., Nthambeleni, R., Jayakuma, J., Kirsten, F., Emedi, B., Meoni, P., 2011. J. Ethnopharmacol., 133:843–849.

Gericke, N., Gericke, O., 2013. Siphonochilone and Related Compounds and Uses Thereof. PCT Patent Application PCT/IB2013/052215.

Gerstner, J., 1939. Bantu Stud., 15:369–383.

Goulding, E., Roberts, O.D., 1915. J. Chem. Soc., 107:314–319.

Holzapfel, C.W., Marais, W., Wessels, P.L., Van Wyk, B.-E., 2002. Phytochemistry, 59:405–407.

Horak, R.M., Wadiwala, E., Fouche, G., Van der Merwe, M.M., Maharaj, V.J., Ackerman, L.G.J., 2010. Preventative Treatment and Remission of Allergic Diseases. United States Patent Application 20100168227.

Igoli, N.P., 2018. Agricultural Research Updates, Vol. 22. Nova Science Publishers Inc., pp. 145–165.

Jäger, A.K., Van Staden, J., 2005. Phytochem. Rev., 4:39–46.

Kress, W.J., Prince, L.M., Williams, K.J., 2002. Am. J. Bot., 89:1682–1696.

Lategan, C.A., Campbell, W.E., Seaman, T., Smith, P.J., 2009. J. Ethnopharmacol., 121:92–97.

Light, M.E., McGaw, L.J., Rabe, T., Sparg, S.G., Taylor, M.B., Erasmus, D.G., Jäger, A.K., Van Staden, J., 2002. S. Afr. J. Bot., 68:55–61.

Lindsey, K.L., 1999. Prostaglandin-synthesis Inhibitory Activity from the Leaves of *Siphonochilus aethiopicus* used in the Treatment of Dysmenorrhoea. MSc dissertation, University of Natal, Pietermaritzburg, South Africa.

Lindsey, K., Jäger, A.K., Raidoo, D.M., Van Staden, J., 1998. J. Ethnopharmacol., 64:9–14.

Lötter, M., Burrows, J.E., Van Staden, L., 2006. National Assessment: Red List of South African Plants version 2017.1. Accessed 17 May 2018.

Malaka, M.S., Naidoo, K., Kabuba, J., 2017. Chem. Eng. Commun., 204:813–819.

Mander, M., 1998. The Marketing of Indigenous Medicinal Plants in South Africa: A Case Study in KwaZulu-Natal. Available from: http://www.fao.org/3/w9195e/w9195e.pdf.

Manzini, T.Z., 2005. Production of Wild Ginger (*Siphonochilus aethiopicus*) under Protection and Indigenous Knowledge of the Plant from Traditional Healers. MSc dissertation, University of Pretoria, Pretoria, South Africa.

Moeng, E.T., Potgieter, M.J., 2011. J. Med. Plant Res., 5:558–564.

Mokgehle, S.N., Tesfay, S.Z., Araya, H.T., Du Plooy, C.P., 2017. Acta Agric. Scand. Sect. B Soil Plant Sci., 67:425–434.
Motsei, M.L., Lindsey, K.L., Jäger, A.K., Van Staden, J., 2003. J. Ethnopharmacol., 86:235–241.
Naudé, Y., Makuwa, R., Maharaj, V., 2016. S. Afr. J. Bot., 106:144–148.
Okimoto, Y., Watanabe, A., Niki, E., Yamashita, T., Noguchi, N., 2000. FEBS Lett. 474:137–140.
Philander, L.A., 2011. J. Ethnopharmacol., 138:578–594.
Reynolds, B., 1966. The Material Culture of the People of the Gwembe Valley. Kariba Studies III. Manchester University Press, Manchester, UK.
Stafford, G.I., Jäger, A.K., Van Staden, J., 2005. J. Ethnopharmacol., 97:107–115.
Steenkamp, V., Grimmer, H., Semano, M., Gulumian, M., 2005. Mutat. Res. Genet. Toxicol. Environ. Mutagen., 581:35–42.
Taylor, J.L.S., Elgorashi, E.E., Maes, A., Van Gorp, U., De Kimpe, N., Van Staden, J., Verschaeve, L., 2003. Environ. Mol. Mutagen., 42:144–154.
Van Wyk, B.-E., 2011. S. Afr. J. Bot., 77:812–829.
Van Wyk, B.-E., Van Oudtshoorn, B., Gericke, N., 2009. Medicinal Plants of South Africa, second ed. Briza Publications, Pretoria, South Africa.
Verschaeve, L., Van Staden, J., 2008. J. Ethnopharmacol., 19:575–587.
Viljoen, A.M., Demirci, B., Baser, K.H.C., Van Wyk, B.-E., 2002. S. Afr. J. Bot., 68:115–116.
Watt, J.M., Breyer-Brandwijk, M.G., 1962. The Medicinal and Poisonous Plants of Southern and Eastern Africa, second ed. E. & S. Livingstone Ltd, Edinburgh and London, UK.
Williams, V.L., Witkowski, T.F., Balkwill, K., 2007. Int. J. Sust. Dev. World, 14:584–603.
Zschocke, S., Rabe, T., Taylor, J.L.S., Jäger, A.K., Van Staden, J., 2000. J. Ethnopharmacol., 71:281–292.

CHAPTER

Terminalia sericea

23

Chinedu Anokwuru and Sandra Combrinck

Department of Pharmaceutical Sciences, Tshwane University of Technology, Pretoria, South Africa

Abstract

Terminalia sericea Burch. ex DC. (Combretaceae), commonly referred to as 'silver cluster-leaf', is a small-to-medium-sized shrub or brush tree of 3–16m in height, although some trees reach a height of 23m. The species is naturally distributed in the Limpopo, Mpumalanga, North West, Gauteng, KwaZulu Natal and Northern Cape provinces of South Africa. The bark is grey to pale brown and coarsely fissured, while the leaves are blueish-green in colour, with silvery hairs. The cream-coloured flowers emit an unpleasant odour. The plant is a very popular traditional medicine for the treatment of coughs, skin infections, diabetes, diarrhoea, gonorrhoea, menorrhagia and infertility. This monograph is a record of the ethnobotany, phytochemistry, in vitro and in vivo biological and pharmacological properties of the plant, as well as its toxicity profile. Chemical profiling of the non-volatile constituents was carried out using semi-automated high-performance thin-layer chromatography (HPTLC) and ultra-performance liquid chromatography coupled to mass spectrometry and photodiode array detection (UPLC–MS–PDA). A characteristic mid-infrared spectrum was obtained for the powdered root. Resveratrol-3-O-β-rutinoside, sericic acid and sericoside were identified as the major constituents and marker compounds of the root based on both HPTLC and UPLC–MS analyses.

Keywords: *Terminalia sericea*, Silver cluster-leaf, Resveratrol-3-*O*-β-rutinoside, Sericic acid, Sericoside, HPTLC, UPLC–MS, MIR spectroscopy

The South African Herbal Pharmacopoeia. https://doi.org/10.1016/B978-0-323-99794-2.00025-8

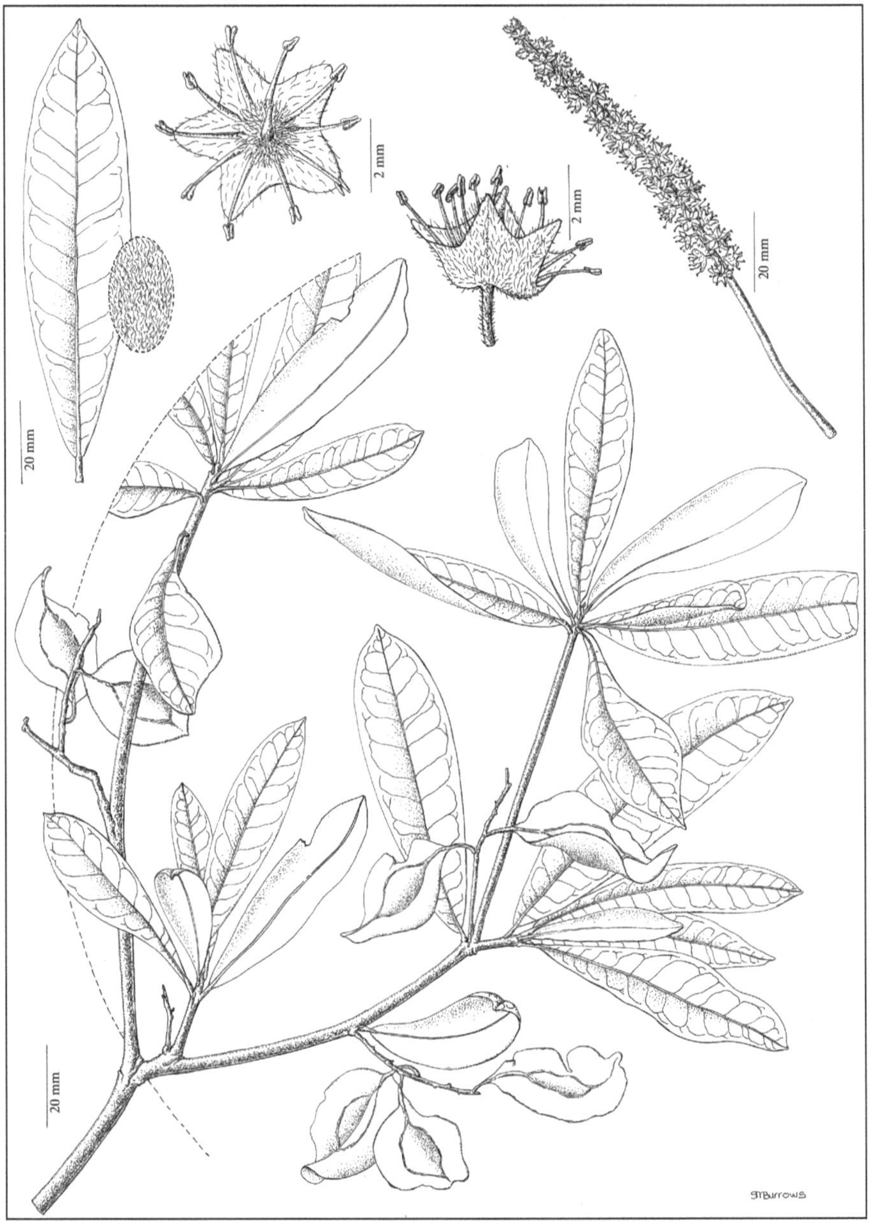
2 mm
2 mm
20 mm
20 mm
20 mm
STBurrows

Part A: General overview

1. Synonyms

Terminalia angolensis O.Hoffm.[a]

2. Common name(s)

Assegai wood, sand yellow wood, Transvaal silver tree, wild quince or silver cluster-leaf (English), '*sandvaalbos*', '*bloubos*', '*sandgeelhout*', '*sandsalie*', '*vaalboom*', '*silwerboom*' (Afrikaans), '*mususu*' (Tshivenda), '*mongonono*', '*Nkonola*' (Tswana), '*amangwe-amhlope*' (isiZulu), '*moxonono*' (Pedi).[b]

3. Conservation status

Least concern.[b]

4. Botany

Terminalia sericea (Combretaceae) is a small-to-medium-sized shrub or brush tree of 3–16 m in height, although some trees reach a height of 23 m (A). The trunk is erect with a characteristic wide, spreading crown. The bark is grey to pale brown and coarsely fissured. Silvery hairs adorn the leaves, which are blueish-green in colour on the adaxial surface and more pale below (B–C). The cream-coloured flowers emit an unpleasant odour (D). Fruiting occurs between January and May. The fruits are about 30 mm long, with two broad papery wings surrounding the thickened central part (C). They range in colour from purple–brown to pink–purple when mature (Likoswe et al., 2008; Chivandi et al., 2013).

[a] World Flora Online (www.worldfloraonline.org).
[b] Red List of South African Plants (http://redlist.sanbi.org).

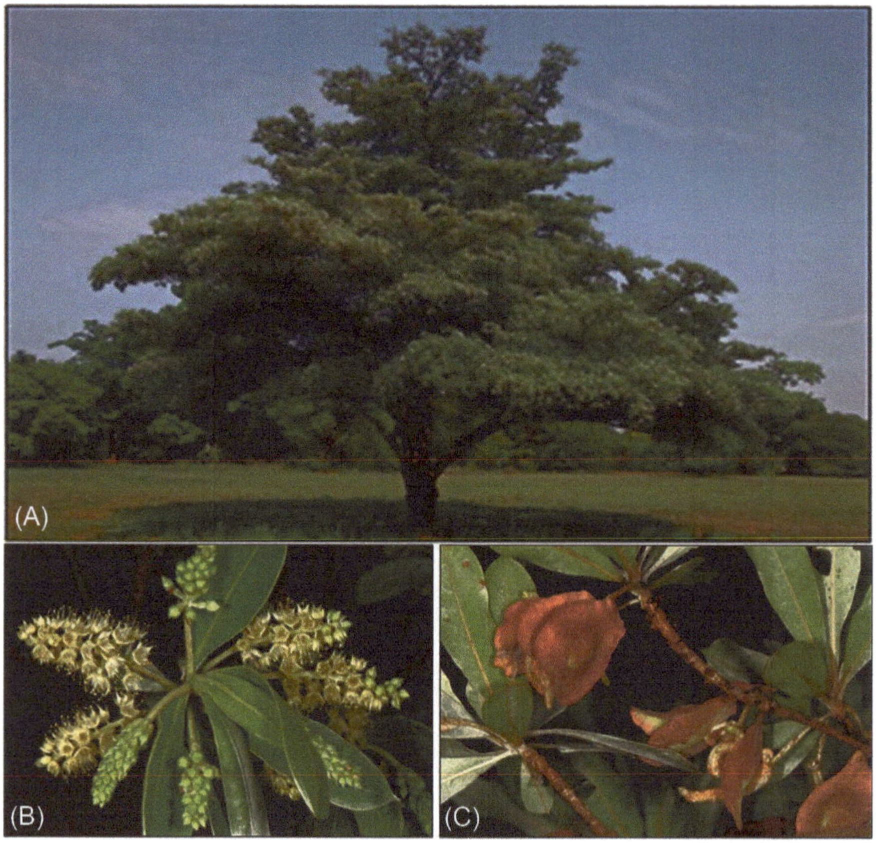

Terminalia sericea tree (A) with dark-green leaves, cream-coloured flowers (B), and purple–brown fruits with papery wings (C).

5. Geographical distribution

Terminalia sericea is found in the savannah woodlands of eastern, central and southern Africa. It is widely distributed throughout Namibia, Botswana, Swaziland (Eswatini) and Zimbabwe. In South Africa, it is abundant in the Limpopo and Mpumalanga provinces and occurs in the North West, Gauteng, KwaZulu Natal and Northern Cape provinces at altitudes of 45–2000 m above sea level (ASL).[c]

[c] http://hdl.handle.net/20.500.12143/818.

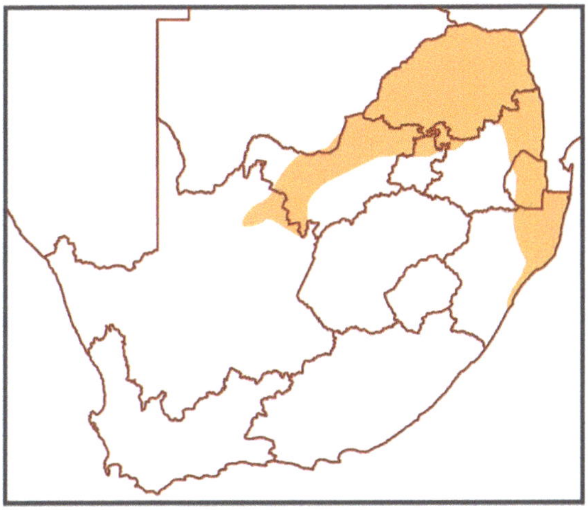

Geographical distribution of *Terminalia sericea* in South Africa.

6. Ethnopharmacology

Ethnomedicinal information revealed that the fruit, leaves, stem-bark and roots of *T. sericea* are commonly used for the treatment of coughs, skin infections, diabetes, diarrhoea and gonorrhoea. The dried leaves and roots are used to treat menorrhagia and infertility, while the powdered dried leaves are applied topically to infected wounds. A decoction of the dried root, prepared as soft porridge with maize flour, is taken for the treatment of diarrhoea. Root decoctions are used to treat stomach disorders, diarrhoea, pneumonia and eye infections (Fyhrquist et al., 2002; Steenkamp et al., 2004; Moshi and Mbwambo, 2005; Eldeen et al., 2006; Chinsembu and Hedimbi, 2010; Ribeiro et al., 2010; Amri and Kisangau, 2012). Leaves of *T. sericea* are also used in ethnoveterinary practice for treating wounds (Luseba and Van der Merwe, 2006). The roots are administered to treat diarrhoea and placenta retention in cows (Gabalebatse et al., 2013).

7. Commercialisation

There are no available records on the commercialisation of *T. sericea*.

8. Pharmacological evaluation

8.1 *In vitro* studies

8.1.1 Antimicrobial activity

Several studies have validated the traditional use of *T. sericea* for the treatment of microbial infections, using the agar well diffusion and microtire plate assays. The organic (dichloromethane:methanol) and aqueous stem-bark extracts displayed noteworthy antibacterial activity towards *Styphylococcus aureus, Bacillus cereus,*

Enterococcus faecalis, Proteus vulgaris, Klebsiella pneumonia and *Shigella flexeneri*, with minimum inhibitory concentration (MIC) values <1 mg/mL (York et al., 2012; Van Vuuren et al., 2015). An ethyl acetate extract of the root displayed noteworthy activity against *Bacillus subtilis* and *K. pneumonia* (Eldeen et al., 2006), while the aqueous stem-bark extract was active towards *B. subtilis, Styphylococcus aureus, K. pneumonia* and *Escherichia coli* (Eldeen et al., 2005). Acetone, hexane, dichloromethane and methanol leaf extracts displayed noteworthy activity towards yeast and fungal strains *Candida albicans, Crytococcus neoformans, Aspergillus fumigatus, Sporothrix schenckii* and *Microsporum canis* (Masoko et al., 2005). The dichloromethane: methanol (1:1) root-bark extracts (42), representing ten populations from three districts in the Limpopo Province of South Africa, were evaluated against eight bacterial pathogens using the microdilution assay (Anokwuru et al., 2020). The same MIC value (1.0 mg/mL) was obtained for the extracts against *B. cereus*, while the MICs of extracts representing different populations varied from 0.25 to 1.0 mg/mL, for *Shigella typhimurium.* Of the nine compounds isolated from the root-bark, many exhibited good activity towards all, or the majority of the pathogens, but the activity did not correspond to the chemical profiles obtained from single samples using ultra-performance liquid chromatography–mass spectrometry (UPLC–MS). Flavogallonic acid dilactone and methyl-flavogallonate, identified in the root-bark, were active towards most of the pathogens, reflecting broad-spectrum activity. A biochemometric analysis was initiated to link the chemistry and the antibacterial activity of the root-bark, however, the model indicated inconsistencies between the concentrations of isolated compounds and the activity of extracts. The authors recommended that further investigation of the compound interactions be undertaken since it was evident that such interactions affect the activity of the extracts.

8.1.2 Other activities

The acetone and methanol extracts of the leaf, stem and roots displayed moderate antimycobacterial activity (Green et al., 2010; Fyhrquist et al., 2014). The root extract displayed good antidiabetic activity through inhibition of α-glucosidase and β-glucoronidase enzymes. The stem extract and isolated compounds, β-sitosterol and lupeol, displayed good activity against α-glucosidase (97% inhibition) (Tshikalange et al., 2008; Nkobole et al., 2011). Sericoside, a saponin isolated from the root, exhibited anti-obesity activity by exerting a strong lipolytic effect on differentiated 3 T3-L1 cells (Mochizuki and Hasegawa, 2007). The leaf and root extracts displayed good anti-HIV activities against HIV-1 reverse transcriptase and polymerase (Bessong et al., 2004; Tshikalange et al., 2008). Stem and root extracts exhibited good anti-oxidant activity (94%), and excellent half-maximal inhibitory concentration (IC_{50} = 0.014 mg/mL) when tested using the 2,2-diphenyl-1-picrylhydrazyl radical (DPPH) assay (Adewusi and Steenkamp, 2011; Nkobole et al., 2011). Noteworthy anti-inflammatory activity was reported for stem and root extracts, using the cyclo-oxygenase (COX-1 and COX-2) assays (Eldeen et al., 2005, 2006).

8.2 *In vivo* studies and clinical trials

Mochizuki and Hasegawa (2007) studied the anti-inflammatory effect of sericoside (30 mg/kg administered over 10 days) and a triterpenoid isolated from the roots of *T. sericea*, using an experimental model of colitis in male rats. The study indicated that sericoside was able to significantly reduce (90%) acute inflammatory colitis induced by ethanolic 2,4,6-trinitrobenzene sulphonic acid.

8.3 Safety

Terminalia sericea root extract exhibited significant toxicity against monkey kidney Vero cells (VK) (Tshikalange et al., 2005), while the stem-bark was reported to exert weak toxicity (Nkobole et al., 2011). Four of eight male captive-bred vervet monkeys (*Chlorocebus pygerythrus*) were fed a maintenance diet comprising stiff maize porridge supplemented with micro- and macro-nutrients and containing 2.14 g/kg of powdered *T. sericea* root-bark (Anokwuru, 2018). The selected dose was 25 times higher than the recommended daily dose of *T. sericea*. After 12 weeks, a washout period ensued, and the feed was replaced with normal feed for another 4 weeks. The control group (four animals) received only the maintenance diet throughout the 16 weeks. Short-term hepatotoxic effects were recorded at week 4, but this was followed by hepatoprotective activity from weeks 8 to 16. Elevated serum creatinine levels reflected the possible kidney toxicity of the root-bark. Reduction of the serum glucose at week 4 indicated that the root-bark has hypoglycemic potential, corresponding with its traditional use. A reduction in the serum haematological parameters was reported, suggesting haematotoxicity. However, the elevated serum platelet count recorded implies possible wound-healing activity. Anokwuru (2018) concluded that no serious toxic effects were observed at a 25 times higher concentration than the normal or expected intake, suggesting that the roots have little toxicity. Further studies to investigate dose-dependent effects were proposed.

9. Phytochemistry

The phytochemistry of *T. sericea* has not been extensively investigated. However, terpenoids (arjunic acid, sericic acid, arjugenin, sericoside, arjunglucoside I, lupeol, β-sitosterol, β-sitosterol-3-acetate and stigma-4-ene-3-one), stilbenes (resveratrol-3-*O*-β-rutinoside), lignans (anolignan b, termilignan b) and tannins (punicalgin, epicatechin, catechin, gallocatechin, epigallocatechin) were isolated from the roots and stem-bark (Mongalo et al., 2016). Anokwuru et al. (2020) isolated nine compounds; sericic acid, sericoside, resveratrol-3-*O*-β-rutinoside, ellagic acid, flavogallonic acid dilactone, methyl-flavogallonate, quercetin-3-(2″-galloylrhamnoside), resveratrol-3-(6″-galloyl)-*O*-D-glucopyranoside and arjunetin, from the root-bark. Chemometric analysis of the UPLC–MS data of the dichloromethane:methanol (1:1) extracts revealed that there were three clusters within the samples, for which sericic acid, sericoside and an unidentified compound (*m/z* 682), were identified as markers. In a further study using the same samples (Mulaudzi et al., 2021), a high-performance thin-layer chromatography (HPTLC) chemical fingerprint of *T. sericea* root-bark was established that can be used as a reference to identify constituents for quality control purposes. An online software, rTLC, was used to perform chemometric analysis of the images obtained from the HPTLC plates. A principal component analysis (PCA) model was constructed and hierarchical cluster analysis (HCA) was performed. The loadings plot generated from the PCA model indicated the presence of two chemotypes, with sericoside associated with Chemotype 1, while sericic acid was revealed as the marker for Chemotype 2.

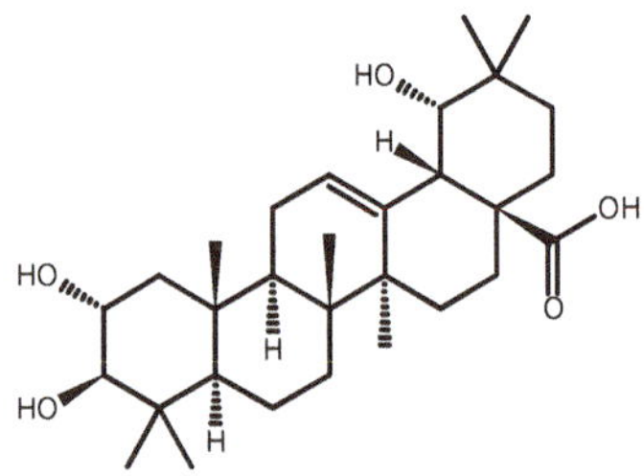

Arjunic acid

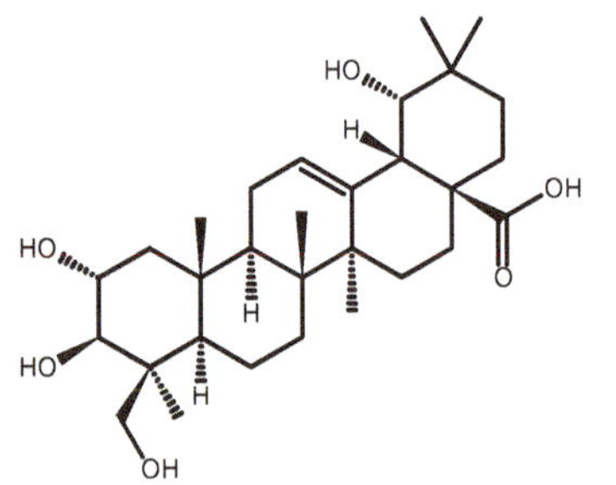

Sericic acid

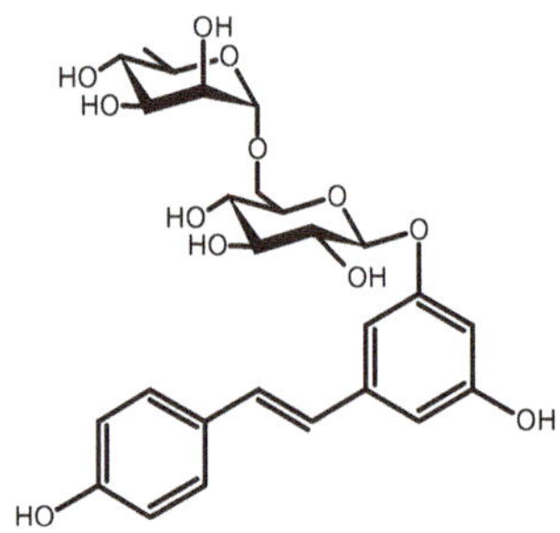

Resveratrol-3-*O*-β-rutinoside

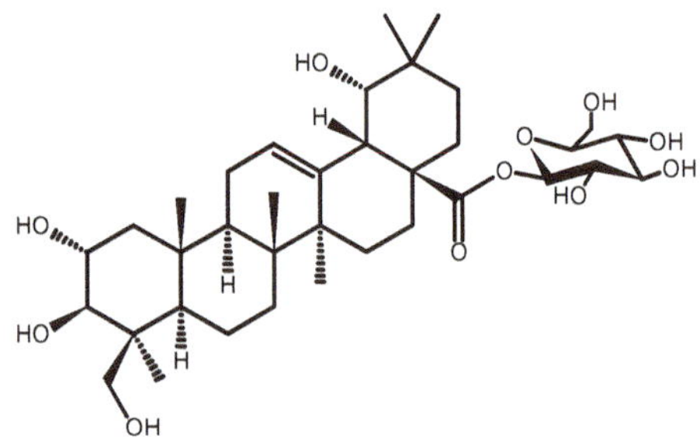

Sericoside

Part B: Chemical profiling and quality control

10. Chromatography analysis

10.1 High-performance thin-layer chromatography (HPTLC) fingerprint analysis

General instrumentation: CAMAG HPTLC instrument consists of an automatic TLC sampler (ATS 4), automatic developing chamber (ADC 2), CAMAG TLC visualiser 2, CAMAG derivatiser, and TLC plate heater. *HPTLC plates:* Silica gel glass plates

60 F_{254} (Merck). *Plant part:* Roots, (dichloromethane:methanol 1:1 v/v). *Sample application:* Application volume of 3 µL extract (10 mg/mL) and standards (1 mg/mL) spotted as 10 mm bands. Plates were developed in a 20 × 10 × 4 cm glass twin-trough chamber to a migration distance of 70 mm. *Tank saturation:* 20 min at 20.8 °C and 30.4% RH, with 25 mL of the mobile phase. *Mobile phase:* Dichloromethane: ethyl acetate: methanol: formic acid (90:10:30:1 v/v/v/v). *Derivatisation:* 10% sulphuric acid in methanol. The plate was sprayed with 3 mL derivatising reagent, heated for 3 min at 100 °C on a TLC plate heater, and then visualised. *Visualisation:* The plate was viewed under white reflectance light.

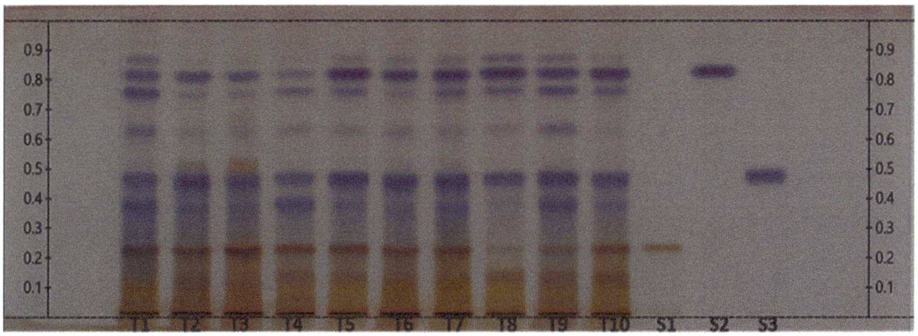

HPTLC plate of *Terminalia sericea* dichloromethane:methanol extracts (n = 10) (T1–T10) and the standards (S1–S3). The samples are characterised by a brown band for resveratrol-3-*O*-β-rutinoside (S1) (R_f = 0.24), and two purple bands for sericic acid (S2) (R_f = 0.83) and sericoside (S3) (R_f = 0.48).

10.2 Ultra-performance liquid chromatography (UPLC) analysis

General instrumentation: Waters Acquity Ultra-Performance Liquid Chromatography system with photodiode array (PDA) detector combined with a Xevo G2QToF mass spectrometer (Waters, United States). *Plant part:* Roots, dichloromethane:methanol extract. *Sample application:* Injection volume of 1.0 µL (full-loop injection) at 1 mg/mL *Column:* Acquity UPLC BEH C_{18} column (150 mm × 2.1 mm, i.d., 1.7 µm particle size, Waters). *Mobile phase:* 0.1% formic acid in water (solvent A) and acetonitrile (solvent B). *Analysis conditions:* Gradient elution at a flow rate of 0.3 mL/min, changing as follows: 95% A: 5% B to 40% A: 60% B in 8 min, to 5% A: 95% B in 7 min, keeping for 1 min and back to initial ratio in 0.5 min, total run time 18 min. *Mass spectrometry*: ESI^- (negative ionisation mode), N_2 used as desolvation gas, desolvation temperature 300 °C at a flow rate of 400 L/h, and source temperature at 100 °C. Capillary and cone voltages, 2500 and 40 V, respectively. Data were collected between *m/z* 100 and 1200.

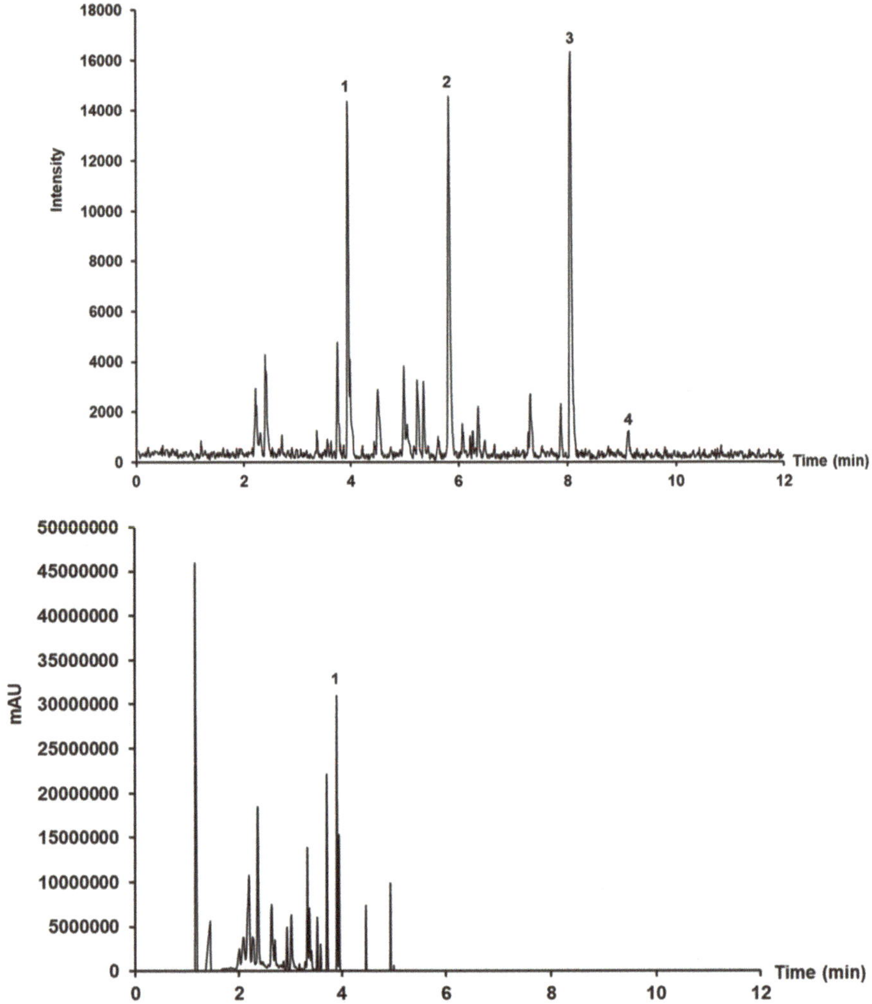

UPLC–ToF–MS ESI$^-$ (upper) and PDA (lower) chromatograms of *Terminalia sericea* dichloromethane:methanol extract: [1] = resveratrol-3-*O*-β-rutinoside *m/z* 535.1803, [2] = sericoside *m/z* 711.3945, [3] = sericic acid *m/z* 503.3368, [4] = arjunic acid *m/z* 487.3399.

11. Mid-infrared (MIR) spectroscopy analysis

General instrumentation: Alpha-P Bruker spectrometer, mounted with an attenuated total reflectance (ATR) diamond crystal. *Spectral acquisition:* Spectrum obtained in absorbance mode, with a spectral resolution of 4 cm^{-1} over the range 4000–550 cm^{-1} and captured using OPUS 6.5 software. *Plant part:* Roots. *Sample preparation:* Roots were powdered, sieved (< 500 µm), and placed directly onto the surface of the diamond crystal.

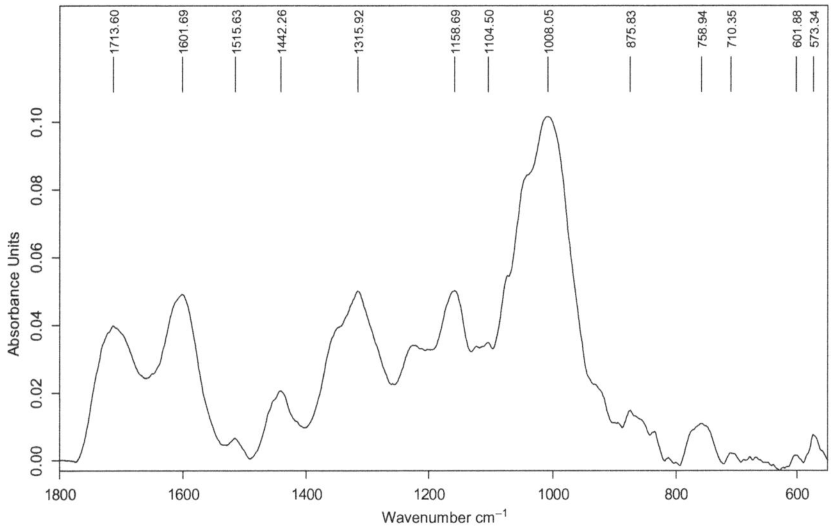

Mid-infrared spectrum of *Terminalia sericea* powder displaying the fingerprint region (1800–550 cm^{-1}).

References

Adewusi, E.A., Steenkamp, V., 2011. Asian Pac. J. Trop. Med., 4:829–835.

Amri, E., Kisangau, D.P., 2012. J. Ethnobiol. Ethnomed., 8:1.

Anokwuru, C.P., 2018. Phytochemical, Biological and Toxicity Studies of *Terminalia sericea* Burch. (Combretaceae). PhD thesis, University of Venda, Thohoyandou, South Africa.

Anokwuru, C.P., Tankeu, S., Van Vuuren, S., Viljoen, A., Ramaite, I.D.I., Taglialatela-Scafati, O., Combrinck, S., 2020. Molecules, 25:3683.

Bessong, P.O., Obi, C.L., Igumbor, E., Andreola, M., Litvak, S., 2004. Afr. J. Biotechnol., 3:555–559.

Chinsembu, K.C., Hedimbi, M., 2010. J. Ethnobiol. Ethnomed., 6:25.

Chivandi, E., Davidson, B.C., Erlwanger, K.H., 2013. S. Afr. J. Bot., 88:96–100.

Eldeen, I., Elgorashi, E.E., Van Staden, J., 2005. J. Ethnopharmacol., 102:457–464.

Eldeen, I.M., Elgorashi, E.E., Mulholland, D.A., Van Staden, J., 2006. J. Ethnopharmacol., 103:135–138.

Fyhrquist, P., Mwasumbi, L., Hggstrm, C., Vuorela, H., Hiltunen, R., Vuorela, P., 2002. J. Ethnopharmacol., 79:169–177.

Fyhrquist, P., Laakso, I., Marco, S.G., Julkunen-Tiitto, R., Hiltunen, R., 2014. S. Afr. J. Bot., 90:1–16.

Gabalebatse, M., Ngwenya, B.N., Teketay, D., Kolawole, O.D., 2013. Afr. J. Trad. Complem. Altern. Med., 10:490–502.

Green, E., Samie, A., Obi, C.L., Bessong, P.O., Ndip, R.N., 2010. J. Ethnopharmacol., 130:151–157.

Likoswe, M.G., Njoloma, J.P., Mwase, W.F., Chilima, C.Z., 2008. Afr. J. Biotechnol., 7:2840–2846.

Luseba, D., Van der Merwe, D., 2006. Onderstepoort J. Vet. Res., 73:115–122.

Masoko, P., Picard, J., Eloff, J.N., 2005. J. Ethnopharmacol., 99:301–308.
Mochizuki, M., Hasegawa, N., 2007. J. Health Sci., 53:329–331.
Mongalo, N.I., McGaw, L.J., Segapelo, T.V., Finnie, J.F., Van Staden, J., 2016. J. Ethnopharmacol., 194:789–802.
Moshi, M.J., Mbwambo, Z.H., 2005. J. Ethnopharmacol., 97:43–47.
Mulaudzi, N., Anokwuru, C.P., Tankeu, S.Y., Combrinck, S., Chen, W., Vermaak, I., Viljoen, A.M., 2021. Molecules, 26:432.
Nkobole, N., Houghton, P.J., Hussein, A., Lall, N., 2011. Nat. Prod. Commun., 6:1–4.
Ribeiro, A., Romeiras, M.M., Tavares, J., Faria, M.T., 2010. J. Ethnobiol. Ethnomed., 6:33.
Steenkamp, V., Mathivha, E., Gouws, M.C., Van Rensburg, C., 2004. J. Ethnopharmacol., 95:353–357.
Tshikalange, T.E., Meyer, J., Hussein, A.A., 2005. J. Ethnopharmacol., 96:515–519.
Tshikalange, T.E., Meyer, J., Lall, N., Muoz, E., Sancho, R., Van de Venter, M., Oosthuizen, V., 2008. J. Ethnopharmacol., 119:478–481.
Van Vuuren, S.F., Nkwanyana, M.N., De Wet, H., 2015. BMC Complement. Altern. Med., 15:53.
York, T., Van Vuuren, S.F., De Wet, H., 2012. J. Ethnopharmacol., 144:118–127.

CHAPTER

Warburgia salutaris

24

Carmen Leonard, Weiyang Chen and Guy Kamatou

Department of Pharmaceutical Sciences, Tshwane University of Technology, Pretoria, South Africa

Abstract

Warburgia salutaris (G.Bertol.) Chiov. is a slender, aromatic, evergreen tree that belongs to the cinnamon family (Canellaceae). This species, found mainly in southern Africa, has the epithet 'salutaris' which means 'salutary to health' or 'health-giving', thus reflecting the initial use of the bark as a general tonic, while the common name, pepper-bark tree, relates to the pungent, peppery taste of the inner bark. Traditionally, the bark of W. salutaris is used as a natural antibiotic for various respiratory tract infections, candidiasis, skin conditions, gastrointestinal ailments, as an analgesic and antipyretic, to combat protozoal diseases, and as a topical treatment for sexually transmitted disease-associated sores and inflammation. This monograph is a record of the conservation status, ethnobotany, phytochemistry, in vitro and in vivo biological activity, safety and commercialisation of the plant. The chemical profiling of the volatile and non-volatile constituents was performed using gas chromatography coupled to mass spectrometry (GC–MS), semi-automated high-performance thin-layer chromatography (HPTLC) and ultra-performance liquid chromatography coupled to mass spectrometry (UPLC–MS). The monoterpenes, myrcene, Z-β-ocimene and E-β-ocimene were dominant in the essential oil of the leaves, as determined by GC–MS analysis. The marker compounds in the non-volatile fraction were the sesquiterpenes, bemadienolide cinnamolide, cinnamolide-3β-acetate and ugandensolide, based on UPLC–MS analysis.

Keywords: *Warburgia salutaris*, Pepper-bark, *Z*–β–Ocimene, Polygodial, Bemadienolide, Cinnamolide, GC–MS, HPTLC, UPLC–MS, MIR spectroscopy

The South African Herbal Pharmacopoeia. https://doi.org/10.1016/B978-0-323-99794-2.00010-6

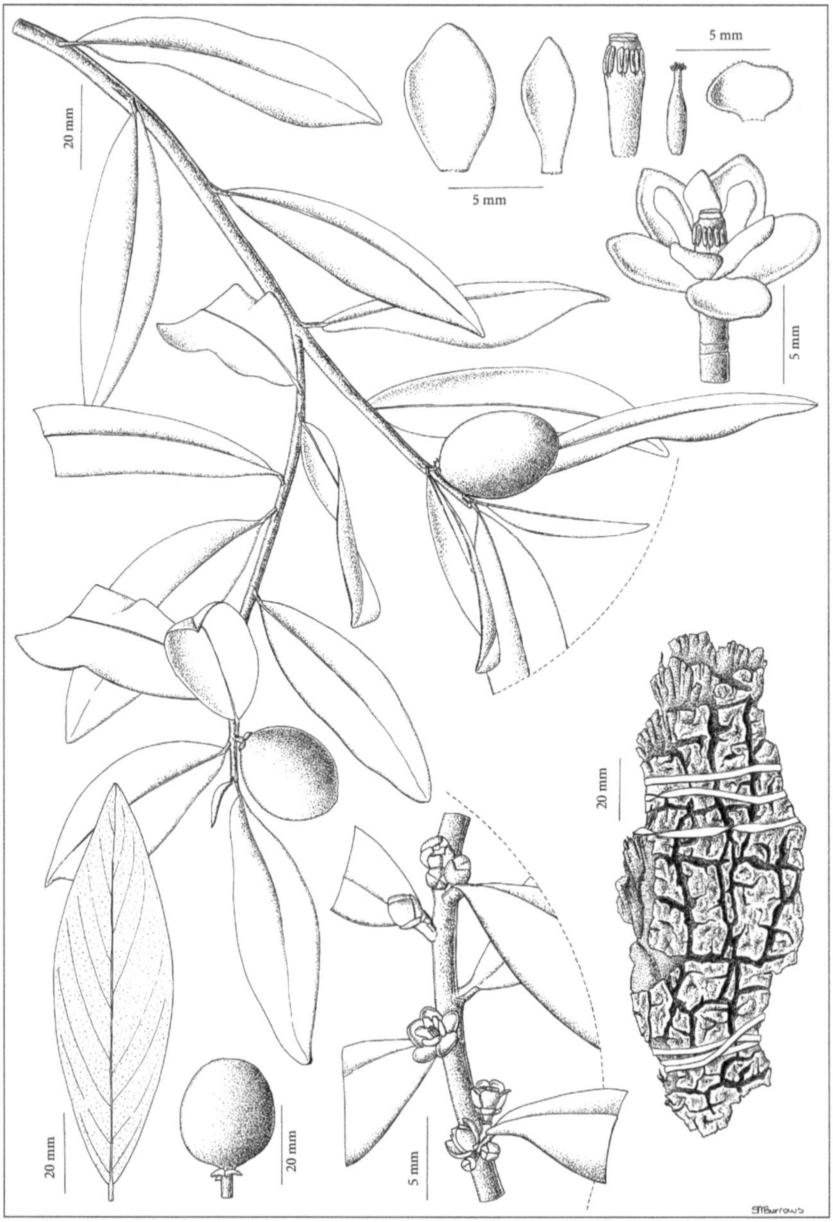
5 mm
20 mm
5 mm
5 mm
20 mm
20 mm
20 mm
5 mm
SMBurrows

Part A: General overview

1. Synonyms

Chibaca salutaris Bertol.f., *Warburgia breyeri* Pott.[a]

2. Common name(s)

Pepper-bark tree, Pepper-root, Pepper-leaf, Fever tree (English); '*Peperbasboom*', '*Peperblaarboom*', '*Koorsboom*' '*Sterkbos*' (Afrikaans); '*Isibhaha*', '*Amazwecehlabayo*' (isiZulu); '*Manaka*', '*Mulanga*' (Tshivenda); '*Shibaha*' (siTsonga); '*Molaka*' (SeSotho); '*Umzungulu*' (isiXhosa); '*Mosokonoi*' (Swahili) (Pooley, 1993; Van Wyk and Gericke, 2000).[a]

3. Conservation status

Warburgia salutaris is an endangered tree in South Africa[a] (Williams et al., 2013) with an estimated 50% decrease in the population, and some subpopulations considered nearly extinct. It is critically endangered in Swaziland (Eswatini) (Dlamini and Dlamini, 2002) and extinct in Zimbabwe (Maroyi, 2008) due to the unsustainable harvesting of the bark, which has led to a sharp decline in the number of trees.

4. Botany

Warburgia salutaris is a slender, aromatic, evergreen tree that belongs to the cinnamon family (Canellaceae). The genus name was given in honour of the German botanist and renowned author, Otto Warburg (1859–1938), who reported on this genus, based on his travels in East Africa and neighbouring regions (Engler, 1895). In July 1917, Dr. H.G. Breyer collected a tree in Pietersburg (now Polokwane) along the Drakensberg mountains. This species, although similar to *Warburgia ugandensis* Sprague (Palmer and Pitman, 1972; Palgrave et al., 2002), was initially known as *Chibaca salutaris* Bertol.f. and *Warburgia breyeri* Pott, but was later renamed *Warburgia salutaris* (Bertol.f.) Chiov. (Pott, 1918; Palgrave et al., 2002). The species epithet '*salutaris*' means 'salutary to health' or 'health-giving', thus reflecting the initial use of the bark as a general tonic, while the common name, pepper-bark tree, relates to the pungent, peppery taste of the inner bark. Many of the *W. salutaris* herbarium voucher specimens collected in South Africa and deposited at the South African National Biodiversity Institute (SANBI) were first incorrectly classified as *Warburgia stuhlmannii*. However, in 1976, Codd reclassified all these specimens as

[a] Red List of South African Plants (http://redlist.sanbi.org).

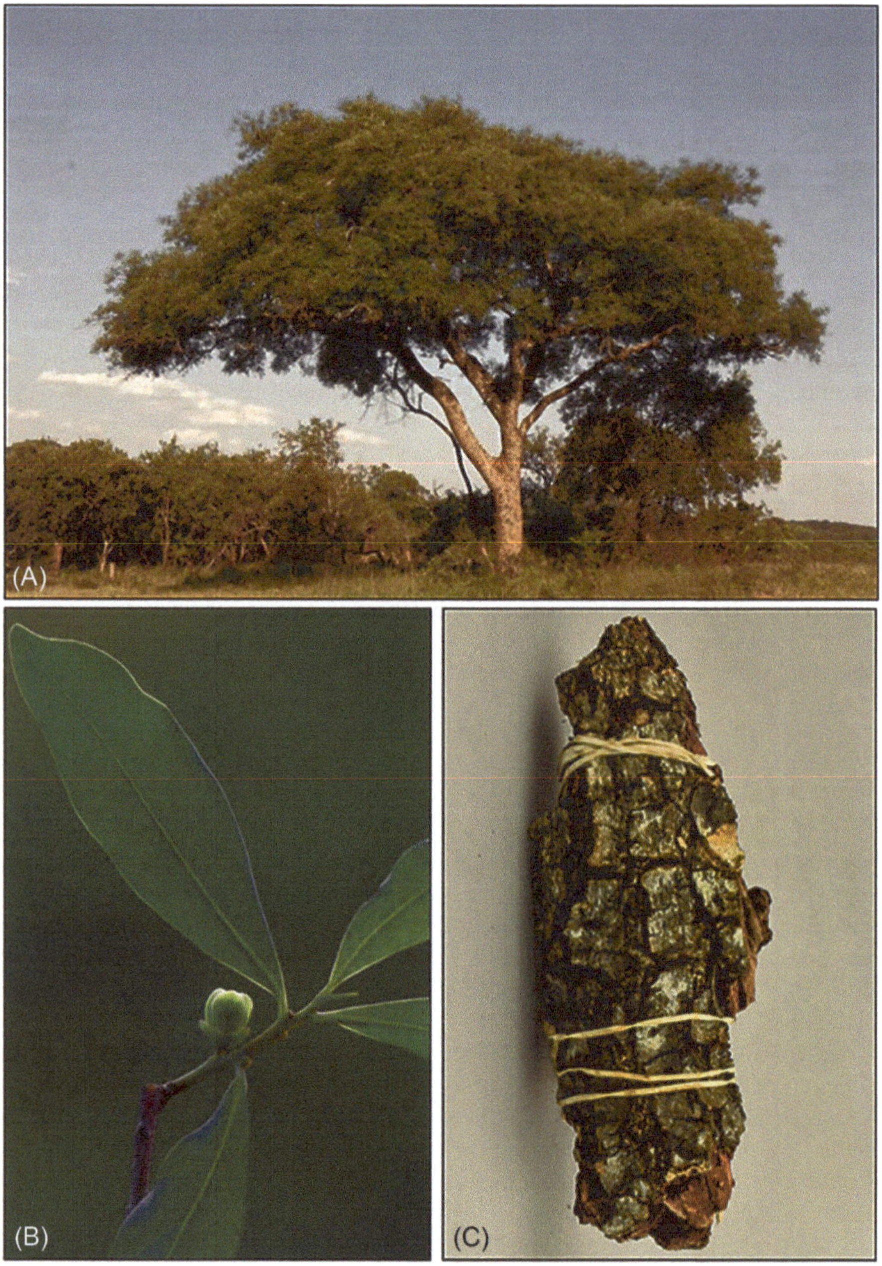

Warburgia salutaris tree (A) with glossy leaves, yellowish-green flowers (B), and a rough, mottled bark (C).

Warburgia salutaris (Leonard and Viljoen, 2015). The tree reaches a height of 10–27 m (A), with the trunk reaching up to 10 m (Pott, 1918). Leaves are simple, alternately arranged, elliptic to lanceolate, and glossy on the upper surfaces, but pale green below with entire margins (B). The midrib is characteristically slightly off-centre with a tapering apex and base. The leaves are distinct, because of their translucent secretory cells, the absence of trichomes, the presence of individual small druse crystals, and the thick cuticles on the epidermal and mesophyll cells (Kotina et al., 2014). The flowers, borne on short strong stalks in autumn to winter (April to June), are small, axillary, solitary or three-flowered cymes, cream in colour, with staminal tubes 3–4 mm in length, presenting 15–20 ovules. The fruits form in winter and early summer, and are green to purple berries of approximately 2.5 cm in diameter that have a leathery appearance (Pott, 1918). The bark (C) is rough and mottled, and red on the inside.

5. Geographical distribution

Warburgia salutaris is widely distributed throughout southern Africa, occurring in Botswana, Lesotho, Malawi, Mozambique, Namibia, South Africa, Swaziland (Eswatini), and Zimbabwe (Dowsett-Lemaire, 1989; Dowsett-Lemaire and White, 1990; Hollmann and Van der Schijff, 1996; Xaba and McVay, 2010). In South Africa, both wild and cultivated populations have been reported in the Limpopo, Mpumalanga and KwaZulu-Natal provinces. Although, *W. ugandensis* is the predominant species found in Tanzania, Kenya and Zambia, the presence of *W. salutaris* has also been reported (Orwa, 2009). It is adjusted to a variety of habitats and occurs in coastal and riverine regions, on dunes and in montane forests, open woodland, thickets and in kloofs. The species is generally slow-growing in the wild. This factor, together with its limited distribution and low abundance, makes it vulnerable to human-induced habitat degradation and over-exploitation as a medicinal plant.

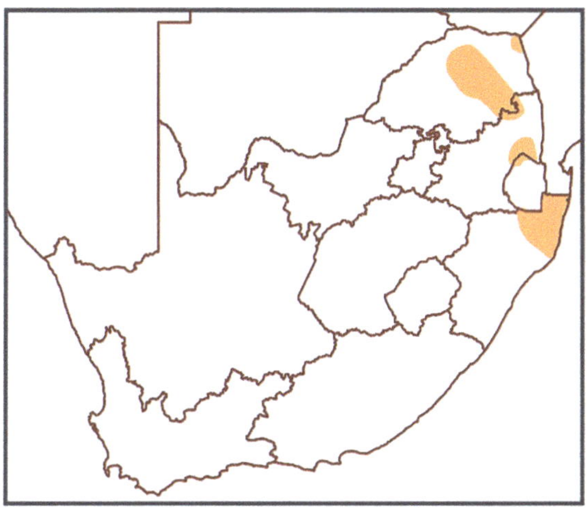

Geographical distribution of *Warburgia salutaris* in South Africa.

6. Ethnopharmacology

Warburgia salutaris is one of the most important medicinal plant species in southern Africa. Initially, this genus was utilised mainly for non-medicinal purposes, namely as a food seasoning, insecticide, for stimulating aggression in bees and dogs, for the crafting of wooden ornaments, and used as firewood (Lovett, 2006; Van Wyk et al., 2009; Van Wyk, 2011). The leaves of *W. salutaris* are used to increase appetite and to improve the organoleptic properties of food, due to its pungent peppery taste (Asfaw and Tadesse, 2001). Maroyi (2014) reported 43 ethnomedicinal uses for *W. salutaris* in countries from the southern African region. The diverse use of various parts of this tree for treating different ailments in traditional medicine has resulted in it being described as the panacea of Africa (Mavi, 1994; Van Wyk and Gericke, 2000). Traditional healers use *W. salutaris* as a natural antibiotic for various respiratory tract infections (coughs, colds and sinusitis), for candidiasis (oral thrush and cystitis), skin conditions, gastrointestinal ailments (stomach aches, constipation, stomach ulcers, as an emetic, and to treat hernias), as an analgesic (arthritis, rheumatism and headaches), antipyretic to combat protozoal diseases (malaria), and as a topical treatment for sexually transmitted disease-associated sores and inflammation. The powdered bark is most often used, but in some cases the leaves, roots and stalks are applied in traditional herbal formulations (Maroyi, 2013). The material is administered most often as a decoction or infusion (Maroyi, 2014), but occasionally through inhalation of the smoke, or as a snuff. Although monotherapy is conventionally used, polyherbal therapy using *W. salutaris* has been described (Maroyi, 2014). For example, in South Africa, *W. salutaris* mixed with fat, and occasionally together with *Hibiscus surattensis*, is applied topically to treat genital sores and inflammation (Hutchings et al., 1996; Van Wyk et al., 2009). Other polyherbal therapies include mixing of the bark of *W. salutaris* with the leaves of *Artemisia afra* and *Acorus calamus*, as an anti-infective agent (Felhaber and Mayeng, 1997), or with *Erythrophleum lasianthum*, as a snuff to treat headaches (Hutchings et al., 1996). As in the case of humans that use *W. salutaris* for traditional medicine, self-medication by various animals, including elephants, hippos and blue monkeys, has also been reported (Wing and Buss, 1970; Butynski, 1990; Maroyi, 2014).

7. Commercialisation

Various international patents have been filed for the use of *Warburgia* species as a chemotherapy agent, as well as for use in the flavour and fragrance industry (Kang et al., 1999; McKee and Karwic, 2009). A patent by Chu et al. (2008) claims various plant-derived bio-active compounds that are anticarcinogenic from *W. salutaris* as an alternative or complementary treatment for cancer (United States patent 0113042A1). A pharmaceutical dosage form was manufactured using organic and alcoholic extracts of *Warburgia* species (Schubert, 2011; EU patent EP2384762). This patent included claims for the development of pharmaceutical dosage forms, and methodology for the development of treatment regimens for microbial diseases and cancers. The most commonly used species in this invention was *W. salutaris* and *W. ugandensis*. In South Africa, Phyto Nova was the first company to produce a tablet containing *W. salutaris* in the form of freeze-dried leaves (Van Wyk, 2011), as a natural antibiotic for the treatment of oral and oesophageal thrush. Nyaba et al. (2018) patented (Patent no. PCT/IB2018/050583) a method for isolating compounds (especially iso-mukaadial acetate) from the stem-bark of *W. salutaris* for the treatment of malaria and for developing associated pharmaceutical dosage forms.

Warburgia salutaris is sold mostly in an uncontrolled manner on the informal market, leading to a sharp decline in wild populations (Maroyi, 2013). Therefore, controlled commercialisation, or large-scale cultivation of *W. salutaris* in a protected environment (e.g. by commercial growers or on game farms) has been initiated to reduce unsustainable harvesting practices. In 1996, when *W. salutaris* was named 'Tree of the Year', the Silverglen Nursery in Durban, South Africa grew large numbers of this tree, provided training on the commercial aspects of growing, and also supplied immature trees and cuttings to traditional healers and herbalists (Symmonds and Crouch, 2000). By 2000, Mr. Rodger Stewart has established a small plantation on a farm north of Durban (Personal communication C. Leonard with R. Stewart). As a result, freeze-dried leaves and bark are now available in small commercial quantities. Leonard and Viljoen (2015) proposed that intercropping with *W. salutaris*, its use as a decorative border, cultivation in provinces where the tree does not naturally occur, and the promotion of the antifeedant properties of the tree could provide additional sustainable material to the informal sector. A specimen of *W. salutaris* in the Kirstenbosch Gardens, Cape Town (Xaba and McVay, 2010) provides justification for the cultivation of the species in areas other than its natural habitat. The possibility of using leaves (with the same pungent taste as the bark) as substitute for the bark has been investigated. Leaves were used to produce the Phyto Nova tablets (marketed in 2000) as a natural antibiotic (Van Wyk, 2011). Due to its importance as a traditional medicine, some healers have started cultivating trees on a small scale for their own use (Botha et al., 2004).

8. Pharmacological evaluation

8.1 *In vitro* studies

8.1.1 Antimicrobial activity

The use of *W. salutaris* as a general 'tonic' is warranted due to its wide range of antimicrobial activities, as well as its widespread use in the treatment of infectious diseases (Van Wyk et al., 2009; Drewes, 2012). In various studies, Kubo and coworkers focussed on the antifungal activity of secondary metabolites (such as polygodial) against both yeasts and filamentous fungi, since most of the promising activity was noted for this group (Kubo et al., 1977; Nakanishi and Kubo, 1977; Taniguchi et al., 1984; Kubo and Taniguchi, 1988; Kubo, 1995; Lunde and Kubo, 2000; Kubo et al., 2001). Compounds such as muzigadial, polygodial and warburganal were highly active against various fungi. Both muzigadial and polygodial displayed strong antifungal activity with a minimum inhibition concentration (MIC) of 3.13 µg/mL reported against *Saccharomyces cerevisiae*, *Candida utilis* and *Sclerotinia libertiana* (Franklin, 1984). When the activities of the three compounds were compared (Taniguchi and Kubo, 1993), polygodial, with MICs ranging from 0.78 to 25 µg/mL, was most consistently potent against a variety of yeasts and filamentous fungi. The mechanism of action for polygodial seems to be the disruption of the hydrogen bonds at the lipid-protein interface, which denatures the protein (Fujita and Kubo, 2003). Another proposed mode of action of polygodial against *S. cerevisiae* is based on the possibility that the compound bypasses pump-based bacterial resistance by not entering the cells (Taniguchi et al., 1984). In contrast, the action of warburganal against the same organism was found to be through inhibition mechanisms, namely inhibition of growth, alcoholic fermentation and alcohol dehydrogenase activity. Cinnamodial and cinnamosmolide, produced by *W. salutaris*, were active against various azole-resistant strains of *Candida albicans* with MICs of 15.6 and 23.4 µg/mL, respectively (Tryvaud-Amiguet et al., 2006). Recently, Machaba and Mahlo (2017) completed an ethnobotanical survey (Limpopo Province, South Africa) *via* semistructured questionnaires and guided field work with traditional healers, to determine the traditional use of *W. salutaris* for fungal treatment. It was found that *W. salutaris* was used in 64.7% of antifungal treatments in the form of an infusion or decoction. Mabona et al. (2013) evaluated organic and aqueous extracts of both the leaves and bark of 47 plants for activity against a range of dermatologically important skin pathogens. The organic bark extract of *W. salutaris* displayed noteworthy antimicrobial activity (MIC range between 0.03 and 1.0 mg/mL) against all the pathogens tested, with the exception of *Brevibacillus agri* and *Microsporum canis.*

The crude extracts of 21 South African plants (including *W. salutaris*) used traditionally for the treatment of sepsis and infection were screened to evaluate their *in vitro* antibacterial ability (Rabe and Van Staden, 1997). Moderate activity (MIC 0.5 mg/mL) was reported for the methanolic extracts against *Bacillus subtilis* and *Staphylococcus aureus*, while *Staphylococcus epidermidis* was inactive (MIC 2.0 mg/mL). Poor results were also obtained for the aqueous extracts. Muzigadial, isolated from *W. salutaris*, was found to be highly active towards Gram-positive bacteria i.e. *S. aureus* (12.5 µg/mL), *B. subtilis* (12.5 µg/mL), *S. epidermis* (100 µg/mL) and *Micrococcus luteus* (50 µg/mL), and also displayed moderate activity towards *Escherichia coli* (100 µg/mL) (Rabe and Van Staden, 2000). Although the antibacterial activity was promising, it was negated by the cytotoxicity revealed in the study (Rabe and Van Staden, 2000). No antibacterial activity was reported for either the aqueous or methanolic extracts for *S. epidermis* or *S. aureus*, when using the zone inhibition assay (Steenkamp et al., 2005). As in the case of yeasts and filamentous fungi, polygodial displayed broad spectrum activity against a variety of organisms, with the best activity reported for *Salmonella choleraesuis* (MIC 50 µg/mL). The proposed mechanism of action was that the lipophilic nature of polygodial, or the terpenes as a collective, results in transport across the lipid-protein bilayer (Wink, 2003; Wink, 2008). At high concentration, it denatures the protein, which in turn affects not only the conformation of the protein, but also its bio-activity. A second proposed mechanism involves binding of the dialdehydes to the free amino-groups of the protein, resulting in the loss of conformation and bio-activity (Wink, 2008). Recently, Soyingbe et al. (2018) reported a zone inhibition of 21.0 mm for *S. aureus* when the acetone extract of the leaves of *W. salutaris* was tested (27.0 mm for positive control, ciprofloxacin and 1% DMSO as negative control were not active). The MIC for *S. aureus* was 160 µg/mL, which was considered noteworthy activity against *S. aureus*. They proposed that this noteworthy antimicrobial activity could be useful in indirectly boosting the immune system and also preventing opportunistic infections from developing in cancer patients. The methanol extract of the leaves showed a 53% inhibition of rhodamine 6G inside both *S. aureus* and *E. coli,* when using the cytosolic lactate dehydrogenase assay. The results suggest that the mechanism of action could be through efflux pumps.

Mohanlall and Odhav (2009) demonstrated that the *W. salutaris* heartwood extract in methanol/ethyl acetate and stem-bark extract in methanol/hexane displayed antifungal activity against *Fusarium moniliforme.* The dichloromethane leaf extract of *W. salutaris* also exhibited antifungal activity against *F. moniliforme*. Kubo and Taniguchi (1988) demonstrated that polygodial, one of the major compounds produced by *Warburgia* species, is fungicidal rather than fungistatic. They found that when *S. cerevisiae* was exposed to polygodial for 10 min, the cell membrane was visibly disrupted and vesicles were evident in the cytoplasm. Furthermore, polygodial was found to have greater potential when combined with other antibiotics. In a study of 30 plants used by Venda traditional healers for the treatment of fungus-related ailments, *W. salutaris* demonstrated antifungal activity (Samie et al., 2010). It was not only inhibitory to fungal growth, but also had fungicidal effects against three fungi tested (MIC/MFC between 0.11 and 7.5 mg/mL). Soyingbe et al. (2018) evaluated both the water and methanol extracts of *W. salutaris* leaves against saprophytic fungi. Noteworthy antifungal activity was observed for the organic extract against *Fusarium oxysporum* (MIC 10 µg/mL after 24 h) and *Aspergillus parasiticus* (20 µg/mL after 48 h). Generally, antimicrobial activity of 10 µg/mL for a crude extract is considered potent and useful for investigating pure compounds responsible for this activity (Kuete, 2010). These authors found that *W. salutaris* was one of the plants warranting further investigation.

8.1.2 Antimycobacterial activity

Mycobacterium tuberculosis, which causes tuberculosis (TB), remains problematic in developing countries. It is of particular concern in South Africa, which has one of the highest rates of infection in the world (McGaw et al., 2008). Plants traditionally used for the treatment of tuberculosis were identified using semistructured questionnaires (Tabuti et al., 2010). The traditional treatments, the majority of which contained *W. salutaris*, were most often administered in the form of decoctions or infusions. The sesquiterpene lactone, 11α-hydroxycinnamosmolide, isolated from *W. salutaris*, was reported to display *in vitro* activity against both *M. tuberculosis* H37Rv and *Mycobacterium bovis* BCG at a concentration of 100 μg/mL over a 10-day period (Madikane et al., 2007). This study indicated that both the crude extract and the isolated compound, 11α-hydroxycinnamosmolide, inhibited the enzyme arylamine *N*-acetyltransferase, thereby blocking mycobacterial cell-wall lipid synthesis. The acetone extract of the leaves of *W. salutaris* were also evaluated for bacterial activity and a noteworthy MIC of 25 μg/mL was reported. The antimycobacterial activity of 14 medicinal plants used in the traditional treatment of TB and other respiratory tract infections were evaluated (Dzoyem et al., 2016). Antimycobacterial activity of the acetone leaf extracts of *W. salutaris* was determined against several fast growing *Mycobacterium* species, namely *Mycobacterium smegmatis*, *Mycobacterium aurum* and *Mycobacterium fortuitum*, as well as towards a field isolate of *M. tuberculosis*. In this study, the MIC and the half-maximal lethal concentration (LC_{50}) for VERO cells were reported. Noteworthy antimycobacterial activity was reported against all the *Mycobacterium* species tested (including the field isolate) with the highest activity against *M. aurum*. Using the tetrazolium-based colorimetric cell proliferation (MTT assay) for the VERO cell-line, the acetone extract yielded a LC_{50} value of 74.67 ± 8.45 μg/mL, in comparison to the approved anticancer drug, doxorubicin, for which an IC_{50} value of 4.51 ± 0.57 μg/mL was reported. This result indicates that the extract is relatively safe to human cells. Although plants used are generally safe for human and animal consumption, certain concentrations may be cytotoxic (Fennell et al., 2004). To safeguard against this, an additional calculation for the selectivity index ($SI = LC_{50}/MIC$), which is the measure of potential efficacy *vs* possible adverse effects, was done. The SI ranged from 0.06 to 0.5 mg/mL for *M. fortuitum*, which indicates that the margin between potential efficacy and cytotoxicity is narrow.

8.1.3 Antiparasitic activity

Malaria, caused by the protozoa, *Plasmodium*, affects approximately 600 million people worldwide, of which approximately 1 million cases are fatal (Lacroix et al., 2011). Although the use of *Warburgia* as traditional treatment for malaria has not been widely reported (Pillay et al., 2008), anecdotal evidence suggests that the inhabitants of various African countries use the stem-bark for this purpose (Felhaber and Mayeng, 1997; Bussmann et al., 2006; Makunga et al., 2008; Graz et al., 2011). The dichloromethane extract of the stem-bark and isomukaadial acetate were found to be effective against a chloroquine-sensitive *Plasmodium* strain (NF54), with half maximal inhibitory concentration (IC_{50}) values of 0.01 ± 0.30 and 0.44 ± 0.10 μg/mL, respectively (Nyaba et al., 2018). These authors concluded that the results justified the traditional use of *W. salutaris* for the treatment of malaria. The root-bark extract of *W. ugandensis* exhibited antiplasmodial activity (IC_{50} value of 4.1 μg/mL; Muthaura et al., 2015). The authors also reported that the methanol stem-bark extract of *W. stuhlmannii* was one of the four plant extracts for which an IC_{50} value of less than 5 mg/mL had been obtained against both chloroquine-resistant (D6) and -sensitive (W2) *Plasmodium falciparum* (Muthaura et al., 2011).

The dichloromethane extract (containing the non-volatile fraction) of the stem-bark was most effective against *Trypanosoma brucei*, with an IC_{50} value of 10.68 µg/mL (Nibret et al., 2010). Further exploration of the antitrypanosomal activity of isolated compounds indicated noteworthy activities for muzigadiolide, mukaadial and 6α,9α-dihydroxy-4(13),7-coloratadiene-11,12-dial, which were attributed to the hydroxyl group at position 9 (Wube et al., 2010). Muzigadial was also reported to be an effective antitrypanosomal agent (Olila et al., 2001). Its activity was attributed to the ability of sesquiterpenes (such as muzigadial, warburganal and polygodial) to form covalent bonds with the amino groups of proteins, thereby affecting a number of cellular activities (Van Wyk and Wink, 2004). Another possible mechanism of action, proposed by Hermann et al. (2011), was the interference of the sesquiterpenes with the trypanothione redox system of trypanosomes. The *in vitro* antitrypanosomal activity of 40 Tanzanian plants, extracted with both dichloromethane and methanol, was evaluated against *Trypanosoma bruce*i (Nibret et al., 2010). The dichloromethane extract of *W. salutaris* had the most potent activity with a corresponding IC_{50} value of 10.68 µg/mL. The researchers reported that *W. salutaris* should be explored for lead compounds, since it was one of five traditional plants investigated that met criteria for efficacy and non-toxicity. Clark and Appleton (1997) evaluated the antimolluscicidal potential of the crude aqueous extracts of six South African indigenous plant species. *Warburgia salutaris* was reported to be one of the three most highly ranked plants investigated, based on the reported toxicity of the crude aqueous extract and cultivation potential (i.e. germination, growth rate and drought resistance).

Bilharzia (schistosomiasis), caused by parasitic worms, is of growing concern in Africa, with 90% of those infected living in sub-Saharan Africa (Olveda et al., 2013). The strategy to eradicate parasitic worms is to kill snails, which are the vectors. *Warburgia salutaris* was one of the southern African trees that met all the determined criteria set for a potential molluscicidal plant (Clark et al., 1997). These plants were evaluated against *Bulinus africanus*, which hosts the parasitic worms that cause urinary bilharzia. The dry leaf material of *W. salutaris* ranked third highest in its antimolluscicidal properties, with 2.48 g/L necessary to kill 50% of the snails over a period of 48 h.

8.1.4 Anti-inflammatory activity

Inflammation and conditions related to an inflammatory response in the body have been widely reported (Weiss, 1979; Dowsett-Lemaire and White, 1990; Johns et al., 1999; Zschocke et al., 2000; Kokwaro, 2009). Based on the ethnomedicinal use of the plant for the treatment of conditions related to inflammatory responses, Frum et al. (2005) evaluated both the *in vitro* anti-inflammatory (5-lipoxygenase inhibitory activity) and anti-oxidant activity of the methanol and aqueous extracts of

W. salutaris leaves using the 2,2-diphenyl-1-picrylhydrazyl radical (DPPH) assay. They reported an IC_{50} value less than 33 µg/mL for the *in vitro* methanol extract, indicating good anti-inflammatory activity, whereas the aqueous extracts were inactive. In contrast, both the aqueous and methanol extracts of the leaves exhibited promising anti-oxidant activities with IC_{50} values of 34.43 and 15.38 µg/mL, respectively. They speculated that the hydroxyl function present on C-6 in warburganal may be responsible for the higher anti-inflammatory activity of the compound as compared to that of mukaadial. The other drimane sesquiterpenes present in *W. salutaris* also contribute to its anti-inflammatory activity, but the anti-oxidant activity is not limited to these compounds. Cock and Van Vuuren (2014) investigated the effects of a variety of traditionally used South African medicinal plants for their effectiveness against *Proteus mirabilis* and *Proteus vulgaris,* which are known microbial triggers of rheumatoid arthritis. Among other plants, the water and methanol extracts of leaves and bark of *W. salutaris* were evaluated for activity against these organisms. The bark extracts were most active against both organisms as reflected by MICs of less than 1 mg/mL. Later, Cock and Van Vuuren (2015) investigated 13 South African plant species with documented traditional use for inflammatory activity against the microbial trigger (*Klebsiella pneumoniae*) involved in the auto-immune disease ankylosing spondylitis. Although the MICs were established for both the bark and leaf extracts (methanol and aqueous), only the bark demonstrated noteworthy activity of 624 and 677 µg/mL, respectively. Promising anti-oxidant activity was reported for both the aqueous and methanol extracts of the leaves, with IC_{50} values of 34.43 and 15.38 µg/mL, respectively (Frum et al., 2005). Kuglerova et al. (2011) attributed the anti-oxidant properties (IC_{50} value of 6.59 µg/mL) of *W. salutaris* to the presence of tannins, which affect the activity of proteins, starches, cellulose and minerals. Flavonoids have the ability to scavenge free radicals, chelate metal ions and inhibit enzymes responsible for free radical generation (Ebenharder and Grünhage, 2003). The free radical scavenging potential of the water and methanol extracts of the stem-bark were reported as 30% and 80%, respectively (Steenkamp et al., 2005). Higher concentrations of phenolic compounds were present in the crude methanol extract of the bark (3.6 mg/g), while the methanol extract of the leaf material contained the most flavonoids (13.8 mg/g) (Steenkamp et al., 2013), which are known to display good anti-oxidant activity.

8.1.5 Anticancer and antiviral activities

Traditionally, Zulu healers use the leaves of *W. salutaris* for the treatment of cancer. In a study by Soyingbe et al. (2018), the MTT assay was used to determine the effect, if any, of the acetone extract of *W. salutaris* towards cancer cell lines, namely MCF-7, Caco-2, A549 and HeLa. All displayed noteworthy activity (IC_{50} value of 34.15 µg/mL). The LD_{50} (10 µg/mL) for methanol leaf extracts of *W. salutaris* indicated toxicity towards VERO cell lines, with SI values between 0.06 and 0.5 mg/mL. Recently, Viol et al. (2016) evaluated the *in vitro* toxicity using the VERO cell lines and the

Brine Shrimp Lethality Test (BSLT or LC_{50}), as well as the antiviral properties of the methanol extracts of the leaves, roots and stem-bark of *W. salutaris* against herpes simplex virus type 2 (sexually transmitted disease that causes genital herpes). In this assay, all three plant parts (leaves, root, and stem-bark) were found to be relatively toxic ($LC_{50} < 500$ μg/mL) with LC_{50} values of 351.41 ± 29.58, 426.10 ± 55.55 and 359 ± 14.33 μg/mL, respectively. The stem-bark [50% cytotoxicity concentration (CC_{50}) 19.53 μg/mL] and leaves (CC_{50} = 78.13 μg/mL) exhibited high cytotoxicity activity against VERO cells. They also yielded a low reduction factor of 1. The methanol extract of the roots was also cytotoxic towards the VERO cell line (CC_{50} = 39.06 μg/mL) and yielded a high viral reduction factor of 10^3. These results indicate that the roots of *W. salutaris* have potential antitumour and antiviral activities that should be further investigated.

8.2 *In vivo* studies and clinical trials

8.2.1 Antimalarial activity

Nyaba et al. (2018) utilised previous reports on the antimalarial activity of the stem-bark of *W. ugandensis* and isolated a new compound (related to mukaadial), namely isomukaadial acetate, from *W. salutaris*. The *in vitro* cytotoxicity of the compound was subsequently evaluated using the MTT assay towards both liver hepatocellular carcinoma (HEPG2) and human embryotic kidney (HEK239) cell lines. The pure compound exhibited only low cytotoxicity (IC_{50} values of 36.7 ± 0.8 and 119.2 ± 8.8 μg/mL) towards the HEK293 and HEPG2 cells, respectively, while very good activity was recorded for the inhibition of the growth of *P. falciparum* (IC_{50} value of 0.44 ± 0.10 μg/mL). The authors indicated that a compound is generally considered successful in the drug discovery process if the IC_{50} value in the presence of the microbe being investigated is less than or equal to 1 μg/mL. Furthermore, the compound must be 10 times more active against the parasite or pathogen than against the human cell lines. In this study, isomukaadial acetate met both these criteria. The *in vitro* IC_{50} (0.01 ± 0.30 μg/mL) for the crude dichloromethane extract was less than that of the pure compound. Thereafter, animal studies were carried out using 16–18 week-old male Sprague–Dawley rats infected with the chloroquine-sensitive *P. berghei* ($n = 36$). The negative control group was infected, but not treated ($n = 12$). The mice in the infected group were treated once a day at a dose of 0.5, 1.5 or 2.5 mg/kg and the positive control group with 5 mg/kg chloroquine. Chloroquine performed the best, followed by the compound isomuzigadial acetate when administered for 5 days. The parasitaemia of the untreated group increased to a maximum of 60% after 12 days. In contrast, the percentage parasitaemia decreased to a negligible amount (after 21 days) for the crude extract, isomukaadial acetate administered once a day for 5 days as well as for the group treated with chloroquine. The pure compound was also able to prevent malaria-associated weight loss. These authors concluded that they had scientifically validated the traditional use of *W. salutaris* for antimalarial treatment and patented the use of this compound accordingly.

8.2.2 Anti-HIV-related infections

A study at a rural community hospital in KwaZulu-Natal Province, South Africa indicated that a large number of patients, especially infants, developed severe HIV-associated oral candidiasis (Motsei et al., 2003). Several plants used traditionally for the treatment of *Candida* infections were evaluated *in vitro* by extracting the appropriate plant parts with water, ethyl acetate, ethanol and hexane. The aqueous bark extract (MIC 6.5 mg/mL) of *W. salutaris* was among the most effective extracts against a clinical isolate from a 5-month-old baby. In addition, the aqueous extracts also showed *in vitro* activity against an isolate from an adult, as well as towards the American Type Culture Collection (ATCC) control (MIC 12.5 mg/mL for both). *Warburgia salutaris* was identified as one of the priority plants for the treatment of HIV-associated oral candidiasis (Lamorde et al., 2010). Researchers evaluated the time-dependent fungicidal effects of *W. salutaris* towards *C. albicans* at 0.4 mg/mL and reported a six-log reduction after 5 h. In a survey, using a structured questionnaire, 25 traditional medicine practitioners were interviewed regarding their knowledge on plants used for the treatment of HIV/AIDS and opportunistic infections associated with these conditions (Lamorde et al., 2010). In this survey, *W. salutaris* was identified in these areas as a priority plant out of the 103 plants reported and, although the symptom was associated with a cough, the practitioner identified it as an HIV/AIDS-associated cough. Devaraj and Roelofson (2015) surveyed the use of complementary medicines or natural products in conjunction with antiretroviral drugs (ARVs) for the treatment of HIV and reported that *W. salutaris* was one of the priority trees to be used in combination with ARVs.

8.2.3 Other activities

Ngure (2014) evaluated the effect of crude extracts of *W. ugandensis*, alone or as adjuvants for *Leishmania* vaccines, in Balb/c mice. Both the hexane and dichloromethane extracts, when injected together with the antigens, were mildly immunostimulatory. However, the combinations slowed down the development of cutaneous lesions and the parasite burden decreased. Efficacy of extractives and isolates from *W. ugandensis* were evaluated for the protection of maize grain against *Sitophilus zeamais*. The oil extract was the most repellent, followed by the hexane extract. The most repellent compounds were mukaadial and polygodial (Opiyo et al., 2015), while the essential oil was the most toxic to the weevils and caused 100% mortality at 21 days. The toxicity levels of the organic extracts ranged from 18.3% to 78.0%, with the hexane extract exhibiting the highest toxicity, followed by the ethyl acetate extract. The oil extract was as active as the actellic dust (control), and completely inhibited the emergence of the insect adults. Polygodial, ugandensolide and warbuganal had the best growth inhibition activity. The results from the present study indicated that *W. ugandensis* could be a useful alternative in the protection of stored grain against maize weevil, and that the isolated compounds are good candidates as phyto-insecticidal agents against insect pests. Ahmed et al. (2014) studied the *in vivo* effect of the ethanol extracts of five plants as an alternative treatment to combat sheep nematodes.

Warburgia species reduced both the nematode egg production and infective larval yields in sheep.

8.3 Safety

The widespread use of *Warburgia* species as a spice to flavour food and in traditional medicine for various diseases, has resulted in this genus being generally regarded as safe for human and animal use. Aqueous stem-bark extracts of *W. ugandensis* had CC_{50} >250 µg/mL and were classified as not cytotoxic. *Warburgia ugandensis* extracts did not cause mortality in BALB/c mice with an LD_{50} >5000 mg/kg body weight in an acute toxicity study. The weights of mice that survived the entire 14 days in all groups increased and were not significantly different from that of controls (Karani et al., 2013). The safety of the pure compounds, as well as various solvent extracts from the stem-bark of *W. salutaris*, remains contentious. Rabe and Van Staden (2000) reported that muzigadial, isolated from the stem-bark of *W. salutaris*, displayed cytotoxic activity, which could possibly explain the potent antimicrobial activity reported earlier (Rabe and van Staden, 1997). Recently, Nyaba et al. (2018) found that isomukaadial acetate, also isolated from the stem-bark of *W. salutaris*, displayed antimalarial activity, but was not cytotoxic towards mammalian cell lines (IC_{50} 0.44 ± 0.1 µg/mL). A similar result was achieved for the dichloromethane crude extracts, which exhibited antimalarial activity, but were not cytotoxic when tested against mammalian cell lines (IC_{50} 0.01 ± 0.3 µg/mL). This absence of cytotoxicity towards mammalian cells, but still having antimycobacterial or antiparasitic activity for the same extract, was also confirmed by Madikane et al. (2007) and Nibret et al. (2010). Steenkamp et al. (2005) and Verschaeve and Van Staden (2008), using the Ames and Vitotox assays, reported that aqueous, methanol and dichloromethane extracts of the stem-bark displayed no genotoxicity or mutagenicity. However, Wan-Ibrahim et al. (2010) reported a direct link between high anti-oxidant activity and mutagenicity. They reported that the aqueous extract of the stem-bark caused moderate (20%–50%) damage to DNA, which they correlated to moderate anti-oxidant activity for this extract. The use of *W. salutaris* by pregnant women is not advised, since it has abortifacient properties or can induce labour (Neuwinger, 2000).

9. Phytochemistry

9.1 Volatile constituents

Volatile organic compounds are produced in both the stem-bark and the leaves. The essential oil profile of *W. salutaris* obtained using one-dimensional gas chromatography was first described by Leonard et al. (2010) and later by Lawal et al. (2014). The volatile fraction of the leaves is dominated by monoterpenes, including myrcene and the *cis*- and *trans*-β-ocimenes. Khumalo et al. (2018) isolated essential oils from the bark of a cultivated tree and reported the isolation of drimenol and *E*-nerolidol.

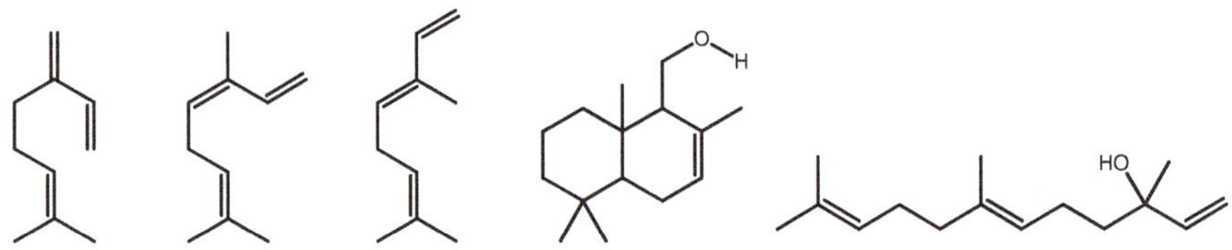

Myrcene | *cis*-β-Ocimene | *trans*-β-Ocimene | Drimenol | *trans*-Nerolidol

9.2 Non-volatile constituents

Since Brooks and Draffen (1969a, b) isolated two novel sesquiterpenoids, warburgin and warburgiadione, as well as drimenol, from the heartwood of *W. ugandensis*, the search for biologically active compounds from *Warburgia* species has continued. In traditional medicine, the use of the stem-bark of *W. salutaris* is well known and therefore most of the research has been focused on this species and plant part. To date, 19 of the 47 compounds (non-volatile fraction) isolated from the stem-bark of other *Warburgia* species have been reported to occur in *W. salutaris* (Leonard and Viljoen, 2015). Szallasi et al. (1998) reported that unsaturated terpenoid dialdehydes, such as polygodial, warburganal, muzigadial and ugandensidial, are pungent compounds present in the bark of *W. ugandensis* and *W. stuhlmannii*. All these compounds are hot tasting to humans. The hot taste of polygodial and epipolygodial was attributed to the presence and configuration of the aldehyde at C-9. The hot taste has also been associated with antifeedant properties in insects. Several antifeedant compounds were isolated from *W. stuhlmannii*; polygodial and the two lactones, cinnamolide and bemadienolide (Kubo et al., 1977). Researchers also isolated 11 drimane sesquiterpenes, of which four were novel compounds from *Warburgia*, namely 3β-hydroxy-cinnamolide, cinnamolide-3β-acetate, diacetyl-ugandensolide and muzigadiolide (Kioy et al., 1990). This was the first report of an oxygenated moiety on the C-3 position of the drimane sesquiterpenes in *Warburgia*. Drimane sesquiterpenes that have been isolated from *W. salutaris* include 11α-hydroxy-cinnamosmolide (Madikane et al., 2007), isopolygodial (isotadeonal), warburganal and polygodial (Mashimbye, 1993), salutarisolide (Mashimbye et al., 1999; Frum et al., 2005; Frum and Viljoen, 2006), muzigadial (cannelal) (Rabe and Van Staden, 2000), ugandensidial (cinnamodial), isopolygodial (Mashimbye et al., 1999) and mukaadial (Mashimbye et al., 1999). The drimane lactone, salutarisolide, was found to be unique to the stem-bark of *W. salutaris*, but similar in structure to muzigadiolide, isolated previously. However, stereochemical differences were evident at C-9, resulting in differences in their optical rotation (Kioy et al., 1990). Muzigadial (Mashimbye et al., 1999; Rabe and Van Staden, 2000; Mohanlall and Odhav, 2009) and ugandensidial (Mashimbye et al., 1999; Khumalo et al., 2018) were also isolated by several researchers from the stem-bark of *W. salutaris*. Seven new and four known drimane and colorane-type sesquiterpenes were identified from the antimycobacterial fraction obtained from the stem-bark of a cultivated specimen using hyphenated nuclear magnetic resonance (NMR) spectroscopy techniques (Clarkson et al., 2007). The presence of the biologically active polygodial and warburganal in both leaf and bark samples was the impetus for Drewes et al. (2001) to propose the interchangeable use of leaves with bark in traditional medicine, for conservation purposes. They reported that there was no significant difference in the ratio of the two sesquiterpenes present, irrespective of the plant part evaluated. Khumalo et al. (2018) isolated 12α-acetyl polygodial, polygodial, ugandensidial and warburganal from a dichloromethane extract of the bark. Mannitol, a sugar alcohol found in most plants, also occurs in the bark of *W. salutaris* (Van Wyk et al., 2009). This polyol is an osmotic diuretic agent and acts as an osmo-regulator in the human body.

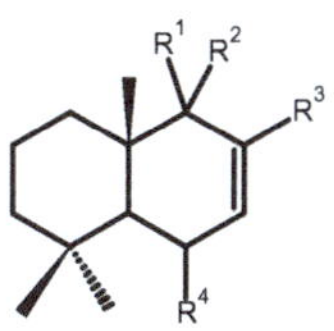

Polygodial: R¹=β-CHO, R²=R⁴=H, R³=CHO
Warburganal: R¹=β-CH, R²=α-OH, R³=CHO, R⁴= H

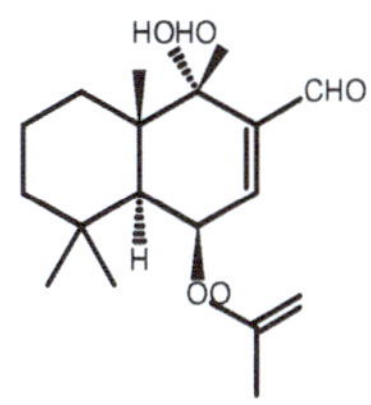

Cinnamodial

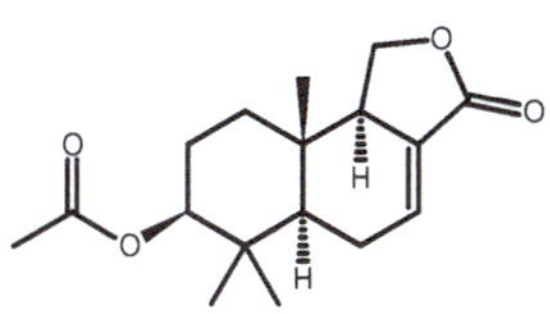

Cinnamolide-3-β-acetate

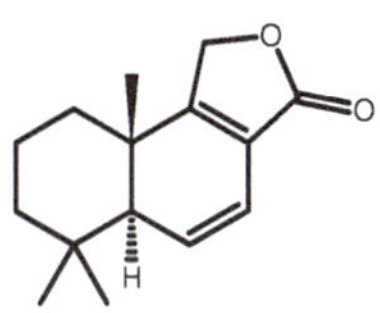

Bemadienolide

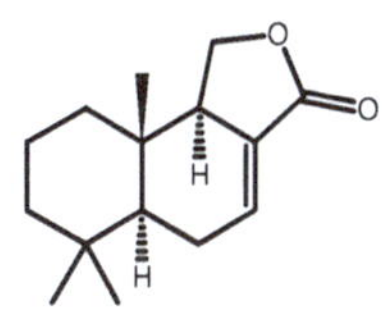

Cinnamolide

Part B: Chemical profiling and quality control

10. Chromatography analysis

10.1 High-performance thin-layer chromatography (HPTLC) fingerprint analysis

General instrumentation: CAMAG HPTLC instrument consisting of an automatic TLC sampler (ATS 4), automatic developing chamber (ADC 2), CAMAG TLC visualiser 2, CAMAG immersion device and TLC plate heater. *HPTLC plates:* Silica gel glass plates 60 F_{254} (Merck).

10.1.1 Non-volatile fraction analysis

Plant part: Bark extracted with methanol:acetic acid (9:1, v/v). *Sample application:* Application volume of 2 μL methanol extract (10 mg/mL) and standard (1 mg/mL) spotted as 10-mm bands. Plates developed in a 20 × 10 × 4 cm glass twin-trough chamber to a migration distance of 85 mm. *Tank saturation:* 20 min at 25 °C and 47% RH, with 25 mL of mobile phase. *Mobile phase:* Dichloromethane:ethyl acetate (90:10, v/v). *Derivatisation:* *p*-Anisaldehyde sulphuric acid reagent. The plate was dipped in reagent and heated for 3 min at 100 °C on a TLC plate heater and then visualised. *Visualisation:* The plate was viewed under 366 nm fluorescent light.

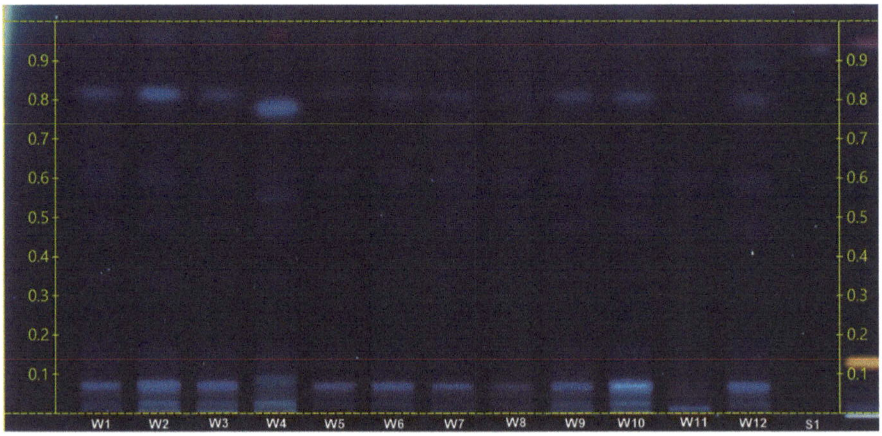

HPTLC plate of *Warburgia salutaris* methanol bark extracts (n = 12), W1–W6 (wild harvested), W7–W12 (cultivated), and the standard (S1). The samples are characterised by a pink band for polygodial (S1) (R_f = 0.95).

10.1.2 Essential oil analysis

Plant part: Leaves, essential oil. *Sample application:* Application volume of 2 μL essential oil (25 μL/mL in toluene) and standard (25 μL/mL in toluene) spotted as 10 mm bands. Plates developed in a 20 × 10 × 4 cm glass twin-trough chamber to a migration distance of 85 mm. *Tank saturation:* 20 min at 20 °C and 47% RH, with 25 mL of mobile phase. *Mobile phase:* Toluene:ethyl acetate:glacial acetic acid (90:10:1, v/v). *Derivatisation:* *p*-Anisaldehyde sulphuric acid reagent. The plate was dipped in reagent and heated for 3 min at 100 °C on a TLC plate heater and visualised. *Visualisation:* The plate was viewed under white reflectance light.

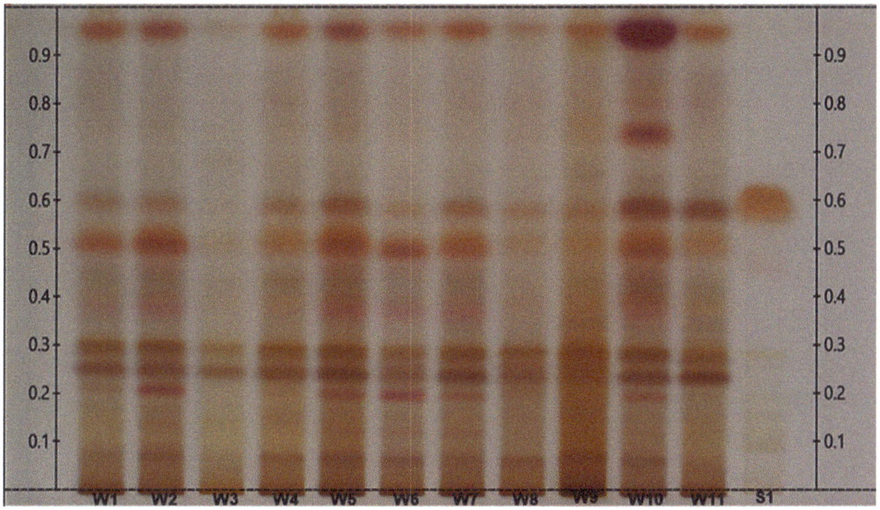

HPTLC plate of *Warburgia salutaris* essential oils ($n = 11$), W1–W6 (wild harvested), W7–W11 (cultivated), and the standard (S1). The samples are characterised by a brown band for myrcene (S1) ($R_f = 0.58$).

10.2 Ultra-performance liquid chromatography (UPLC) analysis

General instrumentation: Waters Acquity Ultra-Performance Liquid Chromatography system with photodiode array (PDA) detector combined with a Xevo G2QToF mass spectrometer (Waters, USA). *Plant part:* Bark, methanol extract. *Sample application:* Injection volume of 2.0 µL (full-loop injection) at 1 mg/mL. *Column:* Acquity UPLC BEH C_{18} column (150 mm × 2.1 mm, i.d., 1.7 µm particle size, Waters). *Mobile phase:* 0.1% formic acid in water (solvent A) and acetonitrile (solvent B). *Analysis conditions:* Gradient elution at a flow rate of 0.3 mL/min, changing as follows: 90% A: 10% B changed to 50% A: 50% B in 4 min, to 25% A: 75% B in 6 min, to 5% A: 95% B in 2.5 min, back to initial ratio in 0.5 min, equilibrating the system for 2 min, total run time 15 min. *Mass spectrometry*: ESI^+ (positive ionisation mode), N_2 used as desolvation gas, desolvation temperature 350 °C at a flow rate of 500 L/h and source temperature at 100 °C. Capillary and cone voltages 3500 and 20 V, respectively. Data collected between *m/z* 100 and 1500.

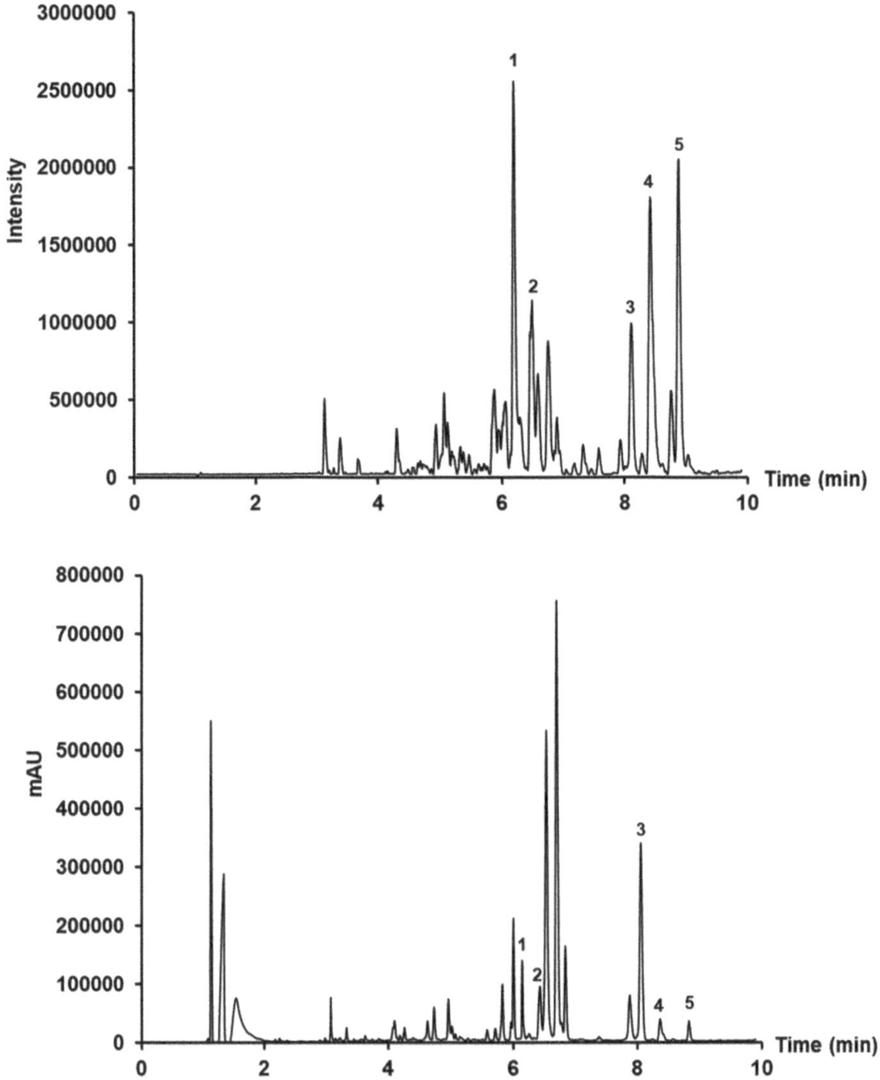

UPLC-ToF-MS ESI$^+$ (upper) and PDA (lower) chromatograms of *Warburgia salutaris* methanol extracts. [1] = ugandensidial *m/z* 309.1702, [2] = cinnamolide-3β-acetate *m/z* 293.1763, [3] = polygodial *m/z* 235.1704, [4] = bemadienolide *m/z* 233.1551, [5] = cinnamolide *m/z* 235.1705.

10.3 Gas chromatography (GC) analysis

General instrumentation: An Agilent 6860N chromatograph (Agilent Technologies, Hanova, USA) fitted with a flame ionisation detector and a mass spectrometer. *Column:* HP-Innowax, 60 m × 250 μm × 0.25 μm (polyethylene glycol column, Agilent Technologies, Hanova, USA). *Plant part:* Aerial parts, essential oil. *Sample application:* Injection volume of 1 μL (split) at 20% (v/v) in hexane. *Analysis conditions:* Inlet temperature 250 °C, split ratio: 1:200, helium carrier gas, flow rate: 1.2 mL/min, pressure: 24.79 psi. Starting oven temperature at 60 °C and then increase to 220 °C at 4 °C/min, holding for 10 min, and increased to 240 °C at 1 °C/min. *Mass spectrometry conditions:* Chromatograms obtained upon electron impact at 70 eV on an Agilent 5973 mass selective detector, scanning range: *m/z* 35 to 550 (Agilent Technologies, Hanova, USA). *Identification:* Authentic standards, NIST®, Mass Finder®.

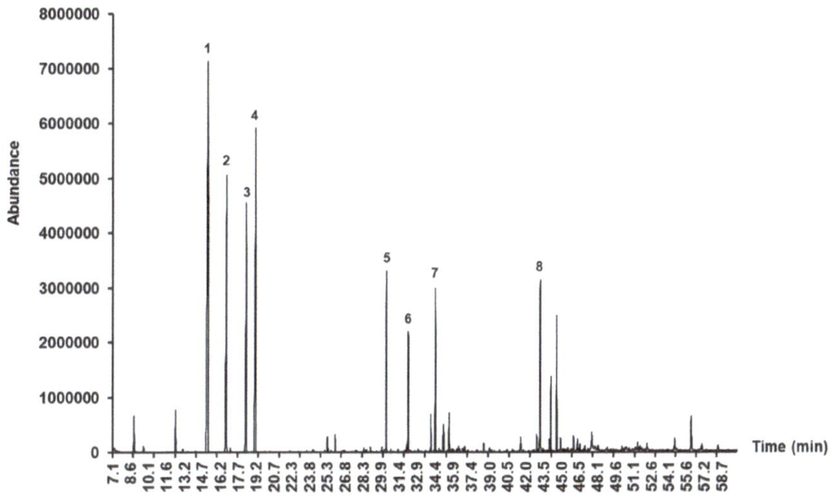

Total ion chromatograms (TIC) of *Warburgia salutaris* essential oil indicating major compounds; [1] = myrcene (R_t 15.13, *m/z* 136.1252), [2] = limonene (R_t 16.72, *m/z* 136.1252), [3] = Z-β-ocimene (R_t 18.41, *m/z* 136.1252), [4] = γ-terpinene (R_t 19.21, *m/z* 136.1252), [5] = linalool (R_t 30.33, *m/z* 154.1358), [6] = β-caryophyllene (R_t 32.16, *m/z* 204.1878), [7] = α-humulene (R_t 34.44, *m/z* 204.1878), [8] = caryophyllene oxide (R_t 43.21, *m/z* 220.1828).

11. Mid-infrared (MIR) spectroscopy analysis

General instrumentation: Alpha-P Bruker spectrometer, mounted with an attenuated total reflectance (ATR) diamond crystal. *Spectral acquisition:* Spectrum obtained in absorbance mode, with a spectral resolution of 4 cm^{-1} over the range 4000–550 cm^{-1} and captured using OPUS 6.5 software.

11.1 Powder analysis

Plant part: Leaf and bark. *Sample preparation:* Plant parts powdered, sieved (< 500 μm) and placed directly onto the surface of the diamond crystal.

11.2 Essential oil analysis

Plant part: Aerial parts, essential oil. *Sample preparation:* Aerial parts, hydro-distillation to obtain essential oil, placed directly onto the surface of the diamond crystal.

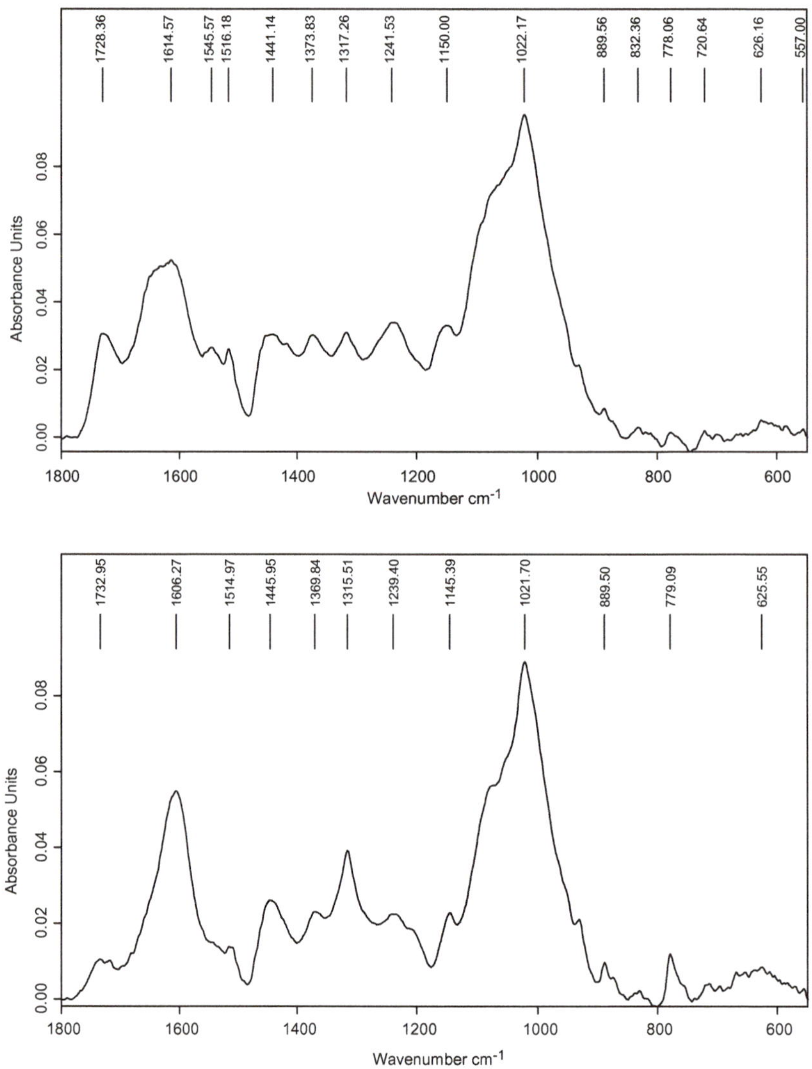

Mid-infrared spectrum of *Warburgia salutaris* leaf (upper) and bark (lower) powder displaying the fingerprint region (1800–550 cm^{-1}).

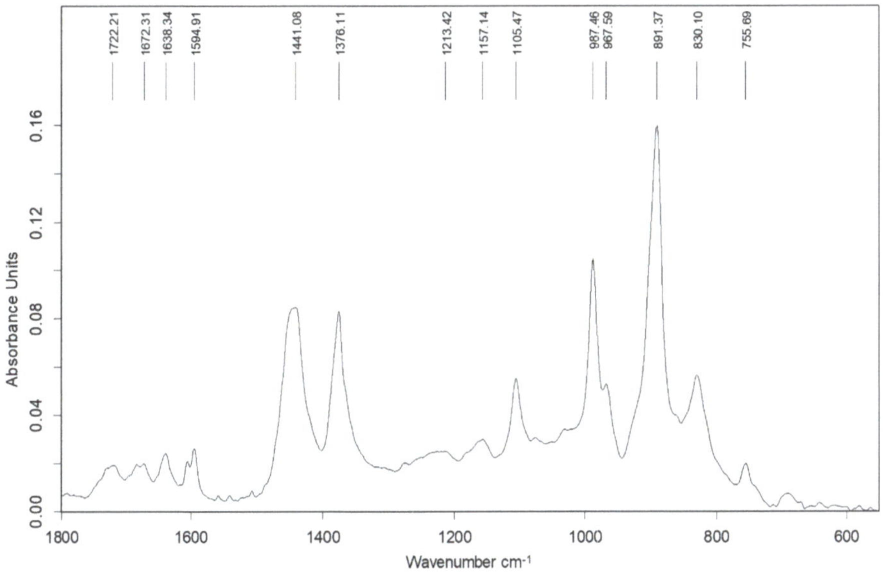

Mid-infrared spectrum of *Warburgia salutaris* essential oil displaying the fingerprint region (1800–550 cm^{-1}).

References

Ahmed, M., Laing, M.D., Nsahlai, I.V., 2014. Trop. Anim. Health Prod., 46:411–417.

Asfaw, Z., Tadesse, M., 2001. Econ. Bot., 55:47–62.

Botha, J., Witkowski, E.T.F., Shackleton, C.M., 2004. Biodivers. Conserv., 13:1675–1698.

Brooks, C.J.W., Draffan, G.H., 1969a. Tetrahedron, 25:2865–2885.

Brooks, C.J.W., Draffan, G.H., 1969b. Tetrahedron, 25:2887–2898.

Bussmann, R., Gilbreath, G.G., Solio, J., Lutura, M., Lutuluo, R., Kunguru, K., Wood, N., Mathenge, S.G., 2006. J. Ethnobiol. Ethnomed., 2:22–29.

Butynski, T.M., 1990. Ecol. Monograph., 60:1–26.

Chu, K.H., Ho, C.Y., Xie, W.D., 2008. Pharmaceutical Composition and Method for Cancer Treatment Based on Combinational Use of Conventional Anticancer Agents and Geranium Oil or Compounds Thereof. Google Patents.

Clark, T.E., Appleton, C.C., 1997. J. Ethnopharmacol., 56:15–30.

Clark, T.E., Appleton, C.C., Drewes, S.E., 1997. J. Ethnopharmacol., 56:1–13.

Clarkson, C., Madikane, E.V., Hansen, S.H., Smith, P.J., Jaroszewski, J.W., 2007. Planta Med., 73:578–584.

Cock, I., Van Vuuren, S., 2014. Inflammopharmacology, 22:1–14.

Cock, I., Van Vuuren, S., 2015. Inflammopharmacology, 23:21–35.

Devaraj, A., Roelofson, M.F., 2015. World J. Pharm. Res., 4:941–946.

Dlamini, T.S., Dlamini, G.M., 2002. Swaziland. In: Golding, J.S. (Ed.), Southern African Plant Red Data Lists. Southern African Botanical Insitute, Pretoria, South Africa.

Dowsett-Lemaire, F., 1989. Bull. Jard. Bot. Natl. Belg/Bull. Natl. Plantentuin Belg., 59:3–131.

Dowsett-Lemaire, F., White, F., 1990. Bull. Jard. Bot. Natl. Belg/Bull. Natl. Plantentuin Belg., 60:73–110.
Drewes, S.E., 2012. S. Afri. J. Sci., 108:17–24.
Drewes, S.E., Crouch, N., Mashimbye, M.J., De Leeuw, B., Horn, M., 2001. S. Afri. J. Sci., 97:383–386.
Dzoyem, J.P., Aro, A.O., McGaw, L.J., Eloff, J.N., 2016. S. Afr. J. Bot., 102:70–74.
Ebenharder, R., Grünhage, D., 2003. Mutat Res. Genet. Toxicol. Environ. Mutagen., 540:1–18.
Engler, A., 1895. Winteranaceae (Canellaceae). Die Pflanzenwelt Ost-Afrikas und der Nachbargebiete C, 276.
Felhaber, T., Mayeng, I., 1997. South African Traditional Healers Primary Health Care Handbook. Kagiso Publishers, Cape Town, South Africa.
Fennell, C., Lindsey, K., Mcgaw, L., Sparg, S., Stafford, G., ElgorashI, E., Grace, O., Van Staden, J., 2004. J. Ethnopharmacol., 94:205–217.
Franklin, D., 1984. Sci. News, 125:375.
Frum, Y., Viljoen, A.M., 2006. Skin Pharmacol. Physiol., 19:329–335.
Frum, Y., Viljoen, A., Drewes, S., 2005. S. Afr. J. Bot., 71:447–449.
Fujita, K.I., Kubo, I., 2003. J. Chem. Ecol., 29:2253–2262.
Graz, B., Kitua, A.Y., Malebo, H.M., 2011. Malar. J., 10:S6.
Hermann, F., Hamoud, R., Sporer, F., Tahrani, A., Wink, M., 2011. Planta Med., 77:1905–1911.
Hollmann, J., Van der Schijff, M., 1996. Veld Flora, 82:115–116.
Hutchings, A., Scott, A.H., Lewis, G., Zululand, U.O., Cunningham, A.B., 1996. Zulu Medicinal Plants: An Inventory. University of Natal Press, Pietermaritzburg, South Africa.
Johns, T., Mahunnah, R.L.A., Sanaya, P., Chapman, L., Ticktin, T., 1999. J. Ethnopharmacol., 66:1–10.
Kang, R.K., Nakatsu, T., Zyzak, L.L., 1999. Flavored Product Additive and Method for Using Same. Google Patents.
Karani, L.W., Tolo, F.M., Karanja, S.M., Khayeka-Wandabwa, C., 2013. S. Afr. J. Bot., 88:183–190.
Khumalo, G., Sadgrove, N., Van Vuuren, S., Van Wyk, B.-E., 2018. S. Afr. J. Bot., 122:547–550.
Kioy, D., Gray, A.I., Waterman, P.G., 1990. Phytochemistry, 29:3535–3538.
Kokwaro, J.O., 2009. Medicinal Plants of East Africa. University of Nairobi Press, Nairobi, Kenya.
Kotina, E.L., van Wyk, B.E., Tilney, P.M., 2014. S. Afr. J. Bot., 94:177–181.
Kubo, I., 1995. Stud. Nat. Prod. Chem., 17:233–249.
Kubo, I., Taniguchi, M., 1988. J. Nat. Prod., 51:22–29.
Kubo, I., Miura, I., Pettei, M.J., Lee, Y.W., Pilkiewicz, F., Nakanishi, K., 1977. Tetrahedron Lett., 18:4553–4556.
Kubo, I., Fujita, K., Lee, Y.W., 2001. J. Agric. Food Chem., 49:1607–1611.
Kuete, V., 2010. Planta Med., 76:1479–1491. https://doi.org/10.1055/s-0030-1250027.
Kuglerova, M., Tesarova, H., Gradé, J.T., Halamova, K., Wanyana-Maganyi, O., Van Damme, P., Kokoska, L., 2011. Afr. J. Biotechnol., 10:3628–3632.
Lacroix, D., Prado, S., Kamoga, D., Kasenene, J., Namukobe, J., Krief, S., Dumontet, V., Mouray, E., Bodo, B., Brunois, F., 2011. J. Ethnopharmacol., 133:850–855.
Lamorde, M., Tabuti, J.R.S., Obua, C., Kukunda-Byobona, C., Lanyero, H., Byakika-Kibwika, P., Bbosa, G.S., Lubega, A., Ogwal-Okeng, J., Ryan, M., Waako, P.J., Merry, C., 2010. J. Ethnopharmacol., 130:43–53.
Lawal, O.A., Ogunwande, I.A., Opoku, A.R., KasalI, A.A., Oyedeji, A.O., 2014. JBAPN, 4:272–277.

Leonard, C.M., Viljoen, A.M., 2015. J. Ethnopharmacol., 165:260–285.
Leonard, C., Van Vuuren, S., Viljoen, A., 2010. Planta Med., 77:PF91.
Lovett, J.C., 2006. Field Guide to the Moist Forest Trees of Tanzania. Society for Environmental Exploration, https://www.cepf.net/sites/default/files/final_lovettruffogereau_fieldguide.pdf.
Lunde, C.S., Kubo, I., 2000. Antimicrob. Agents Chemother., 44:1943–1953.
Mabona, U., Viljoen, A., Shikanga, E., Marston, A., Van Vuuren, S., 2013. J. Ethnopharmacol., 148:45–55.
Machaba, T.C., Mahlo, S.M., 2017. World Acad. Sci. Eng. Technol., 11:390–395.
Madikane, V.E., Bhakta, S., Russell, A.J., Campbell, W.E., Claridge, T.D.W., Elisha, B.G., Davies, S.G., Smith, P., Sim, E., 2007. Bioorg. Med. Chem., 15:3579–3586.
Makunga, N., Philander, L., Smith, M., 2008. J. Ethnopharmacol., 119:365–375.
Maroyi, A., 2008. Int. J. Biodivers. Sci. Manag., 4:148–153.
Maroyi, A., 2013. J. Med. Plant Res., 7:53–60.
Maroyi, A., 2014. Pharm. Biol., 52:378–391.
Mashimbye, M.J., 1993. Chemical Constituents of Plants Native to Venda. PhD thesis, University of Natal, Pietermaritzburg, South Africa.
Mashimbye, M.J., Maumela, M.C., Drewes, S.E., 1999. Phytochemistry, 51:435–438.
Mavi, S., 1994. Strelitzia, 1:169–174.
McGaw, L.J., Lall, N., Meyer, J.J.M., Eloff, J.N., 2008. J. Ethnopharmacol., 119:482–500.
McKee, D., Karwic, A., 2009. Product and Method for Oral Administration of Nutraceuticals. Google Patents.
Mohanlall, V., Odhav, B., 2009. J. Med. Pl. Res., 3:231–240.
Motsei, M.L., Lindsey, K.L., Van Staden, J., Jäger, A.K., 2003. J. Ethnopharmacol., 86:235–241.
Muthaura, C.N., Keriko, J.M., Derese, S., Yenesew, A., Rukunga, G.M., 2011. Exp. Parasitol., 127:609–626.
Muthaura, C.N., Keriko, J.M., Mutai, C., Yenesew, A., Gathirwa, J.W., Irungu, B.N., Nyangacha, R., Mungai, G.M., Derese, S., 2015. J. Ethnopharmacol., 175:315–323.
Nakanishi, K., Kubo, I., 1977. Isr. J. Chem., 16:28–31.
Neuwinger, H.D., 2000. African Traditional Medicine: A Dictionary of Plant Use and Applications. Medpharm GmbH Scientific Publishers, Stuttgart, Germany.
Ngure, P.K., 2014. Pan Afr. Med. J., 17:15.
Nibret, E., Ashour, M.L., Rubanza, C.D., Wink, M., 2010. Phytother. Res., 24:945–947.
Nyaba, Z.N., Murambiwa, P., Opoku, A.R., Mukaratirwa, S., Shode, F.O., Simelane, M.B., 2018. Malar. J., 17:296.
Olila, D., Opuda-Asibo, J., Olwa-Odyek, 2001. Afr. Health Sci., 1:12–15.
Olveda, D.U., Li, Y., Olveda, R.M., Lam, A.K., Chau, T.N.P., Harn, D.A., Williams, G.M., Gray, D.J., Ross, A.G.P., 2013. Trop. Med. Surg., 1:1–9.
Opiyo, S.A., Manguro, L.A.A., Okoth, D.A., Ochung A.A., Ochieng, C.O., 2015. Nat. Prod. J., 5:236.
Orwa, C., 2009. Agroforestree Database: A Tree Reference and Selection Guide, Version 4.0. http://www.worldagroforestry.org/sites/treedbs/treedatabases.asp.
Palgrave, K.C., Drummond, R.B., Moll, E.J., Palgrave, M.C., 2002. Trees of Southern Africa. Struik Publishers, Cape Town, South Africa.
Palmer, E., Pitman, N., 1972. Trees of Southern Africa: Covering All Known Indigenous Species in the Republic of South Africa, South-West Africa, Botswana, Lesotho & Swaziland. Vols. 1 & 2.
Pillay, P., Maharaj, V.J., Smith, P.J., 2008. J. Ethnopharmacol., 119:438–454.

Pooley, E., 1993. The Complete Field Guide to Trees of Natal Zululand and Transkei, first ed. Natal Flora Publication Trust, Natal Herbarium Botanic Gardens, Durban, South Africa.
Pott, P., 1918. Ann. Transvaal Mus., 1:61–63.
Rabe, T., Van Staden, J., 1997. J. Ethnopharmacol., 56:81–87.
Rabe, T., Van Staden, J., 2000. J. Ethnopharmacol., 73:171–174.
Samie, A., Tambani, T., Harshfield, E., Green, E., Ramalivhana, J.N., Bessong, P.O., 2010. Afr. J. Biotechnol., 9:2965–2976.
Schubert, A., 2011. Use of an Extract Obtained From Plants of the Family Canellaceae in the Treatment of Cancer. Google Patents.
Soyingbe, O.S., Mongalo, N.I., Makhafola, T.J., 2018. BMC Complement. Altern. Med., 18:315.
Steenkamp, V., Grimmer, H., Semano, M., Gulumian, M., 2005. Mutat. Res. Genet. Toxicol. Environ., 581:35–42.
Steenkamp, V., Nkwane, O., Van Tonder, J., Dinsmore, A., Gulumian, M., 2013. Afr. J. Pharm. Pharmacol., 7:703–709.
Symmonds, R., Crouch, N., 2000. Plantlife, 22:24–26.
Szallasi, A., Bíró, T., Modarres, S., Garlaschelli, L., Petersen, M., Klusch, A., Vidari, G., Jonassohn, M., De Rosa, S., Sterner, O., Blumberg, P.M., Krause, J.E., 1998. Eur. J. Pharmacol., 356:81–89.
Tabuti, J.R.S., Kukunda, C.B., Waako, P.J., 2010. J. Ethnopharmacol., 127:130–136.
Taniguchi, M., Kubo, I., 1993. J. Nat. Prod., 56:1539–1546.
Taniguchi, M., Adachi, T., Oi, S., Kimura, A., Katsumura, S., Isoe, S., Kubo, I., 1984. Agric. Biol. Chem., 48:73–78.
Treyvaud Amiguet, V., Petit, P., Ta, C.A., Nuñez, R., Sánchez-Vindas, P., Alvarez, L.P., Smith, M.L., Arnason, J.T., Durst, T., 2006. J. Nat. Prod., 69:1005–1009.
Van Wyk, B.E., 2011. S. Afr. J. Bot., 77:812–829.
Van Wyk, B.E., Gericke, N., 2000. People's Plants: A Guide to Useful Plants of Southern Africa. Briza Publications, Pretoria, South Africa.
Van Wyk, B.E., Wink, M., 2004. Medicinal Plants of the World: An Illustrated Scientific Guide to Important Medicinal Plants and their Uses. Briza Publications, Pretoria, South Africa.
Van Wyk, B.E., Van Oudtshoorn, B., Gericke, N., 2009. Medicinal Plants of South Africa. Briza Publications, Pretoria, South Africa.
Verschaeve, L., Van Staden, J., 2008. J. Ethnopharmacol., 119:575–587.
Viol, D.I., Chagonda, L.S., Moyo, S.R., Mericli, A.H., 2016. Am. J. Plant Sci., 7:1538.
Wan-Ibrahim, W.I., Sidik, K., Kuppusamy, U.R., 2010. Food Chem., 122:1139–1144.
Weiss, E.A., 1979. Econ. Bot., 33:35–51.
Williams, V.L., Victor, J.E., Crouch, N.R., 2013. S. Afr. J. Bot., 86:23–35.
Wing, L.D., Buss, I.O., 1970. Wildl. Monogr., 3–92.
Wink, M., 2003. Phytochemistry, 64:3–19.
Wink, M., 2008. Curr. Drug Metab., 9:996–1009.
Wube, A.A., Bucar, F., Gibbons, S., Asres, K., Rattray, L., Croft, S.L., 2010. Phytother Res., 24:1468–1472.
Xaba, P., McVay, R., 2010. Veld Flora, 96:40–41.
Zschocke, S., Rabe, T., Taylor, J.L.S., Jäger, A.K., Van Staden, J., 2000. J. Ethnopharmacol., 71:281–292.

CHAPTER

Xysmalobium undulatum 25

Sowesa Kanama, Weiyang Chen and Thomas Idowu

Department of Pharmaceutical Sciences, Tshwane University of Technology, Pretoria, South Africa

Abstract

Xysmalobium undulatum (L.) Aiton (Apocynaceae), commonly referred to as 'Uzara', is a large perennial herb that grows up to 2 m in height and is widely distributed in the eastern parts of southern Africa. The plant bears creamy-green to yellow flowers, hairy fruits, and fleshy carrot-like roots, characterised by a nauseating smell. Xysmalobium undulatum is one of many South African medicinal plants widely used for the treatment of various diseases by several South African ethnic groups. The root is mostly used to treat different disease conditions, including gastrointestinal disorders, wound healing, hysteria, fevers, headaches and skin diseases. Uzara is one of the highly traded medicinal plants on the informal markets in South Africa, while formulations containing uzara have been successfully marketed by a number of pharmaceutical companies. The plant is also believed to possess diuretic properties and possible cardiotoxicity effects that may manifest due to the presence of cardenolide glycosides with digitalis-like action on the heart. This monograph represents a summary of the ethnobotany, phytochemistry, the in vitro and in vivo biological and pharmacological properties of X. undulatum, and its toxicity profile. Chemical profiling of the non-volatile constituents (methanol extract) was performed using high-performance thin-layer chromatography (HPTLC), ultra-performance liquid chromatography coupled to mass spectrometry (UPLC–MS), and mid-infrared (MIR) spectroscopy. The major compounds reported in the root extract are uzarin and its isomer allouzarin, as well as xysmalorin and alloxysmalorin. The marker compound, uzarin, was identified based on both HPTLC and UPLC–MS analysis and its isomer, xysmalorin, was identified by UPLC–MS in the methanol root extracts.

Keywords: *Xysmalobium undulatum*, Uzara, Root extract, Cardenolide glycosides, Uzarin, Xysmalorin, HPTLC, UPLC–MS, MIR spectroscopy

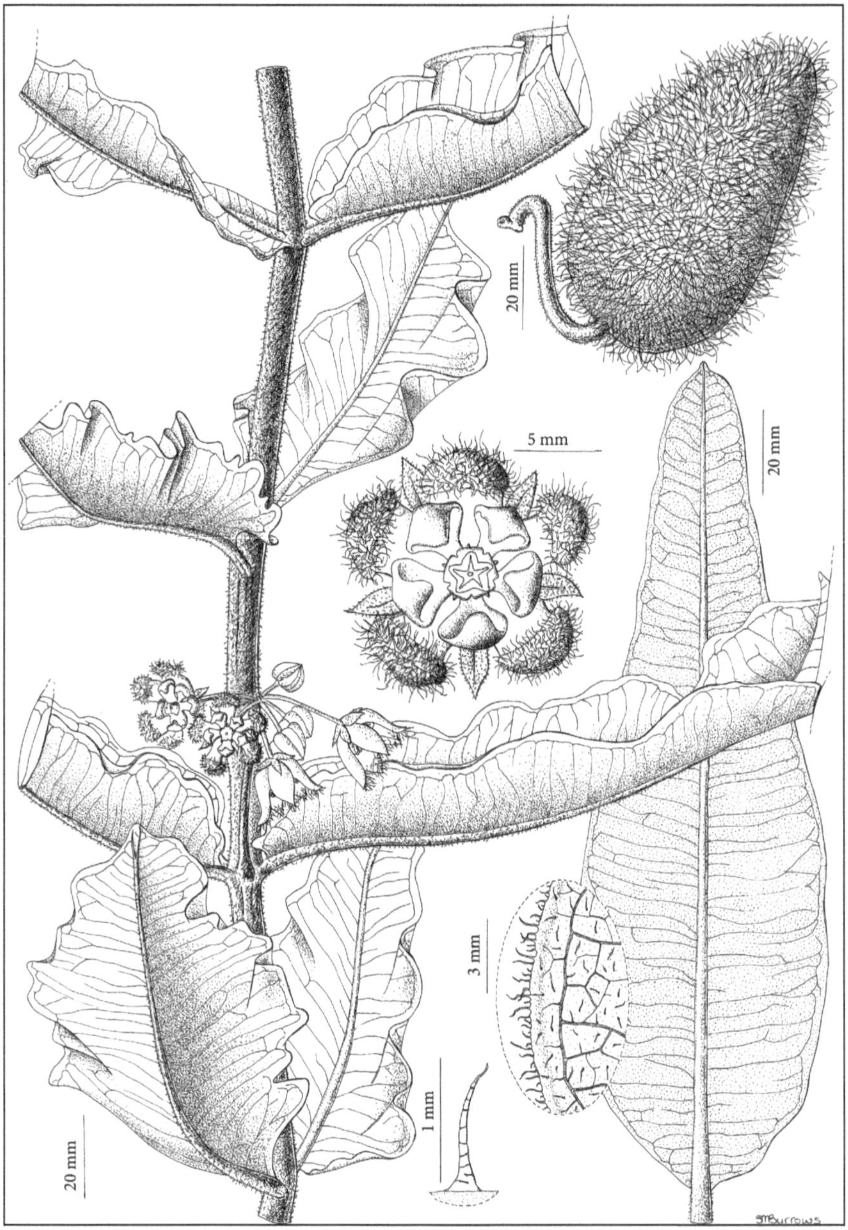
20 mm
5 mm
20 mm
3 mm
1 mm
20 mm

Part A: General overview

1. Synonyms

Asclepias leucotricha Schltr., *Asclepias undulata* L., *Gomphocarpus undulatus* (L.) Schltr., *Woodia trilobata* Schltr., *Xysmalobium ambiguum* N.E.Br., *Xysmalobium amplifolium* Weim., *Xysmalobium angolense* Scott-Elliot, *Xysmalobium barbigerum* N.E.Br., *Xysmalobium dilatatum* Weim., *Xysmalobium dispar* N.E.Br., *Xysmalobium lapathifolium* K.Schum., *Xysmalobium lencotrichum* (Schltr.) N.E.Br., *Xysmalobium prismatostigma* K.Schum., *Xysmalobium trilobatum* (Schltr.) N.E.Br.[a]

2. Common name(s)

Waved-leaved Xysmalobium, uzara, wild cotton, milkwort, milk bush (English), '*bitterhout*', '*bitterhoutwortel*', '*bitterwortel*', '*melkbos*' (Afrikaans), '*ishinga*', '*ishongwane*', '*ishongwe*' (isiZulu), '*ishongwane*', '*iyeza elimhlophe*', '*nwachaba*' (isiXhosa), '*leshokhoa*', '*pohotshehele*' (southern Sotho).[a,b]

3. Conservation status

Least concern.[a]

4. Botany

Xysmalobium undulatum is one of 18 *Xysmalobium* species found in South Africa (Schmelzer, 2011). The genus name *Xysmalobium* is derived from the Greek words '*xysma*' meaning lint/fluff and '*lobion*' meaning small pod, which refers to the hairy fruits. The Latin epithet '*undulatum*' refers to the wavy leaf margins of the plant (Bester, 2009). *Xysmalobium undulatum* is a large perennial herb that grows up to 2 m in height, with erect, thick and hairy branches. The hairy leaves are large, arranged on opposite sides, with prominent veins and wavy margins (A). The plant bears many flowers that occur in dense axillary, embel-like clusters, with colour ranging from cream-green to yellow (A). These stalked inflorescences grow from the leaf axils, with erect lobes that are hairy and curved at the tips. The large, hairy fruit is ovoid-shaped and cream in colour with an inflated appearance (B). The fleshy carrot-like roots have a brown exterior and white interior, characterised by a nauseating smell. The plant exudes milk when damaged (C) (Bester, 2009).

[a] Redlist of South African Plants (http://redlist.sanbi.org).
[b] PlantZAfrica (http://pza.sanbi.org).

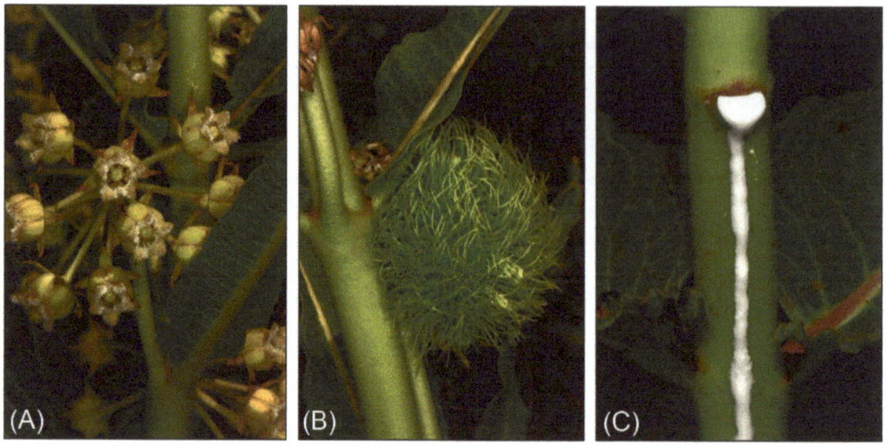

Xysmalobium undulatum with stalked, cream to yellowish-green flowers, large wavy leaves with prominent veins (A), an ovoid, hairy fruit (B), and thick, erect hairy stem (C).

5. Geographical distribution

Xysmalobium undulatum has a widespread distribution in the eastern parts of southern Africa and countries where it occurs include Kenya, Namibia, Botswana, Lesotho, Swaziland (Eswatini) and most provinces of South Africa. The plant grows at altitudes ranging from 84 to 2000 m above sea level, in open grasslands, disturbed areas, wetlands and high rainfall areas (Bester, 2009).

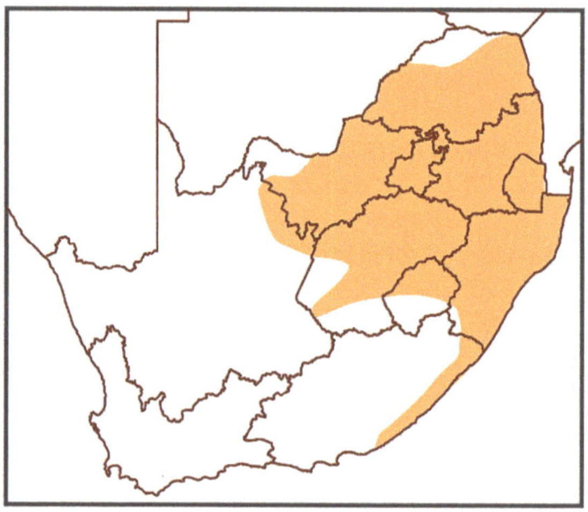

Geographical distribution of *Xysmalobium undulatum* in South Africa.

6. Ethnopharmacology

Reports on the use of *X. undulatum* as a traditional remedy for the treatment of various diseases date back to the 19th century, when the root extract was used as a tonic and the milky sap applied to open wounds to kill maggots (Smith, 1895). Various South African ethnic groups that include the Mpondo and the Nama people, use the plant, specifically the root powder or extract, to treat gastro-intestinal disorders such as diarrhoea, stomach cramps and dysentery (Watt and Breyer-Brandwijk, 1962; Bester, 2009; Schmelzer, 2011). The plant is also believed to possess diuretic effects and it is used in the management of afterbirth cramps, dysmenorrhea, syphilis, urinary tract infections, coughs and headaches (Van Wyk and Wink, 2004). The root in various forms has been used to treat a range of conditions including; (i) topical application on wounds, sores, abscess and snake bites, (ii) as a decoction to manage hysteria by the Xhosa and fevers related to malaria, typhoid and other conditions in Zambia, (iii) chewing the root as antidote to food poisoning by the Tswana, (iv) cold water extract for lumpy skin disease in cattle and (v) as snuff for sedation (Steenkamp et al., 2004; Bester, 2009; Gomes et al., 2009; Schmelzer, 2011). Topical application of the sap has been reported to cure rashes, warts and corns (Schmelzer, 2011).

7. Commercialisation

Uzara is one of the highly traded medicinal plants (no. 51) on the informal markets of the Eastern Cape Province of South Africa (Dold and Cocks, 2002). Commercial cultivation of the plant has been done near Pretoria in South Africa from as early as the 1900s (Schulzke et al., 2011; Van Wyk, 2011). Globally, the plant has received very little attention, with only a few patents filed. Since its introduction into the German market in 1911, uzara has been marketed by Hemopharm GmbH for gastro-intestinal disorders. A tablet formulation, Dysmenurals, containing uzarin (0.05 g) and diamethylaminophenazon (0.30 g), had been on the markets since the1920s, however, its manufacture has since been stopped (Schmelzer, 2011; Schulzke et al., 2011). Another product 'uzarae radix' is marketed in Europe for diarrhoea and menstrual cramps with a daily dose of 90 mg total glycosides, considered as uzarin (Schmelzer, 2011; Schulzke et al., 2011). *Xysmalobium undulatum* is one of the South African plants earmarked for commercialisation (Van Wyk, 2011), however, very little progress has been made in that regard. The research that provided a scientific basis for the traditional use, including extensive phytochemical profiling work on the plants, has been done. The delay in commercialisation is therefore believed to be due to the possible cardiotoxicity effects that may manifest as a result of the presence of cardenolide glycosides with digitalis-like action on the heart (Van Wyk, 2011).

8. Pharmacological evaluation

8.1 *In vitro* studies

8.1.1 Antidiarrhoeal activity

Xysmalobium roots have been reported for use to treat gastro-intestinal disorders. Scientific evidence has documented their contractile effects on smooth muscles of the intestine, uterus, bladder and bronchi (Schulzke et al., 2011). In a study that investigated the *in vitro* effect of uzara on active chloride secretion using a human colon carcinoma cell line (HT-29/B6), the compound (50 mg/mL) inhibited active chloride secretion within 1 h of secretion induction using forskolin (10 mM) (Schulzke et al., 2011). Similarly, uzara caused a 70% partial blockage of cAMP production and increase in human colonic biopsies induced by exposure to forskolin. Both findings led to the conclusion that the antidiarrhoeal effect of uzara is linked to inhibition of active chloride secretion and a reduction in intracellular cAMP responses (Schulzke et al., 2011). The cardenolide, cardiac glycosides of uzarigenin, and other polar cardenolide glycosides present in root extracts exhibited antidiarrhoeal activities *via* an antisecretory mechanism (Schulzke et al., 2011).

8.1.2 Central nervous system activity

To investigate the effect of uzara on the central nervous system (CNS), aqueous and ethanolic extracts of the aerial and root parts were tested separately for their binding affinity to the serotonin transporter (SERT) in a serotonin reuptake transport protein-binding assay (Nielsen et al., 2004). An *ex vivo* whole rat brain tissue suspension was used. The results showed that uzara root extracts had a higher affinity (51% for aqueous extract at 5 mg/mL and 76% for ethanolic extract at 5 mg/mL), compared to the aerial parts (40% at 5 mg/mL and 20% at 5 mg/mL for the aqueous and ethanolic extracts, respectively). At the highest concentrations, the ethanolic leaf extracts displaced more than 50% transport protein bound [^{3}H]-citalopram (Nielsen et al., 2004). In another study, uzara ethyl acetate root extract showed good CNS activity by inhibiting acetylcholinesterase with an IC_{50} value of 125 ng/mL, compared to 0.5 ng/mL for the galanthamine control (Adewusi and Steenkamp, 2011). Stafford et al. (2007) reported weak, non-selective mono-amine oxidase inhibitory activity (IC_{50} value of 849 ± 110 μg/mL) for the same type of extract. The ethanolic root and leaf extracts of uzara displayed weak activities when tested in the ^{3}H-Ro 15–1788 or flumazenil (benzodiazepine agonist)-binding assay in rat cerebral cortices (Stafford et al., 2005, 2008).

8.1.3 Other activities

The anti-infective property of uzara was investigated against a range of pathogens using the broth microdilution assay (Buwa and Van Staden, 2006). The aqueous root extract exhibited weak activity with a minimum inhibitory concentration (MIC) of 12.5 mg/mL towards *Escherichia coli, Klebsiella pneumoniae, Staphylcoccus aureus* and *Candida albicans*, and no activity towards *Bacillus subtilis* at the same concentration. The ethanolic extract exhibited better activity (MIC of 3.125 mg/mL) when tested against the four bacterial pathogens (Buwa and Van Staden, 2006). A dichloromethane:methanol (1:1) extract prepared from the whole plant displayed good antiplasmodial effect, recording an IC_{50} value of 6 µg/mL (Clarkson et al., 2004). A study by Schulzke et al. (2011) reported on the possible digitalis-like effects of high doses of uzara on the heart. Miller et al. (2004) predicted possible addiction if uzara is concomitantly administered with digoxin in cardiovascular patients (Miller et al., 2004). Further work by Melero et al. (2000) suggests that uzara glycosides with the A/B *trans*-configuration may exhibit lower cardiac effects compared to the A/B *cis*-configuration of digitalis-like glycosides.

8.2 *In vivo* studies and clinical trials

Uzara exhibited antidepressant effects in mice in a forced swim test at 250 and 500 mg/kg (Pedersen et al., 2008). The relative immobility following exposure to uzara was 77.6% ± 6.0% and 67.9% ± 8.2% at 250 and 500 mg/kg, respectively, compared to imipramine and desipramine used as controls. A single-blinded, randomised, placebo and verum-controlled clinical trial with three cross-over periods was undertaken on healthy individuals to investigate the cross-reactivity of uzara with digitoxin, as well as the pharmacokinetics and pharmacodynamics of Uzara® Losüng N (40 mg/mL uzara radix dry extract) (Schmiedl et al., 2012). The results did not show any significant cardiovascular or pharmacodynamic changes when the treatments and controls were compared. In a Phase III randomised comparative two-way cross-over pilot study to determine safety and efficacy towards dysmenorrhoea, the results showed comparable efficacy for uzara and ibuprofen (78.3% vs 86.7% of cycles; respectively) (Abd-El-Maeboud et al., 2014). However, Uzara® recorded fewer side effects when compared to ibuprofen (0% vs 8.3%, $P < 0.05$).

8.3 Safety

Few studies have been conducted to determine the toxicity profile of *X. undulatum* to date. The plant has been reported to cause respiratory distress due to its contractile effect on bronchial smooth muscles (Watt, 1930). Possible cardiotoxicity as a result of a digitalis-like action on the heart has been reported for the root extract and compounds that include uzarigenin, uzarigenin rhamnoside, uzarigenin glucoside and uzarin uzaroside (Watt, 1930; Brown et al., 1983).

9. Phytochemistry

Phytochemical profiling studies of the root extract enabled the identification of the following major compounds; uzarin and its isomer allouzarin, as well as xysmalorin and alloxysmalorin (Ghorbani et al., 1997; Schmelzer, 2011).

Other compounds occurring in the plant that are expressed in lower levels include uzarigenin, xysmalogenin allouzarigenin, alloxysmalogenin, ascleposide, coroglaucigenin, corogluaucigenin-3-*O*-glucoside, pachygenol, pachygenol-3β-*O*-glucoside, desglucouzarin, smalogenin, desglucoxysmalorin, uzaroside, pregnenolone and β-sitosterol (Schmelzer, 2011). The glycosidic linkage of the cardinolides is reported to be 1–2, i.e., glucopyranosyl-(1–2)-glucopyranose. However, uncertainty regarding the sugar portion of the major cardenolides has been reported, where the glycosides were reported to be diglucosides (Kuritzkes et al., 1963). The seeds of uzara have been reported to be composed of glycosides that are different from the roots, particularly frugoside (Kuritzkes et al., 1963). Pauli and Fröhlich (2000) isolated two new cardenolides, coroglaucigenin-3-*O*-β-glucoside and pachygenol-3-*O*-β-glucoside. Furthermore, the stereochemical patterns of seven uzara cardenolides, namely uzarigenin, xysmalogenin, ascleposide, coroglaucigenin, coroglaucigenin-3-*O*-β-glucoside, pachygenol and pachygenol-3-*O*-β-glucoside, were elucidated, confirming that the stereogenic centres of these compounds followed regular cardiac glycoside chirality: 3βOH (i.e. non-epi series), 5αH (uzarigenin-type cardenolides), 10βCH_3 (A/B rings exhibiting *trans*-stereochemistry), 13βCH_3 14βOH (C/D rings are *cis*), and 17αH (i.e. non-allo series). Using modern NMR technologies, such as selective TOCSY and pulsed field gradient HMBC experiments, it was possible to determine the stereochemistry and key chiral positions in all the uzara cardenolides as bearing regular equatorial C3-OH groups (non-epi-type aglycones); possessing A/B *trans* ring fusion and thus representing 5α-cardenolides (uzarigenin *trans*-fused A/B), which are diagnostically different from 5β-digitoxigenin-type (*cis*-fused A/B) (cardenolides); Δ5,6 unsaturation for xysmalogenin and pachygenol series (verified by X-ray crystallography); possessing *cis*-C/D ring fusion; and β-orientation of the butenolide ring (Kanama et al., 2016). Modern analytical techniques such as high-performance thin-layer chromatography (HPTLC), ultra-high-performance liquid chromatography-mass spectrometry (UHPLC–MS) and mid-infrared (MIR) spectroscopy, in combination with chemometrics, were proven to be reliable quality control techniques for *X. undulatum* raw material and for the quantification of the major compound uzarin (Kanama et al., 2016).

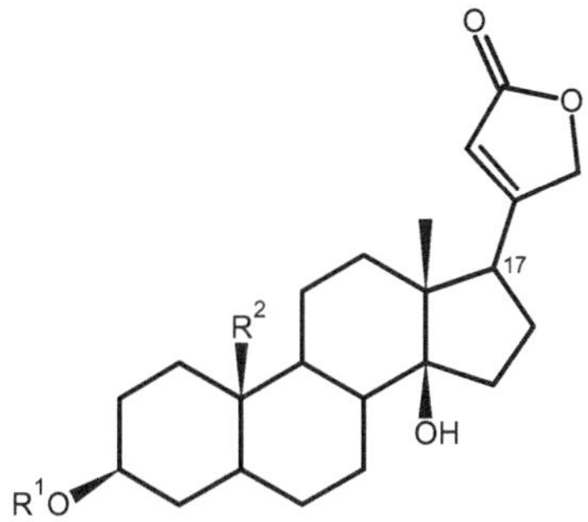

Compound	R1	R2	C17
Uzarigenin	H	CH_3	17αH
Allouzarigenin	H	CH_3	17βH
Coroglaucigenin	H	CH_2OH	17αH
Uzarin	Glucose–glucose[a]	CH_3	17αH
Allouzarin	Glucose–glucose[a]	CH_3	17βH
Desglucouzarin	Glucose[b]	CH_3	17αH
Uzaroxide	Glucose–glucose–glucose[c]	CH_3	17αH

[a]*Sugars conjugated via β-1-2-glucosidic bond.*
[b]*Sugars conjugated with the C-3 hydroxyl of the genin via β-glycosidic linkage.*
[c]*Sugars conjugated via β-1-6-glucosidic bond.*

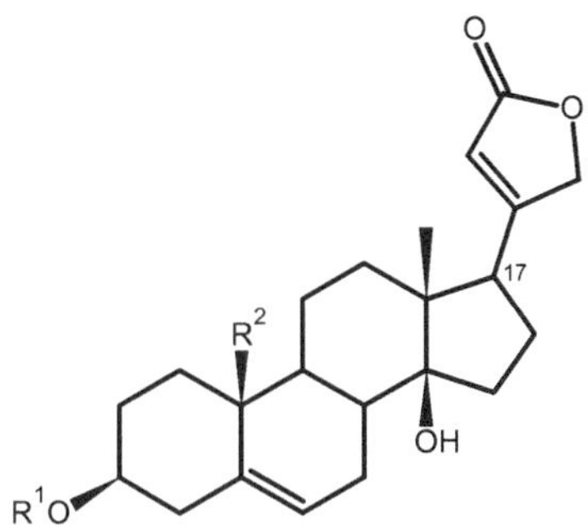

Compound	R1	R2	C17
Xysmalogenin	H	CH_3	17αH
Alloxysmalogenin	H	CH_3	17βH
Xysmalorin	Glucose–glucose[a]	CH_3	17αH
Alloxysmalorin	Glucose–glucose[a]	CH_3	17βH
Desglucoxysmalorin	Glucose[b]	CH_3	17αH
Pachygenol-3β-*O*-glucoside	Glucose[b]	CH_2OH	17αH

[a]*Sugars conjugated via β-1-2-glucosidic bond.*
[b]*Sugars conjugated with the C-3 hydroxyl of the genin via β-glycosidic linkage.*

Part B: Chemical profiling and quality control

10. Chromatography analysis

10.1 High-performance thin-layer chromatography (HPTLC) fingerprint analysis

General instrumentation: CAMAG HPTLC instrument consisting of an automatic TLC sampler (ATS 4), automatic developing chamber (ADC 2), CAMAG TLC visualiser 2, CAMAG derivatiser, and TLC plate heater. *HPTLC plates:* Silica gel glass plates $60 F_{254}$ (Merck). *Plant part:* Roots, methanol extract. *Sample application:* Application volume of 2 µL methanol extract (100 mg/mL) and standards (1 mg/mL) spotted as 10 mm bands. Plates developed in a 20×10×4 cm glass twin-trough chamber to a migration distance of 70 mm. *Tank saturation:* 20 min at 15 °C and 33% RH, with 25 mL of mobile phase. *Mobile phase:* Dichloromethane: methanol: ethyl acetate: formic acid (90:30:10:1, v/v/v/v). *Derivatisation:* *p*-Anisaldehyde sulphuric acid reagent. The plate was sprayed with 3 mL of reagent then heated on a TLC plate heater for 3 min at 100 °C and then visualised. *Visualisation:* The plate was viewed under white reflectance light.

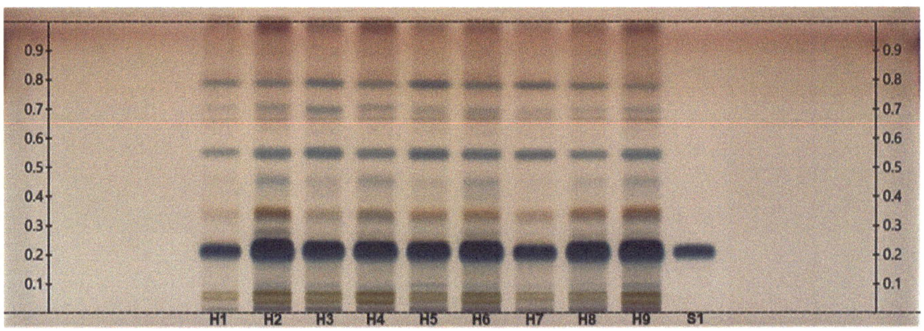

HPTLC plate for *Xysmalobium undulatum* methanol extracts ($n=9$) (H1–H9) and the standard (S1). The samples are characterised by a dark blue band for uzarin (S1) ($R_f = 0.21$).

10.2 Ultra-performance liquid chromatography (UPLC) analysis

General instrumentation: Waters Acquity Ultra-Performance Liquid Chromatography system with photodiode array (PDA) detector combined with a Xevo G2QToF mass spectrometer (Waters, USA). *Plant part:* Roots, methanol extract. *Sample application:* Injection volume of 2.0 µL (full-loop injection) at 1 mg/mL.

Column: Acquity UPLC BEH C_{18} column (150 mm × 2.1 mm, i.d., 1.7 μm particle size, Waters). *Mobile phase:* 0.1% formic acid in water (solvent A) and acetonitrile (solvent B). *Analysis conditions:* Gradient elution at a flow rate of 0.3 mL/min, changing as follows: 85% A: 15% B to 65% A: 35% B in 10 min, to 50% A: 50% B in 0.5 min, held for 1 min, back to initial ratio in 0.5 min, total run time 12 min. *Mass spectrometry*: ESI^+ (positive ionisation mode), N_2 used as desolvation gas, desolvation temperature 350 °C at a flow rate of 500 L/h and source temperature at 100 °C. Capillary and cone voltages 3000 and 35 V, respectively. Data collected between *m/z* 100 and 1200.

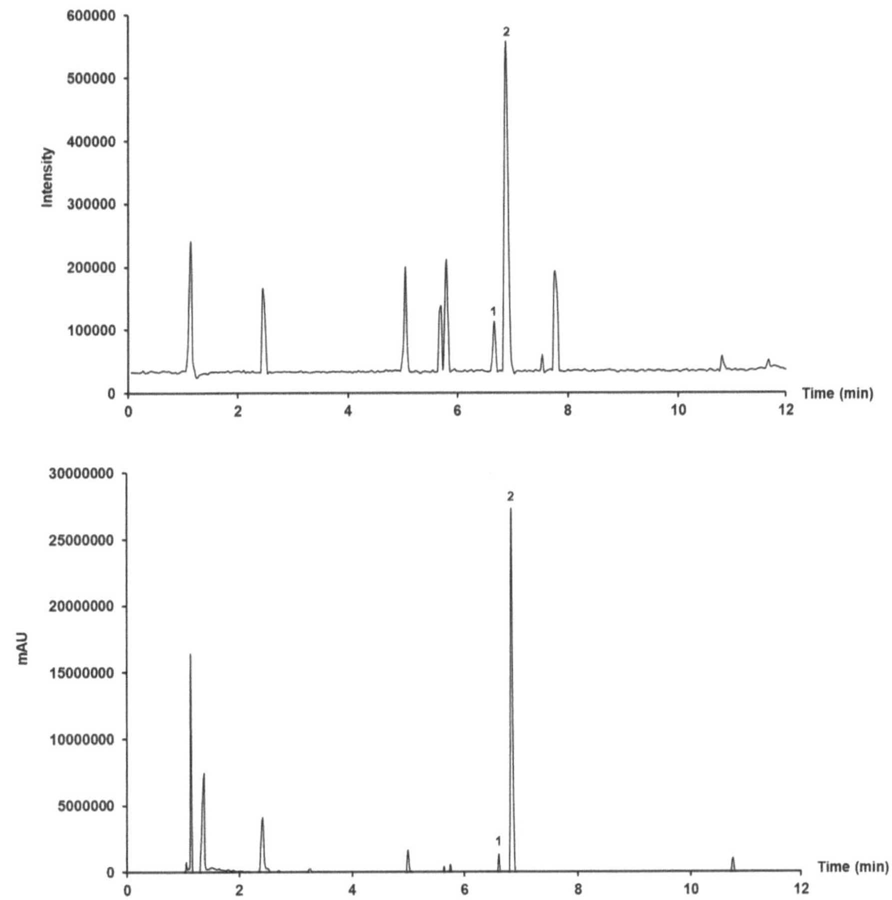

UPLC-ToF-MS ESI^+ (upper) and PDA (lower) chromatograms of *Xysmalobium undulatum* methanol extract: [1] = xysmalorin *m/z* 697.3395, [2] = uzarin *m/z* 699.3561.

11. Mid-infrared (MIR) spectroscopy analysis

General instrumentation: Alpha-P Bruker spectrometer, mounted with an attenuated total reflectance (ATR) diamond crystal. *Spectral acquisition:* Spectrum obtained in absorbance mode, with a spectral resolution of 4 cm^{-1} over the range 4000–550 cm^{-1} and captured using OPUS 6.5 software. *Plant part:* Root parts. *Sample preparation:* Roots powdered, sieved (<500 μm) and placed directly onto surface of diamond crystal.

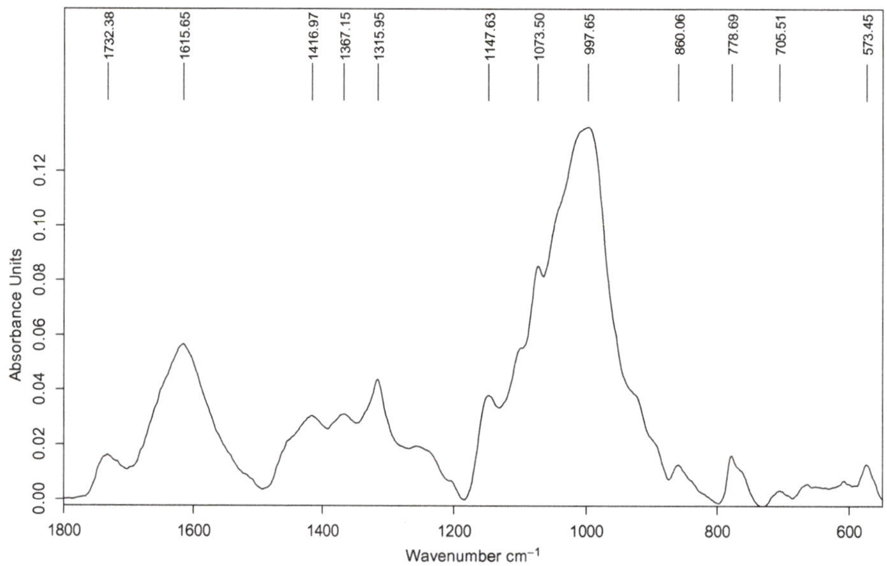

Mid-infrared spectrum of *Xysmalobium undulatum* root powder displaying the fingerprint region (1800–550 cm^{-1}).

References

Abd-El-Maeboud, K.H.I., Kortam, M.A.M.F., Ali, M.S., Ibrahim, M.I., Mohamed, R.M.M.Z., 2014. PLoS One, 9 (8):e104473.

Adewusi, E.A., Steenkamp, V., 2011., Asian Pac. J. Trop. Med., 4:829–835.

Bester, S.P., 2009. *Xysmalobium undulatum* (L.) Aiton f. var *undulatum*. Plantzafrica, Official Website of the South African National Biodiversity Institute (SANBI), Pretoria, South Africa. Available at: http://www.plantzafrica.com/plantwxyz/xysmalobundul.htm.

Brown, L., Erdmann, E., Thomas, R., 1983. Biochem. Pharmacol., 32:2767–2774.

Buwa, L.V., Van Staden, J., 2006. J. Ethnopharmacol., 103:139–142.

Clarkson, C., Maharaj, V.J., Crouch, N.R., Grace, O.M., Pillay, P., Matsabisa, M.G., Bhagwadin, N., Smith, P.J., Folb, P.I., 2004. J. Ethnopharmacol., 92:177–191.

Dold, A.P., Cocks, M.L., 2002. S. Afr. J. Sci., 98:589–597.

Ghorbani, M., Kaloga, M., Frey, H.-H., Mayer, G., Eich, E., 1997. Planta Med., 63:343–346.

Gomes, N.G., Campos, M.G., Orfão, J.M., Ribeiro, C.A., 2009. Prog. Neuro-Psychopharmacol. Biol. Psychiatry, 33:1372–1389.

Kanama, S., Viljoen, A., Enslin, G., Kamatou, G., Chen, W., Sandasi, M., Idowu, T., 2016. Pharm. Biol., 54:1272–1279.

Kuritzkes, A.M., Tamm, C., Hunter, H., Reichstein, T., 1963. Helv. Chim. Acta, 46:8–23.

Melero, C.P., Medarde, M., Feliciano, A.S., 2000. Molecules, 5:51–81.

Miller, K.L., Liebowitz, R.S., Newby, L.K., 2004. Am. Heart J., 147:401–411.

Nielsen, N.D., Sandager, M., Stafford, G.I., Van Staden, J., Jäger, A.K., 2004. J. Ethnopharmacol., 94:159–163.

Pauli, G.F., Fröhlich, R., 2000. Phytochem. Anal., 11:79–89.

Pedersen, M.E., Szewczyk, B., Stachowicz, K., Wieronska, J., Andersen, J., Stafford, G.I., Van Staden, J., Pilc, A., Jäger, A.K., 2008. J. Ethnopharmacol., 119:542–548.

Schmelzer, G.H., 2011. *Xysmalobium undulatum* (L.) W.T. Aiton (Available on:). In: Schmelzer, G.H., Gurib-Fakim, A. (Eds.), Prota 11(2): Medicinal Plants/Plantes Médicinales, PROTA, Wageningen, the Netherlands.

Schmiedl, S., Ritter, A., Szymanski, J., Schneider, F., Plecko, T., Alken, R.G., Theurmann, P.A., 2012. Int. J. Clin. Pharmacol. Ther., 50:729–740.

Schulzke, J.D., Andres, S., Amasheh, M., Fromm, A., Günzel, D., 2011. PLoS One, 6:e18107.

Smith, A., 1895. A Contribution to South African Materia Medica Chiefly From Plants in Use Among the Natives. J.C. Juta & Co., Capetown, South Africa.

Stafford, G.I., Jager, A.K., Van Staden, J., 2005. J. Ethnopharmacol., 100:210–215.

Stafford, G.I., Pedersen, P.D., Jäger, A.K., Van Staden, J., 2007. S. Afr. J. Bot., 73:384–390.

Stafford, G.I., Pedersen, M.E., Van Staden, J., Jäger, A.K., 2008. J. Ethnopharmacol., 119:513–537.

Steenkamp, V., Mathiva, E., Gouws, M.C., Van Rensburg, C.E.J., 2004. J. Ethnopharmacol., 95:353–357.

Van Wyk, B.-E., 2011. S. Afr. J. Bot., 77:812–829.

Van Wyk, B.-E., Wink, M., 2004. Medicinal Plants of the World. Briza Publications, Pretoria, South Africa.

Watt, J.M., 1930. J. Pharmacol. Exp. Ther., 38:261–270.

Watt, J.M., Breyer-Brandwijk, M.G., 1962. The Medicinal and Poisonous Plants of Southern and Eastern Africa, second ed. E. & S. Livingstone Ltd, Edinburgh and London, UK.

Index

Note: Page numbers followed by *f* indicate figures and *t* indicate tables.

B

C

P

Q

R

S

X

Y

Z

FSC
www.fsc.org
MIX
Papier | Fördert gute Waldnutzung
FSC® C083411

Kolibri 360 GmbH
Ferdinand-Jühlke-Straße 7
99095 Erfurt, Deutschland
produktsicherheit@kolibri360.de